Connecting Your Health to Your World

The Technology and Money Edition

GET Hooked ON Learning and Living Well

NEW!
Focus On: Improving Your Financial Health

A new mini-chapter addresses the practical skills students need to capitalize on their financial health, from building a budget to protecting against credit card scams.

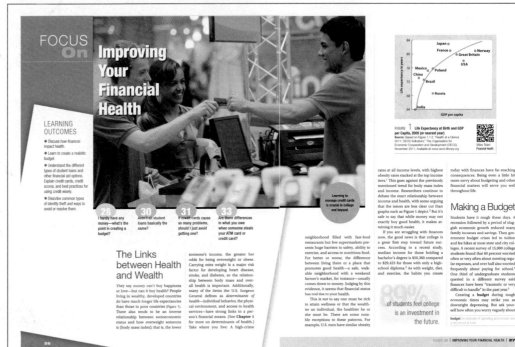

NEW!
Money & Health boxes

The focus on financial health extends throughout the text with new Money & Health feature boxes, giving students the leverage they need to develop a healthy relationship with money. Topics include tips to maximize healthcare benefits while minimizing costs, guidelines to follow when shopping for fitness facilities to ensure you get a good deal, and more.

Money&Health
ARE FRUITS AND VEGGIES BEYOND YOUR BUDGET?

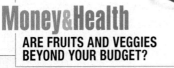

Many people on a tight budget, including college students, think that fruits and vegetables are beyond their budget. Maybe a carton of orange juice and a package of carrots are affordable, but five to nine servings a day? No way.

If that sounds like you, it's time for some facts. In 2011, the U.S. Department of Agriculture published data showing that the average American family spends more money on food than is necessary to consume a nutritious diet—one that includes the recommended servings of fruits and vegetables. The report concluded that, contrary to popular opinion, people on a tight budget can eat healthfully, including plenty of fruits and vegetables, and spend less on food.

So how do you do it? Here are some tips:

✱ Focus on five fresh favorites. Throughout the United States, five of the least expensive, perennially available fresh vegetables are carrots, eggplant, lettuce, potatoes, and summer squash. Five fresh fruit options are apples, bananas, pears, pineapple, and watermelon.

✱ Buy small amounts frequently. Most items of fresh produce keep only a few days, so buy amounts that you know you'll be able to eat or freeze.

✱ Celebrate the season. From apples to zucchini, when fruits and veggies are in season, they cost less. If you can freeze them, stock up. If not, enjoy them fresh while you can.

✱ Do it yourself. Avoid prewashed, precut fruits and vegetables, including salad greens. They cost more and often spoil faster. Also choose frozen 100% juice concentrate and add the water yourself.

✱ Buy canned or frozen on sale, in bulk. Canned and frozen produce, especially when it's on sale, may be much less expensive than fresh. Most frozen items are just as nutritious as fresh, and can be even more so, depending on how long ago the fresh food was harvested. For canned items, choose fruits without added sugars and vegetables without added salt or sauces. Bear in mind that beans are legumes and count as a vegetable choice. Low-sodium canned beans are one of the most affordable, convenient, and nutritious foods you can buy.

✱ Fix and freeze. Make large batches of homemade soup, vegetable stews, and pasta sauce and store them in single-serving containers in your freezer.

✱ Grow your own. All it takes is one sunny window, a pot, soil, and a packet of seeds. Lettuce, spinach, and fresh herbs are particularly easy to grow indoors in small spaces.

Sources: U.S. Department of Agriculture, "Eating Healthy on a Budget: The Consumer Economics Perspective," September 2011, www.choosemyplate.gov; U.S. Department of Agriculture, "Smart Shopping for Veggies and Fruits," Center for Nutrition Policy and Promotion, June 2011, www.choosemyplate.gov; U.S. Centers for Disease Control and Prevention, "30 Ways in 30 Days to Stretch Your Fruit & Vegetable Budget," Fruits & Veggies: More Matters, September 2011, www.fruitsandveggiesmatter.gov

NEW!
Tech & Health boxes

Students can tap into the latest technologies to improve their health with the new Tech & Health boxes throughout the text. Topics range from safety concerns with social media to reviews of various diet- and exercise-monitoring phone apps.

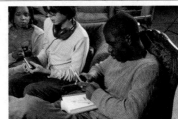

Tech & Health

TAMING TECHNOSTRESS AND iDISORDERS

Are you "twittered out"? Is texting causing your thumbs to seize up in protest? If so, you're not alone. Like millions of others, you may find that the pressure for constant contact is stressing you out! Known as *technostress*, it is defined as stress created by a dependence on technology and the constant state of connection, which can include a perceived obligation to respond, chat, or tweet. When does the constant anxiety over missed messages or an online persona cross the stress load limit?

An increasing number of people would rather hang out online talking to strangers than study, socialize in person, or connect in the real world. There are some clear downsides to all of that virtual interaction.

✳ **Social distress.** Authors Michelle Weil and Larry Rosen describe *technosis*, a very real syndrome in which people become so immersed in technology that they risk losing their own identity. Worrying about checking your e-mail or text messages, constantly switching to Facebook to see updates, perpetually posting to Twitter, and so on can keep you distracted and waste hours of every day.

Technology may keep you in touch, but it can also add to your stress and take you away from real-world interactions.

✳ **Technology dependency.** Increasing research supports the concept that feeling the need to be "wired" 24/7 (while eating, studying, hanging out with friends, in the car, and in nearly every place imaginable) can lead to anxiety, obsessive compulsive disorder, narcissism, sleep disorders, frustration, time pressures, and guilt—some of the negative consequences known as *iDisorders*. When you are more worried about your friends' list on a social media site than you are about spending the time to make real friends, it may be time to rethink your social interactions.

To avoid iDisorders caused by technology overload or technostress, set time limits on your technology usage, and make sure that you devote at least as much time to face-to-face interactions with people you care about. Remember that you don't always need to answer your phone or respond to a text or e-mail immediately.

Make a rule that you cannot turn on your device when out with friends or on vacation. *Tune in* to your surroundings, your loved ones and friends, your job, and your classes by shutting off your devices.

Sources: M. Weil and L. Rosen, *Technostress: Coping with Technology @Work, @Home, @Play* (Hoboken: John Wiley & Sons, 1997); L. D. Rosen et al., "Is Facebook Creating "iDisorders"? The Link Between Clinical Symptoms of Psychiatric Disorders and Technology Use, Attitudes and Anxiety," *Computers in Human Behavior*, in press, http://dx.doi.org/10.1016/j.chb.2012.11.012; National Safety Council, "National Safety Council Estimates That at Least 1.6 Million Crashes Are Caused Each Year by Drivers Using Cell Phones and Texting," press release, January 12, 2010, www.nsc.org; National Highway Traffic Safety Administration, "Blueprint for Ending Distracted Driving," 2012, www.nhtsa.gov

---

NEW! Video Tutors

Video Tutors highlight a book figure or discussion point in an engaging video, covering key concepts such as how drugs act on the brain, reading food labels, and the benefits of regular exercise. Using a QR code reader, students can easily access the Video Tutors on their mobile device—just scan the code and the Video Tutor loads instantly.

food, sleep, and water; at the next level are *security needs*, such as shelter and safety; at the third level are *social needs*, a sense of belonging and affection; at the fourth level are *esteem needs*, self-respect and respect for others; and at the top are needs for *self-actualization* and self-transcendence.[1]

According to Maslow's theory, one's needs must be met at each of these levels before a person can ever truly be healthy. Failure to meet needs at a lower level will interfere with a person's ability to address upper-level needs. For example, someone who is homeless or fearful about personal safety will be unable to focus on fulfilling social, esteem, or actualization needs.[1]

In sum, psychologically healthy people are emotionally, mentally, socially, and spiritually resilient. They usually respond to challenges and frustrations in appropriate ways, despite occasional slips (see Figure 2.3 on page 40). When they do slip, they recognize it and take action to rectify the situation.

Emotional Health

The term **emotional health** refers to the feeling, or tive, side of psychological health. **Emotions** are in feelings or complex patterns of feelings that we ex on a regular basis, including love, hate, frustration, and joy, to name a few. Typically, emotions are d as the interplay of four components: physiological feelings, cognitive (thought) processes, and behaviors. As rational beings, we are responsible for e our individual emotional responses, the environment causing them, and the appropriateness of our action

Emotionally healthy people usually respond ately to upsetting events. Rather than reacting in a fashion or behaving inconsistently or offensively press their feelings, communicate with others, emotions in appropriate ways. In contrast, unhealthy people are much more likely to let their overpower them. They may be highly volatile and unpredictable emotional responses, which lowed by inappropriate communication

A person's **emotional intelligence** to identify, use, understand, and m emotions in positive and constru It is about recognizing state and the Emotion

FIGURE 2.2 Maslow's Hierarchy of Needs
Source: From A. H. Maslow, R. D. Frager, ed., and J. Fadiman, ed., *Motivation and Personality*, 3rd edition. (Upper Saddle River: Pearson Education, 1987). Adapted and Electronically reproduced by permission of Pearson Education, Inc., Upper Saddle River, New Jersey.

Video Tutor: Maslow's Hierarchy

strategies to solve problems, and can carry out personal and professional responsibilities. In addition, a mentally healthy person has the intellectual ability to sort through information, messages, and life events; attach meaning to these events; and appropriately. This is often referred to as *intellectual* a subset of mental health.[2]

CHAPTER 2 | PROMOTING AND PRESERVING YOUR PSYCHOLOGICAL H

emotional intell ability to identify manage emotion and interact positi relationships.

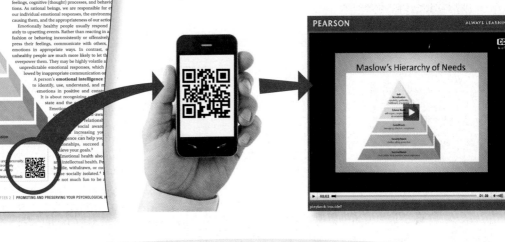

Self-Actualization
creativity, spirituality, fulfillment of potential

Esteem Needs
self-respect, respect for others, accomplishment

Social Needs
belonging, affection, acceptance

Security Needs
shelter, safety, protection

Survival Needs
food, water, sleep, exercise, sexual expression

PEARSON — ALWAYS LEARNING

Maslow's Hierarchy of Needs

NEW! Focus On: Reducing Risks and Coping with Chronic Diseases and Conditions and Focus On: Understanding Complementary and Alternative Medicine are new mini-chapters.

MAKE the Connection between Lecture and Behavior Change

MasteringHealth™

Mastering is the most effective and widely used online homework, tutorial, and assessment system for the sciences. It delivers self-paced tutorials that focus on your course objectives, provide individualized coaching, and responds to each student's progress.

FOR STUDENTS

Proven, assignable, and automatically graded health activities reinforce course learning objectives.

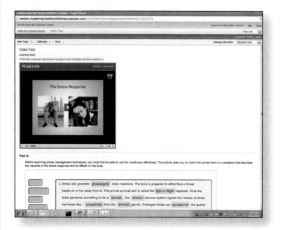

Health and Fitness Coaching Activities

Coaching activities guide students through key health and fitness concepts with interactive mini-lessons that provide hints and feedback.

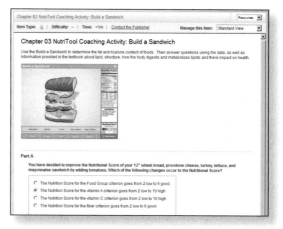

NutriTools Build-A-Meal Activities

These unique activities allow students to combine and experiment with different food options and learn first-hand how to build healthier meals.

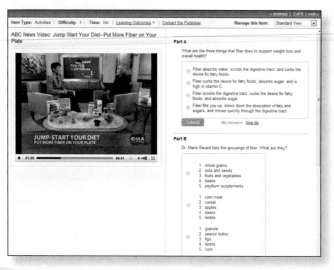

51 *ABC News* Videos

Timely videos, with assessment and feedback, help health come to life and show how it's related to the real world.

Other automatically graded health and fitness activities include:

- Behavior Change Video Activities
- Health Video Tutors
- Chapter Reading Quizzes
- MP3 Tutor Sessions

DO YOUR STUDENTS WANT TO PRACTICE ON THEIR OWN?

MasteringHealth also provides students with the tools to study effectively and practice on their own time at their own pace.

eText

The Pearson eText gives students access to the text whenever and wherever they can access the Internet. The eText can be viewed on PCs, Macs, and tablets, including iPad and Android.

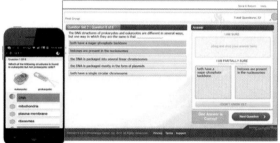

NEW! Dynamic Study Modules

Dynamic Study Modules enable students to study effectively on their own in an adaptive format. Students receive an initial set of questions with a unique answer format asking them to indicate their confidence level. Once completed, reviews include explanations using materials taken directly from the text. These modules can be accessed on smartphones, tablets, and computers.

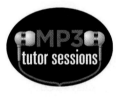

MP3 Tutor Sessions

Downloadable MP3 tutor sessions with rapid review explain the big picture concepts for each chapter and can be downloaded to student smartphones, tablets and computers.

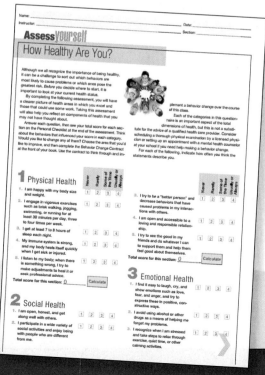

The Study Area

Students can access the Study Area for use on their own or in a study group. Study Area includes: Cumulative Test, RSS Feeds, Audio Case Studies, ABC Videos, and books specific activities.

Labs and Self Assessments

All labs and self assessments are available under the Study Area in an interactive PDF format.

Easy to Get Started, Use, and Make Your Own

MasteringHealth™

FOR INSTRUCTORS

MasteringHealth helps instructors maximize class time with easy-to-assign, customizable, and automatically graded assessments that motivate students to learn outside of the class and arrive prepared for lecture.

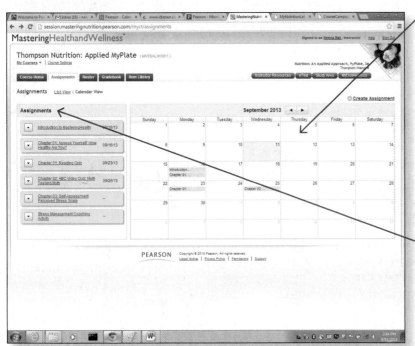

Calendar Feature for Instructors and Students

The Course Home default page now features a Calendar View displaying upcoming assignments and due dates.

- Instructors can schedule assignments by dragging and dropping the assignment onto a date in the calendar.
- The calendar view lets students see at-a-glance when an assignment is due, and resembles a syllabus.

Customize Publisher-provided Problems or Quickly Add Your Own

MasteringHealth™ makes it easy to edit any questions or answers, import your own questions, and quickly add images or links to further enhance the student experience.

Learning Outcomes

Tagged to book content and tied to Bloom's Taxonomy, Learning Outcomes are designed to let Mastering do the work in tracking student performance against your learning outcomes. Mastering offers a data supported measure to quantify students' learning gains and to share those results quickly and easily:

- Add your own or use the publisher-provided learning outcomes.
- View class performance against the specified learning outcomes.
- Export results to a spreadsheet.

Now that students come more prepared to class with MasteringHealth, FLIP YOUR CLASSROOM

NEW! LEARNING CATALYTICS™

Learning Catalytics allows students to use their smart-phones, tablets, or laptops to respond to questions in class.

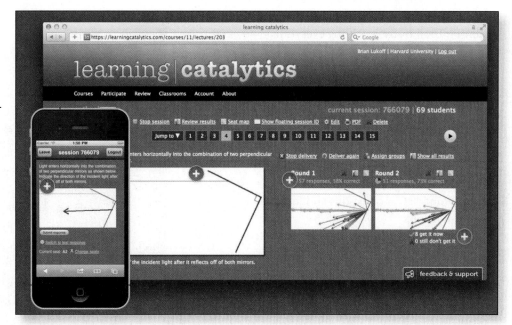

With Learning Catalytics you can:

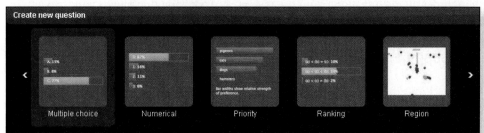

Use a wide variety of question types to engage students: multiple choice, word clouds, sketch a graph, annotate art, high-light a passage, compute a numeric answer, and more.

Use multiple question types to get into the minds of students to understand what they do or don't know and adjust lectures accordingly.

- Access rich analytics to understand student performance.
- Add your own questions to make Learning Catalytics fit your course exactly.
- Assess and improve students' critical-thinking skills, and so much more.

Learning Catalytics is included with the purchase of MasteringHealth.

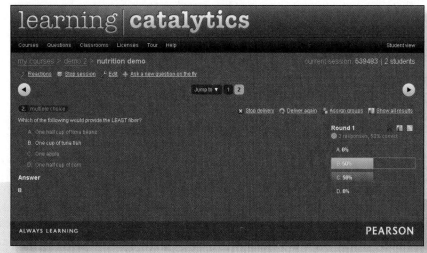

Teaching Toolkit DVD for *Health: The Basics*

The Teaching Toolkit DVD replaces the former printed Teaching Toolbox by providing everything you need to prep for your course and deliver a dynamic lecture in one convenient place. Included on 3 disks are these valuable resources:

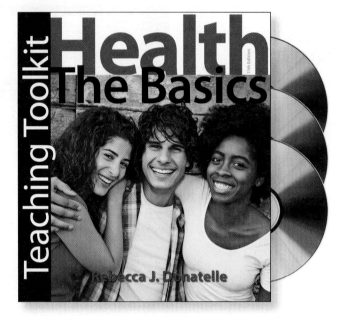

Disk 1: Robust media assets for each chapter:

- 51 *ABC News* Lecture Launcher videos
- PowerPoint® Lecture Outlines
- PowerPoint clicker questions and Jeopardy-style quiz show questions
- Files for all illustrations and tables and selected photos from the text
- Transparency Masters

Disk 2: Comprehensive Test Bank:

- Test Bank in Word and RTF formats
- Computerized Test Bank, which includes all the questions from the test bank in a format that allows you to easily and intuitively build exams and quizzes

Disk 3: Additional innovative supplements for instructors and students:

For Instructors:
- Instructor's Resource Support Manual
- Introduction to MasteringHealth
- Introductory video for Learning Catalytics
- Great Ideas: Active Ways to Teach Health & Wellness
- Teaching with Student Learning Outcomes
- Teaching with Web 2.0

For Students:
- Take Charge of Your Health Worksheets
- Behavior Change Log Book and Wellness Journal
- Eat Right! Healthy Eating in College and Beyond
- Live Right! Beating Stress in College and Beyond
- Food Composition Table

User's Quick Guide for Health: The Basics

This easy-to-use printed supplement accompanies the Teaching Toolkit and offers easy instructions for both experienced and new faculty members to get started with the rich Toolkit content, how to access assignments within MasteringHealth, and how to flip the classroom with Learning Catalytics.

Health
The Basics

11th Edition

REBECCA J. DONATELLE

Oregon State University

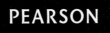

Boston Columbus Indianapolis New York San Francisco Upper Saddle River
Amsterdam Cape Town Dubai London Madrid Milan Munich Paris Montréal Toronto
Delhi Mexico City São Paulo Sydney Hong Kong Seoul Singapore Taipei Tokyo

Executive Editor: Sandra Lindelof

Associate Editor: Erin Schnair

Editorial Manager: Susan Malloy

Development Editors: Marilyn Freedman, Nic Albert, and Erin Strathmann

Production Project Managers: Megan Power and Michael Penne

Editorial Assistant: Tu-Anh Dang-Tran

Assistant Editor: Briana Verdugo

Content Producer: Julia Akpan

Managing Editor: Mike Early

Assistant Managing Editor: Nancy Tabor

Production Management: Thistle Hill Publishing Services

Compositor: Cenveo® Publisher Services/Nesbitt Graphics, Inc.

Interior and Cover Designer: Hespenheide Design

Illustrator: Precision Graphics

Senior Photo Editor: Travis Amos

Manager of Image Resources: Maya Melenchuk

Senior Manufacturing Buyer: Stacey Weinberger

Executive Marketing Manager: Neena Bali

Cover Photo Credit: Peathegee Inc./Blend Images/Corbis

Credits and acknowledgments borrowed from other sources and reproduced, with permission, in this textbook appear on the appropriate page within the text and on p. C-1.

Library of Congress Cataloging-in-Publication Data

Donatelle, Rebecca J., 1950–

   Health : the basics / Rebecca J. Donatelle, Oregon State University.—11th edition.

      pages cm

   Includes bibliographical references and index.

   ISBN-13: 978-0-321-91042-4 (pbk.)

   ISBN-10: 0-321-91042-7 (pbk.)

1. Health—Textbooks. I. Title.

RA776.D663 2015

613—dc23

                                        2013039934

ISBN 10: 0-321-91042-7; ISBN 13: 978-0-321-91042-4 (Student Edition)

ISBN 10: 0-321-95854-3; ISBN 13: 978-0-321-95854-9 (Instructor's Review Copy)

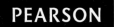

1 2 3 4 5 6 7 8 9 10—CRK—15 14

www.pearsonhighered.com

Brief Contents

Contents

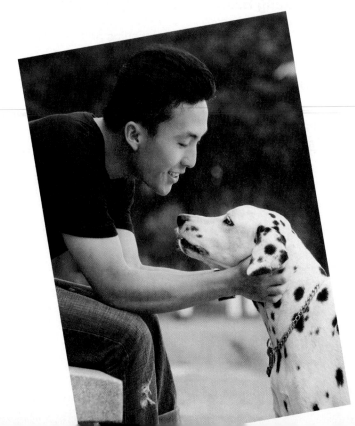

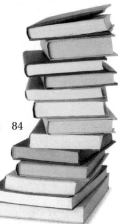

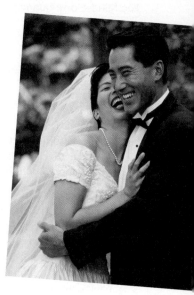

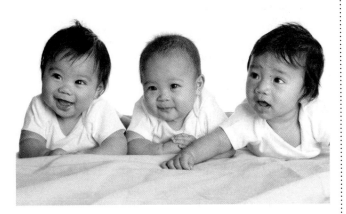

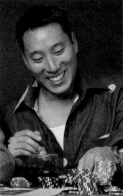

Part Four: Building Healthy Lifestyles

9 Eating for a Healthier You   259

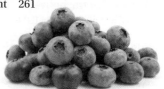

10 Reaching and Maintaining a Healthy Weight   291

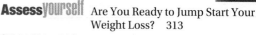

11 Improving Your Personal Fitness 329

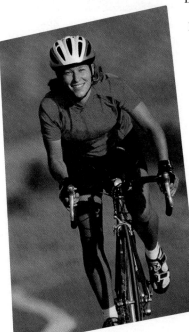

Part Five: Preventing and Fighting Disease

12 Reducing Your Risk of Cardiovascular Disease and Cancer 354

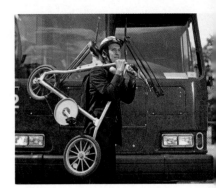

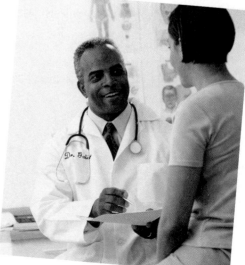

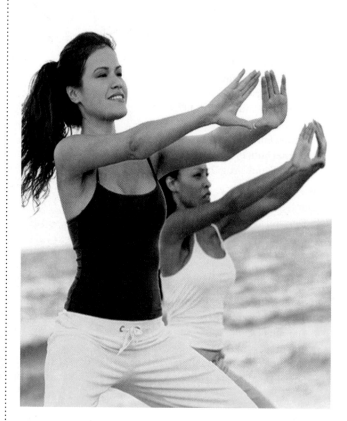

Feature Boxes

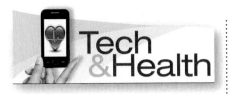
xiii

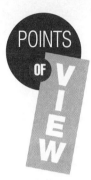
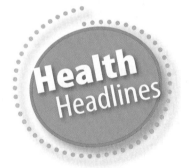
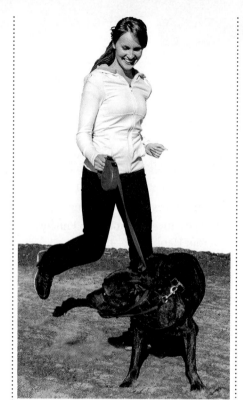

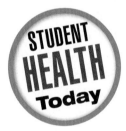
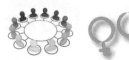
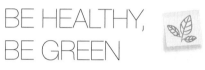
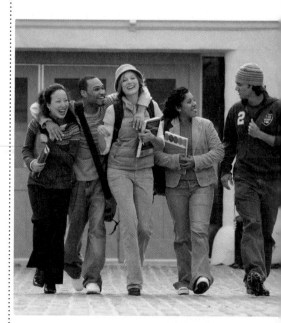

Video Tutors

Preface

In today's world, health is headline news. Whether it is the latest cases of deadly *Escherichia coli* infections from eating infected produce, a new environmental catastrophe, or increasing rates of obesity and diabetes, we are bombarded with a seemingly endless list of potential threats to our health. The issues often seem so huge, so far-reaching, that you may wonder if there is anything you can do to make a difference; to ensure a life that is healthy and long and a planet that is preserved for future generations. You are not alone! Getting healthy and staying healthy is a challenge for many, but the good news is that you *can* do things to improve your health and the health of others. Regardless of your age, sex, race, the environment you live in, or the challenges you face, you can be an agent for healthy change for you, your loved ones, and the greater community.

My goal in writing *Health: The Basics*, 11th Edition, is to empower students to identify their health risks, to examine their behaviors, and to come up with a plan designed to make health a bigger priority in their lives. Because many of today's health concerns know no geographical boundaries, my aim is to challenge students to think globally as they consider health risks and seek creative solutions, both large and small, to address complex health problems. Finding ways to take "baby steps" to change deeply ingrained behaviors is often a key part of successful change. There is no one-size-fits-all recipe for health. This book provides the most scientifically valid information available to help students be smarter in their health decision making, more knowledgeable about personal choices, and more active advocates for healthy changes in their community.

This book is designed to help students quickly grasp the information and understand its relevance to their own lives, both now and in the future. With each new edition of *Health: The Basics*, I am gratified by the overwhelming success that this book has enjoyed through its many revisions and changes. I hope that this edition's rich foundation of scientifically valid information, its wealth of technological tools and resources, and its thought-provoking features will continue to stimulate students to share my enthusiasm for health and to actively engage in health promotion, health behavior, and disease prevention.

New to This Edition

Health: The Basics, 11th Edition, maintains many features that the text has become known for, while incorporating several major revisions and exciting new features. The multimedia created for the 11th Edition is more innovative and robust than ever, and features in the text reflect the exciting, growing connection between multimedia and health. The most noteworthy changes to the text and media as a whole include the following:

- **NEW! MasteringHealth** is an online homework, tutorial, and assessment product designed to improve results by helping students quickly master concepts. Students benefit from self-paced tutorials that feature immediate wrong-answer feedback and hints that emulate the office-hour experience to help keep students on track. With a wide range of interactive, engaging, and assignable activities, students are encouraged to actively learn and retain tough course concepts.
- **NEW! 51 *ABC News* Videos** bring health to life and spark discussion with up-to-date hot topics and include multiple-choice questions that provide wrong-answer feedback to redirect students to the correct answer.
- **NEW! A new mini-chapter, Focus On: Improving Your Financial Health,** covers credit card scams, creating and sticking to a budget, student loans, planning for the future, and other topics related to the practical application of money and finances to health. The chapter follows the first chapter of the book.
- **NEW! Money & Health boxes** cover elements of the financial or economic world that impact personal health. Topics include tips to maximize health care benefits while minimizing costs and guidelines to follow when shopping for fitness facilities to ensure you get a good deal.
- **NEW! Tech & Health boxes** tackle technology advances that make a difference to students. Topics include reviews of various diet- and exercise-monitoring phone apps and a look at whether students who go "tech free" for a time go through the same withdrawal symptoms that drug addicts experience.
- **NEW! Focus On: Reducing Risks and Coping with Chronic Diseases and Conditions** and **Focus On: Understanding Complementary and Alternative Medicine** are new mini-chapters.
- **NEW! Each chapter now includes a Video Tutor** presentation that highlights a book figure or point of discussion in an engaging video (28 total). QR codes placed in the narrative tell students when a video is available. Just scan the QR code with a reader on your smartphone or tablet, and your phone loads up the appropriate Video Tutor.

Chapter-by-Chapter Revisions

The 11th Edition has been updated line by line to provide students with the most current information and references for further exploration. Portions of chapters have been reorganized to improve the flow of topics, and figures, tables, feature boxes, and photos have all been added, improved on, and updated. Throughout the text, all data, statistics, and references have been updated to the most recent possible. The following is a chapter-by-chapter listing of some of the most noteworthy changes, updates, and additions.

Chapter 1: Accessing Your Health

- New **Money & Health** box on maximizing health care and minimizing costs
- New **Tech & Health** box on finding health news on the Internet
- New **Health Headlines** box explaining the Affordable Care Act
- New figure on the transtheoretical model of behavior change

Focus On: Improving Your Financial Health

- New chapter on the basics of financial health, including budgeting, understanding student loans, managing credit cards and debt, and resolving identity theft

Chapter 2: Promoting and Preserving Your Psychological Health

- New **Health Headlines** box covering the causes and effects of too much self-esteem
- New *DSM-5* categories used throughout the discussion of mental illnesses and disorders
- New **Money & Health** box on low-cost options for treating mental health conditions
- Updated discussion of suicide because it has become the leading cause of death on college campuses

Focus On: Cultivating Your Spiritual Health

- New **Skills for Behavior Change** box on community service

Chapter 3: Managing Stress and Coping with Life's Challenges

- New **Health Headlines** box on positive psychology
- New section on shift and persist strategies

Focus On: Improving Your Sleep

- New section describing the impact of technology on sleep patterns
- New photo highlighting the danger of sleepiness among transportation workers
- New graph of U.S. adults who rarely get a good night's sleep

Chapter 4: Preventing Violence and Injury

- New **Tech & Health** box on identity theft, Internet victimization, and social networking safety
- Updated figure showing crime rate statistics

Chapter 5: Building Healthy Relationships and Understanding Sexuality

- New **Tech & Health** box "Love in the Time of Twitter"
- Changed presentation of the figure showing healthy versus unhealthy relationships continuum to enhance readability
- Updated figure of the male reproductive system to identify more organs
- New **Student Health Today** box on social media screening

Chapter 6: Considering Your Reproductive Choices

- New **Tech & Health** box discussing apps for tracking the fertility cycle
- Updated coverage on the most recent innovations in contraception, including statistics on success and failure rates

Chapter 7: Recognizing and Avoiding Addiction and Drug Abuse

- New figure on the cycle of psychological addiction
- New **Tech & Health** box on technology and Internet addiction
- New **Student Health Today** box on gambling and college students
- New section emphasizing the differences between a habit and an addiction
- New photo feature covering recovery from addiction

Chapter 8: Drinking Alcohol Responsibly and Ending Tobacco Use

- New **Tech & Health** box on electronic cigarette risks and concerns
- New **Student Health Today** box on alcohol and energy drinks
- Updated **Health in a Diverse World** box on global alcohol use

Chapter 9: Eating for a Healthier You

- New **Money & Health** box on budgeting for fruits and vegetables
- Expanded information in figure covering foods that provide complementary amino acids
- Updated figure on fats in vegetable oils to enhance readability
- Reorganized section on the recommended intakes for nutrients

Chapter 10: Reaching and Maintaining a Healthy Weight

- New **Tech & Health** box on diet-tracking smartphone apps
- New figure on the world's most and least overweight countries
- Updated table on analyzing popular diet programs

Focus On: Enhancing Your Body Image

- New figures showing the body image and eating issues continuums
- Enhanced information on body image around the world

Chapter 11: Improving Your Personal Fitness

- New **Money & Health** box on choosing a fitness center
- New **Health in a Diverse World** box on how to modify physical activities for people with chronic health conditions
- Reorganized chapter to streamline and enhance the presentation
- Updated discussion of the FITT prescription and associated figure with latest guidelines from the American College of Sports Medicine

Chapter 12: Reducing Your Risk of Cardiovascular Disease and Cancer

- Updated coverage of the risk factors for cardiovascular disease
- Added key term *ideal cardiovascular health*
- Updated **Student Health Today** box on the breast cancer self-examination
- Updated statistics on estimated new cancer cases and cancer deaths
- New figure for the male testicular self-examination
- New table for cancer stages

Focus On: Minimizing Your Risk for Diabetes

- New figure on blood glucose levels
- New **Money & Health** box on the cost of diabetes

Chapter 13: Protecting against Infectious Diseases and Sexually Transmitted Infections

- Revised **Health Headlines** box with more information debunking most anti-vaccination rhetoric
- Updated vaccination recommendations table
- Updated HIV/AIDs infection statistics and recent treatment developments

Focus On: Reducing Risks and Coping with Chronic Diseases and Conditions

- New chapter on key noninfectious diseases, including chronic respiratory diseases, headaches, chronic fatigue syndrome, GI tract problems, back pain, and repetitive motion disorders
- New figures on asthma and the allergic response

Chapter 14: Preparing for Aging, Death, and Dying

- New **Tech & Health** box on hearing loss
- New **Skills for Behavior Change** box with tips for aging well
- New figure on the living arrangements of Americans aged 65 and older

Chapter 15: Promoting Environmental Health

- New **Money & Health** box on food waste
- New **Tech & Health** box on the potential hazards of cell phones
- New **Points of View** box and figure on fracking
- New **Skills for Behavior Change** boxes on shopping to save the planet, avoiding mold, and wasting less water
- Added sections on photochemical smog and acid deposition and acid rain
- Updated coverage of climate change and global warming

Chapter 16: Making Smart Health Care Choices

- New **Money & Health** box on health care spending accounts
- Revised **Points of View** box to reflect recent events in the debate over whether the government should facilitate health care
- Enhanced coverage of issues in today's health care system

Focus On: Understanding Complementary and Alternative Medicine

- Added section on additional forms of energy therapy, including qigong, Reiki, and therapeutic touch

Text Features and Learning Aids

Health: The Basics includes the following special features, all of which have been revised and improved upon for this edition:

- **Chapter learning outcomes** summarize the main competencies students will gain from each chapter and alert students to the key concepts. Focus On mini-chapters now also include learning outcomes.
- **Chapter-opener questions** capture students' attention and engage them in what they will be learning. Questions are repeated and answered in photo legends within the chapter.
- **New! Tech & Health** boxes cover the new technology innovations that can help students stay healthy.
- **New! Money & Health** boxes cover health topics from the financial perspective.
- **What Do You Think?** critical-thinking questions appear throughout the text, encouraging students to pause and reflect on material they have read.
- **Why Should I Care?** features present information on the effects poor health habits have on students in the here and now.
- **What's Working for You?** features call students' attention to the little things they are already doing to improve their health.
- **Assess Yourself** boxes help students evaluate their health behaviors. The **Your Plan for Change** section within each box provides students with targeted suggestions for ways to implement change.
- **Skills for Behavior Change** boxes focus on practical strategies that students can use to improve health or reduce their risks from negative health behaviors.
- **Points of View** boxes present viewpoints on a controversial health issue and ask students *Where Do You Stand?* questions, encouraging them to critically evaluate the information and consider their own opinions.
- **Health Headlines** boxes highlight new discoveries and research, as well as interesting trends in the health field.
- **Student Health Today** boxes focus attention on specific health and wellness issues that relate to today's college students.
- **Health in a Diverse World** boxes expand discussion of health topics to diverse groups within the United States and around the world.
- **Be Healthy, Be Green** boxes offer information on how health topics relate to environmental concerns and suggest ways for students to be both healthy and environmentally friendly.
- A **running glossary** in the margins defines terms where students first encounter them, emphasizing and supporting understanding of material.
- The sections at the ends of chapters focus on student application: **Summary** wraps up chapter content, **Pop Quiz** gives

multiple-choice questions, and **Think about It!** discussion questions encourage students to evaluate and apply new information. **Accessing Your Health on the Internet** and **References** (organized by chapter at the end of the book) offer more opportunities to explore areas of interest.

● A **Behavior Change Contract** for students to fill out is included at the back of the book.

Supplementary Materials

Available with *Health: The Basics,* 11th Edition, is a comprehensive set of ancillary materials designed to enhance learning and to facilitate teaching.

Instructor Supplements

A full resource package accompanies *Health: The Basics* to assist the instructor with classroom preparation and presentation.

● **MasteringHealth** (www.masteringhealthandnutrition.com or www.pearsonmastering.com). MasteringHealth coaches students through the toughest health topics. Instructors can assign engaging tools to help students visualize, practice, and understand crucial content, from the basics of health to the fundamentals of behavior change. **Coaching Activities** guide students through key health concepts with interactive mini-lessons, complete with hints and wrong-answer feedback. **Reading Quizzes** (20 questions per chapter) ensure students have completed the assigned reading before class. *ABC News* **Videos** stimulate classroom discussions and include multiple-choice questions with feedback for students. **NutriTools Coaching Activities** in the nutrition chapter allow students to combine and experiment with different food options and learn firsthand how to build healthier meals. **MP3s** relate to chapter content and come with multiple-choice questions that provide wrong-answer feedback. **Learning Catalytics** provides open-ended questions students can answer in real time. Through targeted assessments, Learning Catalytics helps students develop the critical thinking skills they need for lasting behavior change. For students, the **Study Area** is broken down into learning areas and includes videos, MP3s, practice quizzing, and much more.

● **Teaching Toolkit DVD.** The Teaching Toolkit DVD includes everything an instructor needs to prepare for their course and deliver a dynamic lecture in one convenient place. Resources include: *ABC News* videos, Video Tutor videos, clicker questions, Quiz Show questions, PowerPoint lecture outlines, all figures and tables from the text, transparency masters, PDFs, and Microsoft Word files of the *Instructor Resource and Support Manual* and the Test Bank, the Computerized Test Bank, the User's Quick Guide, *Teaching with Student Learning Outcomes, Teaching with Web 2.0, Great Ideas! Active Ways to Teach Health and Wellness, Behavior Change Log Book and Wellness Journal, Eat Right!, Live Right!,* and *Take Charge of Your Health* worksheets.

● *ABC News* **Videos and Video Tutors.** Fifty-one new *ABC News* videos, each 5 to 10 minutes long, and 28 brand-new brief videos accessible via QR codes in the text help instructors stimulate critical discussion in the classroom. Videos are provided already linked within PowerPoint lectures and are also available

separately in large-screen format with optional closed captioning on the Teaching Toolkit DVD and through MasteringHealth.

● *Instructor Resource and Support Manual.* This teaching tool provides chapter summaries and outlines and a step-by-step visual walk-through of all the resources available to instructors. It includes information on available PowerPoint lectures, integrated *ABC News* video discussion questions, tips and strategies for managing large classrooms, ideas for in-class activities, and suggestions for integrating MasteringHealth and MyDietAnalysis into your classroom activities and homework assignments.

● **Test Bank.** The Test Bank incorporates Bloom's Taxonomy, or the higher order of learning, to help instructors create exams that encourage students to think analytically and critically, rather than simply to regurgitate information. Test Bank questions are tagged to global and book-specific student learning outcomes.

● **User's Quick Guide.** Newly redesigned to be even more useful, this valuable supplement acts as your road map to the Teaching Toolkit DVD.

● *Teaching with Student Learning Outcomes.* This publication contains essays from 11 instructors who are teaching using student learning outcomes. They share their goals in using outcomes, the processes that they follow to develop and refine the outcomes, and provide many useful suggestions and examples for successfully incorporating outcomes into a personal health course.

● *Teaching with Web 2.0.* From Facebook to Twitter to blogs, students are using and interacting with Web 2.0 technologies. This handbook provides an introduction to these popular online tools and offers ideas for incorporating them into your personal health course. Written by personal health and health education instructors, each chapter examines the basics about each technology and ways to make it work for you and your students.

● *Great Ideas! Active Ways to Teach Health & Wellness.* This manual provides ideas for classroom activities related to specific health and wellness topics, as well as suggestions for activities that can be adapted to various topics and class sizes.

● *Behavior Change Log Book and Wellness Journal.* This assessment tool helps students track daily exercise and nutritional intake and create a long-term nutritional and fitness prescription plan. It also includes a Behavior Change Contract and topics for journal-based activities.

Student Supplements

● **The Study Area of MasteringHealth** is organized by learning areas. *Read It* houses the Pearson eText, with which users can create notes, highlight text in different colors, create bookmarks, zoom, click hyperlinked words for definitions, and change page view. Pearson eText also links to associated media files. *See It* includes 51 *ABC News* videos on important health topics and the key concepts of each chapter. *Hear It* contains MP3 Study Tutor files and audio case studies. *Do It* contains critical-thinking questions and Web links. *Review It* contains study quizzes for each chapter. *Live It* will help jump-start students' behavior-change projects with assessments and resources to plan change; students can fill out a Behavior Change Contract, journal and log behaviors, and prepare a reflection piece.

- *Take Charge of Your Health!* **Worksheets.** This pad of 50 self-assessment activities allows students to further explore their health behaviors.
- *Behavior Change Log Book and Wellness Journal.* This assessment tool helps students track daily exercise and nutritional intake and create a long-term nutrition and fitness prescription plan. It includes Behavior Change Contracts and topics for journal-based activities.
- *Eat Right! Healthy Eating in College and Beyond.* This booklet provides students with practical nutrition guidelines, shopper's guides, and recipes.

- *Live Right! Beating Stress in College and Beyond.* This booklet gives students useful tips for coping with stressful life challenges both during college and for the rest of their lives.
- **Digital 5-Step Pedometer** Take strides to better health with this pedometer, which measures steps, distance (miles), activity time, and calories, and provides a time clock.
- **MyDietAnalysis** (www.mydietanalysis.com). Powered by ESHA Research, Inc., MyDietAnalysis features a database of nearly 20,000 foods and multiple reports. It allows students to track their diet and activity using up to three profiles and to generate and submit reports electronically.

Acknowledgments

It is hard for me to believe that *Health: The Basics* is in its 11th edition! Who would have envisioned the evolution of these health texts even a decade ago? With the nearly limitless resources of the Internet, social networking sites, instantaneous access to national databases for statistics, myriads of interesting videos, and late-breaking news reports, there is a media blitz of information to communicate with students. Each step along the way in planning, developing, and translating that information to students and instructors requires a tremendous amount of work from many dedicated people, and I cannot help but think how fortunate I have been to work with the gifted publishing professionals at Pearson. Through time constraints, decision making, and computer meltdowns, this group handled every issue, every obstacle with patience, professionalism, and painstaking attention to detail. From this author's perspective, the personnel personify four key aspects of what it takes to be successful in the publishing world: (1) drive and motivation; (2) commitment to excellence; (3) a vibrant, youthful, forward-thinking and enthusiastic approach; and (4) personalities that motivate an author to continually strive to produce market-leading texts.

In particular, credit goes to the associate editor on this edition, Erin Schnair. Having worked with several outstanding editors over the years, I always wonder if a "new" editor will be as outstanding as the previous one. In this case, Erin's transition to this book was seamless and at the same level of excellence as her fantastic predecessors. I found her to be terrific to work with, highly organized, and thoughtful, and under her guidance, the book has continued to improve. Susan Malloy, the editorial manager for this book, provided overall guidance and expertise to bringing this book to fruition. I have a long history of working with Susan, and she is among the absolute *best* in her field. Marilyn Freedman and Nic Albert used their terrific editorial skills in fine-tuning the diverse chapters of the text. They did amazing work suggesting organizational changes, doing comparative reviews, and merging content and updates with new information and ideas, as well as checking sources for currency and accuracy. A special thanks to them for their behind the scenes efforts! Clearly, I have been very fortunate in having such creative, outstanding individuals leading the editorial direction on my textbooks and an outstanding group of assistants who handle the many details of publishing a textbook. You are fantastic, and your work is much appreciated! Further praise and thanks go to the highly skilled and hard-working, creative, and charismatic Executive Editor Sandra Lindelof, who has helped to catapult this book into a competitive twenty-first century. From searching out and procuring cutting-edge technology to meet the demands of an increasingly savvy student to having her finger on the pulse of what instructors and students need in their classrooms today, Sandy has consistently been a key figure in moving the college/university health text to the next level.

Although these individuals were key contributors to the finished work, there were many other people who worked on this revision of *Health: The Basics*. In particular, I would like to thank Production Project Managers Megan Power and Michael Penne, who skillfully navigated production pitfalls and kept the book moving along. Thanks also to Angela Urquhart, Andrea Archer, and the hard-working staff at Thistle Hill and Cenveo who put everything together to make a polished finished product. The talented artists at Precision Graphics deserve many thanks for making our innovative art program a reality. Gary Hespenheide and his staff at Hespenheide Design worked wonders in bumping up the look and feel of the interior design, and his striking cover is a thing of beauty. Julia Akpan, Content Producer, put together our most innovative and comprehensive media package yet. Additional thanks go to the rest of the team at Pearson, especially Assistant Editor Briana Verdugo, Editorial Assistant Tu-Anh Dang-Tran, and Director of Development Barbara Yien.

The editorial and production teams are critical to a book's success, but I would be remiss if I didn't thank another key group who ultimately helps determine a book's success: the textbook representative and sales group and their leader, Executive Marketing Manager Neena Bali. From directing an outstanding marketing campaign to the everyday tasks of being responsive to instructor needs, Neena does a superb job of making sure that *Health: The Basics* gets into instructors' hands and that adopters receive the service they deserve. In keeping with my overall experiences with Pearson, the marketing and sales staff are among the best of the best. I am very lucky to have them working with me on this project and want to extend a special thanks to all of them!

Contributors to the 11th Edition

Many colleagues, students, and staff members have provided the feedback, reviews, extra time, assistance, and encouragement that have helped me meet the rigorous demands of publishing this book over the years. Whether acting as reviewers, generating new ideas, providing expert commentary, or revising chapters, each of these professionals has added his or her skills to our collective endeavor.

I would like to thank specific contributors to chapters in this edition. In order to make a book like this happen on a relatively short timeline, the talents of many specialists in the field must be combined. Whether contributing creative skills in writing, envisioning areas that will be critical to the current and future health needs of students, using their experiences to make topics come alive for students, or utilizing their professional expertise to ensure scientifically valid information, each of these individuals was carefully selected to help make this text the best that it can be. I couldn't do it without their help! As always, I would like to give particular thanks to Dr. Patricia Ketcham (Oregon State University), who has helped with the *Health: The Basics* series since its earliest beginnings. As Associate Director of health promotion in Student Health Services on campus, with specialties in health promotion and health behavior and substance abuse, Dr. Ketcham provides a unique perspective on the key challenges facing today's students. She contributed to revisions of Chapter 7, Recognizing and Avoiding Addiction and Drug Abuse; Chapter 8, Drinking Alcohol Responsibly and Ending Tobacco Use; Chapter 14, Preparing for Aging, Death, and Dying; and Chapter 16, Making Smart Health Care Choices. Dr. Susan Dobie, Associate Professor in the School of Health, Physical Education, and Leisure Services at University of Northern Iowa, used her background in health promotion and health behavior and in teaching a diverse range of students to provide a fresh approach to revisions of Chapter 2, Promoting and Preserving Your Psychological Health; Chapter 5, Building Healthy Relationships and Understanding Sexuality; and Chapter 6, Considering Your Reproductive Choices. Dr. Erica Jackson, Associate Professor in the Department of Public & Allied Health Sciences at Delaware State University, applied her wealth of fitness knowledge to update and enhance Chapter 11, Improving Your Personal Fitness. With her outstanding background in nutrition science and applied dietary behavior, Dr. Kathy Munoz, Professor in the Department of Kinesiology and Recreation Administration at Humbolt State University, provided an extensive revision and updating of Chapter 9, Eating for a Healthier You. Dr. Karen Elliot, Assistant Professor in the Health Promotion and Health Behavior Program at Oregon State University, contributed to the updating and revision of Focus On: Cultivating Your Spiritual Heath and Focus On: Enhancing Your Body Image. She also provided key updates to the STI and HIV/AIDS sections of Chapter 13. Laura Bonazzoli, who has been a key part of developing and refining many aspects of this book over the last editions, used her considerable knowledge and skills in providing major revisions of Chapter 1, Accessing Your Health and Focus On: Understanding Complementary and Alternative Medicine. Erin Strathmann, who was instrumental in the success of the last edition of this text, provided outstanding suggestions for revisions. Her thorough edits and concise, creative suggestions along the way were instrumental in our ability to meet deadlines and complete a rigorous and thorough update of this text. Importantly, as someone who was key to the success of our innovative financial health text sections, she was able to expand on this important

information by contributing Focus On: Improving Your Financial Health. Thanks also to Debra Smith (Ohio University) for her contribution to the dynamic video tutors and to the talented people who contributed to the supplement package: Elizabeth Barrington (San Diego Mesa College), Karla Rues (Ozarks Technical Community College), Brent Goff, and Nic Albert.

Reviewers for the 11th Edition

With each new edition of *Health: The Basics*, we have built on the combined expertise of many colleagues throughout the country who are dedicated to the education and behavioral changes of students. We thank the many reviewers who have made such valuable contributions to the past nine editions of *Health: The Basics*. For the 11th edition, reviewers who have helped us continue this tradition of excellence include Ari Fisher (Louisiana State University), Tiffany Fuller (North Carolina Agricultural and Technical State University), Michele Hamm (Mesa Community College), Steve Hartman (Citrus College), David Hey (Cal Poly), Jim Ledrick (Grand Valley State University), Donna McGill-Cameron (Woodland Community College), Dana Sherman (Ozarks Technical Community College), Cynthia Smith (Central Piedmont Community College), Cody Trefethen (Palomar College), Glenda Warren (University of the Cumberlands), and the Pearson Campus Ambassadors.

Reviewers for MasteringHealth

We thank the following members of the Faculty Advisory Board, who offered us valuable insights that helped develop MasteringHealth: Steve Hartman (Citrus College), William Huber (County College of Morris), Kris Jankovitz (Cal Poly), Stasi Kasaianchuk (Oregon State University), Lynn Long (University of North Carolina Wilmington), Ayanna Lyles (California University of Pennsylvania), Steven Namanny (Utah Valley University), Karla Rues (Ozarks Technical Community College), Debra Smith (Ohio University), Sheila Stepp (SUNY Orange), and Mary Winfrey-Kovell (Ball State University).

Many thanks to all!
Rebecca J. Donatelle, PhD

About the Author

Rebecca Donatelle is a Professor Emeritus in Public Health at Oregon State University, having served as the department chair, coordinator of the Public Health Promotion and Education Programs, and faculty member and researcher in the College of Health and Human Sciences. She has a doctorate degree in community health/health education, a master of science degree in health education, and a bachelor of science degree with majors in both health/physical education and English. Over the years, she has taught thousands of undergraduate and graduate students in a wide range of health promotion and behavior areas, including courses such as Personal Health, Violence and Public Health, Prevention of Chronic and Infectious Diseases, Health Behaviors, Women's Health, and Health and Aging. Her main research and teaching focus has been on the factors that increase risk for chronic diseases and the use of incentives and social supports in developing behavioral interventions for high-risk populations. She has received several awards for teaching and mentoring students from a wide range of health-related disciplines.

Accessing Your Health

1

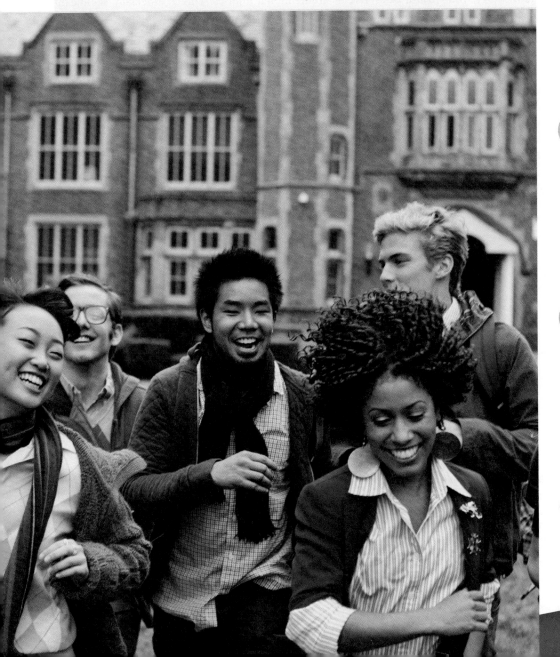

LEARNING OUTCOMES

✱ Describe the immediate and long-term rewards of healthy behaviors and the effects that your health choices may have on others.

✱ Compare and contrast the medical model of health and the public health model, and discuss the six dimensions of health and wellness.

✱ Identify the determinants of health and explain how they influence the health of individuals and communities. Identify several personal factors that influence your health and classify them as modifiable or nonmodifiable.

✱ Compare and contrast the health belief model, the social cognitive model, and the transtheoretical model of behavior change. Identify your own current risk behaviors, the factors that influence those behaviors, and the strategies you can use to change them.

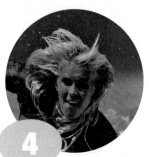

4

How are *health* and *quality of life* related?

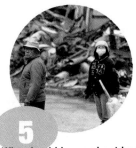

5

Why should I care about health conditions in other places?

15

How can I stay motivated to improve my health habits?

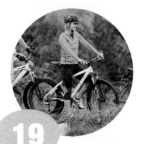

19

How do other people influence my health behaviors?

Got health? That may sound like a simple question, but health is a process, not something we just "get." People who are healthy in their forties, fifties, sixties, and beyond aren't just lucky, wealthy, or the beneficiaries of hardy genes. In most cases, those who thrive in later years prioritized their health early on. You've probably heard from your parents and grandparents that your college years are some of the best of your life. Here the canvas is hung upon which you will paint the story of your life. Whether your story is filled with good health, productive careers, special relationships, and fulfillment of goals is influenced by the health choices you make—beginning right now.

Why Health, Why Now?

In addition to our desire to improve our own health, constant messages via social media, websites, e-mail, television, phone, and other media remind us of health challenges facing the world, the nation, our communities, and our campuses. In the twenty-first century, your health is connected not only to the people with whom you directly interact and the environments in which you spend time, but also to people you've never met and to the well-being of the entire planet.

How does what you do today influence you and those around you? Let's take a look at how your actions and inactions matter.

Choosing Health Now Has Immediate Benefits

Almost everyone knows that overeating leads to weight gain and that drinking and driving increases the risk of motor vehicle accidents. But other choices you make every day may have subtler influences on your well-being in ways you're not aware of. For instance, did you know that the amount of sleep you get each night could affect your weight, your ability to ward off colds, your mood, and even your driving? What's more, inadequate sleep is one of the most commonly reported impediments to academic success (Figure 1.1). Similarly, drinking alcohol reduces your immediate health and your academic performance. It also sharply increases your risk of unintentional injuries. This is especially significant because, for people between the ages of 15 and 44, unintentional injury—whether due to alcohol abuse or any other factor—is the leading cause of death (Table 1.1).

It isn't an exaggeration to say that healthy choices have immediate benefits. When you're well nourished, fit, rested, and free from the influence of nicotine, alcohol, and other drugs, you're more likely to avoid illness, succeed in school, maintain supportive relationships, participate in meaningful work and community activities, and enjoy your leisure time.

Choosing Health Now Leads to Many Long-Term Rewards

The choices you make today are like seeds: Planting good seeds means you're more likely to enjoy the fruits of a longer and healthier life. In contrast, poor choices increase the likelihood of a shorter life, as well as persistent illness, addiction, and other limitations on quality of life. In other words, successful aging begins now.

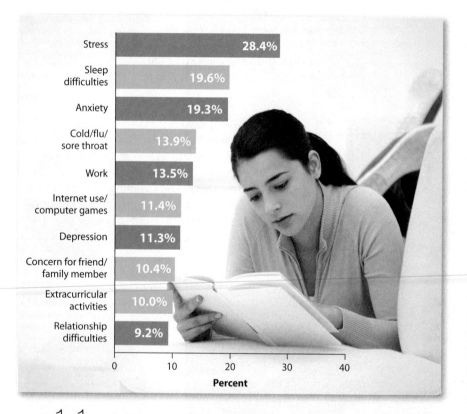

FIGURE 1.1 Top Ten Reported Impediments to Academic Performance—Past 12 Months In a recent survey by the National College Health Association, students indicated that stress, poor sleep, anxiety, and recurrent minor illnesses, among other things, had prevented them from performing at their academic best.

Source: Data from American College Health Association, *American College Health Association—National College Health Assessment II (ACHA-NCHA II) Reference Group Executive Summary*, Fall 2012 (Hanover, MD: American College Health Association, 2013). Available at www.acha-ncha.org

Chart data (Figure 1.1):
- Stress: 28.4%
- Sleep difficulties: 19.6%
- Anxiety: 19.3%
- Cold/flu/sore throat: 13.9%
- Work: 13.5%
- Internet use/computer games: 11.4%
- Depression: 11.3%
- Concern for friend/family member: 10.4%
- Extracurricular activities: 10.0%
- Relationship difficulties: 9.2%

Hear It! Podcasts
Want a study podcast for this chapter? Download **Promoting Healthy Behavior Change** in the Study Area of MasteringHealth™

<table>
<tr><th colspan="2">TABLE 1.1 Leading Causes of Death in the United States, Preliminary Data for 2011, Overall and by Age Group</th></tr>
<tr><td>All Ages</td><td>Number of Deaths</td></tr>
<tr><td>Diseases of the heart</td><td>596,339</td></tr>
<tr><td>Malignant neoplasms (cancer)</td><td>575,313</td></tr>
<tr><td>Chronic lower respiratory diseases</td><td>143,382</td></tr>
<tr><td>Cerebrovascular diseases</td><td>128,931</td></tr>
<tr><td>Accidents (unintentional injuries)</td><td>122,777</td></tr>
<tr><td>Aged 15–24</td><td></td></tr>
<tr><td>Accidents (unintentional injuries)</td><td>12,032</td></tr>
<tr><td>Self-harm (suicide)</td><td>4,688</td></tr>
<tr><td>Assault (homicide)</td><td>4,508</td></tr>
<tr><td>Malignant neoplasms</td><td>1,609</td></tr>
<tr><td>Diseases of the heart</td><td>948</td></tr>
<tr><td>Aged 25–44</td><td></td></tr>
<tr><td>Accidents (unintentional injuries)</td><td>29,424</td></tr>
<tr><td>Malignant neoplasms (cancer)</td><td>15,210</td></tr>
<tr><td>Diseases of the heart</td><td>13,479</td></tr>
<tr><td>Self-harm (suicide)</td><td>12,269</td></tr>
<tr><td>Assault (homicide)</td><td>6,639</td></tr>
<tr><td>Aged 45–64</td><td></td></tr>
<tr><td>Malignant neoplasms (cancer)</td><td>161,072</td></tr>
<tr><td>Diseases of the heart</td><td>105,013</td></tr>
<tr><td>Accidents (unintentional injuries)</td><td>34,621</td></tr>
<tr><td>Chronic lower respiratory diseases</td><td>19,646</td></tr>
<tr><td>Chronic liver disease and cirrhosis</td><td>19,551</td></tr>
<tr><td>Aged 65+</td><td></td></tr>
<tr><td>Diseases of the heart</td><td>476,220</td></tr>
<tr><td>Malignant neoplasms (cancer)</td><td>396,126</td></tr>
<tr><td>Chronic lower respiratory diseases</td><td>122,381</td></tr>
<tr><td>Cerebrovascular diseases</td><td>109,393</td></tr>
<tr><td>Alzheimer's disease</td><td>83,746</td></tr>
</table>

Source: Data from D. L. Hovert and J. Q. Xu, "Deaths: Preliminary Data for 2011, Table 7," *National Vital Statistics Report* 61, no. 6 (Hyattsville, MD: National Center for Health Statistics, 2012), www.cdc.gov

third of all deaths were from infections, and over 40 percent of those deaths were in children under the age of 5.[2] Even among adults, infectious diseases such as tuberculosis and pneumonia were the leading causes of death, and widespread epidemics of infectious diseases such as influenza and polio crossed national boundaries to kill millions.

With the development of vaccines and antibiotics, as well as other public health successes, life expectancy increased dramatically as premature deaths from infectious diseases decreased. As a result, the leading cause of death shifted to **chronic diseases** such as heart disease, cerebrovascular disease (which leads to strokes), cancer, and diabetes. At the same time, advances in diagnostic technologies, heart and brain surgery, radiation and other cancer treatments, as well as new medications, continued the trend of increasing life expectancy into the twenty-first century.

Unfortunately, life expectancy in the United States is several years below that of many other nations, and some researchers believe that our increasing prevalence of extreme obesity may be limiting our gains in life expectancy.[3] A study led by researchers from the Harvard School of Public Health and the University of Washington indicates that smoking, high blood pressure, elevated blood glucose, and overweight/obesity together reduce life expectancy in the United States by 4.9 years in men and 4.1 years in women.[4]

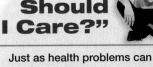

"Why Should I Care?"

Just as health problems can create impediments to success in life, improving your health can lead to better academic performance, greater career success, more relationship satisfaction, and more joy in living.

mortality rate The proportion of deaths to population.

life expectancy Expected number of years of life remaining at a given age, such as at birth.

chronic disease A disease that typically begins slowly, progresses, and persists, with a variety of signs and symptoms that can be treated but not cured by medication.

healthy life expectancy Expected number of years of full health remaining at a given age, such as at birth.

Personal Choices Influence *Healthy* **Life Expectancy** Another benefit of healthful choices is that they increase your **healthy life expectancy**; that is, the number

Personal Choices Influence Life Expectancy

According to current **mortality rates**—which reflect the proportion of deaths within a population—the average **life expectancy** at birth in the United States is projected to be 78.7 years for a child born in 2011.[1] In other words, we can expect that American infants born today will live to an average age of over 78 years—much longer than the 47-year life expectancy for people born in the early 1900s. That's because life expectancy a century ago was largely determined by our susceptibility to infectious diseases. Before the advent of vaccines, antibiotics, and infection control, over a

65 & 67

are the *healthy* life expectancy ages of men and women, respectively, in the United States, while the average total life expectancy ages are 76.3 and 81.1.

of years of full health you enjoy, without disability, chronic pain, or significant illness. One dimension of healthy life expectancy is **health-related quality of life (HRQoL)**, a concept that goes beyond mortality rates and life expectancy and focuses on the impact health status has on physical, mental, emotional, and social function. Closely related to this is **well-being**, which assesses the positive aspects of a person's life, such as positive emotions and life satisfaction.[5]

Choosing Health Now Benefits Others

Our personal health choices don't affect only our own lives. They affect the lives of others because they contribute to global health or the global burden of disease. For example, we've said that overeating and inadequate physical activity contribute to obesity. But obesity isn't a problem only for the individual. Along with its associated health problems, obesity burdens the U.S. health care system and the U.S. economy overall. According to a report from the Brookings Institution, "By some estimates, nearly 21 percent of current medical spending in the U.S. is now obesity related." A significant proportion of these medical costs is paid by Medicaid and Medicare, and one recent analysis concluded that total Medicaid spending would be 12 percent lower in the absence of obesity.[6] In addition, obesity costs the public indirectly. These indirect costs include, for example, reduced tax revenues because of income lost from absenteeism and premature death, increased disability payments because of an inability to remain in the workforce, and increased health insurance rates as claims rise for treatment of obesity itself as well as its associated diseases.

Smoking, excessive consumption of alcohol, and use of illegal drugs also place an economic burden on our communities and our society. Moreover, these behaviors have social and emotional consequences, such as for people who lose loved ones in their prime. The burden on caregivers who must sacrifice personally to take care of those who are disabled by diseases is another part of this problem.

At the root is an ethical question causing considerable debate: To what extent should the public be held accountable for an individual's poor choices? Should we require individuals to somehow pay for their poor choices? Of course, in some cases, we already do. We tax cigarettes and alcohol, 17 states tax candy at a higher rate than other groceries, and 4 states are currently taxing sweetened soft drinks, which have been blamed for rising obesity rates.[7] On the other side of the debate are those who argue that smoking, drinking, and eating certain foods are addictions that require treatment, not punishment, and that obesity is a product of a society of excess. Should individuals be punished for choices that society influenced and the media promoted? And are seemingly personal choices that influence health always entirely within our personal control? Before we explore these questions further, it's essential to understand what health actually is.

health-related quality of life (HRQoL) A multidimensional concept that focuses on the impact health status has on physical, mental, emotional, and social function and quality of life overall.

well-being An assessment of the positive aspects of a person's life, such as positive emotions and life satisfaction.

health The ever-changing process of achieving individual potential in the physical, social, emotional, mental, spiritual, and environmental dimensions.

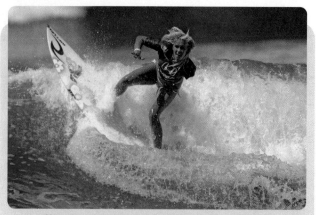

How are *health* and *quality of life* related?

Health-related quality of life is a person's or group's perceived physical and mental health over time. A person with an illness or disability doesn't necessarily have a low quality of life. The Hawaiian surfer Bethany Hamilton lost her arm in a shark attack while surfing at the age of 13, but that hasn't prevented her from achieving her goals and a high quality of life. She returned to surfing just 1 month after the attack and has since competed around the world as a professional surfer.

What Is Health?

Although we use the word **health** almost unconsciously, few people understand the broad scope of the word or how it has evolved over the years.

Models of Health

Over the centuries, different ideals—or models—of human health have dominated. Our current model of health has broadened from a focus on the individual physical body to an understanding of health as a reflection not only of ourselves and our mental and emotional well-being, but also the health and safety of our communities.

Medical Model Prior to the twentieth century, if you made it to your fiftieth birthday, you were regarded as lucky. Survivors were believed to be of hearty, healthy stock—having what we might refer to today as "good genes."

Throughout these years, perceptions of health were dominated by the **medical model**, in which health status focused primarily on the individual and his or her tissues and organs. The surest way to improve health was to cure the individual's disease, either with medication to treat the disease-causing agent or through surgery to remove the diseased body part. Thus, government resources focused on initiatives that led to treatment, rather than prevention, of disease.

Public Health Model Not until the early decades of the 1900s did researchers begin to recognize that entire populations of poor people, particularly those living in certain locations, had higher health risks due to things over which they had little control: polluted water and air, a low-quality diet, poor housing, and unsafe work settings. Slowly, a new, more progressive way of approaching health problems began to evolve, known as the **ecological or public health model**, which viewed diseases and other negative health events as a result of an individual's interaction with his or her social and physical environment.

Recognition of the public health model enabled health officials to prioritize hygiene and sanitation. Communities took action to control contaminants in water, for example, by building

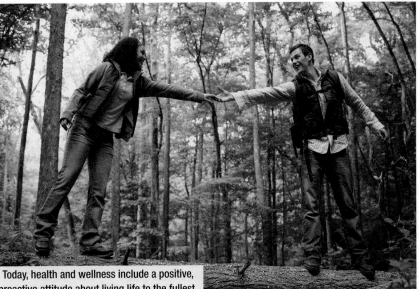

Today, health and wellness include a positive, proactive attitude about living life to the fullest.

adequate sewers, and to control burning and other forms of air pollution. In the early 1900s, colleges began offering courses in health and hygiene, the predecessors of the course you are taking today. And over time, public health officials began to recognize and address many other forces affecting human health, including hazardous work conditions; negative influences in the home and social environment; abuse of drugs and alcohol; stress; mental health; diet; sedentary lifestyle; and cost, quality, and access to health care.

By the 1940s progressive thinkers began calling for even more policies, programs, and services to improve individual health and that of the population as a whole. In other words, their focus shifted from treatment of individual illness to **disease prevention** by reducing or eliminating the factors that cause illness and injury. For example, vaccination programs became widespread, pharmaceutical companies began to manufacture antibiotics to treat bacterial threats, laws governing occupational safety reduced injuries and deaths among American workers, and seatbelts and other vehicle safety standards were mandated. Much of this progress was initiated by a 1947 World Health Organization (WHO) proposal that defined health as more than just a physical state. WHO leaders proposed a more progressive definition of health: "Health is the state of complete physical, mental, and social well-being, not just the absence of disease or infirmity."[8] This new definition definitively rejected the old medical model.

medical model A view of health that focuses primarily on the individual and a biological or diseased organ perspective.

ecological or public health model A view of health in which diseases and other negative health events are seen as a result of an individual's interaction with his or her social and physical environment.

disease prevention Actions or behaviors designed to keep people from getting sick or injured.

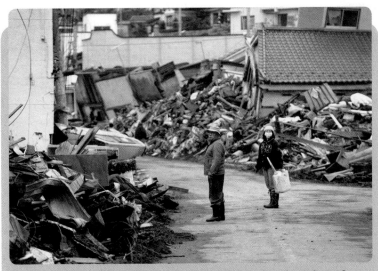

Why should I care about health conditions in other places?

Unhealthy conditions in one location can have far-reaching impacts on the economy and on health. When the 2011 earthquake and tsunami in Japan caused devastation in that country, productivity losses were felt as far away as Europe. The natural disaster damaged the Fukushima Daiichi nuclear power plant, spreading fear of nuclear fallout throughout the world.

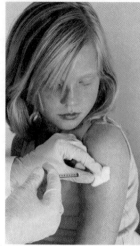

Vaccinations
Motor vehicle safety
Workplace safety
Control of infectious diseases
Reduction in cardiovascular
disease (CVD) and stroke deaths
Safe and healthy foods
Maternal and infant care
Family planning
Fluoridated drinking water
Recognition of tobacco as a
health hazard

FIGURE 1.2 The Top Ten Public Health Achievements of the Twentieth Century

Source: Data from Centers for Disease Control and Prevention, "Ten Great Public Health Achievements—United States, 1900–1999," *Morbidity and Mortality Weekly Report* 48, no. 12 (April 1999).

health promotion The combined educational, organizational, procedural, environmental, social, and financial supports that help individuals and groups reduce negative health behaviors and that promote and maintain positive change.

risk behaviors Actions that increase susceptibility to negative health outcomes.

wellness The dynamic, ever-changing process of trying to achieve one's potential in each of six interrelated dimensions based on one's unique limitations and strengths.

Alongside prevention, the public health model began to emphasize **health promotion**; that is, policies and programs that promote and help maintain behaviors known to support good health. Health-promotion programs identify people who are engaging in **risk behaviors** (those that increase susceptibility to negative health outcomes) and motivate them to change their actions by changing aspects of the larger environment to increase their chances of success.

Over the past 100 years, numerous public policies and services, technological advances, and individual actions have worked together to improve our overall health status. Figure 1.2 lists the ten greatest public health achievements of the twentieth century.

Wellness and the Dimensions of Health

In 1968, biologist, environmentalist, and philosopher René Dubos proposed an even broader definition of health. In his Pulitzer Prize–winning book, *So Human an Animal*, Dubos defined health as "a quality of life, involving social, emotional, mental, spiritual, and biological fitness on the part of the individual, which results from adaptations to the environment."[9] This concept of adaptability, or the ability to cope successfully with life's ups and downs, became a key element in our overall understanding of health.

Eventually the word **wellness** entered the popular vocabulary. This word enlarged Dubos's definition of health by recognizing levels—or gradations—of health within each category (Figure 1.3). To achieve *high-level wellness*, a person must move progressively higher on a continuum of positive health indicators. Those who fail to achieve these levels may slip into ill health, disease, declining quality of life, and premature disability/death.

Today, the words *health* and *wellness* are often used interchangeably to mean the dynamic, ever-changing process of trying to achieve one's potential in each of six interrelated dimensions (Figure 1.4):

● **Physical health.** This dimension includes characteristics such as body size and shape, sensory acuity and responsiveness, susceptibility to disease and disorders, body functioning, physical fitness, and recuperative abilities. Newer definitions of physical health also include our ability to perform normal *activities of daily living (ADL),* or those tasks that are necessary to normal existence in society, such as getting up out of a chair or writing a check.

● **Social health.** The ability to have a broad social network and maintain satisfying interpersonal relationships with friends, family members, and partners is a key part of overall wellness. This implies being able to give and receive love and to be nurturing and supportive in social interactions in a variety of settings. Successfully interacting and communicating with others, adapting to various social situations, and other daily behaviors are all part of social health.

● **Intellectual health.** The ability to think clearly, reason objectively, analyze critically, and use brainpower effectively

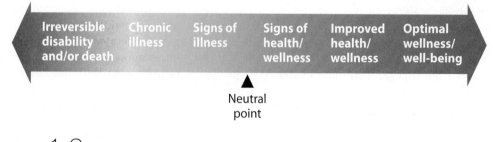

| Irreversible disability and/or death | Chronic illness | Signs of illness | Signs of health/ wellness | Improved health/ wellness | Optimal wellness/ well-being |

Neutral point

FIGURE 1.3 The Wellness Continuum

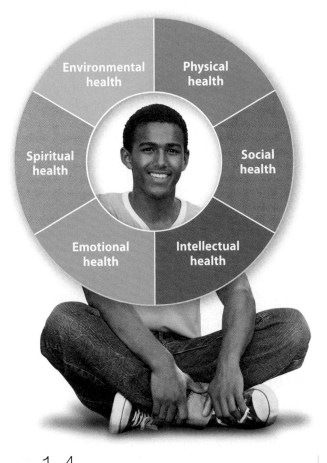

FIGURE 1.4 **The Dimensions of Health**
When all the dimensions are in balance and well developed, they can support your active and thriving lifestyle.

Video Tutor: Dimensions of Health

to meet life's challenges are all part of this dimension. This includes learning from successes and mistakes and making sound, responsible decisions that consider all aspects of a situation. It also includes having a healthy curiosity about life and an interest in learning new things.

● **Emotional health.** This is the feeling component—being able to express emotions when appropriate and to control them when not. Self-esteem, self-confidence, trust, love, and many other emotional reactions and responses are all part of emotional health.

● **Spiritual health.** This dimension involves having a sense of meaning and purpose in your life. This may include believing in a supreme being or following a particular religion's rules and customs. It also may involve the ability to understand and express one's purpose in life; to feel a part of a greater spectrum of existence; to experience peace, contentment, and wonder over life's experiences; and to care about and respect all living things. (For more information on this dimension of health, see Focus On: Cultivating Your Spiritual Health on page 60.)

● **Environmental health.** This dimension entails understanding how the health of the environments in which you live, work, and play can positively or negatively affect you; protecting yourself from hazards in your own environment; and working to preserve, protect, and improve environmental conditions for everyone.

Achieving wellness means attaining the optimal level of well-being for your unique limitations and strengths. For example, a physically disabled person may function at his or her optimal level of performance; enjoy satisfying interpersonal relationships; work to maintain emotional, spiritual, and intellectual health; and have a strong interest in environmental concerns. In contrast, those who spend hours lifting weights to perfect the size and shape of each muscle but pay little attention to their social or emotional health may look healthy but may not maintain a good balance in all dimensions. In short, external trappings reveal very little about a person's overall health. The perspective we need is *holistic,* emphasizing the balanced integration of mind, body, and spirit.

What Influences Health?

If you're lucky, aspects of your world conspire to promote your health: Everyone in your family is slender and fit; there are fresh apples on sale at the neighborhood farmer's market; and a new bike trail opens along the river (and you have a bike!). If you're not so lucky, aspects of your world discourage health: Everyone in your family is overweight, and they eat high-fat diets; there are only cigarettes, alcohol, and junk foods for sale at the corner market; and you wouldn't dare walk or ride alongside the river for fear of being mugged. In short, seemingly personal choices aren't always totally within an individual's control.

Public health experts refer to the factors that influence health as **determinants of health**, a term the U.S. Surgeon General has defined as "the array of critical influences that determine the health of individuals and communities."[10] The Surgeon General's health promotion plan, called *Healthy People,* has been published every 10 years since 1990 with the goal of improving the health-related quality of life and years of life for all Americans. *Healthy People* sets objectives and provides science-based benchmarks to focus efforts and monitor progress on meeting those objectives. The overarching goals set out by the newest version, *Healthy People 2020,* are as follows:

● Attain high-quality, longer lives free of preventable diseases
● Achieve health equity, eliminate disparities, and improve the health of all groups

determinants of health The array of critical influences that determine the health of individuals and communities.

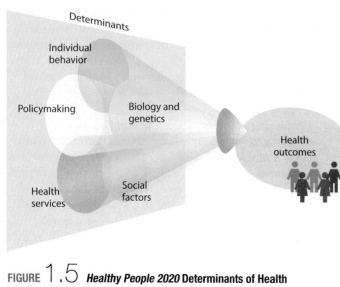

FIGURE 1.5 *Healthy People 2020* **Determinants of Health**
The determinants of health often overlap one another. Collectively, they impact the health of individuals and communities.
Source: Adapted from *Healthy People 2020* Framework, U.S. Department of Health and Human Services, Office of Disease Prevention and Health Promotion.

- Create social and physical environments that promote good health for all
- Promote quality of life, healthy development, and healthy behaviors across all life stages

Healthy People 2020 classifies health determinants into five categories: individual behavior, biology and genetics, social factors, health services, and policymaking (Figure 1.5). A sixth category, health disparities, is equally important.

Individual Behavior

Individual behaviors can help you attain, maintain, or regain good health, or they can deteriorate your health and promote disease. From birth onward, your behaviors are shaped by a multitude of influences. Fortunately, most behaviors are things you can change, so health experts tend to refer to them as *modifiable determinants*. Modifiable determinants significantly influence your risk for chronic disease. Earlier, we said that chronic diseases are the leading causes of death and disability in the United States; indeed, they are responsible for 7 out of 10 deaths.[11] Incredibly, just four modifiable determinants are responsible for most of the illness, suffering, and early death related to chronic diseases (Figure 1.6). They are the following:[12]

- **Lack of physical activity.** Physical inactivity and overweight/obesity are each responsible for nearly 1 in 10 deaths in U.S. adults.

- **Poor nutrition.** Diets high in sodium, saturated fats, and *trans* fats and low in omega-3 fatty acids are the dietary risks with the largest mortality effects.
- **Excessive alcohol consumption.** Alcohol causes 80,000 deaths in adults annually through cardiovascular disease, cancer, other medical conditions, motor vehicle accidents, and violence.
- **Tobacco use.** Tobacco smoking and the cancer, high blood pressure, and respiratory disease it causes are responsible for about 1 in 5 deaths in American adults.

On the flip side, studies have shown that people who drink only in moderation, do not smoke, exercise two or more hours per week, and eat three servings of fruits and vegetables daily live, on average, 12 years longer than those who do not choose these behaviors![13]

Other modifiable determinants include use of vitamins, supplements, caffeine, over-the-counter medications, and illegal drugs; sexual behaviors and use of contraceptives; sleep habits; recycling; and hand washing and other simple infection-control measures.

Biology and Genetics

Biological and genetic determinants are things you can't typically change or modify. Health experts frequently refer to these factors as *nonmodifiable determinants*. They include genetically inherited conditions such as sickle cell disease and hemophilia, as well as inherited predispositions to diseases such as allergies and asthma, certain cancers, and other problems. They also refer to certain innate characteristics such as your age, race, ethnicity, metabolic rate,

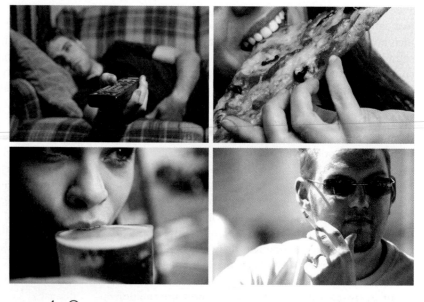

FIGURE 1.6 Four Leading Causes of Chronic Disease in the United States
Lack of physical activity, poor nutrition, excessive alcohol consumption, and tobacco use—all modifiable health determinants—are the four most significant factors leading to chronic disease among Americans today.

and body structure. Your sex is a key biological determinant: As compared to men, women have an increased risk for low bone density and autoimmune diseases (in which the body attacks its own cells), whereas young and middle-aged men have an increased risk for heart disease compared to young and middle-aged women. Your own history of illness and injury also falls within this grouping; if you suffered a serious knee injury in high school, it might cause you to experience pain in walking and exercise, which in turn may predispose you toward weight gain.

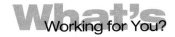

What's Working for You?

Maybe you are already taking strides to live a more healthful life. How many of these healthy behaviors do you practice?

☐ I get a minimum of 7 hours of sleep every night.

☐ I maintain healthy eating habits and manage my weight.

☐ I regularly engage in physical activity.

☐ If I am sexually active, I practice safer sex.

☐ I limit my intake of alcohol and avoid tobacco products.

☐ I schedule regular medical checkups.

Social Factors

Social factors include the social and physical conditions of the environment in which people are born and live. Exposure to crime, violence, mass media, technology, and poverty, as well as availability of educational and job opportunities, healthful foods, transportation, and living wages are social factors. So is the amount of social support available. Physical conditions include the natural environment; conditions such as good lighting, trees, or benches; the state of buildings, such as homes, schools, or workplaces; exposure to toxic substances; and the presence of physical barriers, which can present problems, particularly for people with disabilities.

Economic Factors Among the most powerful of all determinants of health in your social environment are economic factors: Even in affluent nations such as the United States, people who are in lower socioeconomic brackets have substantially shorter life expectancies and more illnesses than do people who are wealthy.[14] Economic disadvantages exert their effects on human health within nearly all domains of life. They include the following:

● Lacking access to quality education from early childhood through adulthood

● Living in poor housing with potential exposure to asbestos, lead, dust mites, rodents and other pests, inadequate sanitation, tap water that's not safe to drink, and high levels of crime

● Being unable to pay for nourishing food, warm clothes, and sturdy shoes; heat and other utilities; medications and medical supplies; transportation; and counseling services, fitness classes, and other wellness measures

See It! Videos

How can a community's cafe help fight hunger? Watch **Hunger at Home** in the Study Area of MasteringHealth™

● Having insecure employment or being stuck in a low-paying job with few benefits

● Having few assets to fall back on in case of illness or injury

Students are likely to face economic challenges. In a recent survey, 33.9 percent of college students report that finances had been "very difficult to handle" in the past year.[15] Even though finances might be difficult, you can develop good financial behaviors that will support your health. (For information on this, see Focus On: Improving Your Financial Health on page 26.)

When you are injured or sick and money is tight, what can you do to get the best health care at the lowest price? Read the **Money & Health** box on page 10 for ideas on maximizing care while minimizing costs.

The Built Environment As the name implies, the built environment includes anything created or modified by human beings and from buildings to roads to recreation areas and transportation systems to electric transmission lines and communications cables.

Researchers in public health have increasingly been promoting changes to the built environment that can improve the health of community members.[16] For example, Walter Willett of the Harvard School of Public Health proposes that sidewalks and bike lanes be part of every federally funded road project.[17] He asserts that when sidewalks are built in neighborhoods and downtowns, people are more apt to start walking and slim down. Similarly, when a supermarket selling fresh produce replaces side-by-side fast-food outlets

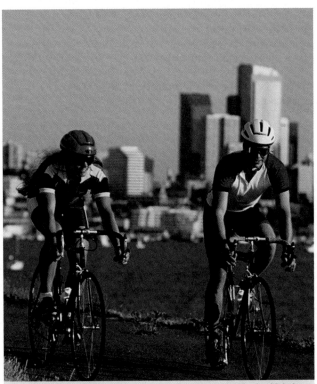

The built environment of your community can promote positive health behaviors. Wide bike paths and thoroughfares closed to automobile traffic encourage residents to incorporate healthy physical activity into their daily lives.

Money&Health
MAXIMIZING CARE WHILE MINIMIZING COSTS

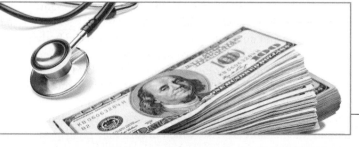

Maybe you're like the 6.3 percent of college students who reported in a 2012 survey that they had no health care insurance. Or maybe you're on your parents' plan or one sponsored by your college or university, but there's a hefty deductible or co-payment, or the test or medication you need isn't covered. Whatever your situation, following a few strategies will help you get the best care for the lowest cost.

❋ **Preserve your health.** Remember that four behaviors—overeating, failing to exercise, smoking, and abusing alcohol—account for the majority of preventable disease. Your most important cost-sparing strategy is to take care of your health in the first place.

❋ **Avoid unnecessary risks.** Unintentional injuries aren't just the top cause of death in young adults, they're also a primary reason young adults seek emergency care.

❋ **Do your research.** If you have health care insurance, read the Summary Plan Description (SPD). This explains what types of care providers, tests, and treatments are covered, and specifies if vision, dental, or prescription benefits are included. The SPD also outlines co-payments, annual deductibles, and in- and out-of-network rules for seeing specialists. When you know the answers to these questions, you're less likely to make decisions that result in large bills.

❋ **Make sure you need health care, not self-care.** The number one reason behind doctor visits is the common cold—for which

Ask your doctor for generic prescriptions to save on your costs, especially if you are uninsured or underinsured.

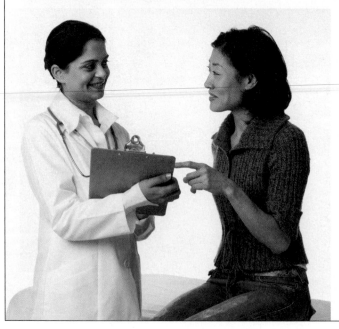

there's no treatment. For many conditions, rest, nutritious fluids, and the passage of time are the only healers. So think before you spend money on health care you don't need.

❋ **Try the least expensive health care options first.** For instance, your student health center may be able to provide exactly the level of care you need for little or no cost. Or call the nurse hotline available on your insurance plan.

❋ **Go prepared.** When you visit your doctor, come with a list of symptoms, concerns, and questions. If you think you need a diagnostic test, request it and explain why. If you're sexually active, ask your doctor what tests you should have for sexually transmitted infections, even if you don't have symptoms.

❋ **Ask your doctor to help you get the lowest cost care.** For instance, generic versions of many prescription medications are available, at a cost that may be 50 to 75 percent lower than that of the brand-name drug. If no generic version is available for a costly drug, ask if a free sample is available.

❋ **Find out what assistance is available to pay for medications.** If you can't afford a medication you need, and you are thinking about not taking it, find out if you qualify for assistance by visiting the website of the Partnership for Prescription Assistance at www.pparx.org. Also talk to your pharmacist. Most large drugstore chains sponsor prescription discount programs, or your pharmacist may be able to direct you to online coupons for commonly prescribed drugs.

❋ **Use the emergency room (ER) only for emergencies.** Studies show that almost 70 percent of ER visits are not really emergencies at all—and care in an ER can cost ten times as much as the same care in a walk-in clinic.

❋ **When you get a bill from your provider, check it for accuracy.** Medical bill errors are common, especially duplicated charges and simple typos. Also review the statements you get from your plan to make sure that you received the care described and the right reimbursements.

❋ **Be aware that if your plan denies coverage for a test or treatment your physician says is necessary, you have the right to appeal the decision.** Check your SPD for your plan's appeals process, which typically involves writing a letter explaining your grievance. Copy both your physician and your state insurance commissioner, and keep a copy for your own records.

Sources: American College Health Association, *American College Health Association-National College Health Assessment II: Reference Group Executive Summary Fall 2012* (Hanover, MD: American College Health Association, 2013), www.acha.org; U.S. Department of Labor, *Top 10 Ways to Make Your Health Benefits Work for You* (September 29, 2010), www.dol.gov; Aetna, *Six Ways to Save Money with Your Aetna Student Health Benefits*, www.aetnastudenthealth.com; CalCPA, *How to Minimize Health Care Costs* (2007), American Institute of Certified Public Accountants, www.calcpa.org

in an inner-city neighborhood, residents' dietary choices improve. Simple changes in community environments can make a difference by enabling you to make better choices.

Pollutants and Infectious Agents Another aspect of the physical environment is the quality of the air we breathe and our land, water, and foods. Exposure to toxins, radiation, irritants, and infectious agents can cause individuals and communities significant harm. The effects are not necessarily limited to the local community. Air pollution can cross continents and oceans, and with the rise of global travel and commerce, infectious diseases can travel the world.

Access to Quality Health Services

The health of individuals and communities is also determined by access to quality health care, including not only services for physical and mental health, but also accurate and relevant health information and products such as eyeglasses, medical supplies, and medications. In 2011, more than 27 percent of young Americans (age 19 to 25) lacked health insurance.[18] Individuals without health insurance may delay going to the doctor for regular preventive care. If they are sick, their disease may not be diagnosed until it is advanced, reducing the chance of recovery and leading to higher rates of hospitalization, longer stays, and more costly health care than for those who have insurance and get preventive screenings and prompt treatment.

In addition to the uninsured is the problem of the millions of "underinsured"—those who have some coverage, but not enough. These individuals cannot afford to pay the difference between what their insurance covers and what their providers and medications cost. Therefore, like the uninsured, they tend to delay care or try other cost-saving measures such as taking only half of the prescribed dose of their medications.

Policymaking

Public policies and interventions can have a powerful and positive effect on the health of individuals and communities. Examples include smoking bans in public places, laws mandating seat belt use, policies that require you to be vaccinated before enrolling in classes, and laws that ban cell phone use while driving. Health policies serve a key role in protecting public health and motivating individuals and communities to change.

Access to health services is also affected by policymaking—including health insurance legislation. Early in 2010, President Obama signed into law a set of health care reforms intended to reduce the nation's health care costs while increasing Americans' access to quality care. These reforms, which are being implemented gradually over

See It! Videos

How can you change your habits and stick with it? Watch **Life-Changing Resolutions** in the Study Area of MasteringHealth™

several years, are discussed in the accompanying **Health Headlines** box on page 12.

Health Disparities

In recognition of the changing demographics of the U.S. population and the vast differences in health status based on racial or ethnic background, *Healthy People 2020* includes strong language about the importance of reducing **health disparities**.[19] (See the **Health in a Diverse World** box on page 13 for examples of groups that often experience health disparities.)

> **health disparities** Preventable differences in the burden of disease, injury, violence, or opportunities to achieve optimal health that are experienced by socially disadvantaged groups.

How Can You Improve Your Health Behaviors?

We've just identified many factors critical to your health status. However, you have the most control over factors in just one category: your individual behaviors. To successfully change a behavior, you need to see change not as a singular *event* but instead as a *process* that requires preparation, has several steps or stages, and takes time to occur.

Models of Behavior Change

Over the years, social scientists and public health researchers have developed a variety of models to reflect this multifaceted process of behavior change. We explore three of those here.

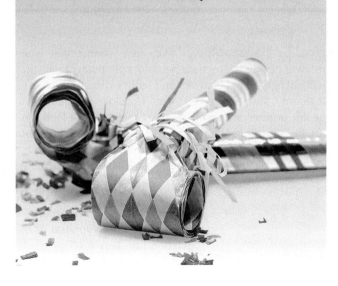

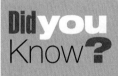 The top resolution for both 2012 and 2013 was to become more physically fit, according to an annual survey by Franklin Covey.

NATIONAL HEALTH CARE REFORM

Four major United States political movements supported national health insurance during the past century, but none succeeded. But on March 23, 2010, after the Obama administration put health care reform at the top of its domestic agenda, the Patient Protection and Affordable Care Act (ACA) became law. The main goal of the ACA is to provide access to health insurance for more than 30 million previously uninsured Americans and to reform some insurance practices and policies deemed unfair or counter to the public good. The legislation is structured to achieve its goals by expanding Medicaid eligibility to include an additional 17 million people. Although individual states could opt out of the expansion, it is largely funded by federal dollars, which few states are expected to refuse. The law also provides tax credits to small businesses to help them pay for coverage for their employees.

One of the most contentious aspects of the ACA is the individual mandate requiring all Americans to carry health insurance (as of 2014) or face an annual (and progressively increasing) fine if they fail to do so. ACA supporters say that the individual mandate is necessary to push young, healthy Americans into the insurance pool and thereby dilute the cost of care overall. Opponents argue that by compelling individuals to purchase an expensive product such as health insurance the federal government is overreaching. In June 2012, the U.S. Supreme Court ruled that Congress could enact the ACA under its authority to raise and collect taxes. This ruling and the reelection of President Obama in November 2012 ended opponents' hopes of overturning the ACA.

Many reforms are already in effect. These include a provision allowing young adults to stay on their parents' health insurance plan up to age 26 if they do not have access to coverage through an employer. In addition, most employer-based and individual plans are now required to cover preventive services such as blood pressure screenings, certain cancer screenings, vaccinations, prenatal care, well-baby care, and smoking-cessation programs with no co-payment or deductible.

Other provisions now in effect ban or place restrictions on certain insurance industry practices such as the following:

✱ Insurers are no longer allowed to deny coverage to individuals with preexisting conditions.
✱ Insurers are not allowed to cancel coverage because the insured made an honest mistake on his or her application.

✱ Insurers now have to publicly justify rate hikes of 10 percent or more and must spend at least 80 percent of premiums on health care as opposed to administration, marketing, etc.
✱ New health insurance plans cannot impose lifetime coverage or annual limits.

Americans can shop for and compare insurance plans with the Health Insurance Marketplace. More information and updates on health care reform can be found at www.healthcare.gov.

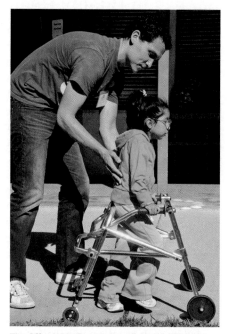

The Affordable Care Act expands health insurance to cover many people currently without insurance, including young adults and children with preexisting conditions.

Health Belief Model We often assume that when rational people realize their behaviors put them at risk, they will change those behaviors and reduce that risk. However, it doesn't always work that way. Consider the number of health professionals who smoke, consume junk food, and act in other unhealthy ways. They surely know better, but their "knowing" is disconnected from their "doing." One classic model of behavior change proposes that our beliefs about our susceptibility to risks may help to explain why this occurs.

A **belief** is an appraisal of the relationship between some object, action, or idea (e.g., smoking) and some attribute of that object, action, or idea (e.g., "Smoking is expensive, dirty, and causes cancer" or "Smoking is sociable and relaxing"). In 1966, psychologist I. Rosenstock developed the **health belief model (HBM)**, which describes when beliefs affect behavior change.[20] The HBM holds that several factors must support a belief before change is likely:

● **Perceived seriousness of the health problem.** The more serious the perceived effects are, the more likely that action will be taken.
● **Perceived susceptibility to the health problem.** People who perceive themselves at high risk are more likely to take preventive action.
● **Perceived benefits.** People are more likely to take action if they believe that this action will benefit them.

belief Appraisal of the relationship between some object, action, or idea and some attribute of that object, action, or idea.

health belief model (HBM) Model that explains when beliefs are likely to affect behavior change.

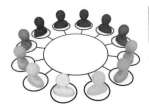
THE CHALLENGE OF HEALTH DISPARITIES

Among the factors that can affect an individual's ability to attain optimal health are the following:

✳ **Race and ethnicity.** Research indicates dramatic health disparities among people of certain racial and ethnic backgrounds. Socioeconomic differences, stigma based on "minority status," poor access to health care, cultural barriers and beliefs, discrimination, and limited education and employment opportunities can all affect health status.

✳ **Sex and gender.** At all ages and stages of life, men and women experience major differences in rates of disease and disability.

✳ **Sexual orientation.** Gay, lesbian, bisexual, or transgender individuals may lack social support, are often denied health benefits due to unrecognized marital status, and face unusually high stress levels and stigmatization by other groups.

✳ **Economics.** One's economic status can influence one's health. For example,

Remote Area Medical (RAM) clinics are one way public health officials attempt to address health disparities due to location, poverty, and lack of insurance. At a RAM clinic, families with little or no insurance wait in line for hours to receive free health care from hundreds of professional doctors, nurses, dentists, and other health workers.

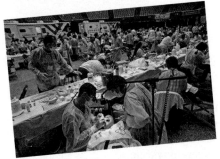

persistent poverty may make it difficult to buy healthy food or to afford preventive medical visits or medication. Economics also influence access to safe, affordable housing, safe places to exercise, and safe working conditions.

✳ **Inadequate health insurance.** People who are uninsured or underinsured may face unaffordable payments or copayments, high deductibles, or limited care in their area.

✳ **Geographic location.** Whether you live in an urban or rural area and have access to high-quality health care facilities and services, public transportation, or your own vehicle can have a huge impact on what you choose to eat, the amount of physical activity you get, and your ability to visit the doctor or dentist.

✳ **Disability.** Disproportionate numbers of disabled individuals lack access to health care services, social support, and community resources that would enhance their quality of life.

Sources: Data from Centers for Disease Control and Prevention, "CDC Health Disparities and Inequalities Report," *Morbidity and Mortality Weekly Report* 60, Supplement (January 14, 2011): 1–116. www.cdc.gov; H. Mead et al., *Racial and Ethnic Disparities in U.S. Health Care: A Chartbook* (Washington, DC: The Commonwealth Fund, 2008).

● **Perceived barriers.** Even if a recommended action is perceived to be effective, the individual may believe it is too expensive, difficult, inconvenient, or time-consuming. These perceived barriers must be overcome, or must be acknowledged as less important than the perceived benefits.

● **Cues to action.** A person who is reminded or alerted about a potential health problem is more likely to take action. These cues to action can range from early symptoms of a disorder to an e-mail from a health care provider.

Why are so many people unable to change a behavior, even in the face of serious threats? Sometimes, the addictive nature of the behavior makes it extremely difficult. Other times, their culture or environment keeps them in a behavioral rut. They also may feel that the immediate pleasure outweighs the long-range cost.

Social Cognitive Model The **social cognitive model (SCM)** developed from the work of several researchers over the past several decades, but it is most closely associated with the work of psychologist Albert Bandura. Fundamentally, the model proposes that three factors interact in a reciprocal

fashion to promote and motivate change. These factors are the *social environment* in which we live; *our inner thoughts and feelings* (*cognition*); and our *behaviors*. We change our behavior in part by observing models in our environments—from childhood to the present moment—reflecting on our observations, and regulating ourselves accordingly.

For instance, if as a child we observed our mother successfully quitting smoking, we are more apt to believe we can do it, too. In addition, when we succeed in changing ourselves, we change our thoughts about ourselves, and this in turn may promote further behavior change: After we've successfully quit smoking, we may feel empowered to increase our level of physical activity. Moreover, as we change ourselves, we change our world; in our example, we become a model of successful smoking cessation for others to observe. Thus, we are not just products of our environments, but producers.

Transtheoretical Model Why do so many New Year's resolutions fail before Valentine's Day? According to Drs. James Prochaska and Carlos DiClemente, it's because we are

social cognitive model (SCM) Model of behavior change emphasizing the role of social factors and cognitive processes (thoughts and feelings) in behavior change.

going about change in the wrong way; fewer than 20 percent of us are really prepared to take action. After considerable research, Prochaska and DiClemente have concluded that behavior changes usually do not succeed if they start with the change itself. Instead, we must go through a series of stages to prepare ourselves for eventual change.[21] According to Prochaska and DiClemente's **transtheoretical model (TTM)** of behavior change (also called the *stages of change model*), our chances of keeping New Year's resolutions will be greatly enhanced if we have proper reinforcement and help during each of the following stages:

1. **Precontemplation.** People in the precontemplation stage have no current intention of changing. They may have tried to change a behavior before and given up, or they may be in denial and unaware of any problem.

2. **Contemplation.** In this phase, people recognize that they have a problem and begin to contemplate the need to change. Despite this acknowledgment, people can languish in this stage for years, realizing that they have a problem but lacking the time or energy to make the change.

3. **Preparation.** Most people at this point are close to taking action. They've thought about what they might do and may even have come up with a plan.

4. **Action.** In this stage, people begin to follow their action plans. Those who have prepared for change appropriately and made a plan of action are more ready for action than those who have given it little thought.

5. **Maintenance.** During the maintenance stage, a person continues the actions begun in the action stage and works toward making these changes a permanent part of his or her life. In this stage, it is important to be aware of the potential for relapses and to develop strategies for dealing with such challenges.

6. **Termination.** By this point, the behavior is so ingrained that constant vigilance may be unnecessary. The new behavior has become an essential part of daily living.

We don't necessarily go through these stages sequentially. They may overlap, or we may shuttle back and forth from one to another—for example, contemplation to preparation, then back to contemplation—for a while before we become truly committed to making a change (Figure 1.7).

Still, it's useful to recognize "where we're at" with a change. The following four-step plan—with ideas from all three behavior change models—gives a simple structure to help you move forward.

Step One: Increase Your Awareness

Before you can decide what to change, you need to learn what researchers know about behaviors that promote and reduce wellness in populations. Each chapter in this book provides a foundation of information focused on different aspects of health.

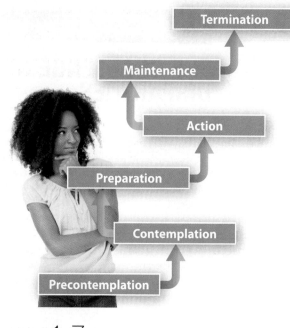

FIGURE 1.7 **Transtheoretical Model**
People don't move through the transtheoretical model stages in sequence. We may make progress in more than one stage at one time, or we may shuttle back and forth from one to another—say, contemplation to preparation, then back to contemplation—before we succeed in making a change.

This is a good time to take stock of your health determinants: What aspects of your biology and behavior support your health, and which are obstacles to overcome? What elements of your social and physical environment could you tap to help you change, and what elements might hold you back? Listing all the health determinants that affect you—both positively and negatively—should greatly increase your understanding of what you might want to change and what you might need to do to make that change happen.

Step Two: Contemplate Change

With increased awareness of the behaviors that contribute to wellness and the specific health determinants affecting you, you may be contemplating change. In this stage, the following strategies may be helpful.

Examine Your Health Habits and Patterns Do you routinely stop at fast-food restaurants for breakfast? Smoke? Party too much on the weekends? Get to bed way past 2 A.M.? When considering a behavior you might want to change, ask yourself the following:

● How long has this behavior existed, and how frequently do you do it?
● How serious are long- and short-term consequences of the habit or pattern?
● What kinds of situations trigger the behavior?

- What are some of the reasons you continue the behavior?
- Are other people involved? If so, how?

As we've explored throughout this chapter, health behaviors involve elements of personal choice, but are influenced by other determinants that make them more or less likely. Some are *predisposing factors*—for instance, if your parents smoke, you're 90 percent more likely to start smoking than someone whose parents don't smoke. Some are *enabling factors*—for example, if your peers smoke, you are 80 percent more likely to smoke. Identifying the factors that may encourage or discourage the habit you're exploring is part of contemplating behavior change.

Various *reinforcing factors* can contribute to your current habits. If you decide to stop smoking but your family and friends smoke, you may lose your resolve. In such cases, it can be helpful to deliberately change aspects of your social environment. For instance, you could spend more time with nonsmoking friends to observe people modeling the positive behavior you want to emulate.

Identify a Target Behavior
To clarify your thinking about the behaviors you might target, ask yourself these questions:

- **What do I want?** What is your goal? To lose weight? Exercise more? Reduce stress? Have a lasting relationship? Whatever it is, you need a clear picture of your target outcome.
- **Which change is the greatest priority at this time?** What behaviors can you change starting today? People often decide to change several things at once. Suppose you are gaining unwanted weight. Rather than saying, "I need to eat less and start exercising," identify one specific behavior that contributes significantly to your greatest problem, and tackle it first.
- **Why is this important to me?** Think through why you want to change. Are you doing it to improve your health? To improve your academic performance? To look better? To win someone else's approval? Targeting a behavior because it's right for you works best, rather than changing to win others' approval.

Successful targeting involves filling in the details. Identifying the specific behavior you would like to change—rather than the general problem—will allow you to set clear goals.

Learn More about the Target Behavior
Once you've clarified what behavior you'd like to change, you're ready to learn more about it. Again, the information in this textbook will help. In addition, this is a great time to learn how to find accurate and reliable health information on the Internet (see the **Tech & Health** box on page 16).

As you conduct your research, don't limit your focus to the behavior and its effects. Also learn all you can about aspects of your world that might pose obstacles to your success. For instance, let's say you decide you want to meditate for 15 minutes a day. You face a big ramp-up learning what meditation is, how it's practiced, and what benefits you might expect from it. But in addition, what might pose an obstacle to meditation? Do you think of yourself as hyper? Do you live in a super-noisy dorm? Are you afraid your friends might think meditating is weird? In short, learn everything you can—positive and negative—about your target behavior now, and you'll be better prepared for change.

Assess Your Motivation and Readiness to Change
On any given morning, many of us get out of bed and resolve to change a given behavior that day. However, most of us soon return to our old behavior patterns.

Wanting to change is an essential prerequisite of the change process, but to achieve change you need more than desire. You need real **motivation**, which isn't just a feeling, but a social and cognitive force that directs your behavior. To understand what goes into motivation, let's return for a moment to two models of change discussed earlier: the health belief model (HBM) and the social cognitive model (SCM).

> **motivation** A social, cognitive, and emotional force that directs human behavior.

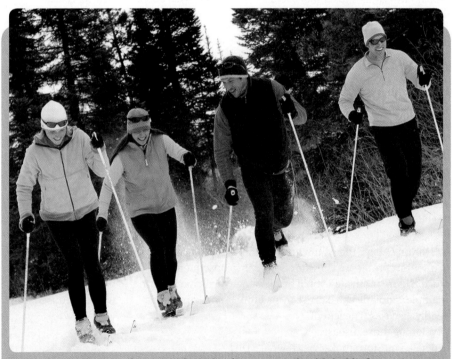

How can I stay motivated to improve my health habits?

Many people find it easiest to keep themselves motivated by planning small, incremental changes; working toward a goal; and rewarding themselves along the way. Your friends can also help you stay motivated by modeling healthy behaviors, offering support, joining you in your change efforts, and providing reinforcement.

The Internet can be a wonderful resource for quickly finding answers to your questions, but it can also be a source of *misinformation*. To ensure that the sites you visit are reliable and trustworthy, follow these tips:

✳ Look for websites sponsored by an official government agency, a university or college, or a hospital/medical center. Government sites are easily identified by their *.gov* extensions (e.g., the National Institute of Mental Health's website is www.nimh.nih.gov). College and university sites typically have *.edu* extensions (e.g., Johns Hopkins University's website is www.jhu.edu). Hospitals often have an extension of *.org* (e.g., the Mayo Clinic's website is www.mayoclinic.org). In addition, national nonprofit organizations, such as the American Heart Association and the American Cancer Society, are often good, authoritative sources of information. Foundations and nonprofits usually have URLs ending with a *.org* extension.

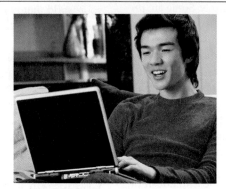

Find reliable health information at your fingertips!

✳ Search for well-established, professionally peer-reviewed journals such as the *New England Journal of Medicine* (http://nejm.org) or the *Journal of the American Medical Association (JAMA;* http://jama.ama-assn.org). Although some of these sites require a fee for access, you can often locate abstracts and information, such as a weekly table of contents, that can help you conduct a search. Check with your college or community library to determine which journals are available to students at no cost.

✳ There are many education-oriented sites, such as WebMD (www.webmd.com), that are independently sponsored and reliable.

✳ The nonprofit health care accrediting organization URAC (www.urac.org) has devised more than 50 criteria that health sites must satisfy to display its seal. Look for the "URAC Accredited Health Web Site" seal on websites you visit.

✳ Check the Accessing Your Health on the Internet section at the end of every chapter of this book for websites that provide accurate, reliable information.

✳ And, finally, don't believe everything you read. Cross-check information to see whether facts and figures are consistent. Be especially wary of websites that try to sell you something. When in doubt, check with your own health care provider, health education professor, or state health division website.

Source: URAC website from URAC homepage, www.urac.org. Reprinted with permission.

Remember that, according to the HBM, your beliefs affect your ability to change. For example, when reaching for another cigarette, smokers sometimes tell themselves, "I'll stop tomorrow," or "They'll have a cure for lung cancer before I get it." These beliefs allow them to continue what they're doing. To put it another way, they dampen motivation. So as you contemplate change, take some time to think about your beliefs and consider whether they are likely to motivate you to achieve lasting change. Ask yourself the following:

● Do you believe that your current pattern could lead you to a serious problem? The more severe the consequences are, the more motivated you'll be to change the behavior. For example, smoking can cause cancer, emphysema, and other deadly diseases. The fear of developing those diseases can help you stop smoking. But what if cancer and emphysema were just words to you? In that case, studying these disorders and the suffering they cause might increase your motivation: In Canada, a recent law requires that graphic images of gangrenous limbs, diseased organs, and chests sawed open for autopsy cover at least half of cigarette packages. The year after the law took effect, 31 percent of smokers who tried to quit cited the images as a motivating factor.[22]

● Do you believe that you are personally likely to experience the consequences of your behavior? For example, losing a loved one to lung cancer could motivate you to work harder to stop smoking. If you can't convince yourself that your behavior will affect you, ask your health care provider to give you an honest assessment of your risk. If that doesn't work, try employing the social cognitive model to help change your belief. For instance, you could interview people struggling with the consequences of the behavior you want to change. Ask them what their life is like, and if, when they were engaging in the behavior, they believed that it would harm them. Your health care provider may be able to put you in touch with patients who would be happy to support your behavior

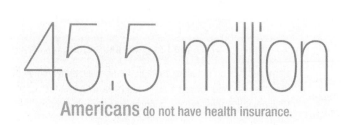

45.5 million
Americans do not have health insurance.

change plan in this way. And don't ignore the motivating potential of positive role models. Do you know people who have successfully lost weight, stopped drinking, or quit smoking? Hang out with them! Finding ways to stay motivated is a key purpose behind many of the behavior change steps and processes we have been describing throughout this section. The **Skills for Behavior Change** box below summarizes some of these tips for maintaining motivation.

Even though motivation is powerful, by itself it's not enough to achieve change. Motivation has to be combined with common sense, commitment, and a realistic understanding of how best to move from point A to point B. *Readiness* is the state of being that precedes behavior change. People who are ready to change possess the knowledge, skills, and external and internal resources that make change possible.[23]

Develop Self-Efficacy **Self-efficacy**—the belief that you are capable of achieving your goals and influencing events in your life—is a critical factor influencing your health status. People who exhibit high self-efficacy are confident that they can succeed, and they approach challenges with a positive attitude. In turn, they may be more likely to succeed. Each success then reinforces expectations of success in the future.

Conversely, people with low self-efficacy doubt what they can achieve. Consequently, they may give up easily or never try to change a behavior.

If you suspect you have low self-efficacy, the contemplation stage is a great time to work on developing it! A technique of cognitive behavioral therapy called *cognitive restructuring* can help. (See **Chapter 3** for information on cognitive restructuring.) Find out more by visiting your campus student counseling services.

what do you think?

Do you have an internal or an external locus of control?

● Can you think of some good friends whom you'd describe as more internally or externally controlled?

● How do people with these different views deal with similar situations?

Cultivate an Internal Locus of Control The conviction that you have the ability to change is a powerful motivator. People who have a strong *internal* **locus of control** believe that they have power over their actions. They are more driven by their own thoughts and are more likely to state their opinions, become their own best health advocates, and act in accordance with their own beliefs.[24] In contrast, people who believe that they have no control over a situation or that others control what they do have an *external* locus of control. They may easily succumb to feelings of anxiety and disempowerment, and give up. For example, a recent review study found that, compared to people with an internal locus of control, people with an external locus of control are likely to suffer more significant symptoms of psychiatric illness following a natural disaster, military service, or other traumatic experience.[25]

A person's locus of control can vary according to circumstance. For instance, someone who learns that diabetes runs in his family may see diabetes as an inevitable part of his life and say that he may as well enjoy himself because he's going to get the disease anyway. As such, he would be demonstrating an external locus of control. However, the same individual might exhibit an internal locus of control when being pressured by friends to smoke. He knows that he does not want to risk the potential consequences of the habit and is confident in his ability to resist the pressure. Developing and maintaining an internal locus of control can help you take charge of your health behaviors.

Step Three: Prepare for Change

You've contemplated change for long enough! Now it's time to set a realistic goal, anticipate barriers, reach out to others, and commit. Here's how.

self-efficacy Belief in one's ability to achieve goals and influence events in life.

locus of control The location, *external* (outside oneself) or *internal* (within oneself), that an individual perceives as the source and underlying cause of events in his or her life.

Skills for Behavior Change

Maintain Your Motivation

❯ **Pick one specific behavior to change.** Trying to change too many things at once can be overwhelming.

❯ **Evaluate your choice.** Ask yourself why it is important to you to make this change. If it doesn't feel important to you, you'll have a hard time finding motivation, and it probably isn't a behavior you should address at this time.

❯ **Set short- and long-term goals.** Take baby steps to improve your chances of accomplishing your goals and staying motivated to move forward.

❯ **Reward yourself.** List things you find rewarding and plan to give yourself specific rewards once you reach specific goals.

❯ **Avoid or anticipate barriers and temptation.** By controlling or eliminating the environmental cues that provoke the behavior you want to change, you'll make it easier for yourself to succeed at lasting change.

❯ **Remind yourself why you are trying to change.** List the benefits you'll realize from making this change, both now and down the road. You can also list the risks you face if you don't make this change. Post the lists where you will see them daily.

❯ **Enlist help and support from others.** Other people can be major motivators for positive change—either as role models, a cheering squad, or partners in change.

❯ **Don't be discouraged by lapses.** A brief lapse doesn't mean the entire cause is lost. Reexamine your plan, look for new strategies to motivate you, set some new short-term goals, and get right back on the horse.

Set a Realistic Goal A realistic goal is one that you truly can achieve—not someday, when other things in your life change, but within the circumstances of your life right now. Knowing that your goal is attainable increases your motivation. This, in turn, leads to a better chance of success and to a greater sense of self-efficacy—which can motivate you to succeed even more.

Use the SMART System Unsuccessful goals are vague and open-ended: for instance, "Get into shape by exercising more." In contrast, successful goals are SMART:

● **S**pecific. A specific goal is "Attend the Tuesday/Thursday aerobics class at the YMCA."
● **M**easurable. A measurable goal is "Reduce my alcohol intake on Saturday nights from three drinks to two."
● **A**ction-oriented. An action-oriented goal is "Volunteer at the animal shelter on Friday afternoons."
● **R**ealistic. A realistic goal is "Increase my daily walk from 15 to 20 minutes."
● **T**ime-oriented. A time-oriented goal is "Stay in my strength-training class for the full 10-week session, then reassess."

Use Shaping **Shaping** is a stepwise process of making a series of small changes. Suppose you want to start jogging 3 miles every other day, but right now you get tired and winded after half a mile. Shaping would dictate a process of slow, progressive steps such as walking 1 hour every other day at a relaxed pace for the first week; walking for an hour every other day at a faster pace the second week; and speeding up to a slow run the third week.

Regardless of the change you plan, remember that current habits didn't develop overnight, and they won't change overnight, either. Start slowly to avoid hurting yourself or causing undue stress. Keep the steps of your program small and achievable, and master one step before moving to the next. Be flexible and ready to change your original plan if it proves to be uncomfortable.

Anticipate Barriers to Change Anticipating *barriers to change*, or stumbling blocks, will help you prepare fully. Various social determinants, aspects of the built environment, or lack of adequate health care can inhibit change. In addition to negative determinants, other barriers to change are as follows:

shaping Using a series of small steps to gradually achieve a goal.

modeling Learning specific behaviors by watching others perform them.

● **Overambitious goals.** Even with the strongest motivation, overambitious goals can derail change. Habits are best changed one small step at a time.
● **Self-defeating beliefs and attitudes.** As the health belief model explains, believing you're too young or fit or lucky to have to worry about the consequences of your behavior can keep you from making a change. Likewise, thinking you are helpless to change your eating, smoking, or other habits can undermine efforts.
● **Failing to accurately assess your current state of wellness.** You might assume that you will be able to walk the 2 miles to campus each morning, for example, only to discover that you're aching and winded after only a mile. Failing to make sure that the planned change is realistic for *you* can be a barrier that leaves you with weakened motivation and commitment.
● **Lack of support and guidance.** If you want to cut down on your drinking, peers who drink heavily may be powerful barriers to change. To succeed, you need to recognize the people in your life who can't support, or might even oppose, your decision to change, and limit your interactions with them.
● **Emotions that sabotage your efforts and sap your will.** Sometimes the best laid plans go awry because you're having a rotten day or are fighting with someone you care about. Emotional reactions to life's challenges aren't inherently bad. However, they can sabotage your efforts to change by distracting you and draining your reserves. Seek help for more severe psychological problems, and recognize that you may need to focus on those before you can effect significant change in other aspects of your health.

Enlist Others as Change Agents The social cognitive model recognizes the importance of our social contacts in successful change. Most of us are highly influenced by the approval or disapproval (real or imagined) of close friends, family members, and our social and cultural groups. In addition, watching others successfully change their behavior can give you ideas and encouragement for your own change. This **modeling**, or learning from role models, is a key component of the social cognitive model of change. Observing a friend who is a good conversationalist, for example, can help you improve your communication skills.

Family Members Strong and positive family units are dedicated to the healthful development of all family members. When a loving family unit does not exist to support your change, you may be able to turn to a coach, teacher, or a caring group of friends.

Take things one step at a time to reach your behavior change goals.

Friends Most of us desire to fit the "norm." If you deviate from what's expected among your friends, you

program. Writing a Behavior Change Contract like the one at the end of this book will help you clarify your goals and make a commitment to change. **Figure 1.8** shows an example of a completed contract.

Step Four: Take Action to Change

It's time to put your plan into action! Behavior change strategies include visualization, countering, controlling the situation, changing your self-talk, rewarding yourself, and journaling. The options don't stop here, but these are a good place to start.

Visualize New Behavior Mental practice can transform unhealthy behaviors into healthy ones. Athletes and others often use a technique known as **imagined rehearsal** to reach their goals. Careful mental and verbal rehearsal of how you intend to act will help you anticipate problems and greatly improve the likelihood of success.

> **imagined rehearsal** Practicing, through mental imagery, to become better able to perform an action in actuality.

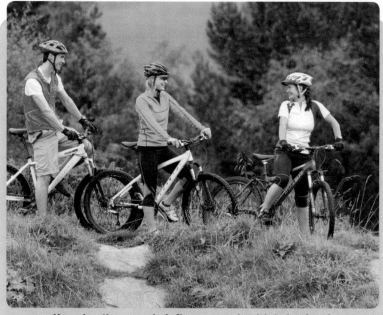

How do other people influence my health behaviors?

Your family, friends, neighbors, coworkers, and society in general can play a huge role in your health choices. The behaviors of the people in your life can predispose you to certain health habits, both enabling and reinforcing them. Seek out the support and encouragement of friends who have similar goals and interests to strengthen your commitment to positive health behaviors.

may suffer negative social consequences. But if your friends offer encouragement, or express interest in joining you in the behavior change, you are more likely to remain motivated. Thus, cultivating and maintaining close friends who share your personal values can greatly increase your success in changing your behaviors.

Professionals Sometimes the change you seek requires more than the help of well-meaning family members and friends. Depending on the type and severity of the problem, you may want to enlist support from professionals such as your health instructor, PE instructor, coach, health care provider, academic adviser, or minister. As appropriate, consider the counseling services offered on campus, as well as community services such as smoking cessation programs, Alcoholics Anonymous support groups, and your local YMCA.

Sign a Contract It's time to get it in writing! A formal *behavior change contract* serves many powerful purposes. It functions as a promise to yourself; as a public declaration of intent; as an organized plan that lays out start and end dates and daily actions; as a list of barriers you may encounter; as a place to brainstorm strategies to overcome barriers; as a list of sources of support; and as a reminder of the benefits of sticking with the

---

Behavior Change Contract

My behavior change will be:
To snack less on junk food and more on healthy foods.

My long-term goal for this behavior change is:
Eat junk food snacks no more than once a week

These are three obstacles to change (things that I am currently doing or situations that contribute to this behavior or make it harder to change):
1. The grocery store is closed by the time I come home from school.
2. I get hungry between classes, and the vending machines only carry candy bars.
3. It's easier to order pizza or other snacks than to make a snack at home.

The strategies I will use to overcome these obstacles are:
1. I'll leave early for school once a week so I can stock up on healthy snacks in the morning.
2. I'll bring a piece of fruit or other healthy snack to eat between classes.
3. I'll learn some easy recipes for snacks to make at home.

Resources I will use to help me change this behavior include:
a friend/partner/relative: my roommates; I'll ask them to buy healthier snacks instead of chips when they do the shopping.
a school-based resource: The dining hall; I'll ask the manager to provide healthy foods we can take to eat between classes.
a community-based resource: The library; I'll check out some cookbooks to find easy snack ideas
a book or reputable website: The USDA nutrient database at www.ars.usda.gov; I'll use this site to make sure the foods I select are healthy choices.

In order to make my goal more attainable, I have devised these short-term goals:
short-term goal Eat a healthy snack 3 times per week   target date September 15   reward new CD
short-term goal Learn to make a healthy snack   target date October 15   reward concert tickets
short-term goal Eat a healthy snack 5 times per week   target date November 15   reward new shoes

When I make the long-term behavior change described above, my reward will be:
ski lift tickets for winter break   target date: December 15

I intend to make the behavior change described above. I will use the strategies and rewards to achieve the goals that will contribute to a healthy behavior change.

Signed: Elizabeth King   Witness: Susan Bauer

FIGURE 1.8 **Example of a Completed Behavior Change Contract**
A blank version of this contract is included at the back of the book and in MasteringHealth for you to fill out.

Learn to "Counter" Countering means substituting a desired behavior for an undesirable one. You may want to stop eating junk food, for example, but quitting cold turkey isn't realistic. Instead, compile a list of substitute foods and places to get them and have this ready before your mouth starts to water at the smell of a burger and fries.

Control the Situation Any behavior has antecedents and consequences. *Antecedents* are aspects of the situation that come beforehand; these cue or stimulate a person to act in certain ways. *Consequences*—the results of behavior—affect whether a person will repeat that action. Both antecedents and consequences can be physical events, thoughts, emotions, or the actions of other people. A diary noting your undesirable behaviors and identifying the settings in which they occur can help you determine the antecedents and consequences involved. Once you recognize the antecedents of a behavior, you can employ **situational inducement** to modify those that are working against you. That is, you can seek settings, people, and other circumstances that support your efforts to change, and avoid those that are likely to derail your change. You can also identify and choose substitute antecedents that can support your change.

Change Your Self-Talk Self-talk, or the way you think to yourself, can also play a role in modifying health-related behaviors. Self-talk can reflect your feelings of self-efficacy, discussed earlier in this chapter. When we don't feel self-efficacious, it's tempting to engage in negative self-talk, which can sabotage our best intentions.

Use Rational, Positive Statements The rational-emotive form of cognitive therapy, or self-directed behavior change, is based on the premise that there is a close connection between what people say to themselves and how they feel. According to psychologist Albert Ellis, most emotional problems and their related behaviors stem from irrational statements that people make to themselves when events in their lives are different from what they would like them to be.[26]

For example, suppose that after doing poorly on a test you say to yourself, "I can't believe I flunked that easy exam. I'm so stupid." By changing this irrational, "catastrophic" self-talk into rational, positive statements about what is really going on, you can increase the likelihood that you will make a positive behavior change. Positive self-talk might be phrased as follows: "I really didn't study enough for that exam. I'm not stupid, I just need to prepare better for the next test." Such self-talk will help you recover quickly from disappointment and take positive steps to correct the situation.

Practice Blocking and Stopping By purposefully blocking or stopping negative thoughts, a person can concentrate on taking positive steps toward behavior change. For example, suppose you are preoccupied with your ex-partner, who has recently left you for someone else. By refusing to dwell on negative images and forcing yourself to focus elsewhere, you can avoid wasting energy, time, and emotional resources and move on to positive change.

Reward Yourself Another way to promote positive behavior change is to reward yourself for it. This is called **positive reinforcement**. Each of us is motivated by different reinforcers:

- *Consumable reinforcers* are edible items that you enjoy, such as your favorite fruit or snack mix.
- *Activity reinforcers* are opportunities to do something enjoyable, such as going on a hike or taking a trip.
- *Manipulative reinforcers* are incentives such as getting a lower rent in exchange for mowing the lawn or the promise of a better grade for doing an extra-credit project.
- *Possessional reinforcers* are tangible rewards such as a new electronic gadget or sports car.
- *Social reinforcers* are signs of appreciation, approval, or love, such as loving looks, affectionate hugs, and praise.

The difficulty with employing positive reinforcement often lies in determining which incentive will be most effective. Your reinforcers may initially come from others (extrinsic rewards), but as you see positive changes in yourself, you will begin to reinforce yourself (intrinsic rewards). Reinforcers should quickly follow a behavior, but beware of overkill. If you reward yourself with a movie every time you go jogging, this reinforcer will soon lose its power. It would be better to give yourself this reward after, say, a full week of adherence to your jogging program.

> **what do you think?**
> What type of reinforcer would most likely get you to change a behavior?
> - Why would it motivate you?
> - Can you think of options to reinforce your behavior changes?

Journal Journaling, or writing down personal experiences, interpretations, ideas for improvement, and results, is an important skill for behavior change. It can help you track your progress, help you identify where your problem areas are, and show you areas of improvement.

Let's Get Started!

After you acquire the skills to support successful behavior change, you're ready to apply those skills to your target behavior. Create a behavior change contract incorporating the goals and skills we've discussed, and place it where you will see it every day and where you can refer to it as you work through the chapters in this text. Consider it a visual reminder that change doesn't "just happen." Reviewing your contract helps you stay alert to potential problems, be aware of your alternatives, maintain a firm sense of your values, and stick to your goals under pressure.

countering Substituting a desired behavior for an undesirable one.

situational inducement Influencing a behavior through seeking out antecedents that support behavior change and avoiding antecedents that derail change.

self-talk The customary manner of thinking and talking to yourself, which can affect your feelings of self-efficacy.

positive reinforcement Presenting yourself with a reward following a behavior change.

How Healthy Are You?

Although we all recognize the importance of being healthy, it can be a challenge to sort out which behaviors are most likely to cause problems or which ones pose the greatest risk. *Before* you decide where to start, it is important to look at your current health status.

Completing the following assessment will give you a clearer picture of health areas in which you excel and those that could use some work. Taking this assessment will also help you reflect on components of health that you may not have thought about.

Answer each question, then total your score for each section and fill it in on the Personal Checklist at the end of the assessment. Think about the behaviors that influenced your score in each category. Would you like to change any of them? Choose the area that you'd like to improve, and then complete the

Live It! Assess Yourself

An interactive version of this assessment is available online in MasteringHealth™

Behavior Change Contract at the back of your book. Use the contract to think through and implement a behavior change over the course of this class.

Each of the categories in this questionnaire is an important aspect of the total dimensions of health, but this is not a substitute for the advice of a qualified health care provider. Consider scheduling a thorough physical examination by a licensed physician or setting up an appointment with a mental health counselor at your school if you need help making a behavior change.

For each of the following, indicate how often you think the statements describe you.

1 Physical Health

	Never	Rarely	Some of the Time	Usually or Always
1. I am happy with my body size and weight.	1	2	3	4
2. I engage in vigorous exercises such as brisk walking, jogging, swimming, or running for at least 30 minutes per day, three to four times per week.	1	2	3	4
3. I get at least 7 to 8 hours of sleep each night.	1	2	3	4
4. My immune system is strong, and my body heals itself quickly when I get sick or injured.	1	2	3	4
5. I listen to my body; when there is something wrong, I try to make adjustments to heal it or seek professional advice.	1	2	3	4

Total score for this section: _____

2 Social Health

	Never	Rarely	Some of the Time	Usually or Always
1. I am open, honest, and get along well with others.	1	2	3	4
2. I participate in a wide variety of social activities and enjoy being with people who are different from me.	1	2	3	4
3. I try to be a "better person" and decrease behaviors that have caused problems in my interactions with others.	1	2	3	4
4. I am open and accessible to a loving and responsible relationship.	1	2	3	4
5. I try to see the good in my friends and do whatever I can to support them and help them feel good about themselves.	1	2	3	4

Total score for this section: _____

3 Emotional Health

	Never	Rarely	Some of the Time	Usually or Always
1. I find it easy to laugh, cry, and show emotions such as love, fear, and anger, and try to express these in positive, constructive ways.	1	2	3	4
2. I avoid using alcohol or other drugs as a means of helping me forget my problems.	1	2	3	4
3. I recognize when I am stressed and take steps to relax through exercise, quiet time, or other calming activities.	1	2	3	4

	Never	Rarely	Some of the Time	Usually or Always
4. I try not to be too critical or judgmental of others and try to understand differences or quirks that I note in others.	1	2	3	4
5. I am flexible and adapt or adjust to change in a positive way.	1	2	3	4

Total score for this section: _____

4 Environmental Health

	Never	Rarely	Some of the Time	Usually or Always
1. I buy recycled paper and purchase biodegradable detergents and cleaning agents, or make my own cleaning products, whenever possible.	1	2	3	4
2. I recycle paper, plastic, and metals; purchase refillable containers when possible; and try to minimize the amount of paper and plastics that I use.	1	2	3	4
3. I try to wear my clothes for longer periods between washing to reduce water consumption and the amount of detergents in our water sources.	1	2	3	4
4. I vote for pro-environment candidates in elections.	1	2	3	4
5. I minimize the amount of time that I run the faucet when I brush my teeth, shave, or shower.	1	2	3	4

Total score for this section: _____

5 Spiritual Health

	Never	Rarely	Some of the Time	Usually or Always
1. I take time alone to think about what's important in life—who I am, what I value, where I fit in, and where I'm going.	1	2	3	4
2. I have faith in a greater power, be it a supreme being, nature, or the connectedness of all living things.	1	2	3	4
3. I engage in acts of caring and goodwill without expecting something in return.	1	2	3	4
4. I sympathize and empathize with those who are suffering and try to help them through difficult times.	1	2	3	4
5. I go for the gusto and experience life to the fullest.	1	2	3	4

Total score for this section: _____

6 Intellectual Health

	Never	Rarely	Some of the Time	Usually or Always
1. I carefully consider my options and possible consequences as I make choices in life.	1	2	3	4
2. I learn from my mistakes and try to act differently the next time.	1	2	3	4
3. I have at least one hobby, learning activity, or personal growth activity that I make time for each week, something that improves me as a person.	1	2	3	4
4. I manage my time well rather than let time manage me.	1	2	3	4
5. My friends and family trust my judgment.	1	2	3	4

Total score for this section: _____

Although each of these six aspects of health is important, there are some factors that don't readily fit in one category. As college students, you face some unique risks that others may not have. For this reason, we have added a section to this self-assessment that focuses on personal health promotion and disease prevention. Answer these questions and add your results to the Personal Checklist in the following section.

7 Personal Health Promotion/ Disease Prevention

	Never	Rarely	Some of the Time	Usually or Always
1. If I were to be sexually active, I would use protection such as latex condoms, dental dams, and other means of reducing my risk of sexually transmitted infections.	1	2	3	4
2. I can have a good time at parties or during happy hours without binge drinking.	1	2	3	4
3. I have eaten too much in the last month and have forced myself to vomit to avoid gaining weight.	4	3	2	1
4. If I were to get a tattoo or piercing, I would go to a reputable person who follows strict standards of sterilization and precautions against bloodborne disease transmission.	1	2	3	4
5. I engage in extreme sports and find that I enjoy the highs that come with risking bodily harm through physical performance.	4	3	2	1

Total score for this section: _____

Personal Checklist

Now, total your scores for each section and compare them to what would be considered optimal scores. Are you surprised by your scores in any areas? Which areas do you need to work on?

	Ideal Score	Your Score
Physical health	20	_____
Social health	20	_____
Emotional health	20	_____
Environmental health	20	_____
Spiritual health	20	_____
Intellectual health	20	_____
Personal health promotion/ disease prevention	20	_____

Scores of 10–14:

Your health risks are showing! Find information about the risks you are facing and why it is important to change these behaviors. Perhaps you need help in deciding how to make the changes you desire. Assistance is available from this book, your professor, and student health services at your school.

Scores below 10:

You may be taking unnecessary risks with your health. Perhaps you are not aware of the risks and what to do about them. Identify each risk area and make a mental note as you read the associated chapter in the book. Whenever possible, seek additional health resources, either on your campus or through your local community, and make a serious commitment to behavior change. If any area is causing you to be less than functional in your class work or personal life, seek professional help. In this book you will find the information you need to help you improve your scores and your health. Remember that these scores are only indicators, not diagnostic tools.

Scores of 15–20:

Outstanding! Your answers show that you are aware of the importance of these behaviors in your overall health. More importantly, you are putting your knowledge to work by practicing good health habits that should reduce your overall risks. Although you received a very high score, you may want to consider areas in which your scores could be improved.

YOUR PLAN FOR CHANGE

The **Assessyourself** activity gave you the chance to gauge your total health status. Now that you have considered these results, you can take steps toward changing certain behaviors that may be detrimental to your health.

Today, you can:

○ Evaluate your behavior and identify patterns and specific things you are doing.

○ Select one pattern of behavior that you want to change.

○ Fill out the Behavior Change Contract at the back of your book. Be sure to include your long- and short-term goals for change, the rewards you'll give yourself for reaching these goals, the potential obstacles along the way, and the strategies for overcoming these obstacles. For each goal, list the small steps and specific actions that you will take.

Within the next 2 weeks, you can:

○ Start a journal and begin charting your progress toward your behavior change goal.

○ Tell a friend or family member about your behavior change goal, and ask him or her to support you.

○ Reward yourself for reaching your short-term goals, and reevaluate your plan if you find they are too ambitious.

By the end of the semester, you can:

○ Review your journal entries and consider how successful you have been in following your plan. What helped you be successful? What made change more difficult? What will you do differently next week?

○ Revise your plan as needed: Are the goals attainable? Are the rewards satisfying? Do you have enough support and motivation?

MasteringHealth™

www.masteringhealthandnutrition.com (or www.pearsonmastering.com)
Build your knowledge—and health!—in the Study Area of MasteringHealth with a variety of study tools.

Summary

✱ Choosing good health has immediate benefits, such as reducing the risk of injury and illnesses and improving academic performance; long-term rewards, such as disease prevention, longevity, and improved quality of life; and societal and global benefits, such as reducing the global disease burden.

✱ For the U.S. population as a whole, the leading causes of death are heart disease, cancer, and chronic lower respiratory diseases. In the 15- to 24-year-old age group, the leading causes are unintentional injuries, suicide, and homicide.

✱ The average life expectancy at birth in the United States is 78.7 years. This has increased greatly over the past century; however, unhealthy behaviors linked to chronic disease may be limiting increases in our total life expectancy and causing a reduction in *healthy* life expectancy.

✱ The definition of *health* has changed over time. The medical model focused on treating disease, whereas the current ecological or public health model focuses on promoting health and preventing disease.

✱ Health can be seen as existing on a continuum and encompassing the dynamic process of fulfilling one's potential in the physical, social, intellectual, emotional, spiritual, and environmental dimensions of life. Wellness means achieving the highest level of health possible in each of the dimensions of health.

✱ Health is influenced by *determinants* that the Surgeon General's health promotion plan, *Healthy People 2020*, classifies as individual behavior, biology and genetics, the social and physical environments, access to health services, and policymaking. Disparities in health among different groups contribute to increased risks.

✱ Models of behavior change include the health belief model, the social cognitive model, and the transtheoretical (stages of change) model. A person can increase the chance of successfully changing a health-related behavior by viewing change as a process containing several steps and components.

✱ When contemplating a behavior change, it is helpful to examine current habits, identify and learn about a target behavior, and assess motivation and readiness to change. Self-efficacy and an internal locus of control are essential for maintaining motivation. When preparing to change, it is helpful to set realistic and incremental goals that employ shaping, anticipate barriers to change, enlist the help and support of others, and sign a behavior change contract. When taking action to change, it is helpful to visualize new behavior, practice countering, control the situation, change self-talk, reward yourself, and keep a blog or journal.

Pop Quiz

1. What statistic is used to describe the number of deaths from heart disease this year?
   a. Morbidity
   b. Mortality
   c. Incidence
   d. Prevalence

2. Everyday tasks, such as walking up the stairs or tying your shoes, are known as
   a. wellness behaviors.
   b. healthy life expectancy.
   c. cues to action.
   d. activities of daily living.

3. Janice describes herself as confident and trusting; she displays both high self-esteem and high self-efficacy. The dimension of health this relates to is the
   a. social dimension.
   b. emotional dimension.
   c. spiritual dimension.
   d. intellectual dimension.

4. *Healthy People 2020* is
   a. a blueprint for health actions designed to improve health in the United States.
   b. a projection of life expectancy rates in the United States in the year 2020.
   c. an international plan for achieving global health priorities for the environment by the year 2020.
   d. a set of specific goals that states must achieve in order to receive federal funding for health.

5. Because Andre's parents smoked, he is 90 percent more likely to start smoking than someone whose parents didn't. This is an example of what factor influencing behavior change?
   a. Circumstantial factor
   b. Enabling factor
   c. Reinforcing factor
   d. Predisposing factor

6. Jake is exhibiting *self-efficacy* when he
   a. believes that he can and will be able to bench-press 125 pounds in his specified time frame.
   b. doubts that his bad shoulder will heal enough to bench-press the weight he is hoping for.
   c. claims he is not good enough to do any physical exercise that will ever allow him to bench-press 125 pounds.
   d. feels he does not possess personal control over this situation.

7. To reach your goal of losing 20 pounds, you take small steps. You start by joining a support group and counting calories. After 2 weeks, you begin an exercise

program and gradually build up to your desired fitness level. What behavior change strategy are you using?

- a. Shaping
- b. Visualization
- c. Modeling
- d. Reinforcement

8. What strategy for change is advised for an individual in the preparation stage of change?
    - a. Following an action plan
    - b. Contemplating a need to change
    - c. Setting realistic goals
    - d. Practicing blocking and stopping

9. The setting events for a behavior that cue or stimulate a person to act in certain ways are called
    - a. antecedents.
    - b. frequency of events.
    - c. consequences.
    - d. cues to action.

10. After Kevin and Heather pay their bills, they reward themselves by watching TV together. The type of positive reinforcement that motivates them to pay their bills is a(n)
    - a. activity reinforcer.
    - b. consumable reinforcer.
    - c. manipulative reinforcer.
    - d. possessional reinforcer.

Answers to these questions can be found on page A-1.

Think about It!

1. How are the words *health* and *wellness* similar? What are important distinctions between these terms? What is health promotion? Disease prevention?
2. How healthy is the U.S. population today? Is our health status better or worse than it has previously been? What factors influence today's disparities in health?
3. What are some of the health disparities existing in the United States today? Why do you think these differences exist? What policies do you think would most effectively address or eliminate health disparities?
4. What is the health belief model? How may this model be working when a young woman decides to smoke her first cigarette? Her last cigarette?
5. Using the transtheoretical model, discuss what you might do (in stages) to help a friend stop smoking. Why is it important that a person be ready to change before trying to change?

Accessing Your Health on the Internet

The following websites explore further topics and issues related to personal health. For links to the websites below, visit the Study Area in MasteringHealth.

1. *CDC Wonder.* This is a clearinghouse for comprehensive information from the Centers for Disease Control and Prevention (CDC). http://wonder.cdc.gov
2. *Mayo Clinic.* This reputable resource for specific information about health topics, diseases, and treatment options is provided by the staff of the Mayo Clinic. www.mayoclinic.org
3. *National Center for Health Statistics.* This is an outstanding place to start for information about health status in the United States. It contains links to key reports; national survey information; and information on mortality by age, race, gender, geographic location, and other important data. www.cdc.gov/nchs
4. *healthfinder.gov.* This is an excellent resource for consumer information about health. www.healthfinder.gov
5. *World Health Organization.* This excellent resource on global health provides information on illness and disease statistics, trends, and illness outbreak alerts. www.who.int/en

Improving Your Financial Health

LEARNING OUTCOMES

✱ Discuss how finances impact health.

✱ Learn to create a realistic budget.

✱ Understand the different types of student loans and other financial aid options. Explain credit cards, credit scores, and best practices for using credit wisely.

✱ Describe common types of identity theft and ways to avoid or resolve them.

28 I hardly have any money—what's the point in creating a budget?

30 Aren't all student loans basically the same?

31 If credit cards cause so many problems, should I just avoid getting one?

33 Are there differences in what you owe when someone steals your ATM card or credit card?

The Links between Health and Wealth

They say money can't buy happiness or love—but can it buy health? People living in wealthy, developed countries do have much longer life expectancies than those in poor countries (Figure 1). There also tends to be an inverse relationship between socioeconomic status and how overweight someone is (body mass index); that is, the lower someone's income, the greater her odds for being overweight or obese. Carrying extra weight is a major risk factor for developing heart disease, stroke, and diabetes, so the relationship between body mass and overall health is important. Additionally, many of the items the U.S. Surgeon General defines as *determinants of health*—individual behavior, the physical environment, and access to health services—have strong links to a person's financial means. (See **Chapter 1** for more on determinants of health.) Take where you live: A high-crime

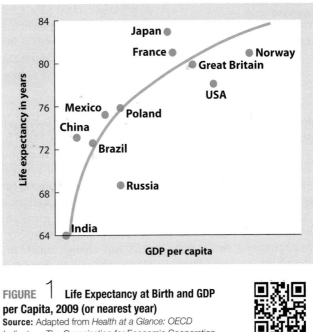

neighborhood filled with fast-food restaurants but few supermarkets presents huge barriers to safety, ability to exercise, and access to nutritious food. For better or worse, the difference between living there or a place that promotes good health—a safe, walkable neighborhood with a weekend farmer's market, for instance—usually comes down to money. Judging by this evidence, it seems that financial status has real ties to your health.

This is *not* to say one must be rich to attain wellness or that the wealthier an individual, the healthier he or she must be. There are some notable exceptions to these patterns. For example, U.S. men have similar obesity

rates at all income levels, with highest obesity rates stacked at the top income tiers.[1] This goes against the previously mentioned trend for body mass index and income. Researchers continue to debate the exact relationship between income and health, with some arguing that the issues are less clear cut than graphs such as Figure 1 depict.[2] But it's safe to say that while money may not exactly buy good health, it makes attaining it much easier.

If you are struggling with finances now, the good news is that college is a great first step toward future success. According to a recent study, median income for those holding a bachelor's degree is $50,360 compared to $29,423 for those with only a high-school diploma.[3] As with weight, diet, and exercise, the habits you create

today with finances have far-reaching consequences. Being even a little bit more savvy about budgeting and other financial matters will serve you well throughout life.

Making a Budget

Students have it rough these days. A recession followed by a period of sluggish economic growth reduced many family incomes and savings. Then government budget crises led to tuition and fee hikes at most state and city colleges. A recent survey of 15,000 college students found that 60 percent worried often or very often about meeting regular expenses, and over half also worried frequently about paying for school.[4] One third of undergraduate students queried in a different survey said finances have been "traumatic or very difficult to handle" in the past year.[5]

Creating a **budget** during tough economic times may strike you as downright depressing. But ask yourself how often you worry vaguely about

budget An estimate of spending and income over a set period of time.

89%
of students feel college is an investment in the future.

Learning to manage credit cards is crucial in college and beyond.

discretionary spending Goods and services that are not life essentials.
budget surplus Money left over for savings after expenses have been paid.
budget deficit Spending more money than your income.

money. If you feel a little guilty or tense every time you open your wallet, then creating a budget may actually be a stress reducer. You will finally know how much you can afford to spend. Use the **Assess Yourself** budget worksheet found at the end of this chapter, or try a personal finance budget phone application or computer program that tracks spending and income. Many universities also offer free spreadsheets for student budgeting. Check your own school's website for options.

Set Goals

Budgeting should be goal oriented. For students, goal number one is to avoid debt as much as possible. If you have more resources, then your goal may be to graduate with no debt at all, or to save for occasional indulgences like a vacation. At other points in life, you may budget to save for a house, a car, or retirement. Whenever your life circumstances change, it is important to draw up a new budget that matches current income level, expenses, and priorities.

Track Expenses

Start by tallying what you owe for things you buy and services you use. Rent, mortgages, utilities, car loan payments, insurance premiums, and (in some cases) phone plans are examples of *fixed expenses*, meaning their cost does not change much in the short term. That makes them fairly easy to track. Add in tuition, books, supplies, and other fees for school. Student loan payments may be deferred, depending on the type of loan, if you are in school at least half time. But other debts such as credit card balances can't be deferred and need to be listed as monthly expenses.

Next, figure out how much you spend on food, clothing, entertainment, and personal products or services. Most of these items are **discretionary spending**, things you like but don't necessarily need. Of course food is essential, but be careful how you classify it. Unless you eat only at a school dining hall that has a fixed fee, chances are you are spending much more on restaurants and store-bought food than you strictly need to.

Track Income

Income is the money you have to spend. It generally includes wages from work or interest payments from investments. It may also include financial aid payments, allowances or stipends from relatives, and other gifts. Some students will also be withdrawing money from college savings accounts to pay for living expenses and tuition.

When you earn more than you spend you have a **budget surplus**. If expenses are greater than income, you have a **budget deficit**. As mentioned before, the goal with budgeting should be to create a surplus and build savings. College is a unique time when many people run budget deficits while earning a degree, trusting that future wage gains from their education make the debt feasible. But sometimes this leads people to feel that because they are already going into debt, they might as well borrow as much as they can to make life easier or more fun in the short term. This should be avoided. Every dollar of debt you take on matters. With compound interest and loan terms, just a few "extra" thousand dollars more at the end of school can take many extra years to pay off.

Making the Budget Numbers Add Up

Both income and expenses may be concentrated at the beginning of each academic term when scholarship and loan money arrive and tuition is due. Students receiving lump sum payments may overspend early on and find themselves unexpectedly broke before finals. Accurate budgets can smooth out spending and avoid that problem.

A recent study found about 35 percent of students used education loans to pay for college.[6] One report also

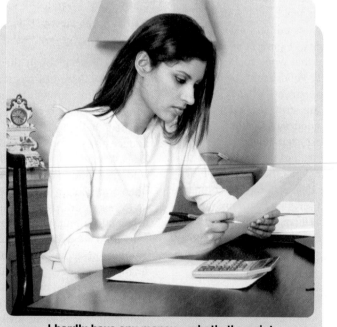

I hardly have any money—what's the point in creating a budget?

The point of a budget is to put limits on spending and save for your goals. No matter the income level, a budget is important.

found nine out of ten families are taking steps to make college more affordable.[7] Figure 2 describes some of things families are doing to make school less expensive.

If you tried to stick to a budget in the past but found the numbers never added up, incomplete tracking of discretionary spending may be the culprit. Say someone creates a budget that shows there should be $150 surplus at the end of each month, but that theoretical surplus never appears. The problem could be something as simple as forgetting to include the purchase of a daily cup of coffee in your expenses. Spending five extra dollars each day equals that missing $150 per month of savings. Five dollars may not be that much money, but little expenses can add up fast.

To track spending accurately it's a good idea to watch expenses for several weeks to a month at a time. Write everything down and keep receipts. Consider using a budget tracking app for your smart phone to make the process easier.

Budget cutting is hard. Nobody enjoys passing on doing things because of money woes. To be happier while reducing spending try to focus on what you gain: self-discipline, control,

Creative Ways to Cut Spending

Little changes in behavior can add up to big savings. Consider some of the following:

❭ **Cut back on the cappuccinos.** A large espresso drink from a coffee shop can cost $4 or $5. Making coffee at home or switching your order to less costly drip varieties saves money.
❭ **Add 2 more weeks between hair cuts.** Book hair appointments every 6 weeks instead of 4. You'll end up paying for three to four fewer haircuts per year than if you scheduled monthly.
❭ **Drive less.** Carpooling saves on bridge tolls and gas. If you live in an area where car sharing or good public transportation exists, getting rid of your car entirely could save thousands of dollars. You can avoid insurance, gas, maintenance, parking fees, and car payments.
❭ **Cook more.** Cooking meals from scratch is often cheaper (and healthier) than eating out. If you live on campus and cannot cook, consider the lower-cost plan options available.
❭ **Use your phone on wifi.** If you don't have an unlimited data plan for your smart phone, texting and downloading on a cellular network gets expensive fast. Avoid charges by using the phone on wifi networks whenever possible. Wifi won't count against your data plan.
❭ **Carry cash instead of credit cards.** Withdraw a set amount of cash each week for daily expenses and reserve the credit cards for less frequent, big-ticket buying.

and more money in your future. Also remind yourself that there are many ways to socialize and entertain yourself that are inexpensive. Make lower-cost options part of your regular routine and reserve higher-cost things for rare treats. Once the period of adjustment is over, you will likely find that your "new financial normal" feels just fine. The **Skills for Behavior Change** box give some examples of little things you can do to help trim spending.

Debt and Credit Basics

It would be nearly impossible for governments, businesses, and individuals to function in the modern world without credit and debt. These tools allow huge projects such as highways and

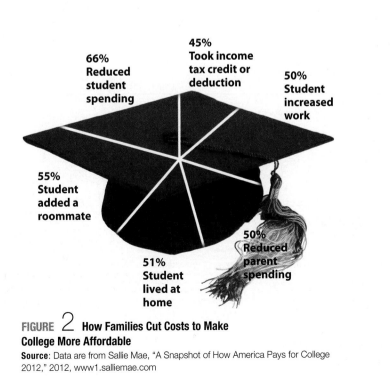

66% Reduced student spending

45% Took income tax credit or deduction

50% Student increased work

55% Student added a roommate

51% Student lived at home

50% Reduced parent spending

FIGURE 2 **How Families Cut Costs to Make College More Affordable**
Source: Data are from Sallie Mae, "A Snapshot of How America Pays for College 2012," 2012, www1.salliemae.com

debt Money owed for goods and services that have been purchased.

credit The ability to buy goods and services in advance of paying for them.

loan Giving money to someone today with an agreement that it will be paid off under certain terms in the future.

principal Either the original loan amount or the amount left outstanding on a loan, excluding interest.

interest A fee paid by the borrower of a loan.

student loans Financial student aid that must be repaid in the future.

grants Financial student aid that does not need to be repaid.

federal work study A type of financial aid in which part-time jobs for students are arranged to help them pay for school.

private student loans Student financial aid loans that are financed by private banks or other institutions.

federal student loans Student financial aid loans that are financed by the government.

airports to be built all at once and then paid for gradually. Families can buy homes and cars or fund college educations, too. Used wisely, credit and debt are incredibly helpful. But overuse of credit and debt are also major contributors to recessions, job losses, and other turmoil such as stress, depression, and relationship conflicts.

Debt is the condition of owing money for something that was purchased. **Credit** is the ability to purchase things in advance of paying for them—put another way, credit is a **loan**, or the ability to incur debt. The original amount borrowed is referred to as the loan **principal**. Loans also include **interest** charges. Interest is sometimes described as "rent" for using someone else's money. *Fixed interest rate loans* have payments that will not fluctuate for the life of the loan. *Variable interest rate loans* have interest rates that fluctuate over time.

Types of Student Aid

The first experience many young adults have with loans comes when reviewing student aid packages. Financial aid options may come from the university itself, from the government, or through private banks or firms. Government aid is often awarded

according to financial need, whereas other aid may be awarded based on achievements in sports or academics.

Student Loans Some people think "aid" and "loans" are exactly the same, but **student loans** refer just to aid options that require repayment. Another type of aid is a **grant**—that's money you don't repay. Most scholarships are grants. You also may have heard of Pell grants, which are issued by the federal government to some undergraduate students. **Federal work study** is another type of aid in which part-time jobs are arranged either on or off campus to help pay for education.

If you take out student loans it is crucial to understand the details regarding repayment, deferrals (situations where you can put off repaying), interest rates, and loan length. The stakes are high. In the past someone who got into financial trouble could declare bankruptcy, which nullified all types of debt and allowed for a fresh financial start. But bankruptcy laws changed over time. They now exclude education loans, meaning debt you incur in college will stick with you for a very long time.[8] In fact, there are cases where senior citizens have student loan payments garnished (deducted) from their retirement social security payments.

The two main categories of student loans are private and federal loans.

Private student loans are issued by banks, credit unions, state agencies, or schools. **Federal student loans** are funded by the federal government. If you have a choice, pick a federal loan. They are almost always more consumer friendly than private loans when it comes to interest rates, deferral options, penalties, tax breaks, and fees. Table 1 compares how both types of loans stack up.

Credit Cards

There are 382 million open credit card accounts in the United States today, which averages to more than one card for every man, woman, and child in the nation.[9] Credit cards are *unsecured loans*, meaning the only thing guaranteeing their repayment is your promise. This differs from *secured loans* such as home mortgages, where the loan giver is allowed to seize an asset (for home mortgages, the house itself) if payments are not made on time.

Getting your first credit card is an important but also potentially dangerous rite of passage. On the positive side, there are some things such as renting a car or booking a hotel that are almost impossible to do without a credit card. Likewise, many high-end cards ("gold" or "platinum" labeled varieties) provide purchase protection programs, so if your new phone falls

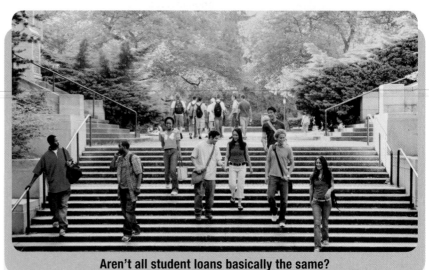

Aren't all student loans basically the same?

No! Usually the government-sponsored loans are a better deal in the long haul than private loans. Be sure you do research before you take on any loans for school.

TABLE 1

Differences in Federal and Private Student Loans

Loan Issue	Federal Student Loans	Private Student Loans
Repayment timeline	You don't start repaying federal student loans until you graduate, leave school, or enroll less than half-time.	Many private student loans require payments while you are still in school.
Interest rate	Fixed interest rates won't change and are often lower than private loans—much lower than credit card interest rates.	May have variable interest rates, some greater than 18%. Variable rates may substantially increase the total amount you repay.
Subsidies	Undergraduates with financial need may qualify for *subsidized loans* for which the government pays the interest if you are in school at least half-time.	Private student loans are not subsidized. No one pays the interest on your loan but you.
Credit checks	You don't need to get a credit check or have a credit history for most federal student loans.	May require a credit record, and the loan cost depends on credit score and other factors.
Interest tax deduction	Interest may be tax deductible.	Interest may not be tax deductible.
Deferrals	If you have trouble repaying your loan, you may be able to temporarily postpone or lower payments.	Private student loans may not offer forbearance or deferment options.
Repayment plans	There are several repayment plans, including an option to tie your monthly payment to your income.	Some, but not all, private loans offer repayment plans.
Loan forgiveness	You may be eligible to have some portion of your loans removed if you work in public service.	It is unlikely that your lender will offer a loan forgiveness program.

Source: Table adapted from "What Types of Aid Can I Get?," Federal Student Aid, an Office of the U.S. Department of Education, 2013, http://studentaid.ed.gov

into the bathtub, your card may actually compensate for the loss. But the danger of credit cards is that they make shopping too easy and pain free. Once spending is out of control, extra fees and compounding interest can make your debt balloon fast.

Interest and Fees Because credit cards are loans, banks and firms that issue them make money by charging interest on what you owe (your *account balance*) as well as other fees. Common fee types include *cash advance fees,* for when you withdraw money from a credit card at an ATM; *annual fees,* charged once every 12 months; and *late fees,* for when you pay off your monthly balance late.

Credit card interest is calculated in a variety of ways. Some cards have variable rates, others have fixed (though fixed rates can change; lenders just need to inform you in writing before they alter anything.) Add in a dizzying array of fees, and you get widespread confusion about which card is a good deal. The rule of thumb is that you want a card with as low an interest rate as possible, and fewer fees. A good

starting point for comparison shopping is the **annual percentage rate (APR),** which is the officially quoted interest rate you pay over a year-long period. The Truth in Lending Act makes all credit cards clearly state the APR.

Card APRs vary greatly: One person may have a card featuring a 10 percent rate and another a card charging 22 or 23 percent. Think about it: A person with a 10 percent APR is charged less than *half* the interest than is someone with the higher APR. It literally pays to get the best credit card deal possible.

What counts as your official "first credit card" is one created in your name only, with no cosigner who is guaranteeing that charges will be covered. The first card you have independently likely has a small **credit limit.** This is good. It allows you to build credit history without getting far into debt. Start with a single account. Most people get into trouble when they run up balances on multiple cards.

Another important issue is whether a card has an interest rate *grace period.* Many cards do not charge interest if you pay the balance off in full each month. Knowing what day of the month your payment is due (it's not

annual percentage rate (APR) The yearly cost of a credit card account, including interest and certain fees, expressed as a percentage.

credit limit The maximum amount a person can charge on a credit card account.

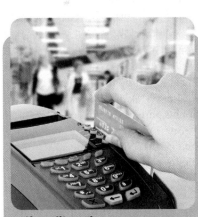

If credit cards cause so many problems, should I just avoid getting one?

Responsible credit card use is necessary to build a credit history that will allow you to rent apartments, obtain car loans, and be approved for home mortgages. So do get a credit card, just be careful how you use it.

always the first) as well as your grace period can allow you to avoid most interest charges and other fees.

Credit Scores

Although your first credit card may have a low credit limit, it will almost certainly have a high APR. That's because you don't have any credit history yet, and that makes it hard for companies to judge how much of a risk it is to loan to you. To compensate for this, credit cards charge you high interest. Others who hold cards with high interest rates may do so because they have low **credit scores**. A credit score is a calculation done by firms such as FICO and VantageScore. It is an evaluation of how likely a person is to default on his or her debt. Scores are based on factors such as length of credit history, how much current debt you have, total credit available, and how often you've recently applied for credit. General payment history of bills is also factored in, so if you forgot to mail the electrical bill on time a few months back, it could hurt your score. Age is part of the calculation, but it is illegal for companies to use race, sex, marital status, national origin, or religion as parameters for scoring.[10]

You may have heard people say their credit score is in the 600s or 700s. They were probably referring to FICO, a company has a scale running from 300 to 850. The higher the number, the better. A FICO score in the mid- to high 600s will get you approved for

$15,422

is the average amount of U.S. credit card debt.

most credit cards. However, scores in the mid-700s or higher receive the best (lowest) interest rates.

Credit Score Accuracy

Since so much rides on credit scores, it's important that the information that goes into the calculation, known as your **credit report**, is accurate. Three companies, Equifax, Experian, and TransUnion, keep credit report records. You can get free copies of reports once a year by going to www.annualcreditreport.com or by calling 1-877-322-8228. Be aware there are lots of imposter credit report websites. Since you input name, social security number, and other personal information to get a real report, scammers set up shop trying to trick you into divulging identity details to them. Double check that the website or phone number you connect with is valid before you give any sensitive information. The Fair Credit Reporting Act (FCRA) also gives you the right to buy your own credit score for a reasonable fee.

If you find errors on your credit report, you must dispute them in writing. The U.S. Federal Trade Commission has a website that includes a sample dispute letter, and a step by step walk through of that process. You can find it by searching for "disputing errors on credit reports" at www.consumer.ftc.gov.

Know Your Consumer Credit Rights

If your credit card application is rejected, you have the right to find out why. Being rejected should be investigated, since it may indicate identity theft or a credit report mistake. After rejection you can always apply for a credit card somewhere else. A "no" at one company doesn't automatically mean "no" elsewhere.

For many years credit card companies were criticized for unfair practices related to young adults. Firms paid universities for easy access to students on campus. Students received mugs, tee shirts, and other items in exchange for filling out brief applications. People of limited financial means could rapidly get multiple cards. Interest rates and fees were high,

and penalties for missed payments extreme. In 2009 the Credit Card Accountability Responsibility and Disclosure (CARD) Act was enacted. It included rules to prevent predatory practices aimed at young consumers. New rules state the following:[11]

- Credit card issuers who set up on or near campus can't give students gifts in exchange for applying for cards.
- Colleges must publicly disclose marketing contracts with credit card companies.
- Those under age 21 must provide proof of ability to repay charges by themselves in card applications. Otherwise, the card must be cosigned by someone over age 21 who has financial means to cover potential debts.
- If a card is cosigned, then credit limits cannot be raised without written permission of the cosigner.

The CARD Act also banned retroactive rate increases and limited fees, removed certain limits on store gift cards (like expiration dates), and required "plain language" disclosure of fees and rates.

In 2010 the Consumer Financial Protection Bureau (CFPB) was created. It is a new agency whose goal is to educate, conduct research, and enforce federal laws that protect consumers. The CFPB is still in the process of being built, but it's now the place to look for any recent developments in credit card rules. You can find their website at www.consumerfinance.gov.

Protect Against Fraud and Identity Theft

Identity theft occurs when someone steals personal information (name, address, social security number, credit card or bank account numbers) and uses it without permission. Identity crimes always existed but exploded when credit cards, computers, and

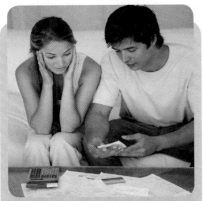

Are there differences in what you owe when someone steals an ATM card or credit card?

Big differences. Bank ATM or debit card fraud pulls money out of your personal account, and unless you detect and report the fraud immediately, you are quickly on the hook for $500 or more in losses. You are unlikely to be responsible for more than $50 for a stolen credit card.

online banking became widespread. In 2011 identity theft cost Americans about $37 billion and impacted about 1 in 25 people.[12] According to the non-profit group Identity Theft Assistance Center, those 18 to 24 years old are at greatest risk. In 2011 the average victim suffered over $600 in out-of-pocket costs related to the crime.[13]

Identity theft may involve a utility account at a stranger's house being set up in your name, theft of your tax refund, or someone committing crimes and getting arrested in your name, so you get a criminal record and the imposter does not.[14] Other common theft types are described below.

Credit Card Theft

If you see unfamiliar charges on your statement, call the fraud number on the back of your card immediately. You will not be held responsible for charges if they happen after you report the card theft. After the first few days, you may be liable for up to $50 in charges.

It's a hassle when someone steals your credit card number and charges up a storm on the internet, but if they use your main card, chances are you

will discover it quickly. Worse is when a thief sets up new bank accounts and credit cards in your name, sends the bills to a different address, and never pays them. It can take a while to discover this, and in the meantime your credit gets wrecked.

Debit Card Theft

As with credit cards, if you report theft of ATM or debit cards before any charges have occurred, you won't be liable for any charges. Reporting a theft within two business days will only cost you $50. But reporting bank card fraud 2 to 60 days after a crime leaves you liable for up to $500 of losses, and if you discover the problem after 60 days, you will be unable to recover *any* lost money.[15] Watch those bank cards and balances carefully!

Medical Account Theft

Because health care is extremely expensive, some thieves steal medical insurance numbers. Your account information is sold to someone who uses it to pay for medical care. If the person using your account lives in the same locale, this can be more than a financial crime. Incorrect medical records could endanger your own health when you seek treatment.

Protecting Personal Information and Avoiding Scams

Sometimes accounts are compromised through data breaches from hacker attacks at credit card and banking facilities. The companies in question should notify you of the problem and, if necessary, close the compromised accounts and transfer your balances to new accounts. Monitor your credit report for signs of identity theft after a data breach.

phishing A scam in which someone lies in an e-mail in an attempt to gain your financial account numbers or other personal information so that they can steal from you.

You don't have control over breaches, but there are other types of fraud you can help prevent.

Steer Clear of Phishers Phishing is an e-mail scam where someone impersonates a bank, credit card company, or other entity in an attempt to trick you into divulging account numbers or passwords. Ever get an e-mail from a Nigerian prince who wanted to borrow your bank account and give you a hefty fee as thanks? That's a classic phish scam. Most financial institutions will not contact you via e-mail asking for personal information. Never supply personal information without verifying the request is genuine—and verifying is not clicking on a link or calling a number listed in the suspicious e-mail. Look up contact information independently to check the requester out.

$631 is the average out-of-pocket expense for an identity theft victim.

Update Smart Phone Operating Systems and Computer Software Regularly When security vulnerabilities are discovered, programmers bug patch them quickly to resolve threats. But you remain open to attack if you don't update to newer versions.

Remove Key Information from Social Media Accounts A recent study found that LinkedIn, Google+, and Facebook users had much higher rates of fraud than survey respondents who weren't on social networks.[16] That's not to say social networks directly cause extra fraud. Instead, it's been observed people on social networks share birth

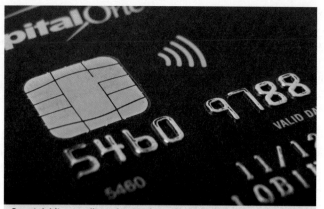
Smart debit or credit cards contain a microchip and are much more secure from fraud than are cards that only have a magnetic strip.

dates and other life details commonly used for passwords, such as names of pets, home towns, and high schools. Be aware of similarities between profile information and passwords. Passwords should not contain words or dates a stranger can easily look up.

Get a Smart Card Traditional credit and debit cards have magnetic strip technology that is fairly easy to steal from. New smart cards contain

fraud alert A 90-day warning placed on a credit report or account that notifies potential lenders of potential identity theft.

microchips that make it harder to hijack account information. Merchants and banks in the United States have been slow to adopt smart cards, but increased fraud means they are likely to become more widely available soon.

Password Lock Your Smart Phone and PC If you don't put a password on the home screen of your PC or other devices they become a goldmine of names, numbers, and other information for identity thieves when stolen.

Shred Anything with Your Credit Card Number on It Don't throw away old card statements or communications unless the account numbers have been rendered unreadable.

Cleaning Up Identity Theft Messes

Once you discover identity theft, you should take the following four steps as quickly as possible:

1. Place a **fraud alert** on your credit reports and ask for report copies to review for problems.

2. Close any accounts that were misused or set up fraudulently. Also, fill out dispute forms so related debts won't be held against you. (Once disputes are settled, get a letter from each company stating this; it provides proof of fraud and legal protection.)

3. File a police report to document the crime.

4. File a complaint with the Federal Trade Commission (FTC). The FTC is the clearinghouse for identity theft issues in the United States. To find victim resources, from complaint forms to sample dispute letters and information on how to correct credit reports, search for "identify theft" on www.ftc.gov.

Budgeting for College Students

Knowing how much money you have coming in and going out each month is essential for long-term financial health. Use this budgeting worksheet as a starting point for tallying your income, expenses, and net income (total income minus total expenses).

	Monthly Budget	Monthly Actual	Annual Budget
INCOME			
Wages from jobs			
Stipends (from parents or others)			
Student loan aid			
Scholarship awards			
Gifts			
Other/miscellaneous			
TOTAL INCOME			
EXPENSES			
Tuition			
Textbooks			
Supplies			
School fees			
Computer, tablet, wifi, etc.			
Rent or mortgage			
Utilities: gas, electric, water			
Insurance: car, health, residence			
Car: parking, gas, loan payments, maintenance, registration			
Public transportation			
Airfare (if flying to/from school regularly in the year)			

	Monthly Budget	Monthly Actual	Annual Budget
EXPENSES *continued*			
Cell phone			
Internet/other			
Dining plan or groceries			
Eating out			
Entertainment			
Clothing			
Personal products and services			
Miscellaneous			
TOTAL EXPENSES			
NET INCOME			

YOUR PLAN FOR CHANGE

The **Assessyourself** activity allowed you to begin tracking spending, income, and saving. If you face a budget deficit then consider some of the following steps to fix it:

Today, you can:

○ Calculate a dollar amount you need to reduce spending by eliminating your budget shortfall. Knowing that makes spending cuts more constructive.

○ Reduce purchases of new clothing, switch to less expensive brands for food or personal products, and go to the movies and restaurants less often.

○ Unless something is broken postpone purchases of phones, cars, or computers.

Within the next month, you can:

○ Research lower cost options for internet service providers, and consider downgrading or eliminating cable TV service.

○ If utility bills are high, be more mindful of your water, electricity, or gas usage.

○ Weigh costs and benefits of getting a part-time job or increasing current work hours so there is more money coming in.

○ Look up your phone plan details. See if it is possible to switch to a lower-cost option without incurring penalties or fees.

By the end of the semester, you can:

○ Ditch car loans. Sell the vehicle, pay off the loan, and buy a car you can afford outright. If you live on campus you might sell the car and not replace it.

○ Reduce housing expenses. If you rent a residence near family, consider moving home. If that's not possible, find a cheaper apartment or a roommate to reduce costs.

Promoting and Preserving Your Psychological Health

2

LEARNING OUTCOMES

✱ Define each of the four components of psychological health, and identify the basic traits shared by psychologically healthy people.

✱ Learn what factors affect your psychological health.

✱ Describe the interactions between emotions and health.

✱ Discuss the positive steps you can take to enhance psychological well-being.

✱ Describe psychological disorders, such as mood disorders, anxiety disorders, personality disorders, and schizophrenia, and explain their causes and treatments.

✱ Discuss warning signs of suicide and actions that you can take to help suicidal individuals.

✱ Explain the different types of mental health professionals and treatments, and examine the role they play in managing mental health issues and disorders.

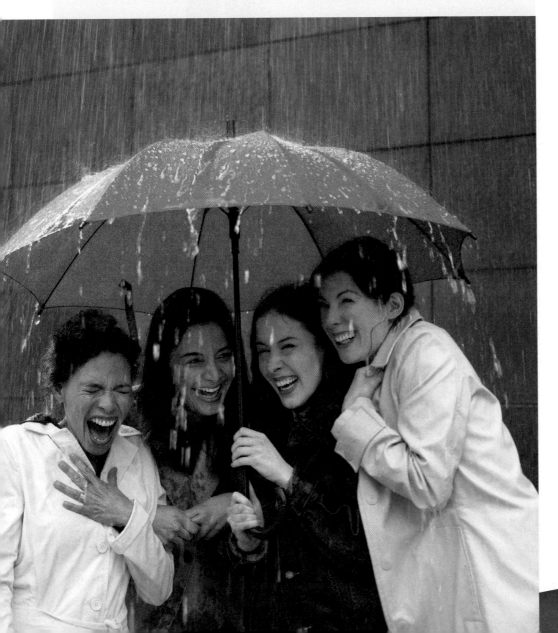

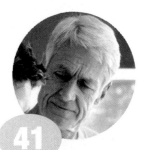

41

How do others influence my psychological well-being?

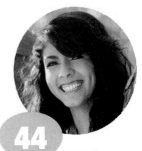

44

Is laughter really the best medicine?

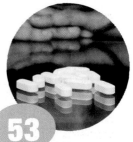

53

What should I do if someone I know is suicidal?

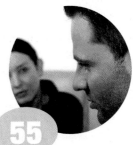

55

How can I choose the right therapist for me?

Most college students describe their college years as among the best of their lives, but many find the pressure of grades, finances, and relationships, along with the struggle to find themselves, to be extraordinarily difficult. Psychological distress caused by relationship issues, family concerns, academic competition, and adjusting to college life runs rampant on campuses today. Experts believe that the anxiety-inducing campus environment is a major contributor to poor health decisions such as high levels of alcohol consumption and unhealthy food choices and, in turn, to health problems that can ultimately affect academic success and success in life.

Fortunately, humans possess a resiliency that enables us to cope, adapt, and thrive, regardless of life's challenges. How we feel and think about ourselves, those around us, and our environment can tell us a lot about our psychological health.

What Is Psychological Health?

Psychological health is the sum of how we think, feel, relate, and exist in our day-to-day lives. Our thoughts, perceptions, emotions, motivations, and behaviors are a product of our experiences and the skills we have developed to meet life's challenges. **Psychological health** includes mental, emotional, social, and spiritual dimensions (Figure 2.1).

psychological health The mental, emotional, social, and spiritual dimensions of health.

Most experts identify several basic elements shared by psychologically healthy people:

- **They feel good about themselves.** They are typically not overwhelmed by positive or negative emotions, such as fear, love, anger, jealousy, guilt, or worry. They know who they are, have a realistic sense of their capabilities, and respect themselves even though they realize they aren't perfect.
- **They feel comfortable with other people and feel respect and compassion for others.** They enjoy satisfying and lasting personal relationships and do not take advantage of others or allow others to take advantage of them. They accept that there are others whose needs are greater than their own and take responsibility for their fellow human beings. They can give love, consider others' interests, take time to help others, and respect personal differences.
- **They control tension and anxiety.** They recognize the underlying causes and symptoms of stress and anxiety in their lives and consciously avoid irrational thoughts, hostility, excessive excuse making, and blaming others for their problems. They use resources and learn skills to control reactions to stressful situations.
- **They meet the demands of life.** They try to solve problems as they arise, accept responsibility, and plan ahead. They set realistic goals, think for themselves, and make independent decisions. Acknowledging that change is inevitable, they welcome new experiences.

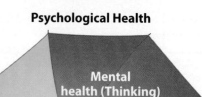

Psychological Health

Mental health (Thinking)

Spiritual health (Being)

Emotional health (Feeling)

Social health (Relating)

FIGURE 2.1 **Psychological Health**
Psychological health is a complex interaction of the mental, emotional, social, and spiritual dimensions of health. Possessing strength and resiliency in these dimensions can maintain your overall well-being and help you weather the storms of life.

- **They curb hate and guilt.** They acknowledge and combat tendencies to respond with anger, thoughtlessness, selfishness, vengefulness, or feelings of inadequacy. They do not try to knock others aside to get ahead, but rather reach out to help others.
- **They maintain a positive outlook.** They approach each day with a presumption that things will go well. They look to the future with enthusiasm rather than dread. Fun and making time for themselves are integral parts of their lives.
- **They value diversity.** They do not feel threatened by those of a different gender, religion, sexual orientation, race, ethnicity, age, or political party. They are nonjudgmental and do not force their beliefs and values on others.
- **They appreciate and respect the world around them.** They take time to enjoy their surroundings, are

conscious of their place in the universe, and act responsibly to preserve their environment.

Psychologists have long argued that before we can achieve any of the above characteristics of psychologically healthy people we must have certain basic needs met in our lives. In the 1960s, human theorist Abraham Maslow developed the classic *hierarchy of needs* to describe this idea (Figure 2.2). At the bottom of his hierarchy are basic *survival needs,* such as food, sleep, and water; at the next level are *security needs,* such as shelter and safety; at the third level are *social needs,* a sense of belonging and affection; at the fourth level are *esteem needs,* self-respect and respect for others; and at the top are needs for *self-actualization* and self-transcendence.

According to Maslow's theory, one's needs must be met at each of these levels before a person can ever truly be healthy. Failure to meet needs at a lower level will interfere with a person's ability to address upper-level needs. For example, someone who is homeless or fearful about personal safety will be unable to focus on fulfilling social, esteem, or actualization needs.[1]

In sum, psychologically healthy people are emotionally, mentally, socially, and spiritually resilient. They usually respond to challenges and frustrations in appropriate ways, despite occasional slips (see Figure 2.3 on page 40). When they do slip, they recognize it and take action to rectify the situation.

Mental Health

The term **mental health** is used to describe the "thinking" or "rational" dimension of our health. A mentally healthy person perceives life in realistic ways, can adapt to change, can develop rational strategies to solve problems, and can carry out personal and professional responsibilities. In addition, a mentally healthy person has the intellectual ability to sort through information, messages, and life events; attach meaning to these events; and respond appropriately. This is often referred to as *intellectual health,* a subset of mental health.[2]

Emotional Health

The term **emotional health** refers to the feeling, or subjective, side of psychological health. **Emotions** are intensified feelings or complex patterns of feelings that we experience on a regular basis, including love, hate, frustration, anxiety, and joy, to name a few. Typically, emotions are described as the interplay of four components: physiological arousal, feelings, cognitive (thought) processes, and behavioral reactions. As rational beings, we are responsible for evaluating our individual emotional responses, the environment that is causing them, and the appropriateness of our actions.

Emotionally healthy people usually respond appropriately to upsetting events. Rather than reacting in an extreme fashion or behaving inconsistently or offensively, they express their feelings, communicate with others, and show emotions in appropriate ways. In contrast, emotionally unhealthy people are much more likely to let their feelings overpower them. They may be highly volatile and prone to unpredictable emotional responses, which may be followed by inappropriate communication or actions.

A person's **emotional intelligence** is the ability to identify, use, understand, and manage one's emotions in positive and constructive ways. It is about recognizing your own emotional state and the emotional states of others. Emotional intelligence consists of four core abilities: self-awareness, self-management, relationship management, and social awareness. Developing or increasing your emotional intelligence can help you build strong relationships, succeed at work, and achieve your goals.[3]

Emotional health also affects social and intellectual health. People who feel hostile, withdrawn, or moody may become socially isolated.[4] Because they are not much fun to be around, their

mental health The thinking part of psychological health; includes your values, attitudes, and beliefs.
emotional health The feeling part of psychological health; includes your emotional reactions to life.
emotions Intensified feelings or complex patterns of feelings we regularly experience.
emotional intelligence A person's ability to identify, understand, use, and manage emotional states effectively and interact positively with others in relationships.

FIGURE 2.2 Maslow's Hierarchy of Needs

Self-Actualization
creativity, spirituality, fulfillment of potential

Esteem Needs
self-respect, respect for others, accomplishment

Social Needs
belonging, affection, acceptance

Security Needs
shelter, safety, protection

Survival Needs
food, water, sleep, exercise, sexual expression

Source: From A. H. Maslow, R. D. Frager, ed., and J. Fadiman, ed., *Motivation and Personality,* 3rd edition. (Upper Saddle River: Pearson Education, 1987). Adapted and Electronically reproduced by permission of Pearson Education, Inc., Upper Saddle River, New Jersey.

Video Tutor: Maslow's Hierarchy of Needs

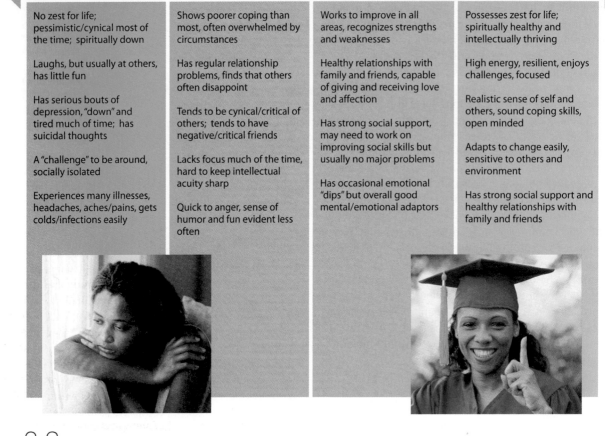

| Psychologically unhealthy | | | Psychologically healthy |

No zest for life; pessimistic/cynical most of the time; spiritually down

Laughs, but usually at others, has little fun

Has serious bouts of depression, "down" and tired much of time; has suicidal thoughts

A "challenge" to be around, socially isolated

Experiences many illnesses, headaches, aches/pains, gets colds/infections easily

Shows poorer coping than most, often overwhelmed by circumstances

Has regular relationship problems, finds that others often disappoint

Tends to be cynical/critical of others; tends to have negative/critical friends

Lacks focus much of the time, hard to keep intellectual acuity sharp

Quick to anger, sense of humor and fun evident less often

Works to improve in all areas, recognizes strengths and weaknesses

Healthy relationships with family and friends, capable of giving and receiving love and affection

Has strong social support, may need to work on improving social skills but usually no major problems

Has occasional emotional "dips" but overall good mental/emotional adaptors

Possesses zest for life; spiritually healthy and intellectually thriving

High energy, resilient, enjoys challenges, focused

Realistic sense of self and others, sound coping skills, open minded

Adapts to change easily, sensitive to others and environment

Has strong social support and healthy relationships with family and friends

FIGURE 2.3 Characteristics of Psychologically Healthy and Unhealthy People
Where do you fall on this continuum?

friends may avoid them at the very time they are most in need of emotional support.

For students, a more immediate concern is the impact of emotional trauma on academic performance. Have you ever tried to study for an exam after a fight with a friend or family member? Emotional turmoil can seriously affect your ability to think, reason, and act rationally.

Social Health

Social health includes your interactions with others on an individual and group basis, your ability to use social resources and support in times of need, and your ability to adapt to a variety of social situations. Socially healthy individuals enjoy a wide range of interactions with family, friends, and acquaintances and are able to have healthy interactions with an intimate partner. Typically, socially healthy individuals can listen, express themselves, form healthy attachments, act in socially acceptable and responsible ways, and find the best fit for themselves in society. Numerous studies have documented the importance of positive relationships with family members, friends, and significant others in overall well-being and longevity.[5]

Social bonds reflect the level of closeness and attachment that we develop with individuals and are the very foundation of human life. They provide intimacy, feelings of belonging, opportunities for giving and receiving nurturance, reassurance of one's worth, assistance, and guidance. Social bonds take multiple forms, the most common of which are social support and involvement in a community.

The concept of **social support** is more complex than many people realize. In general, it refers to the networks of people and services with whom and with which you interact and share social connections. These ties can provide *tangible support,* such as babysitting services or money to help pay the bills, or *intangible support,* such as encouraging you to share what's on your mind. Sometimes, support can be the knowledge that someone would be there for you in a crisis. Generally, the closer and the higher the quality of the social bond, the more likely a person is to ask for and receive social support. For example, if

social health Aspect of psychological health that includes interactions with others individually and in groups, ability to use social supports, and ability to adapt to various situations.

social bonds The level of closeness and attachment with other individuals.

social support Networks of people and services with whom you share ties and from whom you get support.

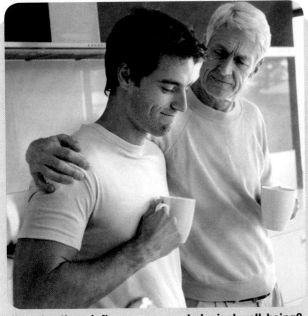

How do others influence my psychological well-being?

Your family members play an important role in your psychological health. As you were growing up, they modeled behaviors and skills that helped you develop cognitively and socially. Their love and support can contribute to your sense of self-worth and encourage you to treat others with compassion and care.

your car broke down on a dark country road in the middle of the night, who could you call for help and know that the person would do everything possible to help you? Common descriptions of strong social support include the following:[6]

- Being cared for and loved, with shared understanding
- Being esteemed and valued
- Sharing companionship, communication, and mutual obligations with others; having a sense of belonging
- Having "informational" support, that is, having access to information, advice, community services, and guidance from others

Social health also reflects the way we react to others. (Look for more information on interpersonal relationships in **Chapter 5.**)

Spiritual Health

It is possible to be mentally, emotionally, and socially healthy and still not achieve optimal psychological well-being. What is missing? For many people, the difficult-to-describe element that gives purpose to life is the spiritual dimension of psychological health.

Spirituality is broader in meaning than is religion: It is defined as an individual's sense of peace, purpose, and connection to others and beliefs about the meaning of life.[7] Spirituality may be practiced in many ways, including through religion; however, religion does not have to be part of a

spiritual person's life. **Spiritual health** refers to the sense of belonging to something greater than the purely physical or personal dimensions of existence. For some, this unifying force is nature; for others, it is a feeling of connection to other people; for still others, the unifying force is a god or other higher power. (Focus On: Cultivating Your Spiritual Health, starting on page 60, will help you explore your spiritual health in more detail and better understand the role spirituality plays in your overall psychological health.)

Factors That Influence Psychological Health

Most of our reactions to life are a direct result of our experiences and social and cultural expectations. Our psychological health is based, in part, on how we perceive life experiences.

Family

Families have a significant influence on psychological development. Healthy families model and help develop the cognitive and social skills necessary to solve problems, express emotions in socially acceptable ways, manage stress, and develop a sense of self-worth and purpose. Children raised in healthy, nurturing homes are more likely to become well-adjusted, productive adults. In adulthood, family support is one of the best predictors of health and happiness.[8]

Children raised in **dysfunctional families**—in which there is violence; distrust; anger; dietary deprivation; drug abuse; parental discord; or sexual, physical, or emotional abuse—may have a harder time adapting to life and may run an increased risk of psychological problems. In dysfunctional families, love, security, and unconditional trust may be in such short supply that children become psychologically damaged. Yet not all people raised in dysfunctional families become psychologically unhealthy, and not all people from healthy environments become well-adjusted.

Support System

Our initial social support may be provided by family members, but as we grow and develop, the support of peers and friends becomes more and more important. We rely on friends to help us figure out who we are and what we want to do with our lives. We often check in with friends to bounce ideas off them and see if they think we are being logical or smart or fair. Recent research shows that college students with adequate social support have improved overall well-being.[9] Having people in your life who provide positive support, who are nurturing, and who are reliable is important to your psychological health.

spiritual health The aspect of psychological health that relates to having a sense of meaning and purpose to one's life, as well as a feeling of connection with others and with nature.

dysfunctional families Families in which there is violence; physical, emotional, or sexual abuse; parental discord; or other negative family interactions.

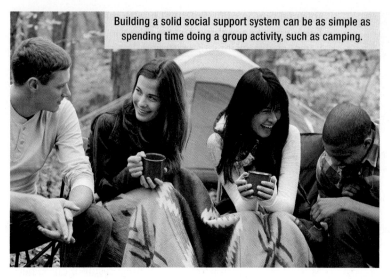

Building a solid social support system can be as simple as spending time doing a group activity, such as camping.

box on page 43 describes what happens when people never fail and have extremely high self-esteem.

Our self-esteem is a result of the relationships we have with our parents and family during our formative years; with our friends as we grow older; with our significant others as we form intimate relationships; and with our teachers, coworkers, and others throughout our lives. How can you strengthen your self-esteem?

Learned Helplessness versus Learned Optimism Psychologist Martin Seligman has proposed that people who continually experience failure may develop a pattern of responding known as **learned helplessness** in which they give up and fail to take any action to help themselves. Seligman ascribes this response in part to society's tendency toward *victimology*—blaming one's problems on other people and circumstances.[10] Although viewing ourselves as victims may make us feel better temporarily, it does not address the underlying causes of a problem. Ultimately, it can erode self-efficacy by making us feel that we cannot do anything to improve the situation.

Community

The communities we live in can have a positive impact on our psychological health through collective actions. For example, neighbors may join together to clean up trash on the street, participate in a neighborhood watch to keep children safe, help each other with home repairs, or initiate a community picnic. Likewise, you are a part of a campus community. That community can support and care for your psychological health by creating a safe environment to explore and develop your mental, emotional, social, and spiritual dimensions.

64 million

Americans volunteer through or for an organization at least once a year.

Today, many self-help programs have been developed that use elements of Seligman's principle of **learned optimism.** The basis for these programs is the thought that just as we learn to be helpless, so can we teach ourselves to be optimistic. By changing our self-talk, examining our reactions, and blocking negative thoughts, we can "unlearn" negative thought processes that have become habitual. Some programs practice positive affirmations with clients, teaching them the sometimes difficult task of learning to acknowledge positive things about themselves. Often we are our own worst critics, and learning to be kinder to ourselves can be difficult.

Self-Efficacy and Self-Esteem

During our formative years, successes and failures in school, athletics, friendships, intimate relationships, jobs, and every other aspect of life subtly shape our beliefs about our personal worth and abilities. These beliefs become internal influences on our psychological health.

Self-efficacy describes a person's belief about whether he or she can successfully engage in and execute a specific behavior. In contrast, **self-esteem** refers to one's sense of self-respect or self-worth. It can be defined as one's evaluation of oneself and one's personal worth as an individual. People with high levels of self-efficacy and self-esteem tend to express a positive outlook on life. People with low self-esteem may demean themselves and doubt their ability to succeed. Although self-esteem is important for psychological health, you can have too much of a good thing. The **Health Headlines**

Personality

Your personality is the unique mix of characteristics that distinguish you from others. Heredity, environment, culture, and experience influence how each person develops. Personality determines how we react to the challenges of life, interpret our feelings, and resolve conflicts.

Most recent schools of psychological theory promote the idea that we have the power to understand our behavior and change it, thus molding our own personalities. Although this is more difficult if social environments are inhospitable, there may be opportunities for making positive changes. One way to examine personality is by looking at traits that are associated with psychological health. In general, the following personality traits are often related to psychological well-being:[11]

self-efficacy Belief in one's own ability to perform a task successfully.

self-esteem Sense of self-respect or self-worth.

learned helplessness Pattern of responding to situations by giving up because of repeated failures in the past.

learned optimism Teaching oneself to think positively.

OVERDOSING ON SELF-ESTEEM?

Fostering self-esteem in children has been seen as key to keeping them away from drugs and violence and to ensuring well-adjusted lives. While it is true people tend to thrive when praised for hard work and accomplishments, society is now seeing a possible downside to handing out trophies just for showing up. There is a point at which *healthy self-esteem* hits the slippery slope of vanity and narcissism, leading some to have an exaggerated investment in self-image, a need for constant compliments, and a sense of feeling entitled to special treatment.

According to a growing list of critics, Generation Y may have overdosed on self-esteem by growing up in an environment in which nobody fails and everyone is considered gifted. Dr. Jean Twenge, author of "Generation Me: Why Today's Young Americans are More Confident, Assertive, Entitled and More Miserable Than Ever," discusses a study of over 16,000 college students who took the Narcissistic

Personality Inventory between 1982 and 2006. Average scores for college students progressively increased over time—with the most recent students showing a 30 percent increase in narcissism over their peers from the early 1980s.

Preliminary research indicates that people who never fail and have extremely high levels of self-esteem might be more prone to anger, aggression, and other negative behaviors when others don't praise them or meet their needs for instant gratification. A recent University of Michigan study sounded an interesting new alarm about just how important self-esteem may be to the self-esteem generation. Although the sample size was small, students reported liking and wanting moments that boost their self-esteem more than having sex, eating a favorite food, drinking, or nearly all other pleasurable events!

Psychologists continue to support the idea that self-esteem is important for positive growth and development. However, the exact criteria for healthy self-esteem remain elusive. More research is needed

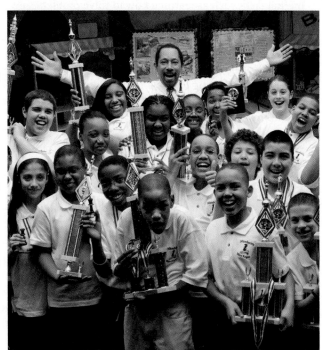

It's common for everyone on a team to receive a trophy for participation, whatever the actual outcome of the competition.

to examine potential risks of too much self-esteem and the best ways to deal with it once it occurs.

Sources: "Narcissistic and Entitled to Everything—Does Gen Y Have Too Much Self-Esteem?" Aspen Educational Group, 2011, http://aspeneducation.crchealth.com; J. M. Twenge et al., "Egos Inflating Over Time: A Cross Temporal Meta-Analysis of the Narcissistic Personality Inventory," *Journal of Personality* 76, no. 4 (2008): 875–902; B. J. Bushman, S. J. Moeller, and J. Crocker, "Sweets, Sex, or Self-Esteem? Comparing the Value of Self-Esteem Boosts with Other Pleasant Rewards," *Journal of Personality* (2011), doi: 10.1111/j.1467-6494.2011.00712.

● **Extraversion**—the ability to adapt to a social situation and demonstrate assertiveness as well as power or interpersonal involvement

● **Agreeableness**—the ability to conform, be likable, and demonstrate friendly compliance and love

● **Openness to experience**—the willingness to demonstrate curiosity and independence (also referred to as *inquiring intellect*)

● **Emotional stability**—the ability to maintain emotional control

● **Conscientiousness**—the qualities of being dependable and demonstrating self-control, discipline, and a need to achieve

● **Resiliency**—the ability to adapt to change and stressful events in healthy and flexible ways

Life Span and Maturity

Although our temperaments are largely determined by genetics, as we age we learn to control the volatile emotions of youth and channel our feelings in more acceptable ways. For example, as children we might have screamed, thrown things, or hit people when upset, but as we mature we learn to control angry outbursts. People who have not completed early developmental tasks, however, may find their lives interrupted by recurrent crises left over from earlier stages.[12] For example, if you did not learn to trust others in childhood, you may have difficulty establishing trusting intimate relationships as an adult.

The college years mark a critical transition period as young adults move away from families and establish themselves as independent adults. This transition is easier for those who have successfully accomplished earlier developmental tasks such as learning how to solve problems, evaluate alternatives and make decisions, define and adhere to personal values, and establish both casual and intimate relationships. For many, graduating from college is another transition to further independence. Anticipating an adjustment period and exploring campus resources available to recent graduates can be helpful with adjusting and developing autonomy after graduation.[13]

The Mind–Body Connection

Can negative emotions make us physically ill? Can positive emotions help us stay well? Researchers are exploring the interaction between emotions and health, especially in conditions of uncontrolled, persistent stress. At the core of the mind–body connection is the study of **psychoneuroimmunology,** or how the brain and behavior affect the body's immune system.

One factor that appears to be particularly promising in enhancing physical health is *happiness*—a collective term for several positive states in which individuals actively embrace the world around them.[14] Scientists examining the characteristics of happy people have found that this emotion can have a profound impact on the body. Happiness, or related mental states such as hopefulness, optimism, and contentment, appears to reduce the risk or limit the severity of cardiovascular disease, pulmonary disease, diabetes, hypertension, colds, and other infections. Laughter can increase heart and respiration rates and reduce levels of stress hormones in much the same way as light exercise can. For this reason, laughter has been promoted as a possible risk reducer for people with hypertension and other forms of cardiovascular disease.[15]

Subjective well-being is that uplifting feeling of inner peace or an overall "feel-good" state, which includes happiness. Subjective well-being is defined by three central components: satisfaction with present life, relative presence of positive emotions, and relative absence of negative emotions.[16] You do not have to be happy all the time to achieve overall subjective well-being. Everyone experiences disappointments, unhappiness, and times when life seems unfair. However, people with a high level of subjective well-being are typically resilient, able to look on the positive side and get back on track fairly quickly, and are less likely to fall into despair over setbacks.

Scientists suggest that some people may be biologically predisposed to happiness. One study of more than 2,500 Americans showed that two variants of a gene actually influenced how satisfied or dissatisfied people were with their lives. This marks an advance toward explaining why some people seem naturally happier than others. However, researchers are careful to point out that happiness is only partially influenced by genetics.[17]

Other psychologists suggest that we can develop happiness by practicing positive psychological actions.[18] The **Skills for Behavior Change** box on page 45 suggests ways to enhance your happiness by incorporating positive psychology into your life.

psychoneuroimmunology The science that examines the relationship between the brain and behavior and how this affects the body's immune system.

subjective well-being An uplifting feeling of inner peace.

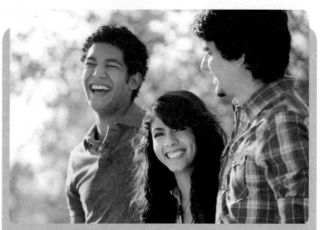

Is laughter really the best medicine?

Although research on laughter is inconclusive, we've all experienced the sense of well-being that a good laugh can bring. Regardless of whether it actually increases blood flow, boosts immune response, lowers blood sugar levels, or facilitates better sleep, sharing laughter and fun with others can strengthen social ties and bring joy to your everyday life.

Strategies to Enhance Psychological Health

As we have seen, psychological health involves four dimensions. Attaining self-fulfillment is a lifelong, conscious process that involves enhancing each of these components. Strategies include building self-efficacy and self-esteem, understanding and controlling emotions, maintaining support networks, and learning to solve problems and make decisions.

● **Develop a support system.** One of the best ways to promote self-esteem is through a support system of peers and others who share your values. Members of your support system can help you feel good about yourself and force you to take an honest look at your actions and choices. Keeping in contact with old friends and important family members can provide a foundation of unconditional love that will help you through life transitions.

● **Complete required tasks.** A good way to boost your sense of self-efficacy is to learn new skills and develop a history of success. Most college campuses provide study groups and

Using Positive Psychology to Enhance Your Happiness

To enhance happiness and employ a more positive outlook on life:

❯ **Check yourself.** Throughout the day, stop and evaluate what you're thinking. If your thoughts are mainly negative, try to stop them and substitute a positive thought.

❯ **Use your sense of humor.** Give yourself permission to smile or laugh, especially during difficult times. When you can laugh at life, you feel less stressed.

❯ **Follow a healthy lifestyle.** Exercise at least three times a week to positively affect mood and reduce stress. Follow a healthy diet to fuel your mind and body. Learn to manage your stress.

❯ **Surround yourself with positive people.** Make sure those in your life are positive, supportive people who give helpful advice and feedback. Negative people may increase your stress level and may make you doubt your ability to manage stress in healthy ways.

❯ **Practice positive self-talk.** Start by following one simple rule: Don't say anything to yourself that you wouldn't say to anyone else.

Source: Adapted from MayoClinic.com, "Positive Thinking: Reduce Stress by Eliminating Negative Self-Talk," March 22, 2013. Copyright © 2011 by Mayo Foundation for Medical Education and Research. Reprinted with permission.

---

learning centers that can help you manage time, improve study and writing skills, and prepare for tests, all actions that promote academic success.

● **Form realistic expectations.** If you expect top grades, a steady stream of Saturday-night dates, and the perfect job, you may be setting yourself up for disappointment. Assess your current resources and the direction in which you are heading. Set small, incremental goals that you can actually meet.

● **Make time for you.** Taking time to enjoy your life is another way to boost your self-esteem and psychological health. View a new activity as something to look forward to and an opportunity to have fun.

● **Maintain physical health.** Regular exercise fosters a sense of well-being. Research repeatedly supports the role of exercise and good nutrition in improved mental health.

● **Examine problems and seek help when necessary.** Know when to seek help from friends, support groups, family, or professionals. Sometimes you can handle life's problems alone; at other times, you need assistance.

● **Get adequate sleep.** Getting enough sleep daily is a key factor in physical and psychological health. Rest allows our bodies to conserve energy for our daily activities and provides time for restoring supplies of the **neurotransmitters** that we use up during our waking hours.

When Psychological Health Deteriorates

Sometimes circumstances overwhelm us to such a degree that we need help to get back on track. Stress, abusive relationships, anxiety, loneliness, financial upheavals, and other traumatic events can derail our coping resources, causing us to turn inward or act in ways that are outside of what might be considered normal. Chemical imbalances, drug interactions, trauma, neurological disruptions, and other physical problems may also contribute to these behaviors.

Mental illnesses are disorders that disrupt thinking, feeling, moods, and behaviors, and cause varying degrees of impaired functioning in daily living. They are believed to be caused by a variety of biochemical, genetic, and environmental factors.[19] Risk factors for developing or triggering mental illness include the following: having biological relatives with a mental illness; malnutrition or exposure to viruses while in the womb; stressful life situations, such as financial problems, a loved one's death, or a divorce; chronic medical conditions, such as cancer; combat; taking psychoactive drugs during adolescence; childhood abuse or neglect; and lack of friendships or healthy relationships.[20] As with physical disease, mental illnesses can range from mild to severe and can exact a heavy toll on quality of life, both for people with the illnesses and those who interact with them.

neurotransmitters Chemicals that relay messages between nerve cells or from nerve cells to other body cells.

mental illnesses Disorders that disrupt thinking, feeling, moods, and behaviors, and that impair daily functioning.

Mental disorders are common in the United States and worldwide. The basis for diagnosing mental disorders in the United States is the *Diagnostic and Statistical Manual of Mental Disorders,* Fifth Edition, (*DSM-5*). An estimated 20 percent of Americans aged 18 and older—almost 1 in 5 adults—suffer from a diagnosable mental disorder in a given year, and nearly half of them have more than one mental illness at the same time. About 5 percent of adults, or 1 in 20, suffer from a serious mental illness requiring close monitoring, residential care in many instances, and medication.[21] Mental disorders are the leading cause of disability in the United States and Canada for people aged 15 to 44, costing more than $100 billion annually.[22]

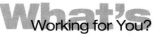

What's Working for You?

Maybe you already are doing things to enhance your psychological health. Are any of the following true for you?

☐ I have a network of friends and advisers I can go to when I need to talk about a problem.

☐ I know where to find psychological counseling on campus should I need it.

☐ I have healthy outlets for dealing with my emotions when I'm upset.

☐ I volunteer regularly in my college community, an activity that not only helps the community, but gives me a sense of purpose as well.

Mental Health Threats to College Students

Mental health problems are common among college students, and they appear to be increasing in number and severity.[23] The most recent National College Health Assessment survey found that nearly 1 in 3 undergraduates reported "feeling so depressed it was difficult to function" at least once in the past year. Seven percent of students reported that they seriously considered attempting suicide in the past year.[24] In another study with over 3,000 participants, 41 percent of students met the criteria for moderate to severe depression.[25] Although those study results may seem alarming, it is important to note that increases in help-seeking behavior, in addition to increases in the actual prevalence of mental disorders, may contribute to these trends. Figure 2.4 shows the mental health concerns of American college students.

Although there are many forms of mental illness, we will focus here on disorders that are most common among college students: mood disorders, anxiety disorders, personality disorders, and schizophrenia. The **Health Headlines** box on page 47 provides information on another growing mental health concern among young adults, attention-deficit/hyperactivity disorder.

chronic mood disorder Experience of persistent emotional states, such as sadness, despair, hopelessness, or euphoria.

major depression Severe depressive disorder that entails chronic mood disorder, physical effects such as sleep disturbance and exhaustion, and mental effects such as the inability to concentrate; also called *clinical depression.*

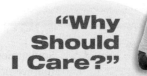

"Why Should I Care?"

Mental health problems can affect people of any age and have a huge impact on your life—including your success in academics, career, and relationships, and your general ability to function and enjoy life. Because mental health concerns are prevalent among college students, your roommate or a friend could have a problem and need your help and support.

feeling beaten and bruised. How do we know if these emotions are really signs of **major depression**? Major or clinical depression is not the same as having a bad day or feeling down after a negative experience. It is also not something that can be wished away or ignored for the sake of "growing a thicker skin." Major depression is the most common mood disorder, affecting approximately 8.6 percent of the U.S. population.[27]

Major depression is characterized by a combination of symptoms that interfere with work, study, sleep, appetite, relationships, and enjoyment of life. Symptoms can last for weeks, months, or years and vary in intensity.[28] Common signs include the following:

- Sadness and despair
- Loss of motivation or interest in pleasurable activities

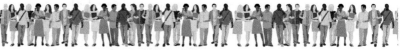

Felt overwhelmed by all they needed to do 85.2%

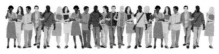

Felt things were hopeless 44.6%

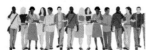

Felt so depressed that it was difficult to function 29.5%

Seriously considered suicide 7.0%

Intentionally injured themselves 5.6%

Attempted suicide 1.3%

= 2%

FIGURE 2.4 Mental Health Concerns of American College Students, Past 12 Months

Source: Data from American College Health Association, *American College Health Association–National College Health Assessment II (ACHA-NCHA II) Reference Group Data Report Fall 2012* (Hanover, MD: American College Health Association, 2013).

Mood Disorders

Chronic mood disorders are disorders that affect how you feel, such as persistent sadness or feelings of euphoria. They include major depression, dysthymic disorder, bipolar disorder, and seasonal affective disorder. In any given year, approximately 9.4 percent of Americans aged 18 or older suffer from a mood disorder.[26]

Major Depression

Sometimes life throws us a curveball. We experience loss, pain, disappointment, or frustration, and we can be left

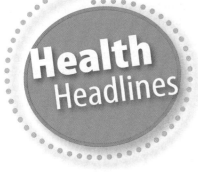

WHEN ADULTS HAVE ADHD

Attention-deficit/hyperactivity disorder (ADHD) is often associated with school-aged children, but for many people, symptoms persist into adulthood. About 4 percent of the adult population, or 8 million adults, are living with ADHD.

EFFECTS OF ADULT ADHD

Left untreated, ADHD can disrupt everything from careers to relationships to financial stability. Key areas of disruption might include the following:

✱ **Health.** Impulsivity and trouble with organization can lead to health problems, such as compulsive eating, alcohol and drug abuse, or forgetting to take medication for a chronic condition.

✱ **Work and finances.** Difficulty concentrating, completing tasks, listening, and relating to others can lead to trouble at work and school. Managing finances may also be a concern because a person with ADHD may struggle to pay bills on time, lose paperwork, miss deadlines, or spend impulsively, resulting in debt.

✱ **Relationships.** If you have ADHD, you might wonder why loved ones constantly nag you to tidy up, get organized, and take care of business. If your romantic partner has ADHD, you might be hurt that your loved one doesn't seem to listen to you, blurts out hurtful things, and leaves you with the bulk of organizing and planning.

GET EDUCATED ABOUT ADHD

If you suspect you or someone close to you has ADHD, learn as much as you can about adult ADHD and treatment options. The organization Children and Adults with Attention-Deficit/Hyperactivity Disorder (CHADD) is a good source of information and support (www.chadd.org). Adult ADHD can be a challenge to diagnose; there is no simple test for it, and it often occurs concurrently with other conditions, such as depression or anxiety. To ensure that you have the best treatment, secure a diagnosis and treatment plan from a qualified professional with experience in ADHD. ADHD can be treated, and getting the needed help can improve health, relationships, finances, and grades.

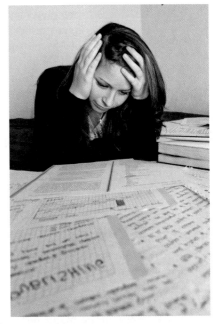

Disorder and chaos can be headaches for us all, but ADHD sufferers may find them to be insurmountable obstacles.

Sources: Centers for Disease Control and Prevention, "Attention-Deficit Hyperactivity Disorder," www.cdc.gov/ncbddd/adhd/facts.html, Updated May 2010; Helpguide.org, "Adult ADD/ADHD: Signs, Symptoms, Effects, and Treatment," June 2011, www.helpguide.org; AdultADHD.net, "Symptoms," Updated December 2012, www.adultadhd.net; R. C. Kessler et al., "The Prevalence and Correlates of Adult ADHD in the United States: Results from the National Comorbidity Survey Replication," *The American Journal of Psychiatry* 163, no. 4 (2006): 716–723.

● Preoccupation with failures and inadequacies; concern over what others are thinking
● Difficulty concentrating; indecisiveness; memory lapses
● Lost sex drive or interest in close interactions with others
● Fatigue and loss of energy; slow reactions
● Sleeping too much or too little; insomnia
● Feeling agitated, worthless, or hopeless
● Withdrawal from friends and family
● Diminished or increased appetite
● Significant weight loss or weight gain
● Recurring thoughts that life isn't worth living; thoughts of death or suicide

Depression in College Students Mental health problems, particularly depression, can be a major obstacle to academic success and healthy adjustment. Students who have weak communication skills; who find that college isn't what they expected; or who lack motivation often have difficulties adjusting to college life, increasing the risk of a depressive episode. Stressors such as anxiety over relationships, pressure to get good grades and win social acceptance, abuse of alcohol and other drugs, poor diet, and lack of sleep can create a toxic cocktail that can overwhelm even the most resilient students. In the most recent American College Health Association survey, 11.3 percent of college students reported having been diagnosed with or treated for depression in the past 12 months.[29]

Being far from home without the security of family and friends can exacerbate problems. Most campuses have counseling centers and other services available; however, some students do not use them because of persistent stigma associated with going to a counselor.

Dysthymic Disorder

Some people suffer from **dysthymic disorder (dysthymia),** a syndrome of chronic, less severe, mild depression. Dysthymia can be harder to recognize than major

dysthymic disorder (dysthymia) A type of depression that is milder and harder to recognize than major depression, is chronic, and is often characterized by fatigue, pessimism, or a short temper.

depression. Dysthymic individuals may appear to function well, but they may lack energy or fatigue easily; be short-tempered, overly pessimistic, and ornery; or just not feel quite up to par while not displaying any significant, overt symptoms. People with dysthymia may cycle into major depression over time. For a diagnosis, symptoms must persist for at least 2 years in adults (1 year in children). This disorder affects approximately 0.5 percent of the adult population in the United States in a given year.[30]

Bipolar Disorder

People with **bipolar disorder** (also called *manic depression*) often have severe mood swings, ranging from extreme highs (mania) to extreme lows (depression). Sometimes these swings are dramatic and rapid; other times they are slow and gradual. When in the manic phase, people may be overactive, talkative, and filled with energy; in the depressed phase, they may experience some or all of the typical symptoms of major depression.

Although the cause of bipolar disorder is unknown, biological, genetic, and environmental factors, such as drug abuse and stressful or psychologically traumatic events, seem to trigger episodes of the illness. Once diagnosed, persons with bipolar disorder have several counseling and pharmaceutical options, and most will be able to live a healthy, functional life while being treated. Bipolar disorder affects approximately 1.8 percent of the adult population in the United States.[31]

Seasonal Affective Disorder (SAD)

Another form of depression, **seasonal affective disorder (SAD),** strikes during the winter months and is associated with reduced exposure to sunlight. People with SAD suffer from irritability, apathy, carbohydrate craving and weight gain, increased sleep time, and general sadness. Several factors are implicated in SAD development, including disruption in the body's natural circadian rhythms and changes in levels of the hormone melatonin and the brain chemical serotonin.[32]

Spending time in the fresh air with your best friend is a simple way to enhance your psychological health.

The most beneficial treatment for SAD is light therapy, which exposes patients to lamps that simulate sunlight. Eighty percent of patients experience relief from their symptoms within 4 days. Other treatments for SAD include diet changes (such as eating more complex carbohydrates), increased exercise, stress-management techniques, sleep restriction (limiting the number of hours slept in a 24-hour period), psychotherapy, and prescription medications.

What Causes Mood Disorders?

Mood disorders are caused by the interaction between multiple factors, including biological differences, hormones, inherited traits, life events, and early childhood trauma.[33] The biology of mood disorders is related to individual levels of brain chemicals called neurotransmitters. Several types of depression, including bipolar disorder, appear to have a genetic component. Depression can be triggered by a serious loss, difficult relationships, financial problems, and pressure to succeed. Early childhood trauma, such as loss of a parent, may cause permanent changes in the brain, making one more prone to depression.

Changes in the body's physical health can be accompanied by mental changes, particularly depression. Stroke, heart attack, cancer, Parkinson's disease, chronic pain, type 2 diabetes, certain medications, alcohol, hormonal disorders, and a wide range of other afflictions can cause us to become depressed, frustrated, or angry. When this happens, recovery is often more difficult. A person who feels exhausted and defeated may lack the will to fight illness and do what is necessary to optimize recovery.

Anxiety Disorders

Anxiety disorders include generalized anxiety disorder, panic disorders, phobic disorders, obsessive-compulsive disorder, and post-traumatic stress disorder. They are characterized by persistent feelings of threat and worry.

Anxiety disorders are the number one mental health problem in the United States, affecting more than 21.3 percent of all adults.[34] Anxiety is also a leading mental health problem among adolescents, affecting 25.2 percent of Americans aged 13 to 17.[35] Twelve percent of U.S. undergraduates report being diagnosed with or treated for anxiety in the past year.[36]

Generalized Anxiety Disorder (GAD)

One common form of anxiety disorder, **generalized anxiety disorder (GAD),** is severe enough to interfere significantly with daily life. Generally, a person with GAD is a consummate worrier who develops a debilitating level of anxiety. To be diagnosed with GAD, one must exhibit at least three of the following symptoms for more days than not during a 6-month period: restlessness or feeling keyed up or on edge, being easily fatigued, difficulty concentrating or mind going blank, irritability, muscle tension, and/or sleep disturbances.[37] Generalized anxiety disorder often runs in families, but it is readily treatable.

Panic Disorders

Panic disorders are characterized by the occurrence of **panic attacks,** a form of acute anxiety reaction that brings on an intense physical reaction. You may dismiss the feelings as the jitters from too much stress, or the reaction may be so severe that you fear you will have a heart attack and die. Approximately 3.1 percent of Americans aged 18 and older experience panic attacks, usually in early adulthood.[38] Panic attacks and disorders are increasing in incidence, particularly among young women.

Although highly treatable, panic attacks may become debilitating and destructive, particularly if they happen often and cause the person to avoid going out in public or interacting with others. A panic attack typically starts abruptly, peaks within 10 minutes, lasts about 30 minutes, and leaves the person tired and drained.[39] Symptoms include increased respiration, chills, hot flashes, shortness of breath, stomach cramps, chest pain, difficulty swallowing, and a sense of doom or impending death.

Although researchers aren't sure what causes panic attacks, heredity, stress, and certain biochemical factors may play a role. Your chances of having a panic attack increase if a close relative has them. Some researchers believe that people who suffer panic attacks are experiencing an overreactive fight-or-flight physical response.

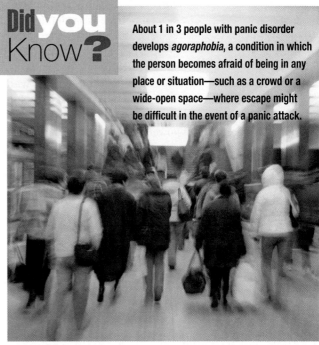

Source: Data from Anxiety and Depression Association of America, "Panic Disorder & Agoraphobia," 2012, www.adaa.org

Phobic Disorders

Phobias, or phobic disorders, involve a persistent and irrational fear of a specific object, activity, or situation, often out of proportion to the circumstances. Phobias result in a compelling desire to avoid the source of the fear. About 10.1 percent of U.S. adults suffer from specific phobias, such as fear of spiders, snakes, or public speaking.[40]

Another 7.4 percent of U.S. adults suffer from **social phobia**, also called *social anxiety disorder*.[41] Social phobia is an anxiety disorder characterized by the persistent fear and avoidance of social situations. Essentially, the person dreads these situations for fear of being humiliated, embarrassed, or even looked at. These disorders vary in scope. Some cause difficulty only in specific situations, such as getting up in front of a class to give a presentation. In extreme cases, a person avoids all contact with others.

generalized anxiety disorder (GAD) A constant sense of worry that may cause restlessness, difficulty in concentrating, tension, and other symptoms, and that interferes with daily life.

panic attack Acute anxiety reaction in which a particular situation, often for unknown reasons, causes terror.

phobia A deep and persistent fear of a specific object, activity, or situation that results in a compelling desire to avoid the source of the fear.

social phobia A phobia characterized by fear and avoidance of social situations; also called *social anxiety disorder*.

Obsessive-Compulsive Disorder (OCD)

People who feel compelled to perform rituals over and over again; who are fearful of dirt or contamination; who have an unnatural concern about order, symmetry, and exactness; or who have persistent intrusive thoughts that they can't shake may

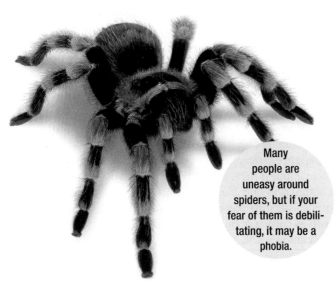

Many people are uneasy around spiders, but if your fear of them is debilitating, it may be a phobia.

be suffering from **obsessive-compulsive disorder (OCD).** Approximately 1.3 percent of Americans aged 18 and over have OCD.[42]

Not to be confused with being a perfectionist, a person with OCD often knows the behaviors are irrational, yet is powerless to stop them. According to the *DSM-5,* for a person to be diagnosed with OCD, the obsessive behaviors must consume more than 1 hour per day and interfere with normal social or life activities. Although the exact cause is unknown, genetics, biological abnormalities, learned behaviors, and environmental factors have all been considered. Obsessive-compulsive disorder usually begins in adolescence or early adulthood; the median age of onset is 19.[43]

Post-Traumatic Stress Disorder (PTSD)

People who have experienced or witnessed a traumatic event, such as a natural disaster, serious accident, or combat, may develop **post-traumatic stress disorder (PTSD).** The lifetime risk of PTSD is 10.1 percent in the United States, with rates as high as 30 percent in strife-torn regions of the world.[44] Sustained combat soldiers have high rates of PTSD, ranging from about 20 percent of those who fought in Iraq to over 30 percent of soldiers who returned from Vietnam.[45]

Symptoms of PTSD include the following:

- Dissociation, or perceived detachment of the mind from the emotional state or even the body
- Intrusive recollections of the traumatic event, such as flashbacks, nightmares, and recurrent thoughts or visual images
- Acute anxiety or nervousness, in which the person is hyperaroused, cries easily, or experiences mood swings
- Insomnia and difficulty concentrating
- Intense physiological reactions, such as shaking or nausea, when something reminds the person of the traumatic event

Although these symptoms may be appropriate as initial responses to traumatic events, PTSD may be diagnosed if a person experiences them for at least 1 month following the event. However, in some cases, symptoms don't appear until months or even years later.

What Causes Anxiety Disorders?

Because anxiety disorders vary in complexity and degree, scientists have yet to find clear reasons why one person develops them and another doesn't. The following factors are often cited as possible causes:[46]

obsessive-compulsive disorder (OCD) A form of anxiety disorder characterized by recurrent, unwanted thoughts and repetitive behaviors.

post-traumatic stress disorder (PTSD) A collection of symptoms that may occur as a delayed response to a serious trauma.

personality disorder One of a class of mental disorders characterized by inflexible patterns of thought and beliefs that lead to socially distressing behavior.

- **Biology.** Some scientists trace the origin of anxiety to the brain and its functioning. Using sophisticated positron-emission tomography (PET) scans, scientists can analyze areas of the brain that react during anxiety-producing events. Families appear to display similar brain and physiological reactivity, so we may inherit tendencies toward anxiety disorders.
- **Environment.** Anxiety can be a learned response. Although genetic tendencies may exist, experiencing a repeated pattern of reaction to certain situations programs the brain to respond in a certain way. For example, if your mother or father screamed whenever a large spider crept into view, or if other anxiety-raising events occurred frequently, you might be predisposed to react with anxiety to similar events later in life.
- **Social and cultural roles.** Cultural and social roles also may be risk factors for anxiety. Because men and women are taught to assume different roles in society (such as man as protector, woman as victim), women may find it more acceptable to scream, shake, pass out, or otherwise express extreme anxiety. Men, in contrast, may have learned to repress such anxieties rather than act on them.

Personality Disorders

According to the *DSM-5,* a **personality disorder** is an "enduring pattern of inner experience and behavior that deviates markedly from the expectation of the individual's culture and is pervasive and inflexible."[47] About 9 percent of adults in the United States have some form of personality disorder.[48] People who live, work, or are in relationships with individuals suffering from personality disorders often find interactions with them challenging and destructive.

Narcissistic personality disorders involve an exaggerated sense of self-importance and self-absorption. Persons with narcissistic personalities are fascinated with themselves and are preoccupied with fantasies of how wonderful they are. Typically, they are overly needy and demanding and believe that they are entitled to nothing but the best.

Persons with *antisocial personality disorders* display a long-term pattern of manipulation and taking advantage of others, often in a criminal manner. Symptoms include disregard for the safety of others and lack of remorse, arrogance, and anger. Far more men than women are affected, and it is one of the most difficult personality disorders to treat.[49]

Borderline personality disorder (BPD) is characterized by impulsiveness and risky behaviors such as gambling sprees, unsafe sex, use of illicit drugs, and daredevil driving.[50] Sufferers have trouble stabilizing their moods and can experience erratic mood swings. Other characteristics of this mental illness include reality distortion and the tendency to see things in only black-and-white terms. Seventy to 80 percent of persons diagnosed with BPD engage in self-injury, such as cutting or burning themselves, as a way to cope with their emotions.[51]

Schizophrenia

Perhaps the most frightening psychological disorder is **schizophrenia,** which affects about 1 percent of the U.S. population.[52] Schizophrenia is characterized by alterations of the senses (including auditory and visual hallucinations); the inability to sort out incoming stimuli and make appropriate responses; an altered sense of self; and radical changes in emotions, movements, and behaviors. Typical symptoms include fluctuating courses of delusional behavior, hallucinations, incoherent and rambling speech, inability to think logically, erratic movement and odd gesturing, and difficulty with normal activities of daily living.[53] The net effect is that society often regards such individuals as odd; viewed that way, they have difficulties in social interactions and may withdraw.

For decades, scientists believed that schizophrenia was a form of madness provoked by the environment in which a child lived. They blamed abnormal family interactions or early childhood traumas. Since the mid-1980s, however, when magnetic resonance imaging and PET scans began allowing us to study brain function more closely, scientists have determined that schizophrenia is a biological disease of the brain. The brain damage occurs early in life, possibly as early as the second trimester of fetal development. Fetal exposure to toxic substances, infections, and medications has been studied as a possible risk. Hereditary links are also being explored. Symptoms usually appear in men in their late teens and twenties and in women in their late twenties and early thirties.[54]

Even though old theories of schizophrenia have been discarded in favor of theories less focused on blaming the patient's family life, a stigma remains attached to this disease. Families of people with schizophrenia frequently experience anger and guilt. They often need information, family counseling, and advice on how to meet the schizophrenic person's needs for shelter, medical care, vocational training, and social interaction.

At present, schizophrenia is treatable but not curable. Treatments usually include some combination of hospitalization, medication, and supportive psychotherapy. Supportive psychotherapy, as opposed to psychoanalysis, can help a patient acquire skills for living in society. With proper medication, public understanding, support of loved ones, and access to therapy, many schizophrenics lead normal lives.

schizophrenia A mental illness with biological origins that is characterized by irrational behavior, severe alterations of the senses, and often an inability to function in society.

Suicide: Giving Up on Life

Suicide is the fourth leading cause of death for 5- to 14-year-olds and the second leading cause for 15- to 24-year-olds in the United States.[55] It has recently become the leading cause of death on college campuses, now ranking higher than alcohol-related deaths or car crashes.[56] The pressures, joys, disappointments, challenges, and changes of the college environment are believed to be partially responsible for the emotional turmoil that can lead a young person to contemplate suicide. However, young adults who choose not to go to college but who are searching for direction in careers, relationships, and other life goals are also at risk; in fact, suicide rates are higher in the general population than among college students. Specific risk factors include a family history of suicide, previous suicide attempts, excessive drug and alcohol use, prolonged depression, financial difficulties, serious illness in oneself or a loved one, and loss of a loved one through death or rejection. Lesbian, gay, bisexual, and transgender (LGBT) students face a unique set of challenges. The **Student Health Today** box on page 52 discusses the suicide rates of LGBT youth.

Recent studies indicate that suicide has become the leading cause of death by injury (both unintentional and intentional) among adults.[57] Whether they are more likely to attempt suicide or are more often successful in their attempts, nearly four times as many men die by suicide as women.[58] Overall, firearms, suffocation, and poison are the most common methods of suicide. However, men are almost twice as likely as women to commit suicide with firearms, whereas women are almost three times as likely as men to commit suicide by poisoning.[59]

Warning Signs of Suicide

Most people who commit suicide indicate their intentions, though others do not always recognize the warning.[60] Anyone who expresses a desire to kill himself or herself or who

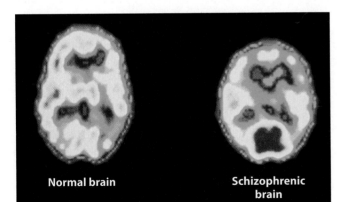

Normal brain **Schizophrenic brain**

These brain images reveal the difference in brain activity in persons with and without schizophrenia. The yellow and red correspond to areas of the greatest activity and the blue signifies areas with reduced activity.

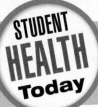

LGBT YOUTH AND SUICIDE PREVENTION

Lesbian, gay, bisexual, and transgender (LGBT) youth are up to four times more likely to attempt suicide than are their heterosexual peers. More than one third of LGBT youth report having made a suicide attempt, and nearly half of young transgender people have seriously thought about taking their lives. LGBT youth who come from highly rejecting families are much more likely to have attempted suicide than are their LGBT peers who reported no or low levels of family rejection. Furthermore, those that have experienced bullying in school are at greater risk for suicide.

Many factors that reduce suicide attempts have been identified and include the following:

✳ Support through ongoing medical and mental health care relationships
✳ Coping, problem-solving, and conflict-resolution skills
✳ Restricted access to highly lethal means of suicide
✳ Strong connections to family

✳ Family and parental acceptance of sexual orientation and/or gender identity
✳ School safety, support, connectedness, and peer groups such as gay-straight alliances
✳ Cultural and religious beliefs that discourage suicide and support self-preservation

Nationally, there is growing awareness of the need to address LGBT suicide risk and possible interventions, including providing resources and training to school personnel, organizing peer-based support groups, and implementing policies to prevent violence and bullying.

Sources: A.P. Haas et al., "Suicide and Suicide Risk in Lesbian, Gay, Bisexual, and Transgender Populations: Review and Recommendations," *Journal of Homosexuality* 58, no. 1 (2011): 10–51; Suicide Prevention Research Center, "Suicide Risk among LGBT Youth," 2011, www.sprc.org; D. Reynolds and P. Schneider, "An Overview of Suicide Risks among Lesbian, Gay, Bisexual, Transgender and Questioning (LGBTQ) Youth," Social Workers Help Starts Here (blog), February 8, 2013, www.helpstartshere.org

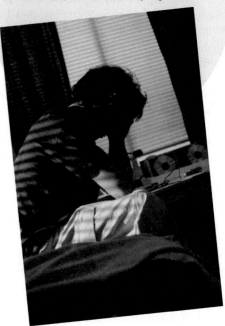
LGBT youth can face unique challenges that can lead to depression or attempting suicide.

---

has made an attempt is at risk. Common signs that a person may be contemplating suicide include the following:[61]

● Recent loss and a seeming inability to let go of grief
● A history of depression
● Change in personality, such as sadness, withdrawal, irritability, anxiety, tiredness, indecisiveness, or apathy
● Change in behavior, such as inability to concentrate, loss of interest in classes or work, or unexplained demonstration of happiness following a period of depression
● Sexual dysfunction (such as impotence) or diminished sexual interest
● Expressions of self-hatred and excessive risk-taking, or an "I don't care what happens to me" attitude
● Change in sleep patterns and/or eating habits
● A direct statement about committing suicide, such as "I might as well end it all"
● An indirect statement, such as "You won't have to worry about me anymore"
● Final preparations such as writing a will, giving away prized possessions, or writing revealing letters

● A preoccupation with themes of death
● Marked changes in personal appearance

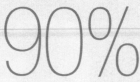

Of people who kill themselves

90% have a diagnosable mental disorder, most commonly depression or a substance abuse disorder.

Preventing Suicide

Most people who attempt suicide really want to live but see death as the only way out of an intolerable situation. Crisis counselors and suicide hotlines may help temporarily, but the best way to prevent suicide is to get rid of conditions and substances that may precipitate attempts, including alcohol, drugs, loneliness, isolation, and access to guns.

If someone you know threatens suicide or displays warning signs of doing so, get involved—ask questions and seek help. Specific actions you can take include the following:[62]

- **Monitor the warning signals.** Keep an eye on the person or see that there is someone around the person as often as possible. Don't leave him or her alone.
- **Take threats seriously.** Don't brush them off as "just talk."
- **Let the person know how much you care.** State that you are there to help.
- **Listen.** Try not to discredit or be shocked by what the person says. Empathize, sympathize, and keep the person talking.
- **Ask questions.** Ask directly, "Are you thinking of hurting or killing yourself?"
- **Do not belittle the person's feelings.** Don't tell the person that he or she doesn't really mean it or couldn't succeed at suicide. To some people, these comments offer the challenge of proving you wrong.
- **Help the person think about alternatives to suicide.** Offer to go for help along with the person. Call your local suicide hotline, and use all available community and campus resources.
- **Tell your friend's spouse, partner, parents, siblings, or counselor.** Do not keep your suspicions to yourself. Don't let a suicidal friend talk you into keeping your discussions confidential. If your friend succeeds in a suicide attempt, you may find that others will question your decision, and you may blame yourself.[61]

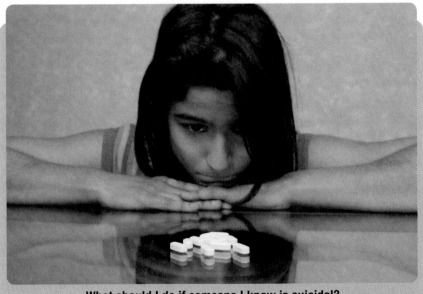

What should I do if someone I know is suicidal?

If you notice warning signs of suicide in someone you know, you must take action. Suicidal people urgently need professional assistance. Your willingness to talk to the person about depression and suicide in a nonjudgmental way can be the encouragement he or she needs to seek help. Remember: Always take thoughts of or plans for suicide seriously—a life may depend on it.

Seeking Professional Help for Psychological Problems

A physical ailment will readily send most of us to the nearest health professional, but some people view seeking professional help for psychological problems as an admission of personal failure. Although estimates show that 20 percent of adults have some kind of mental disorder, only 6 to 7 percent of adults use mental health services.[63]

Researchers view breakdowns in support systems, high societal expectations, and dysfunctional families as three major reasons why more people are asking for assistance than ever before.

Consider seeking help if:

- You feel that you need help or feel out of control
- You experience wild mood swings or inappropriate emotional responses to normal stimuli
- Your fears or feelings of guilt frequently distract your attention
- You begin to withdraw from others
- You have hallucinations
- You feel inadequate or worthless or that life is not worth living
- Your daily life seems to be nothing but a series of repeated crises
- You are considering suicide
- You turn to drugs or alcohol to escape your problems

Low-cost or free counseling sessions or support groups are often available on college campuses to help students deal with all types of issues, including mental illness. See the **Money & Health** box on page 54 for tips on how to get good mental health care on a tight budget.

Mental Illness Stigma

Stigmas are negative stereotypes about groups of people. Common stigmas about people with mental illness are that they are dangerous, irresponsible, childlike and requiring constant care, or that they "just need to get over it."

The reality is that very few people with a mental illness are dangerous. Most live independently, go to school, hold jobs, and are productive members of society. A mental illness is like any other chronic disease. You can't decide just to "get over it."

The stigma of mental illness often leads to feelings of shame, guilt, loss

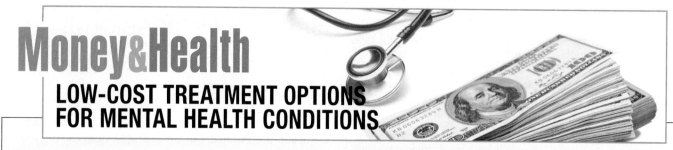

Money&Health

LOW-COST TREATMENT OPTIONS FOR MENTAL HEALTH CONDITIONS

Mental health disorders are treatable, yet people don't always seek help. Often the cost of therapy and prescription drugs is a major barrier; many insurance plans may provide only limited coverage of mental health services. If you are on a tight budget and struggle with depression, anxiety, or other mental health issues, it's always a good idea to speak with your family physician about low-cost treatment resources in your region and state. Here is a roundup of possible treatment options one can pursue, along with tips on easing the expense.

THERAPY

Cognitive-behavioral therapy can cost $100 or more per hour. However, some therapists or federally funded clinics offer therapy on a sliding scale, which means the fee varies based on income. Some colleges and universities also offer low-cost therapy for mental health problems through the health center.

PRESCRIPTION DRUGS

Medication can help reduce symptoms of certain mental health disorders, including anxiety and depression, but for many people drugs can be very expensive. Most pharmaceutical companies offer patient-assistance programs for low-income patients. These programs provide prescribed medication at little to no cost. Also ask your doctor if a generic (non-brand-name) drug might work for you as well as a brand-name drug. Additionally, your doctor might have medication samples he or she could give you for free.

Note that if you are considering medication, it must be prescribed and monitored by your physician. Even if cost is a factor, do not adjust the dosage or frequency or stop taking it abruptly without first discussing it with your doctor.

Sources: ADAA, Low Cost Treatment, 2011, www.adaa.org; Partnership for Prescription Assistance, 2011, Patient Frequently Asked Questions, www.pparx.org; J. Grohol, "Finding Low-Cost Psychotherapy," PsychCentral, January 2012, http://psychcentral.com; Psych Central Staff, "Mental Health Care Benefits Under Affordable Care Act," July 2012, http://psychcentral.com.

what do you think?

Do you notice social stigma against mental illness in your community?

● How often do you hear terms like "crazy" or "whacko" used to describe people who appear to have a mental health problem? Why are those words harmful to others?

● Why are mental illnesses perceived to be different from physical ones such as diabetes?

of self-esteem, and a sense of isolation and hopelessness. Many people who have successfully managed their mental illness report that the stigma they faced was more disabling at times than the illness itself.[64] The stigma may cause people who are struggling with mental illness to delay seeking treatment or avoid care that could dramatically improve their symptoms and quality of life.

Getting Evaluated for Treatment

If you are considering treatment for a psychological problem, schedule a complete evaluation first. Consult a credentialed health professional for a thorough examination, which should include three parts:

1. *A physical checkup,* which will rule out thyroid disorders, viral infections, and anemia—all of which can result in depression-like symptoms—and a neurological check of coordination, reflexes, and balance to rule out brain disorders.

2. *A psychiatric history,* which will trace the course of the apparent disorder, genetic or family factors, and any past treatments.

3. *A mental status examination,* which will assess thoughts, speaking processes, and memory, and include an in-depth interview with tests for other psychiatric symptoms.

Once physical factors have been ruled out, you may decide to consult a professional who specializes in psychological health.

Mental Health Professionals

Several types of mental health professionals are available to help you; Table 2.1 on page 55 compares several of the most common. When choosing a therapist, the most important criterion is not how many degrees the person has, but whether you feel you can work with him or her. A qualified mental health professional should be willing to answer all your questions during an initial consultation. Questions to ask the therapist and yourself include the following:

● **Can you interview the therapist before starting treatment?** An initial meeting will help you determine whether this person will be a good fit for you.

● **Do you like the therapist as a person?** Can you talk to him or her comfortably?

Mental Health Professionals

What Are They Called?	What Kind of Training Do They Have?	What Kind of Therapy Do They Do?	Professional Association
Psychiatrist	Medical doctor degree (MD), followed by 4 years of mental health training	Can prescribe medications and may have admitting privileges at a local hospital.	American Psychiatric Association www.psych.org
Psychologist	Doctoral degree in counseling or clinical psychology (PhD), plus several years of supervised practice to earn license	Various types, such as cognitive-behavioral therapy, and specialties including family or sexual counseling.	American Psychological Association www.apa.org
Clinical/psychiatric social worker	Master's degree in social work (MSW), followed by 2 years of experience in a clinical setting to earn license	May be trained in certain specialties, such as substance abuse counseling or child counseling.	National Association of Social Workers www.socialworkers.org
Counselor	Master's degree in counseling, psychology, educational psychology, or related human service; generally must complete at least 2 years of supervised practice before obtaining a license	Many are trained to provide individual and group therapy; may specialize in one type of counseling, such as family, marital, relationship, children, or drug abuse.	American Counseling Association www.counseling.org
Psychoanalyst	Postgraduate degree in psychology or psychiatry (PhD or MD), followed by 8–10 years of training in psychoanalysis, which includes undergoing analysis themselves	Based on theories of Freud and others, focuses on patterns of thinking and behavior and recalling early traumas that block personal growth. Treatment lasts 5–10 years, with 3–4 sessions per week.	American Psychoanalytic Association www.apsa.org
Licensed marriage and family therapist (LMFT)	Master's or doctoral degree in psychology, social work, or counseling, specializing in family and interpersonal dynamics; generally must complete at least 2 years of supervised practice before obtaining a license	Treat individuals or families who want relationship counseling. Treatment is often brief and focused on finding solutions to specific relational problems.	American Association for Marriage and Family Therapy www.aamft.org

● **Is the therapist watching the clock or easily distracted?** You should be the focus of the session.

● **Does the therapist demonstrate professionalism?** Be concerned if your therapist is frequently late or breaks appointments, suggests social interactions outside your therapy sessions, talks inappropriately about himself or herself, has questionable billing practices, or resists releasing you from therapy.

● **Will the therapist help you set your own goals and timetables?** A good professional should evaluate your general situation and help you set small goals to work on between sessions.

Please note, in most states, the use of the title *therapist* or *counselor* is unregulated. Make your choice carefully.

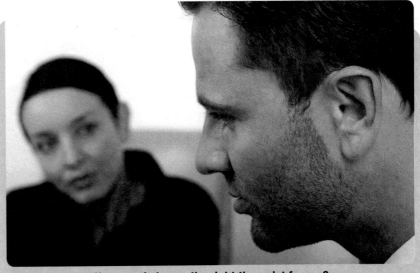

How can I choose the right therapist for me?

When you begin seeing a mental health professional, you enter into a relationship with that person, and just as with any person, you will connect better with some therapists than others. If one person doesn't "feel right" to you, trust your instincts and look for someone else.

What to Expect in Therapy

The first trip to a therapist can be difficult. That first visit is a verbal and mental sizing up between you and the therapist. If you decide that this professional is not for you, you will at least have learned how to present your problem and what qualities you need in a therapist.

Before meeting, briefly explain your needs and ask what the fee is. Dress however you feel most comfortable, arrive on time, and expect your visit to last about an hour. The therapist will want to take down your history and details about the problems that have brought you to therapy. Answer honestly and do not be embarrassed to acknowledge your feelings. It is critical to the success of your treatment that you trust this person enough to be open and honest.

Do not expect the therapist to tell you what to do or how to behave. The responsibility for improved behavior lies with you. If after your first visit (or even after several visits), you feel you cannot work with this person, say so. You have the right to find a therapist with whom you feel comfortable.

Treatment Models Many different types of counseling exist, including psychodynamic therapy, interpersonal therapy, and cognitive-behavioral therapy.

Psychodynamic therapy focuses on the psychological roots of emotional suffering. This type of therapy involves self-reflection, self-examination, and the use of the relationship between therapist and patient as a window into problematic relationship patterns in the patient's life. Its goal is not only to alleviate the most obvious symptoms, but also to help people lead healthier lives.[65]

Interpersonal therapy focuses on social roles and relationships. The patient works with a therapist to evaluate specific problem areas in the patient's life, such as conflicts with family and friends or significant life changes or transitions. Although past experiences help inform the process, interpersonal therapy focuses mainly on improving relationships in the present.[66]

Treatment for mental disorders can include various cognitive-behavioral therapies. *Cognitive therapy* focuses on the impact of thoughts and ideas on feelings and behavior. It helps a person to look at life rationally and correct habitually pessimistic or faulty thinking patterns. *Behavioral therapy* focuses on what we do. Behavior therapy uses the concepts of stimulus, response, and reinforcement to alter behavior patterns. With cognitive-behavioral therapy, you work with a mental health professional (psychotherapist) in a structured way, attending a limited number of sessions to become aware of inaccurate or negative thinking. Cognitive-behavioral therapy enables you to view challenging situations more clearly and respond to them in a more effective and positive way. Cognitive-behavioral therapy can be a very helpful tool in treating anxiety or depression.[67]

Pharmacological Treatment

It is not uncommon for psychotherapeutic treatment to combine talk therapy with drug therapy. Psychotropic drugs require a doctor's prescription and have been approved by the U.S. Food and Drug Administration (FDA). These medications are not, however, without side effects and risks. Common side effects include dry mouth, headaches, nausea, sexual dysfunction, and weight gain, among others. Additionally, the FDA requires warnings for antidepressant medications, including labeling that warns of increased risks of suicidal thinking and behavior during initial treatment in young adults aged 18 to 24.[68]

Potency, dosage, and side effects of drugs can vary greatly, even within the same drug category. It is vital to talk to your health care provider and completely understand the risks and benefits of any medication you may be prescribed. Likewise, your doctor needs to be aware as soon as possible of any adverse effects you may experience. With some drug therapies, such as antidepressants, you may not feel the therapeutic effects for several weeks, so patience is important. Finally, be sure to follow your doctor's recommendations for beginning or ending a course of any medication.

Staying Psychologically Healthy: Test Your Coping Skills

How do you stay psychologically healthy and well? There are many ways, but one particularly effective method is improving your coping skills. This assessment will help you identify how well you cope. It will also help you learn about some beneficial and healthy ways to cope, which will, in turn, help you stay psychologically healthy.

Carefully assess yourself by scoring each item according to how often each statement applies to you.

	Always	Often	Sometimes	Rarely	Never
1. I seek out emotional support from others.	1	2	3	4	5
2. In light of new developments, I am willing to change my opinions.	1	2	3	4	5
3. I find myself so overwhelmed that I completely shut down.	1	2	3	4	5
4. If I think there is some research or other information about a problem I have, I will seek it out.	1	2	3	4	5
5. I try to keep the situation in perspective.	1	2	3	4	5
6. I refuse to give up.	1	2	3	4	5
7. I remind myself that eventually things will get better.	1	2	3	4	5
8. It is difficult to forget about my problems and worries and just have fun.	1	2	3	4	5
9. I experience difficulty sleeping because my mind is racing.	1	2	3	4	5
10. I manage to find an outlet to express my emotions (writing a journal, drawing, exercising, etc.).	1	2	3	4	5

Interpreting Your Score

Add up your score for numbers 3, 8, and 9. A perfect score is 15. The higher your score, the stronger your coping skills.

Add up your score for numbers 1, 2, 4, 5, 6, 7, and 10. A perfect score is 7. The lower your score here, the greater your ability to cope with stress in an effective, healthy manner. The higher the score, the more you need to improve your coping skills. To see where you need the most improvement, look at your answers to these questions. For example, if your score for question 1 is "4, rarely," or "5, never," reaching out to others for emotional support will improve your psychological health.

Source: Psych Tests AIM Inc., "Coping and Stress Management Skills Test—Abridged/10 Questions, 5 Mins," http://testyourself.psychtests.com/testid/3111. Reprinted by permission.

YOUR PLAN FOR CHANGE

The **Assess yourself** activity gave you the chance to assess your coping abilities. After considering the results, you can take steps to change behaviors that may be detrimental to your psychological health.

Today, you can:

◯ Evaluate your behavior and identify patterns and specific things you are doing that negatively affect your psychological health. What can you change now? What can you change in the near future?

◯ Start a journal and note your moods. Look for trends and think about ways you can address them.

◯ List the things that bring you joy. Commit yourself to making more room for these joy-givers in your life.

Within the next 2 weeks, you can:

◯ Visit your campus health center and learn about the counseling services they offer. If you are feeling overwhelmed, depressed, or anxious, make an appointment with a counselor.

◯ Pay attention to the negative thoughts that pop up throughout the day. Being aware of these thoughts gives you an opportunity to stop, evaluate them, and choose a different thought.

By the end of the semester, you can:

◯ Make a commitment to an ongoing therapeutic practice aimed at improving your psychological health. Depending on your current situation, this could mean anything from seeing a counselor or joining a support group to practicing meditation or attending religious services.

◯ Volunteer regularly with a local organization you care about. Focus your energy and gain satisfaction by helping to improve others' lives or the environment.

MasteringHealth™

Build your knowledge—and health!—in the Study Area of MasteringHealth with a variety of study tools.

Summary

* Psychological health is a complex phenomenon involving mental, emotional, social, and spiritual dimensions.

* Many factors influence psychological health, including life experiences, family, the environment, other people, self-esteem, self-efficacy, and personality.

* The mind–body connection is an important link in overall health and well-being. Positive psychology emphasizes happiness as a key factor in determining reactions to life's challenges.

* Developing self-esteem and self-efficacy, making healthy connections, understanding and controlling emotions, and learning to solve problems and make decisions are keys to enhancing psychological health.

* The college years are a high-risk time for developing depression or anxiety disorders because of high stress levels, pressures for grades, and financial strain.

* Mood disorders include major depression, dysthymic disorder, bipolar disorder, and seasonal affective disorder. Anxiety disorders include generalized anxiety disorder, panic disorders, phobic disorders, obsessive-compulsive disorder, and post-traumatic stress disorder. Personality disorders include paranoid, narcissistic, antisocial, and borderline personality disorders.

* Schizophrenia is a biological disease of the brain, with brain damage possibly occurring as early as during the prenatal period. It is characterized by alterations of the senses, an inability to sort out stimuli and respond appropriately, an altered sense of self, and radical changes in emotions, movement, and behavior.

* Suicide is a result of negative psychological reactions to life. People intending to commit suicide often give warning signs of their intentions and can often be helped. It is important to pay attention if an individual exhibits any of the warning signs of suicide. Suicide prevention involves getting rid of the conditions that may lead to attempts.

* Mental health professionals include psychiatrists, psychologists, clinical/psychiatric social workers, counselors, psychoanalysts, and licensed marriage and family therapists. Many therapy methods exist, including psychodynamic, interpersonal, and cognitive-behavioral therapy.

* Treatment of mental disorders can combine talk therapy and drug therapy using psychotropic drugs, such as antidepressants.

Pop Quiz

1. All of the following traits have been identified as characterizing psychologically healthy people *except*
   a. they like themselves.
   b. they do not need social relationships for support.
   c. they meet life's demands.
   d. they have positive outlooks.

2. The term that most accurately refers to the feeling or subjective side of psychological health is
   a. social health.
   b. mental health.
   c. emotional health.
   d. spiritual health.

3. A person with high self-esteem
   a. possesses feelings of self-respect and self-worth.
   b. believes he or she can successfully engage in a specific behavior.
   c. believes external influences shape one's psychological health.
   d. has a high altruistic capacity.

4. People who have experienced repeated failures at the same task may eventually give up and quit trying altogether. This pattern of behavior is termed
   a. post-traumatic stress disorder.
   b. learned helplessness.
   c. self-efficacy.
   d. introversion.

5. Subjective well-being includes all of the following components *except*
   a. psychological hardiness.
   b. satisfaction with present life.
   c. relative presence of positive emotions.
   d. relative absence of negative emotions.

6. Which statement below is *false*?
   a. One in 4 adults in the United States suffers from a diagnosable mental disorder in a given year.
   b. Mental disorders are the leading cause of disability for 15- to 44-year-olds in the United States.
   c. Dysthymia is an example of an anxiety disorder.
   d. Bipolar disorder can also be referred to as manic depression.

7. Every winter, Stan suffers from irritability, apathy, weight gain, and sadness. He most likely has
   a. panic disorder.
   b. generalized anxiety disorder.
   c. seasonal affective disorder.
   d. chronic mood disorder.

8. What is the most common mental health problem in the United States?
   a. Depression
   b. Anxiety disorders
   c. Alcohol dependence
   d. Schizophrenia

9. This disorder is characterized by a need to perform rituals over and over again; fear of dirt or contamination; or an unnatural concern with order, symmetry, and exactness.
   a. Personality disorder
   b. Obsessive-compulsive disorder
   c. Phobic disorder
   d. Post-traumatic stress disorder

10. A person with a PhD in counseling psychology and training in various types of therapy is a
    a. psychiatrist.
    b. psychologist.
    c. social worker.
    d. psychoanalyst.

Answers to these questions can be found on page A-1.

Think about It!

1. What is psychological health? What indicates that a person is or is not psychologically healthy? Why might the college environment provide a challenge to psychological health?
2. Consider the factors that influence your overall level of psychological health. Which factors can you change? Which ones may be more difficult to change?
3. Which psychological dimensions do you need to work on? Which are most important to you, and why? What actions can you take today?
4. Why are college students particularly at risk for suicide? What are the warning signs of suicide? Of depression? What would you do if you heard a friend in the cafeteria say to no one in particular that he was going to "do the world a favor and end it all"?
5. Review the different types of health professionals and therapies. If you felt depressed about breaking off a long-term relationship, which professional and which therapy do you think would be most beneficial to you?

Accessing Your Health on the Internet

The following websites explore further topics and issues related to psychological health. For links to the websites below, visit the Study Area in MasteringHealth.

1. *American Foundation for Suicide Prevention.* This group provides resources for suicide prevention and support for family and friends of those who have committed suicide. www.afsp.org
2. *Veterans Crisis Line.* This is a site and help line that provides information on suicide and connects veterans and their families to qualified responders through online chat, text, or phone. www.veteranscrisisline.net or 1-800-273-8255
3. *National Suicide Prevention Lifeline.* Help is available from NSPL 24 hours a day for people in crisis via online chat, text, or phone. www.suicidepreventionlifeline.org or 1-800-273-8255
4. *American Psychological Association Help Center.* This site includes information on psychology at work, the mind–body connection, psychological responses to war, and other topics. www.apa.org/helpcenter
5. *National Alliance on Mental Illness.* This group is a support and advocacy organization of families and friends of people with severe mental illnesses. www.nami.org
6. *National Institute of Mental Health (NIMH).* The NIMH provides an overview of mental health information and new research relating to mental health. www.nimh.nih.gov
7. *Helpguide.* You can find resources here for improving mental and emotional health as well as specific information on topics such as self-injury, sleep, depression, and anxiety disorders. www.helpguide.org
8. *Active Minds.* This campus education and advocacy organization was formed to combat the stigma of mental illness, encourage students who need help to seek it early, and prevent tragedies related to untreated mental illness. www.activeminds.org

Cultivating Your Spiritual Health

LEARNING OUTCOMES

✳ Define spirituality and describe its three facets, and distinguish between religion and spirituality.

✳ Discuss the evidence that spiritual health has physical benefits, has psychological benefits, and lowers stress.

✳ Describe three ways you can develop your spiritual health.

61 How many college students focus on their spiritual health?

62 Is spirituality the same as religion?

64 Does spirituality influence health?

67 How can I stick with a meditation routine?

Lia's favorite spot on campus is the secluded Japanese garden on the south side of the library. Whether she's feeling stressed about exams or is mulling over an important decision, a few minutes alone in the garden always seem to help. Sometimes she sits quietly and watches the birds come and go. Sometimes she gets out her camera and photographs particularly brilliant blossoms. Often she simply rests, eyes closed, feeling the sun's warmth on her face, and lets her thoughts turn to gratitude for her health, her loving family, and her opportunity to study. However she spends it, her "garden break" leaves Lia feeling refreshed and refocused, with greater confidence in her ability to tackle the challenges of her day.

Lia's desire to find a sense of purpose, meaning, and harmony in her life is shared by a majority of American college students. According to UCLA's Higher Education Research Institute (HERI), incoming undergraduate students have a wide spectrum of spiritual, social, and ethical concerns.[1] More than 203,967 students at more than 270 colleges and universities were surveyed as they entered college in the fall of 2012. The data showed that,

of college students say they are "searching for meaning and purpose in life."

important focus of her daily life, bringing her greater awareness and serenity. If you're feeling as if you could use a little more of these qualities in your own life, read on: This chapter will help you explore ways to sharpen your spiritual focus.

What Is Spirituality?

From one day to the next, many of us attempt to satisfy our needs for belonging and self-esteem by acquiring material possessions. But at some point we come to realize that new gadgets, clothes, or concert tickets don't necessarily make us happy or improve our sense of self-worth. That's when many of us begin to contemplate another side of ourselves: our spirituality.

But what is spirituality? It isn't easy to define. Although part of the universal human experience, it's highly personal and involves feelings and senses that are often intangible. As such, it tends to defy the boundaries that strict definitions would impose. Let's begin by exploring its root, *spirit,* which in many cultures refers to *breath,* or the force that animates life. When you're "inspired," your energy flows. You're not held back by doubts about the purpose or meaning of your work and life. Indeed, many definitions of spirituality incorporate this sense of transcendence. For example, the National

A quiet meadow can be an ideal spot for contemplation and spiritual renewal.

compared to their peers, 35.9 percent of incoming freshman students rated themselves above average in spirituality, 51.5 percent in emotional health, and 79.6 percent in being able to work with a diverse population.[2]

Also, researchers found that 87.4 percent reported volunteering in the past year and 57.2 percent reported participating in community service as part of a class. Lastly, 73 percent of students reported high levels of being tolerant of diverse beliefs.[3]

Spiritual health is one of six key dimensions of health (see **Figure 1.4** on page 7). Lia's sense of wonder and respect for the natural world and her gratitude for the good things in her life suggest that spiritual health is an

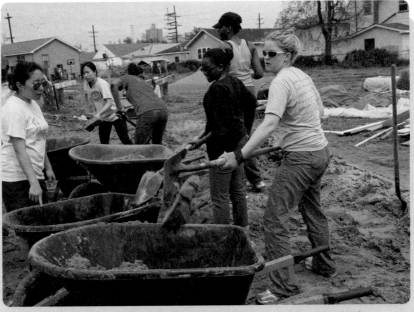

How many college students focus on their spiritual health?

Spiritual and ethical concerns are important to a majority of American college students. One of the ways college students express their spirituality is by working to reduce suffering in the world; many contribute their time and skills to volunteer organizations, as these students are doing by working to build homes for Habitat for Humanity.

spirituality An individual's sense of peace, purpose, and connection to others and beliefs about the meaning of life.

religion A system of beliefs, practices, rituals, and symbols designed to facilitate closeness to the sacred or transcendent.

Characteristics Distinguishing Religion and Spirituality	
Religion	**Spirituality**
Community focused	Individualistic
Observable, measurable, objective	Less measurable, more subjective
Formal, orthodox, organized	Less formal, less orthodox, less systematic
Behavior oriented, outward practices	Emotionally oriented, inwardly directed
Authoritarian in terms of behaviors	Not authoritarian, little accountability
Doctrine separating good from evil	Unifying, not doctrine oriented

Source: National Center for Complementary and Alternative Medicine (NCCAM), "Prayer and Spirituality in Health: Ancient Practices, Modern Science," *CAM at the NIH* 12, no. 1 (2005): 1–4.

Cancer Institute defines **spirituality** as an individual's sense of peace, purpose, and connection to others, and beliefs about the meaning of life.[4] Similarly, Harold G. Koenig, MD, one of the foremost researchers of spirituality and health, defines *spirituality* as the personal quest for understanding answers to ultimate questions about life, about meaning, and about our relationship with the sacred or transcendent.[5] The sacred or transcendent could be a higher power or it could relate to our relationship with nature or forces we cannot explain.

Religion and Spirituality Are Distinct Concepts

Spirituality may or may not lead to participation in organized **religion;** that is, a system of beliefs, practices, rituals, and symbols designed to facilitate closeness to the sacred or transcendent.[6] In other words, although spirituality and religion share some common elements, they are not the same thing. Most Americans consider spirituality to be important in their lives, but not necessarily in the form of religion: A recent national survey revealed that 73 percent of Americans 30 years and older believe in God, but not all of these respondents identified themselves as being affiliated with a particular religion.[7] Thus, it's clear that religion does not have to be part of a spiritual person's life. Table 1 identifies some characteristics that can help you distinguish between religion and spirituality.

Another finding of the same survey was that 74 percent of Americans affiliated with a religious tradition agreed that other religions are also valid.[8] Perhaps this is because all major religions express a belief in a unifying spiritual concept, a oneness with a greater power. It seems that a majority of Americans recognize and respect this underlying unity of spiritual ideas, expressed in different religious and spiritual practices.

Spirituality Integrates Three Facets

Brian Luke Seaward, a professor at the University of Northern Colorado and author of several books on spirituality and mind–body healing, identifies three facets of human existence that together constitute the core of human spirituality: relationships, values, and purpose in life (Figure 1, page 63).[9] Questions arising in these three domains prompt many of us to look for spiritual answers. At the same time, spiritual well-being is characterized by healthy relationships, strong personal values, and a sense that we have a meaningful purpose in life.

Relationships Have you ever wondered if someone you were attracted to is really right for you? Or, conversely,

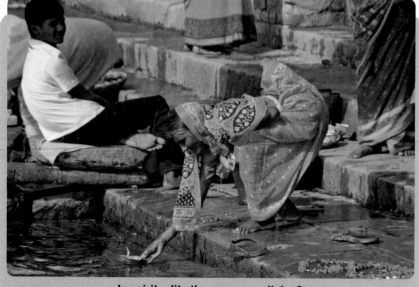

Is spirituality the same as religion?

Spirituality and religion are not the same. Many people find that religious practices, such as attending services or making offerings—such as the small lamp this Hindu woman is placing in the sacred Ganges River—help them to focus on their spirituality. However, religion does not have to be part of a spiritual person's life.

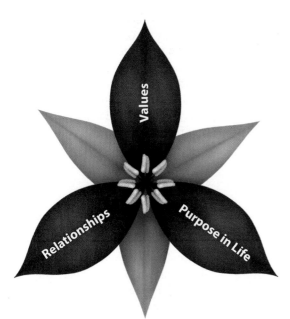

FIGURE 1 Three Facets of Spirituality
Most of us are prompted to explore our spirituality because of questions relating to our relationships, values, and purpose in life. At the same time, these three facets together constitute spiritual well-being.

Video Tutor: Facets of Spirituality

if you should break off a long-term relationship? Have you ever wished you had more friends, or that you were a better friend to yourself? Have you ever tried to make a connection with some sort of Presence or Higher Self? For many people, such questions and yearnings are natural triggers for spiritual growth: As we contemplate whom we should choose as a life partner or how to mend a quarrel with a friend, we begin to foster our own inner wisdom. At the same time, healthy relationships are a sign of spiritual well-being. When we treat ourselves and others with respect, honesty, integrity, and love, we are manifesting our spiritual health.

Values Our personal **values** are our principles—not only the things we say we care about, but also the things that cause us to behave the way we do. For instance, if you value honesty, then you are not likely to call in sick for work when you intend to spend the day at the beach. In other words, our value system is the set of fundamental rules by which we conduct our lives. It's what we stand for. When we attempt to clarify our values, and then to live according to those values, we're engaging in spiritual work. Spiritual health is characterized by a strong personal value system.

Meaningful Purpose in Life What career do you plan to pursue after you graduate? Do you hope to marry? Do you plan to have or adopt children? What things will make you happy and feel "complete"? How do these choices reflect what you hold as your purpose in life? At the end of your days, what things would you want people to say about how you've lived your life and what your life has meant to others? Contemplating these questions fosters spiritual growth. People who are spiritually healthy are able to articulate their purpose, and to make choices that manifest that purpose. In thinking about your own purpose, avoid the temptation to get too ambitious, as in, "I'm here to eradicate world hunger!" Instead, try to articulate just what you see as your unique contribution to the world—something you can actually do, starting now.

Spiritual Intelligence Is an Inner Wisdom

Our relationships, values, and sense of purpose together contribute to our overall **spiritual intelligence (SI).** This term was introduced by physicist and philosopher Danah Zohar, who defined it as "an ability to access higher meanings, values, abiding purposes and unconscious aspects of the self."[10] Zohar includes qualities such as the ability to think outside the box, humility, and an access to energies that come from a source beyond the ego in her definition of *spiritual intelligence,* explaining that SI helps us use meanings, values, and purposes to live a richer and more creative life.

Since Zohar's introduction of SI, dozens of clerics, psychologists, and even business consultants have expanded on the definition. For example, Rabbi Yaacov Kravitz of the Center for Spiritual Intelligence explains that SI helps us find a moral and ethical path to help guide us through life. SI also helps us in the search for meaning and purpose in life. Would you like to find out your own spiritual IQ? See the **Assess Yourself** box on page 70.

The Benefits of Spiritual Health

The importance of the mind–body connection and spiritual health to overall health and wellness has been documented by a broad range of large-scale surveys.[11]

Physical Benefits

The emerging science of mind–body medicine is a research focus of the National Center for Complementary and Alternative Medicine (NCCAM) and an important objective in NCCAM's 2011–2015 Strategic Plan. One area under study is the association between spiritual health and general health. The NCCAM cites evidence that spirituality can have a positive influence on health and suggests that the connection may be due to improved immune function, cardiovascular function, other physiological changes, or a combination of all three. More and more studies are showing that certain spiritual practices, such as yoga, deep meditation, and prayer, can affect the mind, brain,

values Principles that influence our thoughts and emotions and guide the choices we make in our lives.

spiritual intelligence (SI) The ability to access higher meanings, values, abiding purposes, and unconscious aspects of the self, a characteristic that helps each of us find a moral and ethical path to guide us through life.

body, and behavior in ways that have potential to treat many health problems and to promote healthy behavior.[12] Ongoing research is investigating the use of spirituality in treating specific pain conditions, irritable bowel syndrome, insomnia, and more.[13]

Some researchers believe that a key to understanding the improved health and longer life of spiritually healthy people is mindfulness training. In a recent study, participants who practiced mindfulness meditation showed measurable changes in brain regions associated with memory and stress. These changes indicate that they may be more likely to cope better with stress on a daily basis.[14]

The National Cancer Institute (NCI) contends that when we get sick, spiritual or religious well-being may help restore health and improve quality of life in the following ways:[15]

- By decreasing anxiety, depression, anger, discomfort, and feelings of isolation
- By decreasing alcohol and drug abuse
- By decreasing blood pressure and the risk of heart disease
- By increasing the person's ability to cope with the effects of illness and with medical treatments
- By increasing feelings of hope and optimism, freedom from regret, satisfaction with life, and inner peace

Several studies show an association between spiritual health and a person's ability to cope with a variety of physical illnesses as well as with cancer.[16] For example, a study of people living with chronic pain and neurological conditions showed a benefit to using spiritual health and mind–body techniques.[17] Researchers have also looked into the overall association between spiritual practices and mortality, and a review of over a decade of research studies indicated that individuals who incorporate spiritual practices regularly have a significant reduction in mortality and risk of cardiovascular events.[18]

Psychological Benefits

Current research also suggests that spiritual health contributes to psychological health. For instance, the NCI and independent studies have found that spirituality reduces levels of anxiety and depression.[19]

People who have found a spiritual community also benefit from increased social support among members. Participation in religious services, charitable organizations, and social gatherings can help members avoid isolation. At such gatherings, clerics and other members may offer spiritual support for challenges that participants may be facing. Or a community may have retired members who offer child care for harried parents, meals for members with disabilities, or transportation to those needing to get to medical appointments. All such measures can contribute to members' overall feelings of security and belonging.

Benefits from Lowered Stress

The NCI cites stress reduction as one probable mechanism among spiritually healthy people for improved health and longevity and for better coping with illness.[20] In addition, several small studies support the contention that positive religious practices support effective stress management.[21] And a recent study suggests that increasing mindfulness through meditation reduces stress levels not only in people with physical and mental disorders, but also in healthy people.[22]

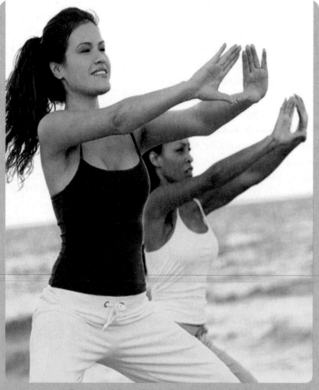

Does spirituality influence health?

Spirituality is widely acknowledged to have a positive impact on health and wellness. The benefits range from reductions in overall morbidity and mortality to improved abilities to cope with illness and stress. These students are using the movement techniques of tai chi to improve their spiritual health.

What Can You Do to Focus on Your Spiritual Health?

Cultivating your spiritual side takes just as much work as becoming physically fit or improving your diet. Ways to develop your spiritual health include training your body, expanding your mind, tuning in, and reaching out.

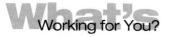
Working for You?

Maybe you're already focusing on enhancing your spiritual health. Do you incorporate any of the following behaviors into your daily life?

☐ I practice yoga.
☐ I meditate.
☐ I do volunteer work.
☐ I maintain healthy relationships.

Train Your Body

For thousands of years, in regions throughout the world, spiritual seekers have cultivated transcendence through physical means. One of the foremost examples is the practice of various forms of **yoga**. Although in the West we think of yoga as involving controlled breathing and physical postures, traditional forms also emphasize meditation, chanting, and other practices that are believed to cultivate unity with the *Atman,* or spiritual life principle of the universe.

If you are interested in exploring yoga, sign up for a class on campus, at your local YMCA, or at a dedicated yoga center. Make sure you choose a form that seems right for you: Some, such as *hatha yoga,* focus on developing flexibility, deep breathing, and tranquility, whereas others, such as *ashtanga yoga,* are fast-paced and demanding, and thus focus more on developing physical fitness. For your first class, dress comfortably in somewhat close fitting, relaxed fabrics so that when you bend at the waist or lift your leg you won't feel constricted or exposed. No shoes or socks are worn. At the beginning of the class, the instructor will likely lead you through some gentle warm-up poses (called *asanas*) and then add more challenging poses with coordinated inhalations and exhalations to align, stretch, and invigorate each region of your body. Most classes provide yoga mats to cushion your joints as you work through the postures. Your class will probably conclude with several minutes of relaxation and deep breathing.

Training your body to improve your spiritual health doesn't necessarily require you to engage in a formal practice such as yoga. By energizing your body and sharpening your mental focus, jogging, biking, aerobics, or any other exercise you do every day can contribute to your spiritual health. The ancient Eastern meditative movement

yoga A system of physical and mental training involving controlled breathing, physical postures *(asanas)*, meditation, chanting, and other practices that are believed to cultivate unity with the *Atman,* or spiritual life principle of the universe.

techniques of tai chi or qigong can also increase physical activity, mental focus, and deep breathing. Both have been shown to have beneficial effects on bone health, cardiopulmonary fitness, balance, and quality of life.[23] To transform an exercise session into a spiritual workout, begin by acknowledging gratitude for your body's strength and speed, then, throughout the session, try to maintain mindfulness of your breathing. We'll say more about mindful breathing in the discussion of meditation below.

You can also cultivate spirituality through fully engaging your body's senses. In fact, you can think of vision, hearing, taste, smell, and touch as five portals to spiritual health. Viewing an engaging piece of artwork or listening to beautiful music can calm the mind and soothe the spirit. The flip side of cultivating your senses is depriving them! Closing your eyes and sitting in silence removes the distraction of visual and auditory stimuli, helping you to focus within. To take advantage of silence, turn off your cell phone and take a long, solitary walk. You might even spend a weekend at one of the many retreat centers throughout the United States. To find one, see the state-by-state listing at www.SpiritSite.com.

Expand Your Mind

For many people, psychological counseling is a first step toward improving spiritual health. Therapy helps you let go of the hurts of the past, accept your limitations, manage stress and anger, reduce anxiety and depression, and take control of your life—all of which are also steps toward spiritual growth. If you've never engaged in therapy, making the first appointment can feel daunting. Your campus health department can usually help by providing a referral.

Yoga incorporates a variety of poses (called *asanas*), from energetic to restful. This yoga student is performing a restful asana known as the *child's pose.*

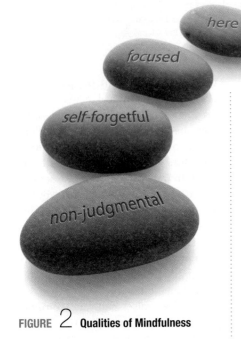

FIGURE 2 Qualities of Mindfulness

Another practical way to expand your mind is to study the sacred texts of the world's major religions and spiritual practices. Many seekers find guidance in the writings of great spiritual teachers. Libraries and bookstores are filled with volumes that explore the diverse approaches humans take to achieve spiritual fulfillment.

Finally, you can expand your awareness of different spiritual practices by exploring on-campus meditation groups, taking classes in spirituality or comparative religions, attending meetings of student organizations where different religious tenets are explored, visiting different religious organizations in your local area and noting what spiritual elements they hold in common, attending public lectures and critically evaluating whether the speakers demonstrate a spiritual bent or reflect bias or exclusion in their lectures, and checking out the official websites of spiritual and religious organizations.

contemplation A practice of concentrating the mind on a spiritual or ethical question or subject, a view of the natural world, or an icon or other image representative of divinity.

mindfulness A practice of purposeful, nonjudgmental observation in which we are fully present in the moment.

Tune in to Yourself and Your Surroundings

Focusing on your spiritual health has been likened to tuning in a radio station: Inner wisdom is perpetually available to us, but if we fail to tune our "receiver," we won't be able to hear it for all the "static" of daily life. Fortunately, four ancient practices still used throughout the world can help you tune in. These are contemplation, mindfulness, meditation, and prayer, which you can think of as studying, observing, quieting, and communing with the Divine.

Contemplation In a dictionary, the word *contemplation* means a study of something—whether a candle flame or a theory of quantum mechanics. In the domain of spirituality, **contemplation** usually refers to a practice of concentrating the mind on a spiritual or ethical question or subject, a view of the natural world, or an icon or other image representative of divinity. For instance, a Zen Buddhist might contemplate a riddle, called a *koan,* such as, what is the sound of one hand clapping? A Sufi might contemplate the 99 names of God. A Roman Catholic might contemplate an image of the Virgin Mary. Spiritual people with no religious affiliation might contemplate the natural world, a favorite poem, or an ethical question such as, what is the origin of

evil? In addition, most religious and spiritual traditions advocate engaging in the contemplation of gratitude, forgiveness, and unconditional love.

When practicing contemplation, it can be helpful to keep a journal to record any insights that arise. In addition, journaling itself can be a form of contemplation. For example, you might want to make a list of 20 things in your life that you are grateful for or write a poem of forgiveness for yourself or a loved one. You might also use your journal to record inspirational quotations that you encounter in your readings.

Mindfulness A practice of focused, nonjudgmental observation, **mindfulness** is the ability to be fully present in the moment (Figure 2). If you have ever been immersed in a moment, experiencing it completely by using all your senses—sight, hearing, taste, smell, touch—this is mindfulness. Examples can be watching the sun set over a mountain, or listening to a great pianist playing Bach, or even performing a challenging calculation in math. In other words, mindfulness is an awareness of present-moment reality—a holistic sensation of being totally involved in the moment rather than being focused on some past worry or being on "automatic pilot."[24]

So how do you practice mindfulness? The range of opportunities is as infinite as the moments of our everyday lives. Living mindfully means to allow ourselves to become more deeply and completely aware of what it is we are sensing in each moment.[25]

Even the most mundane activities—such as peeling an orange—can have spiritual value if done mindfully.

BE HEALTHY, BE GREEN

DEVELOPING ENVIRONMENTAL MINDFULNESS

We know that the Earth's oil reserves won't last forever, yet in 2011, many American automakers saw their biggest sales increases in large pickups and SUVs. We know that beef production releases gobs of greenhouse gases, yet each year Americans consume 26 billion pounds of beef. Why do we make such choices? We want to "go green," so what's in our way?

If the environmental movement seems to be running out of steam, many activists say that it's due to an overemphasis on our external choices, whereas the real challenge is to change our state of mind. They argue that until we confront the mental habits and identities that fuel our consumption patterns, meaningful change won't happen. In short, they advocate mindfulness.

When we pay attention to our thoughts as we make choices, we might notice

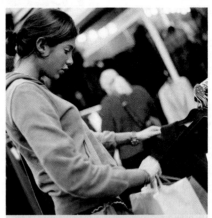

To be mindfully green requires us to ask ourselves some tough questions, such as, what is my fair share? And how much do I really need?

guilt, insecurity, disparagement of ourselves or others, or even righteous claims to entitlement. Only by becoming aware

of these "inner demons" can we begin to take action to expel them.

So how do we cultivate environmental mindfulness? In her book *Mindfully Green*, environmentalist Stephanie Kaza advises us to ask ourselves a set of troubling questions, such as: What do I actually need? What is my fair share? Am I willing to witness suffering? She explains that mindfulness requires us to stay present with our actions moment by moment, always asking, "What is the kind thing to do now?"

Source: D. Drubin and T. Krishner, "SUVs, Trucks Lift Auto Sales," Associated Press, October 3, 2011; Economic Research Service, U.S. Department of Agriculture, "U.S. Beef and Cattle Industry," May 2011, www.ers.usda.gov; E. Nichtern, *The Psychology of Ecology: Exploring the Internal Landscape of Consumption* (Stockbridge, MA: Kripalu Center, 2008); S. Kaza, *Mindfully Green* (Boston, MA: Shambhala Publications, 2008).

For instance, the next time you get ready to eat an orange, pay attention! What does it feel like to pierce the skin with your thumbnail? Do you smell the fragrance of the orange as you peel it? What does the rind really look like? How do the drops of juice splatter as you separate the orange into segments? And finally, what does it taste like, and how does the taste change from the first bite to the last?

Pursuing almost any endeavor that requires close concentration can

help you develop mindfulness. For instance, think of physical and mental challenges, such as a competitive diver leaping from the board or a physician attempting a difficult diagnosis. Or consider creative and performing arts such as sculpting, painting, writing, dancing, or playing a musical instrument. Even household activities such as cooking or cleaning can foster mindfulness—as long as you pay attention while you do them.

In this era of global environmental concerns, we can also cultivate mindfulness by paying attention to how our choices affect our world. This doesn't only mean mindfulness about recycling our soda cans and taking the subway instead of our car. Those are the easy examples. Instead, mindfulness of our environment calls on us to examine our values and behaviors as we share our Earth every moment of each day. The **Be Healthy, Be Green** box will help you begin.

what do you think?

Why do you think mindfulness practices are gaining more recognition?

● What are the benefits of mindfulness?

● In today's fast-paced, multitasking world, do you think it is challenging to practice mindfulness on a regular basis?

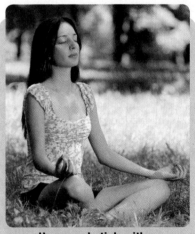

How can I stick with a meditation routine?

Professor Adam Burke, Director of San Francisco State's Institute for Holistic Health Studies, says that the key to sticking with meditation is choosing a technique that you like. He points out that there are a variety of different meditation techniques, and it is important to pick the one that works best for you.

See It! Videos

Is meditation a key to happiness? Watch **Meditating to Happiness** in the Study Area of MasteringHealth™

Meditation *Meditation* is a practice of cultivating a still or quiet mind. Although the precise details vary with different schools of meditation, the fundamental task is the same: to quiet the mind's noise (variously referred to as "chatter," "static," or "monkey mind").

Why would you want to cultivate the stillness of meditation? For thousands of years, human beings of different cultures and traditions have found that achieving periods of meditative stillness each day enhances their spiritual health. Today, researchers are beginning to discover why. The NCCAM reports that researchers using brain-scanning techniques have found that experienced meditators show a significantly increased level of *empathy*, the ability to understand and share another person's experience.[26] Similarly, another recent study found that participants who practiced a specific form of meditation, known as compassion-meditation, increased their levels of compassion toward others.[27]

There are physical benefits, too. Studies suggest that meditation reduces stress, anxiety, and depression.[28] The physiological processes that produce these effects are only partially understood. One theory suggests meditation works by reducing the body's stress response. When under stress, the body reacts by raising heart rate, increasing breaths, and constricting blood vessels. Over the long run, too much stress can lead to both increased wear and tear on the body and a harried, exhausted outlook on life.[29] By practicing deep, calm contemplation, people who meditate seem to promote activity in the body's systems, which leads to slower breathing, lower blood pressure, and easier digestion, along with the spiritual benefits.

So how do you meditate? Detailed instructions are beyond the scope of this text, but most teachers advise beginning by sitting in a quiet place with low lighting where you can be certain you won't be interrupted. Many advocate assuming a "full lotus" position, with both legs bent fully at the knees and each ankle over the opposite knee. However, this position can be painful for beginners, people with poor flexibility, and people with joint pain. Thus, you may want to assume a modified lotus position, in which your legs are simply crossed in front of you. Lying down is not recommended because you may fall asleep. Rest your hands palm upward on your knees. This position uncrosses the two bones of the forearm. Your eyes can be open, half-open, or closed, but if you are a beginner, you may find it easier to meditate with your eyes closed.

Once you're in a position conducive to meditation, it's time to start quieting your mind. Different schools of meditation teach different methods to achieve this.

- **Mantra meditation.** Focus on a *mantra*, a single word such as *Om, Amen, Love,* or *God.* Repeat this word silently to yourself. When a distracting thought arises, simply set it aside. It may help to imagine the thought as a leaf, and mentally let it fall on a gently flowing stream that carries it away. Do not fault yourself for becoming distracted. Simply notice the thought, release it, and return to your mantra.
- **Breath meditation.** Count each breath: Pay attention to each inhalation, the brief pause that follows, and the exhalation. Together, these equal one breath. When you have counted ten breaths, return to one. As with mantra meditation, as distractions arise, release them and return to following the breath.
- **Color meditation.** When your eyes are closed, you may perceive a field of color, such as a deep, restful blue. Focus on this color. Treat distractions as in the other forms of meditation.

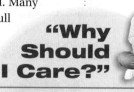

"Why Should I Care?"

Practicing meditation can improve your brain's ability to process information, reduce your stress level, and improve your sleep, all important factors when trying to manage your classes and handle daily demands.

- **Candle meditation.** With your eyes open, focus on the flame of a candle. Allow your eyes to soften as you meditate on this object. Treat distractions as in the other forms of meditation.

After several minutes of meditation, and with practice, you may come to experience a sensation sometimes described as "dropping down," in which you feel yourself release into the meditation. In this state, which can be likened to a wakeful sleep, distracting thoughts are far less likely to arise, and yet you may suddenly receive surprising insights.

When you're beginning, try meditating for 10 to 20 minutes a session, once or twice a day. In time, you can increase your sessions to 30 minutes or more. As you meditate for longer periods, you will likely find yourself feeling more rested and less stressed throughout your day, and you may begin to experience the increased levels of empathy reported among expert meditators.

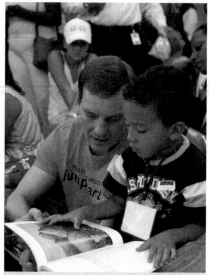

Volunteering can be a fun and fulfilling way to broaden your experience, connect with your community, and focus on your spiritual health.

26%

of young adults under the age of 30 reported that they meditate at least once a week.

Prayer

In **prayer,** an individual focuses the mind in communication with a transcendent Presence. Spiritual traditions throughout the world distinguish several forms that this communication can take. For many, prayer offers a sense of comfort; a sense that we are not alone; and an avenue for expressing concern for others, for admission of transgressions, for seeking forgiveness, and for renewing hope and purpose. Focusing on the things we can be grateful for in life can move people to look to the future with hope and give them the strength to get through the most challenging times.

Reach Out to Others

Altruism, the giving of oneself out of genuine concern for others, is a key

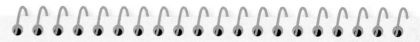

Finding Your Spiritual Side through Service

Recognizing that we are all part of a greater system and that we have responsibilities to and for others is a key part of spiritual growth. Volunteering your time and energy is a great way to connect with others and help make the world a better place while improving your own health. Here are a few ideas:

❭ Offer to help elderly neighbors by providing lawn care or helping with simple household repairs.

❭ Volunteer with Meals on Wheels, a local soup kitchen, food bank, or other program that helps neighbors obtain adequate food.

❭ Organize or participate in an after-school or summertime activity for neighborhood children.

❭ Participate in a highway, beach, or neighborhood cleanup; restoration of park trails and waterways; or other environmental preservation projects.

❭ Volunteer at the local humane society walking dogs, caring for cats, helping with cleaning, or raising money for shelter programs.

❭ Become a Big Brother or Big Sister and mentor a child who may face significant challenges or have poor role models.

❭ Join an organization working on a cause such as global warming or hunger, or start one yourself.

❭ Spend time volunteering in a neighborhood challenged by poverty, low literacy levels, or a natural disaster. Or volunteer with an organization such as Habitat for Humanity to build homes or provide other aid to developing communities.

aspect of a spiritually healthy lifestyle. Volunteering to help others, working for a nonprofit organization, donating money or other resources to a food bank or other program—even spending an afternoon picking up litter in your neighborhood—are all ways to serve others and simultaneously enhance your own spiritual and overall health. Researchers have referred to the benefits of volunteering as a "helpers high," or a distinct physical sensation associated with helping. About half of participants in one study reported that they

feel stronger and more energetic after helping others; many also reported feeling calmer and less depressed, with increased feelings of self-worth.[30]

Community service can also take the form of **environmental stewardship,** which the Environmental Protection Agency (EPA) defines as the responsibility for environmental quality shared by all those whose actions affect the environment. Responsibility manifests in action. Simple actions such as reducing and recycling packaging, turning off lights, making sure the heat or air-conditioning maintains an ecofriendly temperature, using energy-efficient lightbulbs and appliances, and taking shorter showers can make a difference.

For more strategies to enhance your spiritual health, refer to the **Skills for Behavior Change** box.

prayer Communication with a transcendent Presence.

altruism The giving of oneself out of genuine concern for others.

environmental stewardship Responsibility for environmental quality shared by all those whose actions affect the environment.

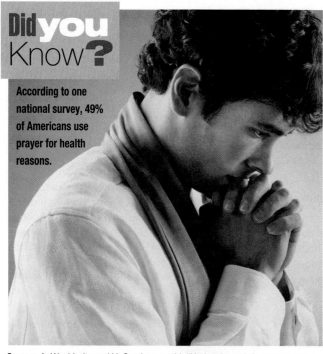

Did you Know?

According to one national survey, 49% of Americans use prayer for health reasons.

Source: A. Wachholtz and U. Sambamoorthi, "National trends in prayer use as a coping mechanism for health concerns: Changes from 2002 to 2007," *Psychology of Religion and Spirituality* 3, no. 2 (2011): 67, doi 10.1037/a0021598.

Assess yourself

What's Your Spiritual IQ?

Many tools are available for assessing your spiritual intelligence. Although each differs significantly according to its target audience (therapy clients, business executives, church members, etc.), most share certain underlying principles reflected in the questionnaire below. Answer each question as follows:

0 = not at all true for me
1 = somewhat true for me
2 = very true for me

_____ 1. I frequently feel gratitude for the many blessings of my life.

_____ 2. I am often moved by the beauty of Earth, music, poetry, or other aspects of my daily life.

_____ 3. I readily express forgiveness toward those whose missteps have affected me.

_____ 4. I recognize in others qualities that are more important than their appearance and behaviors.

_____ 5. When I do poorly on an exam, lose an important game, or am rejected in a relationship, I am able to know that the experience does not define who I am.

_____ 6. When fear arises, I am able to know that I am eternally safe and loved.

_____ 7. I meditate or pray daily.

_____ 8. I frequently and fearlessly ponder the possibility of an afterlife.

_____ 9. I accept total responsibility for the choices that I have made in building my life.

_____ 10. I feel that I am on Earth for a unique and sacred reason.

Scoring

The higher your score on this quiz, the higher your spiritual intelligence. To improve your score, apply the suggestions for spiritual practices from this chapter.

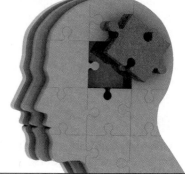

YOUR PLAN FOR CHANGE

The **Assess yourself** activity gave you the chance to evaluate your spiritual intelligence, and the chapter introduced you to practices used successfully by millions of people over many generations to enhance their spiritual health. If you are interested in cultivating your own spirituality further, consider taking some of the small but significant steps listed below.

Today, you can:

◯ Find a quiet spot; turn off your cell phone; close your eyes; and contemplate, meditate, or pray for 10 minutes. Or spend 10 minutes in quiet mindfulness of your surroundings.

◯ In a journal or on your computer, begin a numbered list of things you are grateful for. Today, list at least ten things. Include people, pets, talents and abilities, achievements, favorite places, foods … whatever comes to mind!

Within the next 2 weeks, you can:

◯ Explore the options on campus for beginning psychotherapy, joining a spiritual or religious student group, or volunteering with a student organization working for positive change.

◯ Think of a person in your life with whom you have experienced conflict. Spend a few minutes contemplating forgiveness toward this person and then write him or her an e-mail or letter apologizing for any offense you may have given and offering your forgiveness in return. Wait for a day or two before deciding whether you are truly ready to send the message.

By the end of the semester, you can:

◯ Develop a list of several spiritual texts that you would like to read during your break.

◯ Begin exploring options for volunteer work next summer.

Managing Stress and Coping with Life's Challenges

3

LEARNING OUTCOMES

* Define *stress* and examine its potential impact on health, relationships, and success in college and life.

* Explain the phases of the general adaptation syndrome and the physiological changes that occur during them.

* Examine the physical and psychological health risks that may occur with chronic stress.

* Examine the intellectual health risks that may occur due to high levels of stress.

* Discuss sources of stress and examine the unique stressors that affect college students.

* Explore stress-management and stress reduction strategies, ways you can cope more effectively with stress, and ways you can enrich your life experiences to protect against the effects of stress.

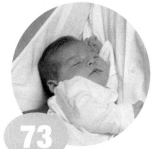

73
Isn't some stress healthy?

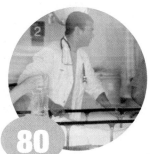

80
Who is most prone to stress?

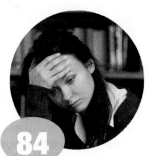

84
Are college students more stressed out than other groups?

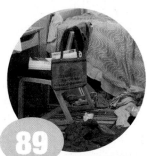

89
Can reducing clutter help me de-stress in college?

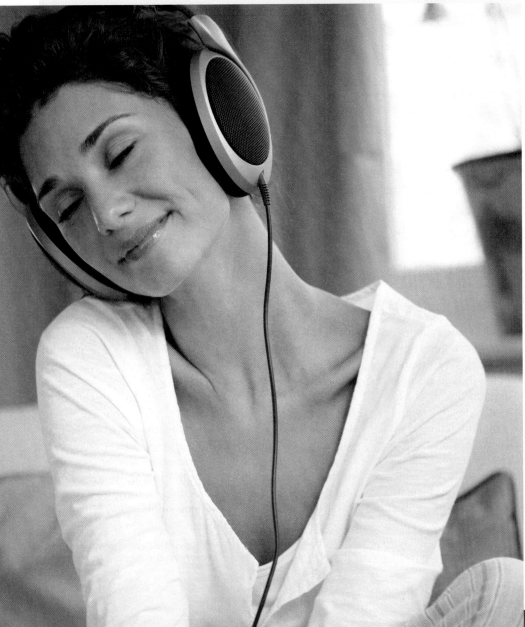

Skyrocketing tuition, roommates and friends who bug you, anxiety over fitting in, dating, pressure to get good grades, money, and worries about getting a job after graduation—they all lead to STRESS! In today's fast-paced, 24/7-connected world, stress can cause us to feel overwhelmed and zap our energy. It can also cause us to push ourselves to improve performance, bring excitement, and help us thrive.

According to a recent American Psychological Association study, chronic stress that interferes with our ability to function normally over an extended period has become a public health crisis, particularly among caregivers and people living with a chronic illness such as obesity or depression. Key findings from the study indicate the following[1]:

- Although reported stress levels are down slightly in the last 5 years, Americans consistently report high stress levels (22% report extreme stress).
- Adults ages 18–46 report the highest levels of stress and the greatest increases in stress levels.
- Biggest sources of stress for adults ages 18–32 are money (80%), work (72%), and housing costs (49%). Individuals aged 66 and older were more likely to cite their families' health problems as a key source of stress (63%).

Huge gender differences exist in how men and women experience and cope with stress, with women being more vulnerable to negative effects of stress. Although men may recognize and report stress, they are much less likely to take action to reduce it.)[2]

Stress levels have increased

10% to 30%

since 1983.

The exact toll stress exerts on us during a lifetime is unknown, but we know stress is a significant health hazard. It can rob the body of needed nutrients, damage the cardiovascular system, raise blood pressure, increase our risks for cancer and diabetes, and dampen the immune system's defenses. In addition, it can drain our emotional reserves and contribute to depression, anxiety, fatigue, and irritability, impacting relationships with friends, family, and coworkers. It can also leave us sleep deprived and functioning at a fraction of our normal capacity. Importantly, research indicates that being "stressed out" can take a major toll among even the young, with youth suffering from stress-related headaches, stomachaches, difficulty sleeping, or other illnesses at increasing rates. Stress seems to be a particular threat to youth who are overweight. The higher the stress, the greater the chances of overeating,

stress A series of mental and physiological responses and adaptations to a real or perceived threat to one's well-being.

stressor A physical, social, or psychological event or condition that upsets homeostasis and produces a stress response.

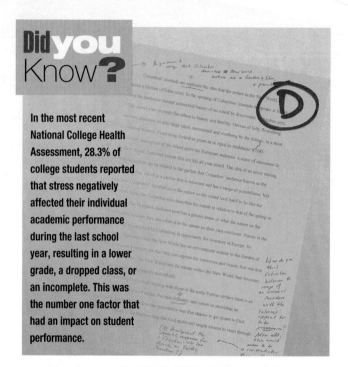

Source: Data from American College Health Association, *American College Health Association—National College Health Assessment II, Reference Group Report, Fall 2012* (Hanover, MD: American College Health Association, 2013).

sleeping too much, and too much television, which in turn contributes to weight gain and more stress.[3]

Is too much stress inevitably negative? Fortunately, the answer is no. How we react to real and perceived threats often is key to whether stressors are enabling or debilitating. Learning to assess our perceptions and to anticipate, avoid, and develop skills to reduce or better manage those stressors is key. First, we must understand what stress is.

What Is Stress?

Most current definitions state that **stress** is the mental and physical response and adaptation by our bodies to real or perceived change and challenges. A **stressor** is any real or perceived physical, social, or psychological event or stimulus that causes our bodies to react or respond.[4] Several factors influence one's response to stressors, including *characteristics of the stressor* (How traumatic is it? Can you control it? Does it occur often?); *biological factors* (e.g., your age or gender); and *past experiences* (e.g., things that have happened to you, their consequences, and your response). Stressors may be *tangible*, such as a failing grade on a test, or *intangible*, such as the angst associated with meeting your significant other's parents for the first time. Importantly, stress is in the eye of the beholder: Your unique combination of heredity, life experiences, personality, and ability to cope influence your perceptions and the meaning you attach to them. What "stresses you out" may not even bother others.

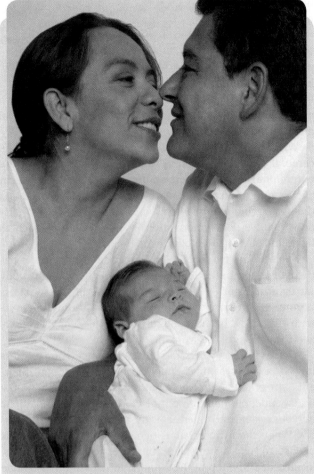

Isn't some stress healthy?

Stress isn't necessarily bad for you. Events that cause eustress, such as the birth of a child, can have positive effects on your growth and well-being.

with wild, acute stress. Individuals experiencing episodic acute stress may be "repeaters" and talk continually about stressors. They may be worrywarts who see the world not as a place of "what is," but rather as one of "what-ifs" where bad things are always lurking. These "awfulizers" are often reactive and anxious, but these patterns can be so habitual, they don't realize that there is anything wrong. Acute and episodic acute stress both can cause physical and emotional problems. But **chronic stress,** which may not appear as intense but can linger indefinitely, wreaks silent havoc on your body systems. Losing your mother after her long battle with breast cancer can cause the stress response to reverberate in you for months after her death, causing you to struggle to balance emotions such as anger, grief, loneliness, and guilt while trying to keep up with classes and life. Another type of stress, **traumatic stress,** is experienced when events such as major accidents, war, shootings, assault, or natural disasters occur and you may be hurt or witness horrible things. Effects of traumatic stress may be felt for years after the event and cause significant disability, which may lead to post-traumatic stress disorder or PTSD (see **Chapter 2** for a discussion of PTSD).[6]

eustress Stress that presents opportunities for personal growth; positive stress.

distress Stress that can have a detrimental effect on health; negative stress.

acute stress The short-term physiological response to an immediate perceived threat.

episodic acute stress The state of regularly reacting with wild, acute stress about one thing or another.

chronic stress An ongoing state of physiological arousal in response to ongoing or numerous perceived threats.

traumatic stress A physiological and mental response that occurs for a prolonged period of time after a major accident, war, assault, natural disaster, or an event in which one may be seriously hurt, killed, or witness horrible things.

homeostasis A balanced physiological state in which all the body's systems function smoothly.

adaptive response The physiological adjustments the body makes in an attempt to restore homeostasis.

Generally, positive stress is called **eustress.** Eustress presents the opportunity for personal growth and satisfaction and can actually improve health. It can energize you, motivate you, and raise you up when you are down. Getting married or winning a major competition can give rise to the pleasurable rush associated with eustress.

Distress, or negative stress, is caused by events that result in debilitative tension and strain, such as financial problems, the death of a loved one, academic difficulties, or ending a relationship.

There are several kinds of distress. The most common type, **acute stress,** comes from demands and pressures of the recent past and anticipated demands and pressures of the near future.[5] Usually, acute stress is intense, lasts for a short time, and disappears quickly without permanent damage to your health. A major class presentation or meeting the person you've been chatting with online for the first time could cause trembling, nausea, headache, cramping, or diarrhea, along with a galloping heartbeat. A second type of stress is **episodic acute stress,** which describes the state of regularly reacting

Your Body's Stress Response

The body's physiological responses to stressors evolved to protect humans from harm. Thousands of years ago, if you didn't respond by fighting or fleeing, you might have been eaten by a saber-toothed tiger or killed by a marauding enemy clan. Today, these same responses must be managed rather than causing us to lash out at others. Continually having to "stuff" our reactions rather than letting our physiological responses run their course can harm our health over time.

The General Adaptation Syndrome

When stress levels are low, the body is often in a state of **homeostasis** or balance; all body systems are operating smoothly to maintain equilibrium. Stressors trigger a crisis-mode physiological response, after which the body attempts to return to homeostasis by means of an **adaptive response.** First characterized by Hans Selye in 1936, the

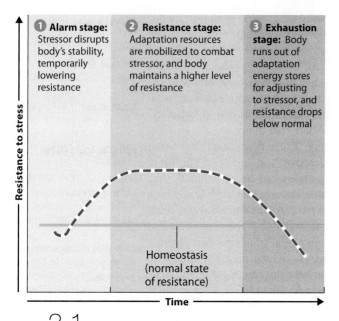

Hear It! Podcasts

Want a study podcast for this chapter? Download the podcast **Managing Stress: Coping with Life's Challenges** in the Study Area of MasteringHealth™

1 Alarm stage: Stressor disrupts body's stability, temporarily lowering resistance

2 Resistance stage: Adaptation resources are mobilized to combat stressor, and body maintains a higher level of resistance

3 Exhaustion stage: Body runs out of adaptation energy stores for adjusting to stressor, and resistance drops below normal

Resistance to stress

Homeostasis (normal state of resistance)

Time

FIGURE 3.1 **The General Adaptation Syndrome (GAS)**
The GAS describes the body's method of coping with prolonged stress.

internal fight to restore homeostasis in the face of a stressor is known as the **general adaptation syndrome (GAS)** (Figure 3.1). The GAS has three distinct phases: alarm, resistance, and exhaustion.[7]

general adaptation syndrome (GAS) The pattern followed in the physiological response to stress, consisting of the alarm, resistance, and exhaustion phases.

fight-or-flight response Physiological arousal response in which the body prepares to combat or escape a real or perceived threat.

autonomic nervous system (ANS) The portion of the central nervous system that regulates body functions that a person does not normally consciously control.

sympathetic nervous system Branch of the autonomic nervous system responsible for stress arousal.

parasympathetic nervous system Branch of the autonomic nervous system responsible for slowing systems stimulated by the stress response.

hypothalamus A structure in the brain that controls the sympathetic nervous system and directs the stress response.

epinephrine Also called *adrenaline*, a hormone that stimulates body systems in response to stress.

cortisol Hormone released by the adrenal glands that makes stored nutrients more readily available to meet energy demands.

Regardless of whether you are experiencing distress or eustress, similar physiological changes will occur in your body. In addition, the GAS can occur in varying degrees of intensity, last varying amounts of time, and be experienced differently by different individuals.

Alarm Phase Suppose you are walking to your residence hall after a night class on a dimly lit campus. As you pass a particularly dark area, you hear a cough and feel someone approaching rapidly behind you. You walk faster, only to hear the quickened footsteps of the other person. Your senses become increasingly alert, your breathing quickens, your heart races, and you begin to perspire. In desperation you wheel around and let out a blood-curdling yell. To your surprise, the only person you see is a classmate: She has been trying to stay close to you out of her own anxiety about walking alone in the dark. She screams and jumps backward, and you

both burst out laughing in startled embarrassment. You have just experienced the alarm phase of GAS. Also known as the **fight-or-flight response,** this physiological reaction is one of our most basic, innate survival instincts[8] (see Figure 3.2 on page 75).

When the mind perceives a real or imaginary stressor, the cerebral cortex, the region of the brain that interprets the nature of an event, triggers an **autonomic nervous system (ANS)** response that prepares the body for action. The ANS is the portion of the nervous system that regulates body functions that we do not normally consciously control, such as heart and glandular functions and breathing.

The ANS has two branches: sympathetic and parasympathetic. The **sympathetic nervous system** energizes the body for fight or flight by signaling the release of several stress hormones. The **parasympathetic nervous system** slows systems stimulated by the stress response—in effect, it counteracts the actions of the sympathetic branch.

The responses of the sympathetic nervous system to stress involve a series of biochemical exchanges between different parts of the body. The **hypothalamus,** a structure in the brain, functions as the control center of the sympathetic nervous system and determines the overall reaction to stressors. When the hypothalamus perceives that extra energy is needed to fight a stressor, it stimulates the adrenal glands, located near the top of the kidneys, to release the hormone **epinephrine,** also called *adrenaline.* Epinephrine causes more blood to be pumped with each beat of the heart, dilates the airways in the lungs to increase oxygen intake, increases the breathing rate, stimulates the liver to release more glucose (which fuels muscular exertion), and dilates the pupils to improve visual sensitivity. It revs the body for action.

In addition to the fight-or-flight response, the alarm phase can trigger a longer-term reaction to stress. The hypothalamus uses chemical messages to trigger the pituitary gland within the brain to release a powerful hormone, *adrenocorticotropic hormone (ACTH).* ACTH signals the adrenal glands to release **cortisol,** a hormone that makes stored nutrients more readily available to meet energy demands. Finally, other parts of the brain and body release *endorphins,* which relieve pain that a stressor may cause.

Resistance Phase In the resistance phase of the GAS, the body tries to return to homeostasis by resisting the alarm responses. However, because some perceived stressor still exists, the body does not achieve complete calm or rest. Instead, the body stays activated or aroused at a level that causes a higher metabolic rate in some organ tissues. For example, you get a lockdown alert because a shooter is on campus, and your fear response triggers an acute alarm reaction. As you hear that the shooter has been subdued, you may calm down a bit, but your body may not return to normal until the all clear has sounded and you are safe at home.

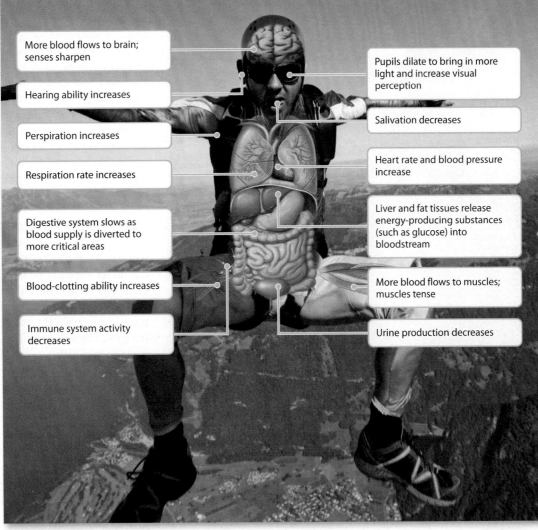

Labels on figure:

More blood flows to brain; senses sharpen

Hearing ability increases

Perspiration increases

Respiration rate increases

Digestive system slows as blood supply is diverted to more critical areas

Blood-clotting ability increases

Immune system activity decreases

Pupils dilate to bring in more light and increase visual perception

Salivation decreases

Heart rate and blood pressure increase

Liver and fat tissues release energy-producing substances (such as glucose) into bloodstream

More blood flows to muscles; muscles tense

Urine production decreases

FIGURE 3.2 **The Body's Acute Stress Response**
Exposure to stress of any kind causes a complex series of involuntary physiological responses.

Video Tutor: Body's Stress Response

Exhaustion Phase A prolonged effort to adapt to an acute, episodic, or chronic stress response leads to **allostatic load,** or exhaustive wear and tear on the body. In the exhaustion phase of GAS, the physical and emotional energy used to fight a stressor has been depleted. You may feel tired or drained. When stress is chronic or unresolved, the body typically begins to adjust by prompting the adrenal glands to continue releasing cortisol and other stress hormones, which remain in the bloodstream, keeping you wired for longer periods of time as a result of slower metabolic responsiveness. Over time, excessive cortisol can reduce **immunocompetence,** or the ability of the immune system to protect you from infectious diseases and other threats to health.[9]

allostatic load Wear and tear on the body caused by prolonged or excessive stress responses.

immunocompetence The ability of the immune system to respond to attack.

50% of older U.S. men who have had moderate to high levels of stress in their lives over the years have an **increased risk of death.**

Lifetime Effects of Stress

Stress is often described as a "disease of prolonged arousal" that leads to a cascade of negative health effects. The longer you are chronically stressed, the more likely there will be

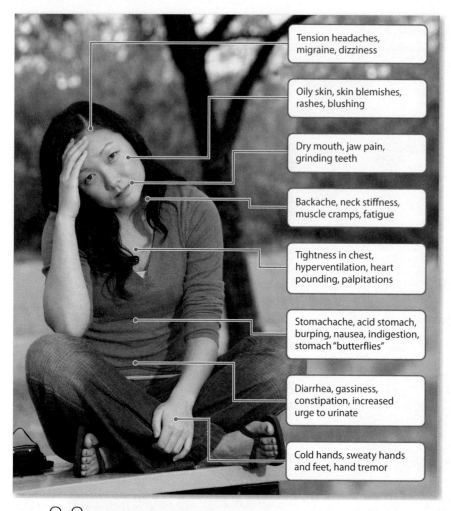

FIGURE 3.3 **Common Physical Symptoms of Stress**
Sometimes you may not even notice how stressed you are until your body starts sending you signals. Do you frequently experience any of these physical symptoms of stress?

Labels on figure:
- Tension headaches, migraine, dizziness
- Oily skin, skin blemishes, rashes, blushing
- Dry mouth, jaw pain, grinding teeth
- Backache, neck stiffness, muscle cramps, fatigue
- Tightness in chest, hyperventilation, heart pounding, palpitations
- Stomachache, acid stomach, burping, nausea, indigestion, stomach "butterflies"
- Diarrhea, gassiness, constipation, increased urge to urinate
- Cold hands, sweaty hands and feet, hand tremor

negative health effects. Look at the stress symptoms shown in **Figure 3.3**.

Physical Effects of Stress

The higher the levels of stress you experience and the longer that stress continues, the greater the likelihood of damage to your physical health.[10] In addition to the physical disease threats we've discussed, increases in rates of suicide, homicide, hate crimes, alcohol and drug abuse, and domestic violence are symptoms of a nation that is chronically stressed.

Stress and Cardiovascular Disease Perhaps the most studied and documented health consequence of unresolved stress is cardiovascular disease (CVD). Research on CVD demonstrates the impact of chronic stress on heart rate, blood pressure, heart attack, and stroke.[11]

Historically, the increased risk of CVD from chronic stress has been linked to increased arterial plaque buildup due to elevated cholesterol, hardening of the arteries, increases in inflammatory responses in the body, alterations in heart rhythm, increased and fluctuating blood pressures, and difficulties in cardiovascular responsiveness due to all of the above.[12] In the past two decades, research into the relationship between stress and CVD contributors has shown direct links between the incidence and progression of CVD and stressors such as job strain, caregiving, bereavement, and natural disasters.[13] (For more information about CVD, see **Chapter 12**.)

Stress and Weight Gain Are you a *"stress"* or *"emotional eater"*? Do you run for the refrigerator when you are under pressure or feeling anxious or down? If you think that when you are extremely stressed, you tend to eat more and gain weight, you didn't imagine it. We comfort ourselves with things we love; hence that bag of chips or ice cream sundae may be just the thing to distract us. But there is more to stress eating than soothing our emotions.

Higher stress levels may drive us toward food because they may increase cortisol levels in the bloodstream. Because cortisol contributes to increased hunger and seems to activate fat-storing enzymes, people who are stressed may get a double whammy of risks from higher-circulating cortisol levels. High cortisol may also increase cravings for salty and sweet foods. Animal and human studies, including those in which subjects suffer from post-traumatic stress, seem to support the theory that cortisol plays a role in laying down extra belly fat and increasing eating behaviors.[14]

Stress and Alcohol Dependence New research has found that a specific stress hormone, the *corticotropin-releasing factor (CRF)*, is key to the development and maintenance of alcohol dependence in animals. CRF is a natural substance involved in the body's stress response, stimulating the secretion of various stress hormones. If proven to be true in humans, options for dealing with stress and alcohol may increase dramatically.[15]

Stress and Hair Loss Too much stress can lead to thinning hair, and even baldness, in men and women. The most common type of stress-induced hair loss is *telogen effluvium*. Often seen in individuals who have lost a loved one or experienced severe weight loss or other trauma, this condition pushes colonies of hair into a resting phase. Over time, hair begins to fall out. A similar stress-related condition known as *alopecia areata* occurs when stress triggers white blood cells to attack and destroy hair follicles, usually in patches.[16]

Stress and Diabetes Controlling stress levels is critical for preventing weight gain and other risk factors for type 2 diabetes, as well as for successful short- and long-term diabetes management.[17] People under lots of stress often don't get enough sleep, don't eat well, and may drink or take other drugs to help them get through a stressful time. All of these behaviors can alter blood sugar levels and promote development of diabetes. (For full information on diabetes, see **Focus On: Minimizing Your Risk for Diabetes** beginning on page 386.)

Stress and Digestive Problems Digestive disorders are physical conditions for which the causes are often unknown. It is widely assumed that an underlying illness, pathogen, injury, or inflammation is already present when stress triggers nausea, vomiting, stomach cramps and gut pain, or diarrhea. Although stress doesn't directly cause these symptoms, it is clearly related and may actually make your risk of having symptoms worse.[18] For example, people with depression or anxiety, or who feel tense, angry, or overwhelmed, are more susceptible to dehydration, inflammation, and other digestive problems. Irritable bowel syndrome may be more likely, in part, because stress stimulates colon spasms by means of the nervous system. Some relaxation techniques and mindfulness training (found later in this chapter) may be helpful in coping with stressors that irritate your digestive system. These relaxation techniques reduce the activity of the sympathetic nervous system, leading to decreases in heart rate, blood pressure, and other stress responses. They also appear to reduce gastrointestinal reactivity and decrease your risks of gastrointestinal tract flare-ups.[19]

Stress and Impaired Immunity A growing area of scientific investigation known as **psychoneuroimmunology (PNI)** analyzes the intricate relationship between the mind's response to stress and the immune system's ability to function effectively. (We also discussed PNI in **Chapter 2.**) Several recent reviews of research linking stress to adverse health consequences suggest that too much stress over a long period can negatively affect various aspects of the cellular immune response. This increases risks for upper respiratory infections and certain chronic conditions, increases adverse fetal development and birth outcomes, and exacerbates problems for children and adults suffering from post-traumatic stress.[20] More prolonged stressors, such as the loss of a loved one, caregiving, living with a handicap, and unemployment, also have been shown to impair the natural immune response among various populations over time.[21]

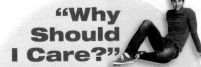
Intellectual Effects of Stress

In a recent national survey of college students, more than half of the respondents said that they had felt overwhelmed by all that they had to do within the past 2 weeks, 48.3 percent reported being exhausted, and 19.2 percent felt overwhelmed by anxiety in the same time period. About 37 percent of students felt they had been under more-than-average stress in the past 12 months, whereas over 10 percent reported being under tremendous stress during that same time period. Not surprisingly, these same students rated stress as their number one impediment to academic performance, followed by lack of sleep and anxiety.[22] Stress can play a huge role in whether students stay in school, get good grades, and succeed on their career path. It can also wreak havoc on students' ability to concentrate, affect memory, and decrease ability to understand and retain information.

Stress, Memory, and Concentration Although the exact reasons stress can affect grades and job performance are complex, new research has provided possible clues. Animal studies have provided compelling indicators of how glucocorticoids—stress hormones released from the adrenal cortex—are believed to affect memory. In humans, acute stress has been shown to impair short-term memory, particularly verbal memory.[23] Recent laboratory studies with rats have linked prolonged exposure to cortisol (a key stress hormone) to actual shrinking of the hippocampus, the brain's major memory center.[24]

psychoneuroimmunology (PNI) The study of the interrelationship between mind and body, and on immune system functioning.

Psychological Effects of Stress

Stress may be one of the single greatest contributors to mental disability and emotional dysfunction in industrialized nations. Studies have shown that the rates of mental disorders, particularly depression and anxiety, are associated with various environmental stressors.[25] College students not only face pressure to get good grades, they also face additional new stressors stemming from housing searches, becoming financially independent, career choices and employment (or the lack thereof), relationships, interactions with family and peers, and perceived environmental threats. Coping skills and social support from family, friends, and community services can buffer the negative effects of stress overload.[26]

See It! Videos

Can a test identify your risk for stress-related illnesses? Watch **Stress Can Damage Women's Health** in the Study Area of MasteringHealth™

What Causes Stress?

On any given day, we all experience eustress and distress, usually from a wide range of sources. One of the most comprehensive studies examining sources of stress among various populations is conducted annually by the American Psychological Association (Figure 3.4). The 2012 survey found that concerns over money, work, the economy, and relationships were the biggest reported causes of stress for Americans.[27] College students, in particular, face stressors that come from internal sources, as well as external pressures to succeed in a competitive environment. Awareness of the sources of stress can do much to help you develop a plan to avoid, prevent, or control the things that cause you stress.

Psychosocial Stressors

Psychosocial stressors refer to the factors in our daily routines and in our social and physical environments that cause us to experience stress. Key psychosocial stressors include adjustment to change, hassles, interpersonal relationships, academic and career pressures, frustrations and conflicts, overload, and stressful environments.

Adjustment to Change Anytime change, whether good or bad, occurs in your normal routine, you experience stress. The more changes you experience and the more adjustments you must make, the greater the chances are that stress will have an impact on your health. Unfortunately, although your first days on campus can be exciting, they can also be among the most stressful you will face in your life. Moving away from home, trying to fit in and make new friends from diverse backgrounds, adjusting to a new schedule, and learning to live with strangers in housing that is often lacking in the comforts of home can all cause sleeplessness and anxiety and keep your body in a continual fight-or-flight mode.

Hassles: Little Things That Bug You Some psychologists have proposed that the little stressors, frustrations, and petty annoyances, known

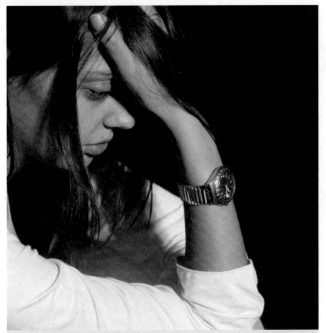

Stress and depression have complicated interconnections based on emotional, physiological, and biochemical processes. Prolonged stress can trigger depression in susceptible people, and prior periods of depression can leave individuals more susceptible to stress.

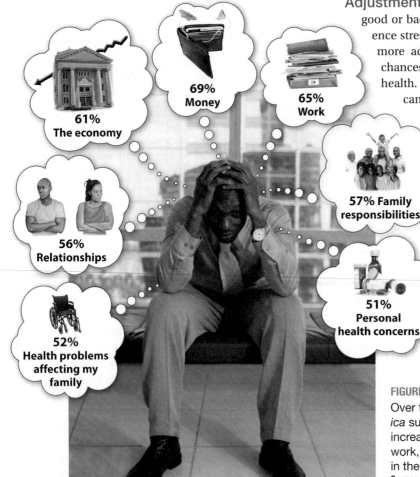

61% The economy

69% Money

65% Work

57% Family responsibilities

56% Relationships

51% Personal health concerns

52% Health problems affecting my family

FIGURE 3.4 **What Do We Say Stresses Us?**
Over the past few years, the annual *Stress in America* survey has indicated that American adults are increasingly experiencing concerns over money, work, and the economy as major sources of stress in their lives.
Source: Data from American Psychological Association, *2012 Stress in America, Key Findings,* 2013, www.apa.org

Tech & Health

TAMING TECHNOSTRESS AND iDISORDERS

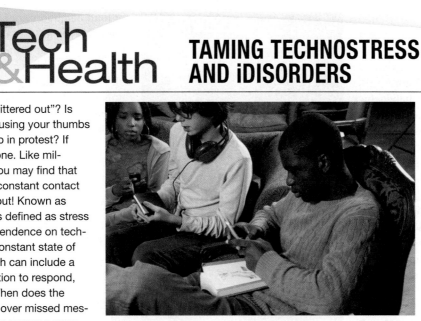

Technology may keep you in touch, but it can also add to your stress and take you away from real-world interactions.

Are you "twittered out"? Is texting causing your thumbs to seize up in protest? If so, you're not alone. Like millions of others, you may find that the pressure for constant contact is stressing you out! Known as *technostress*, it is defined as stress created by a dependence on technology and the constant state of connection, which can include a perceived obligation to respond, chat, or tweet. When does the constant anxiety over missed messages or an online persona cross the stress load limit?

An increasing number of people would rather hang out online talking to strangers than study, socialize in person, or connect in the real world. There are some clear downsides to all of that virtual interaction.

✴ **Social distress.** Authors Michelle Weil and Larry Rosen describe *technosis,* a very real syndrome in which people become so immersed in technology that they risk losing their own identity. Worrying about checking your e-mail or text messages, constantly switching to Facebook to see updates, perpetually posting to Twitter, and so on can keep you distracted and waste hours of every day.

✴ **Technology dependency.** Increasing research supports the concept that feeling the need to be "wired" 24/7 (while eating, studying, hanging out with friends, in the car, and in nearly every place imaginable) can lead to anxiety, obsessive compulsive disorder, narcissism, sleep disorders, frustration, time pressures, and guilt—some of the negative consequences known as *iDisorders*. When you are more worried about your friends' list on a social media site than you are about spending the time to make real friends, it may be time to rethink your social interactions.

To avoid iDisorders caused by technology overload or technostress, set time limits on your technology usage, and make sure that you devote at least as much time to face-to-face interactions with people you care about. Remember that you don't always need to answer your phone or respond to a text or e-mail immediately.

Make a rule that you cannot turn on your device when out with friends or on vacation. *Tune in* to your surroundings, your loved ones and friends, your job, and your classes by shutting off your devices.

Sources: M. Weil and L. Rosen, *Technostress: Coping with Technology @Work, @Home, @Play* (Hoboken: John Wiley & Sons, 1997); L. D. Rosen et al., "Is Facebook Creating "iDisorders"? The Link Between Clinical Symptoms of Psychiatric Disorders and Technology Use, Attitudes and Anxiety," *Computers in Human Behavior*, in press, http://dx.doi.org/10.1016/j.chb.2012.11.012; National Safety Council, "National Safety Council Estimates That at Least 1.6 Million Crashes Are Caused Each Year by Drivers Using Cell Phones and Texting," press release, January 12, 2010, www.nsc.org; National Highway Traffic Safety Administration, "Blueprint for Ending Distracted Driving," 2012, www.nhtsa.gov

collectively as *hassles,* can add up and be just as stressful as major life changes.[28] Put another way, cumulative hassles add up. They tax the physiological systems of the body and cause stress-related wear and tear, known as an *allostatic load,* on the body. Listening to others monopolize class time, not finding parking on campus, continual drops on your cell phone connections, and a host of other irritants can push your buttons and trigger an acute fight-or-flight response.[29] For many people, electronic devices that are supposed to be fun can cause anxiety and zap time. See the **Tech & Health** box for more on technostress.

The Toll of Relationships Let's face it, relationships can trigger some of the biggest fight-or-flight reactions of all time. Although romantic relationships are the ones we often think of first—the wild, exhilarating feeling of new love and the excruciating pain of breakups—relationships with friends, family, and coworkers can be sources of struggles, just as they can be sources of support. These relationships can make us strive to be the best that we can be and give us hope for the future, or they can diminish our self-esteem and leave us reeling from destructive interactions. A recent comparison of nearly 80 studies of stress and work provides strong evidence that work situations with high demands, little control, and coworkers who are difficult to get along with increase the likelihood of employee complaints about gastrointestinal ailments and sleep difficulties. Competition for rewards and systems that favor certain classes of employees or pit workers against one another are among the most stressful job situations.[30]

Academic and Financial Pressure It isn't surprising that today's college and university students face mind-boggling amounts of pressure while competing for grades, internships, athletic positions, and jobs. Challenging classes can be tough enough, but many students must juggle studies with work to pay the bills, and an economic downturn can make student dreams seem unobtainable. (For tips on how to head off some financial stressors before they start, see **Focus On: Improving Your Financial Health** on page 26.) Increasing reports of mental health problems on college campuses may be one result of too much stress and no clear way of finding relief.

Frustrations and Conflicts Whenever there is a disparity between our goals (what we hope to obtain in life) and our behaviors (actions that may or may not lead to these goals), frustration can occur. For example, you realize that you must get good grades in college to enter graduate school, which is your ultimate goal. If your social life is cutting into your studying time, you may find your goals slipping away, leading to increased stress.

Conflicts occur when we are forced to decide among competing motives, impulses, desires, and behaviors (for example, go out partying or study) or when we are forced to face pressures or demands that are incompatible with our own values and sense of importance (for example, get good grades or play on an all-star sports team). College students who are away from their families for the first time may face a variety of conflicts among parental values, their own beliefs, and the beliefs of others who are very different from themselves.

Overload We've all experienced times in our lives when the demands of work, responsibilities, deadlines, and relationships all seem to be pulling us underwater. **Overload** occurs when we are overextended and, try as we might, there are not enough hours in the day to do what we must get done. Students suffering from overload may experience depression, sleeplessness, mood swings, frustration, anxiety, or a host of other symptoms. Binge drinking, high consumption of junk food, lack of money, and arguments can all add fuel to the overload fire. Unrelenting stress and overload can lead to a state of physical and mental exhaustion known as *burnout*.

overload A condition in which a person feels overextended and overly pressured by demands.

background distressors Environmental stressors of which people are often unaware.

Stressful Environments For many students, where they live and the environment around them cause significant levels of stress. Perhaps you cannot afford quality housing, a bad roommate is producing major environmental stress, or loud neighbors are keeping you up at night. Maybe it isn't safe to walk to your car after dark on campus, or you have to leave your bicycle in a prime "rip-off" location during classes. Seemingly unending inconveniences and minor threats can wear you down.

Unexpected natural disasters that affect you or others can cause great emotional upset. Superstorm Sandy and Hurricane Katrina; the Sumatra, Japan, and Haiti earthquakes; killer tornadoes in Oklahoma, Iowa, and Kansas; as well as human disasters such as the Gulf Oil Spill have threatened millions with mayhem and death, disrupted lives, and damaged ecosystems for the foreseeable future. Even after the initial images of suffering pass and the crisis has subsided, shortages of vital resources such as gasoline, clean water, food, housing, health care, sewage disposal, and other necessities, as well as electricity outages and transportation problems, can wreak havoc in local communities and on campuses. Although not as newsworthy as major disasters, **background distressors** in the environment, such as noise, air, and water pollution; allergy-aggravating pollen and dust; unsafe food; or environmental tobacco

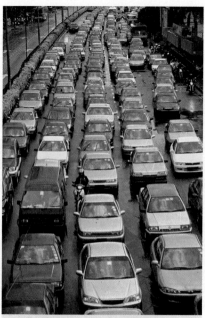
Traffic jams and noise pollution are examples of daily hassles that can add up and jeopardize our health.

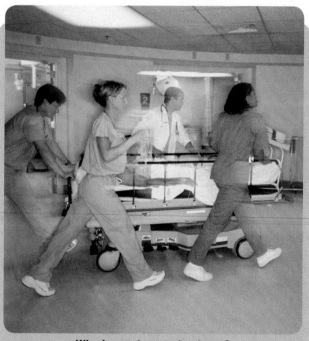

Who is most prone to stress?

Some people have careers or life circumstances that impose external pressures on them. Doctors and nurses face long work hours and a high-stakes work environment that make them especially prone to stress, overload, and burnout.

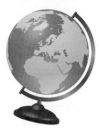

INTERNATIONAL STUDENT STRESS

International students experience unique adjustment issues related to language barriers, cultural barriers, financial issues, and a lack of social support, among other challenges. Academic stress may pose a particular problem for the nearly 765,000 international students who left their native countries to study in the United States in 2011–2012. Accumulating evidence suggests that seeking emotional support from others is a particularly effective way to cope with stressful and upsetting situations. Yet, many international students refrain from doing so because of cultural norms, feelings of shame, and the belief that seeking support is a sign of weakness that calls inappropriate attention to both the individual and the respective ethnic group. This reluctance, coupled with language barriers, cultural conflicts, and the pressure to succeed, can lead international students to suffer significantly more stress-related illnesses

Language barriers, cultural conflicts, racial prejudices, and a reluctance to seek social support all contribute to a significantly higher rate of stress-related illnesses among international students studying in the United States.

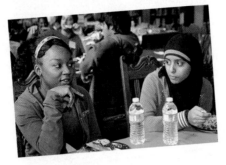

than their American counterparts. Many universities are responding to this extra stress by hosting stress management workshops each term that are geared toward the needs of international students and that encourage them to share stress management techniques from

their home countries. Both American and international students can help each other reduce stress with simple actions: Share companionship and communication, and lend a helping hand. When you make another person's life less stressful, you reap benefits yourself by participating in a support network, reaching out to others, and embracing altruism. To paraphrase a popular Hindu proverb: "Help thy neighbor's boat across and thine own boat will also reach the shore."

Sources: P. Hoffman, *Examining Factors of Acculturative Stress on International Students as They Affect Utilization of Campus-Based Health and Counseling Services at Four-Year Public Universities in Ohio*, doctoral dissertation, Ohio State University, 2010; S. Seda, *International Students' Psychological and Sociocultural Adaptation in the United States*, doctoral dissertation, Georgia State University, 2009; Institute of International Education, "Record Numbers of International Students in U.S. Higher Education," press release, November 16, 2009, http://opendoors .iienetwork.org

---

smoke can also be incredibly stressful. Campus violence, shootings, and highly charged political clashes on campus can also be sources of anxiety as students worry about safety.

Bias and Discrimination Racial and ethnic diversity of students, faculty members, and staff enriches everyone's educational experiences. It also challenges us to examine our personal attitudes, beliefs, and biases. As campuses become more internationalized, a diverse cultural base of vastly different life experiences, languages, and customs is emerging. Often, those perceived as dissimilar may become victims of subtle and not-so-subtle forms of bigotry, insensitivity, harassment, or hostility, or they may simply be ignored. Race, ethnicity, religious affiliation, age, sexual orientation, gender, or other differences may hang like a dark cloud over these students.[31] See **Health in a Diverse World** above for more on stress and international students.

Evidence of the health effects of excessive stress in minority groups abounds. For example, African Americans suffer higher rates of hypertension, CVD, and most cancers than do whites.[32] Poverty and socioeconomic status have been blamed for much of the spike in hypertension rates

for African Americans and other marginalized groups. Instead, chronic, physically debilitating stress among these groups may reflect the real and perceived effects of institutional racism. More research is necessary to show direct associations between racism, stress, and hypertension; however, it is important to realize that all types of "isms" may influence stress-related hypertension and make it more difficult for those affected to engage in healthy lifestyle behaviors. [33]

Internal Stressors

Although stress can come from the environment and other external sources, it can result from internal factors as well. Internal stressors such as negative appraisal, low self-esteem, and low self-efficacy can affect your health.

what do you think?

Do you get stressed out by things in your home or school environment?

● Which environmental stressors bug you the most?

● When you encounter these environmental stressors, what actions do you take, if any?

Appraisal and Stress Throughout life, we encounter many different types of demands and potential stressors. It is our appraisal of these demands, not the demands themselves, that results in our experiencing stress. **Appraisal** is defined as the interpretation and evaluation of information provided to the brain by the senses. Typically, it isn't a conscious activity, but rather a natural process whereby the brain sizes up a situation. Appraisal helps us recognize stressors, evaluate them on the basis of past experiences and emotions, and decide how to cope with them.

How daunting that pile of books and homework is depends on your appraisal of it.

Self-Esteem and Self-Efficacy

Self-esteem refers to how you feel about yourself (as we learned in **Chapters 1** and **2**). Self-esteem can and does continually change.[34] When you feel good about yourself, you are less likely to view an event as stressful and more likely to be able to cope.[35] Of particular concern, research with high school and college students has found that low self-esteem and stressful life events significantly predict **suicidal ideation,** a desire to die and thoughts about suicide. On a more positive note, research has also indicated that it is possible to increase an individual's ability to cope with stress by increasing self-esteem.[36] (In **Chapter 2** we discussed several ways to develop and maintain self-esteem.)

Self-efficacy, or confidence in one's skills and ability to cope with life's challenges, appears to be a key buffer in preventing negative stress effects. Research has shown that people with high levels of self-efficacy tend to have a greater sense or feeling of being in control of stressful situations and, as such, report fewer stress effects.[37] Self-efficacy is considered one of the most important personality traits that influences psychological and physiological stress responses.[38] Developing self-efficacy is also vital to coping with and overcoming academic pressures and worries.[39] For example, by learning to handle anxiety around testing situations, you will feel more capable of handling testing situations, and your sense of academic self-efficacy will grow. For tips on how to deal with test-taking anxiety, see the **Skills for Behavior Change** box on page 83. (For more information about self-efficacy, see **Chapters 1** and **2.**)

appraisal The interpretation and evaluation of information provided to the brain by the senses.

suicidal ideation A desire to die and thoughts about suicide.

self-efficacy Belief in one's ability to achieve goals and influence events in life.

hostility The cognitive, affective, and behavioral tendencies toward anger, distrust, and cynicism.

Type A and Type B Personalities

It should come as no surprise to you that personality can have an impact on whether you are happy and socially well-adjusted or sad and socially isolated. However, your personality may affect more than just your social interactions: It may be a critical factor in your stress levels.

In 1974, physicians Meyer Friedman and Ray Rosenman published a book indicating that Type A individuals had a greatly increased risk of heart disease.[40] *Type A* personalities are defined as hard-driving, competitive, time-driven perfectionists. In contrast, *Type B* personalities are described as being relaxed, noncompetitive, and more tolerant of others.

Today, most researchers recognize that none of us will be wholly Type A or Type B all of the time, and we may exhibit either type in selected situations. In addition, recent research indicates that not all Type A people experience negative health consequences; in fact, some Type A individuals thrive on their supercharged lifestyles. Often Type A's who exhibit a "toxic core," that is, who have disproportionate amounts of anger; are distrustful of others; and have a cynical, glass-half-empty approach to life—a set of characteristics referred to as **hostility**—are at increased risk for heart disease.[41]

Type C and Type D Personalities

In addition to CVD, personality types have often been linked to increased risk for a variety of other illnesses, ranging from asthma to cancer, even though much of this research remains in question. A type commonly discussed today is the *Type C* personality, characterized as stoic, with a tendency to stuff feelings down and conform to the wishes of others (or be "pleasers"). Preliminary research suggests that Type C individuals may be more susceptible to illnesses such as asthma, multiple sclerosis, autoimmune disorders, and cancer; however, more research is necessary to support this relationship.[42]

A more recently identified personality type is *Type D* (distressed), which is characterized by a tendency toward excessive negative worry, irritability, gloom, and inability to express these feelings due to social inhibition. Several recent studies have indicated that Type D people may be up to eight times more likely to die of a heart attack or sudden death.[43]

Are Internal Stressors Inescapable?

For most people most of the time, enough exposure to stressors will evoke the stress response. With the long list of stressors we've just reviewed, especially for people prone to Type A behavior, it might seem like stress is a given. But two factors seem to break the cycle and offer some protection

Overcoming Test-Taking Anxiety

Testing well is a skill needed in college and beyond. Try these tips on your next exam.

BEFORE THE EXAM

❭ Manage your study time. Keep up with reading during the term. Make sure your preparation for the test is a review rather than an initial reading of material. Don't wait until the last minute to cram. At least 1 week before your test, start studying for a set amount of time each day. Do a limited review the night before, get a good night's sleep, and arrive for the exam early.

❭ Think about how much time you might need to answer different types of test questions. If you know how much time will be available for the test, make a general strategy for using the time that you can and quickly refine at the beginning of the test.

❭ Eat a balanced meal before the exam. Avoid sugar and rich or heavy foods, as well as foods that might upset your stomach. You want to feel your best.

❭ Wear a watch to class on the day of the test, in case there is no clock.

DURING THE EXAM

❭ Manage your time during the test. Look at how many questions there are and what each is worth. Prioritize the high-point questions, allow a certain amount of time for each, and make sure that you leave some time for the rest. Hold to this schedule.

❭ Slow down and pay attention. Focus on one question at a time. Check off each part of multipart questions to make sure your answers are complete.

from stress: psychological hardiness and the shift-and-persist strategy.

Psychological Hardiness According to psychologist Susanne Kobasa, **psychological hardiness** may negate self-imposed stress associated with Type A behavior. Psychologically hardy people are characterized by *control, commitment,* and willingness to embrace *challenge.*[44] People with a sense of control are able to accept responsibility for their behaviors and change those that they discover are debilitating. People with a sense of commitment have good self-esteem and understand their purpose in life. Those who embrace challenge see change as an opportunity for growth.

The concept of hardiness has evolved to include a person's ability to cope with stress and adversity.[45] In recent years, it has become common for people to think of this general hardiness concept in terms of **psychological resilience.** Essentially, resilience refers to our capacity to maintain or regain psychological well-being in the face of challenge.[46] Resilient individuals are often able to do well in the face of adversity because of "protective factors" such as strong support networks of family, friends, and healthy communities and their own coping skills. Resilience has been studied extensively and appears to be a key indicator of good psychological and social development.[47]

Shift and Persist Even though they face extreme poverty, abuse, and unspeakable living conditions as they grow up, some youth seem to thrive when their conditions are bleak. Why? An exciting, emerging body of sociological research proposes that in the midst of extreme, persistent adversity, youth—often with the help of positive role models in their lives—are able to reframe appraisals of current stressors more positively (*shifting*), while *persisting* in focusing on a future that has something to offer them. These youth are able to endure the present by adapting, holding on to meaningful things in their lives, and staying optimistic and positive. These **"shift and persist"** strategies are among the most recently identified factors that protect against the negative effects of too much stress in our lives.[48]

Managing Stress in College

College students thrive under a certain amount of stress, but excessive stress can overwhelm many. Studies have indicated that first-year students report not only more problems with stress, but also more emotional reactivity in the form of anger, hostility, frustration, and a greater sense of being out of control.[49] Sophomores and juniors reported fewer problems with these issues, and seniors reported the fewest problems. This may indicate students' progressive emotional growth through experience, maturity, increased awareness of support services, and more social connections.[50]

Students generally report using health-enhancing methods to combat stress, but research has found that students sometimes resort to health-compromising activities to escape the stress and anxiety of college.[51] Numerous researchers have found stress among college students to be correlated to unhealthy behaviors such as substance abuse, lack of physical activity, poor psychological and physical health, lack of social problem solving, and infrequent use of social support networks.[52]

psychological hardiness A personality trait characterized by control, commitment, and the embrace of challenge.

psychological resilience The capacity to maintain or regain psychological well-being in the face of adversity, trauma, tragedy, threats, or significant sources of stress.

shift and persist A strategy of reframing appraisals of current stressors and focusing on a meaningful future that protects a person from the negative effects of too much stress.

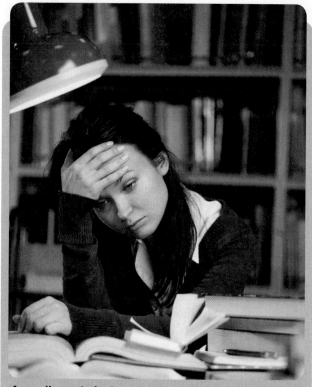

Are college students more stressed than other groups?

Studies suggest yes. The combination of a new environment; peer and parental pressure; financial pressures; and the many demands of course work, campus activities, and social life likely contributes to this problem.

coping Managing events or conditions to lessen the physical or psychological effects of excess stress.

stress inoculation Stress-management technique in which a person consciously anticipates and prepares for potential stressors.

cognitive restructuring The modification of thoughts, ideas, and beliefs that contribute to stress.

Being on your own in college may pose challenges, but it also lets you take control of and responsibility for your life. Although you can't eliminate all life stressors, you can train yourself to recognize the events that cause stress and to anticipate your reactions to them. **Coping** is the act of managing events or conditions to lessen the physical or psychological effects of excess stress.[53] One of the most effective ways to combat stressors is to build coping strategies and skills, known collectively as *stress-management techniques*, such as those discussed in the following sections.

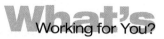
Working for You?

Maybe you're already on your way to a less-stressed life. Below is a list of some things you can do to cope with stress. Which of these are you already incorporating into your life?

☐ I listen to relaxing music.

☐ I exercise regularly.

☐ I get 8 hours of sleep each night.

☐ I practice deep breathing.

Practicing Mental Work to Reduce Stress

Stress management isn't something that just happens. It calls for getting a handle on what is going on in your life, taking a careful look at yourself, and coming up with a personal plan of action. Because your perceptions are often part of the problem, assessing your self-talk, beliefs, and actions are good first steps. Why are you so stressed? How much of it is due to perception rather than reality? What's a realistic plan of action for you? Think about your situation and map out a strategy for change. The tools in this section will help you.

Assess Your Stressors and Solve Problems

Assessing what is really going on in your life is an important first step to solving problems and reducing your stress. Here's how:

- Make a list of the major things that you are worried about right now.
- Examine the causes of the problems and worries.
- Consider how big each problem is. What are the consequences of doing nothing? Of taking action?
- List your options, including ones that you may not like very much.
- Outline an action plan, and then *act*. Remember that even little things can sometimes make a big difference and that you shouldn't expect immediate results.
- After you act, evaluate. How did you do? Do you need to change your actions to achieve a better outcome next time? How?

One useful way of coping with your stressors, once you have identified them, is to consciously anticipate and prepare for specific stressors, a technique known as **stress inoculation.** For example, suppose speaking in front of a class scares you. Practice in front of friends or in front of a video camera to banish panic and prevent your freezing up on the day of the presentation.

Change the Way You Think and Talk to Yourself

As noted earlier, our appraisal of a situation is what makes things stressful. Several types of negative self-talk can make things more stressful. Among the most common are *pessimism,* or focusing on the negative; *perfectionism,* or expecting superhuman standards; *"should-ing,"* or reprimanding yourself for things that you should have done; *blaming* yourself or others for circumstances and events; and *dichotomous thinking,* in which everything is either black or white (good or bad) instead of somewhere in between. To combat negative self-talk, we must first become aware of it, then stop it, and finally replace the negative thoughts with positive ones—a process called as **cognitive restructuring.** Once you realize that some of your thoughts may be negative, irrational, or overreactive, interrupt this self-talk by saying, "Stop" (under your breath or aloud), and make a conscious

Rethink Your Thinking Habits

❱ **Reframe a distressing event from a positive perspective.** *Reframing* is a technique that helps you change your perspective to focus on the positive. For example, if you feel perpetually frustrated that you can't be the best in every class, reframe the issue to highlight your strengths.

❱ **Break the worry habit.** If you are preoccupied with what-ifs and worst-case scenarios, the following suggestions can help slow the worry drain:

  ❱ If you must worry, create a 20-minute "worry period" when you can journal or talk about it each day. After that, move on and block the worry if it pops up again.

  ❱ When you worry, **stop**. Think about something else.

  ❱ Try to focus on the many things that are going right, rather than the one thing that *might* go wrong.

  ❱ Learn to accept what you cannot change. Chronic worriers want to be in control, but each of us must learn to live with some uncertainty.

  ❱ If your worries seem to be out of control, seek help. Talk with a trusted friend or family member or make an appointment with a counselor.

❱ **Tolerate mistakes.** Rather than getting upset by mishaps, evaluate what happened and learn from it. Try to laugh at mistakes. Take yourself less seriously.

---

continually drain you with their own issues or negative outlooks on life. If supportive friends or family are unavailable, most colleges and universities offer counseling services at no cost for short-term crises. Clergy, instructors, and residence hall supervisors also may be excellent resources. Most communities also offer low-cost counseling through mental health clinics.

Invest in Your Loved Ones As our lives get busy and obligations become overwhelming, we often don't make time for the very people who are most important to us: our friends, family, and other loved ones. In order to have a healthy social support network, we have to invest time and energy. Cultivate and nurture the relationships that matter: those built on trust, mutual acceptance and understanding, honesty, and genuine caring. In addition, treating others empathically provides them with a measure of emotional security and reduces *their* anxiety. If you want others to be there for you to help you cope with life's stressors, you need to be there for them.

Cultivating Your Spiritual Side

One of the most important factors in reducing stress in your life is taking the time and making the commitment to cultivate your spiritual side: finding your purpose in life and living your days more fully. (For information on spirituality and how it can affect your overall health, see **Focus On: Cultivating Your Spiritual Health**, beginning on page 60.)

Managing Emotional Responses

Have you ever gotten all worked up about something only to find that your perceptions were totally wrong? We often get upset not by realities, but by our faulty perceptions.

---

effort to think positively. See the **Skills for Behavior Change** box for other suggestions of ways to rethink your thinking habits.

Developing a Support Network

As you plan a stress-management program, remember the importance of social networks and social bonds. Studies of college students have demonstrated the importance of social support in *buffering* individuals from the effects of stress.[54] Different friends often serve different needs, so having more than one is usually beneficial.

Find Supportive People Family members and friends can be a steady base of support when the pressures of life seem overwhelming. People who are positive, help you to see the realities of your situation, and offer constructive suggestions can help you get through even the toughest times. Avoid "debby-downers" who

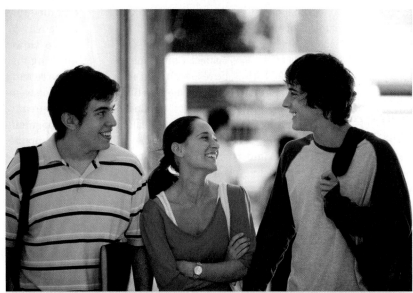

Spending time communicating and socializing can be an important part of building a support network and reducing your stress level.

Stress management requires that you examine your emotional responses to interactions with others. With any emotional response to a stressor, you are responsible for the emotion and the resulting behaviors. Learning to tell the difference between normal emotions and emotions based on irrational beliefs or expressed and interpreted in an over-the-top manner can help you stop the emotion or express it in a healthy and appropriate way.

Fight the Anger Urge Anger usually results when we feel we have lost control of a situation or are frustrated by a situation that we can do little about. Major sources of anger include (1) perceived *threats* to self or others we care about; (2) *reactions to injustice*, such as unfair actions, policies, or behaviors; (3) *fear,* which leads to negative responses; (4) *faulty emotional reasoning,* or misinterpretation of normal events; (5) *low frustration tolerance,* often fueled by stress, drugs, lack of sleep, and other factors; (6) *unreasonable expectations* about ourselves and others; and (7) *people rating,* or applying derogatory ratings to others.

Each of us has learned by this point in our lives that we have three main approaches to dealing with anger: *expressing it, suppressing it,* or *calming it.* You may be surprised to find out that, in the long run, expressing your anger is probably the healthiest thing to do, if you express anger in an assertive rather than an aggressive way. However, it's a natural reaction to want to respond aggressively, and that is what we must learn to keep at bay. To accomplish this, there are several strategies you can use:[55]

● **Identify your anger style.** Do you express anger passively or actively? Do you hold anger in, or do you explode? Do you throw the phone, smash things, or scream at others?

● **Learn to recognize patterns in your anger responses and how to de-escalate them.** For 1 week, keep track of everything that angers you or keeps you stewing. What thoughts or feelings lead up to your boiling point? Keep a journal and listen to your anger. Try to change your self-talk. Explore how you can interrupt patterns of anger, such as counting to 10, getting a drink of water, or taking some deep breaths.

● **Find the right words to de-escalate conflict.** Communicate to de-escalate. When conflict arises, be respectful and state your needs or feelings rather than shooting zingers at the other person. Avoid "you always" or "you never" and instead say, "I feel_____ when you_____" or "I would really appreciate it if you could_____." Another approach would be to say, "I really need help understanding . . . or . . . figuring out a way to_____." If you find you are continually revved up for a battle, consider taking a class or workshop on assertiveness training or anger management.

● **Plan ahead.** Explore options to minimize your exposure to anger-provoking situations such as traffic jams. Give yourself an extra 15 minutes, and learn to "chill" when unexpected delays occur.

● **Vent to your friends.** Find a few close friends you can confide in. They can provide insight or another perspective. But, don't wear down your supporter with continual rants.

● **Develop realistic expectations of yourself and others.** Anger is often the result of unmet expectations, frustrations, resentments, and impatience. Are your expectations of yourself and others realistic? Try talking about your feelings with those involved at a time when you are calm.

● **Turn complaints into requests.** When frustrated or angry with someone, try reworking the problem into a request. Instead of screaming and pounding on the wall because your neighbors are blaring music at 2:00 A.M., talk with them. Try to reach an agreement that works for everyone. Again, think ahead about the words you will use.

● **Leave past anger in the past.** Learn to resolve issues and not bring them up over and over. Let it go. If you can't, seek the counsel of a professional to learn how.

Learn to Laugh, Be Joyful, and Cry Have you ever noticed that you feel better after a belly laugh or a good cry? Adages such as "laughter is the best medicine" and "smile and the world smiles with you" didn't evolve out of the blue. Humans have long recognized that smiling, laughing, singing, dancing, and other actions can elevate our moods, relieve stress, make us feel good, and help us improve our relationships. Learning to take yourself less seriously and laugh at yourself is a good starting place. Crying can have similar positive physiological effects in relieving tension. Several studies have indicated that laughter and joy may increase endorphin levels, increase oxygen levels in the blood, decrease stress levels, relieve pain, enhance productivity, and reduce risks of chronic disease; however, the evidence for *long-term* effects on immune functioning and protective effects for chronic diseases is only just starting to be understood.[56] For ideas on how to find more joy and laughter in your daily life, see the **Health Headlines** box on page 87.

Taking Physical Action

Feeling unbearably tense and ready to explode? Remember that the human stress response is intended to end in physical activity. Yet in today's world we usually aren't able to fight or flee. However, exercise can "burn off" stress hormones by directing them toward their intended metabolic function.[57] Exercise can also help combat stress by raising levels of endorphins—mood-elevating, painkilling hormones—in the bloodstream, increasing energy, reducing hostility, and improving mental alertness. Go for a brisk walk, a quick run, or a dash up the stairs. Get up and get moving. (For more information on the beneficial effects of exercise, see **Chapter 11.**)

Get Enough Sleep Adequate amounts of sleep allow you to refresh your vital energy, cope with multiple stressors more effectively, and be productive when you need to be. In fact, sleep is one of the biggest stress busters of them all. (These benefits and others are discussed in much more depth in **Focus On: Improving Your Sleep** beginning on page 98.)

Practice Self Nurturing Make time to relax and practice relaxation techniques discussed later in this chapter.

HAPPINESS: THE MAGIC STRESS ELIXIR?

In the past few decades, a field of research called *positive psychology* has emerged to study how people can become happier. Some positive psychologists have found that people who are generally more optimistic or happier have fewer mental and physical health problems, and less stress! If happiness and optimism are keys to stress reduction, how can *you* find them?

✱ **Set realistic goals.** Psychologist Alice Donner says that striving for a 100 percent dose of contentment and perfection is unrealistic. She suggests that managing your expectations is key. Decide what is realistic for you and work toward that place.

✱ **Remember that money doesn't buy happiness.** Too much focus on acquiring things rather than on relationships and connections may be a major cause of discontent. Also, people who have to pay for a lot of material things tend to work longer hours, vacation less, and not take time for themselves.

✱ **Lose yourself in the moment.** Finding your *flow*, a state of effortless concentration and enjoyment, should be a daily goal. What energizes you, makes time fly, and causes you to concentrate fully on the present? The more often you find and follow that, the happier you'll be.

✱ **Count your blessings.** Although we all can find time to complain, focusing on our many positive attributes and being thankful for the good things in our lives should become a daily ritual. This might include daily journaling, creating a time to contemplate all of the good things about the day.

✱ **Try new things and reinvigorate.** For example, try new recipes, find new ways of exercising, plan a fun outing, find a new place on campus to study, learn a new skill, or volunteer your time.

✱ **Forgive and forget.** Rather than ruminating over some slight or indiscretion, try to understand what may have caused someone to act in a hurtful manner, and then move on.

✱ **Remember to prioritize *you.*** Your own happiness is as important as that of others in your life. Limit the time you spend with people who bring you down. Instead, find time for breaks, fun interludes, and time alone.

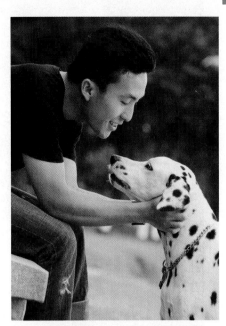

Don't forget to make time for joy and beauty in your life.

Sources: R. Kobau et al., "Mental Health Promotion in Public Health: Perspectives and Strategies from Positive Psychology," *American Journal of Public Health* 101, no. 8 (2011): e1–e9; S. Algoe, B. Fredrickson, and L. Barbara, "Emotional Fitness and the Movement of Affective Science from Lab to Field," *American Psychologist* 66, no. 1 (2011): 35–42; M. E. P. Seligman, *Authentic Happiness: Using the New Positive Psychology to Realize Your Potential for Lasting Fulfillment* (New York: Free Press/Simon & Schuster, 2002).

Find time each day for something fun—something that you enjoy and that calms you. Take a hot bath, get a massage, and allow yourself a set amount of guilt-free time texting or chatting with friends. Turn on your iPod or MP3 and listen to your favorite songs. Remember that taking time out for you should be a part of every day. Like exercise, relaxation can help you cope with stressful feelings, preserve your energy, and refocus your energies.

Eat Healthfully
It is clear that eating a balanced, healthy diet will help provide the stamina you need to get through problems and will stress-proof you in ways that are not fully understood. It is also known that undereating, overeating, and eating the wrong kinds of foods can create distress in the body. In particular, avoid **sympathomimetics,** substances in foods that produce (or mimic) stresslike responses, such as caffeine. (For more information about the benefits of sound nutrition, see **Chapter 9.**)

Managing Your Time

Ever put off writing a paper until the night before it was due? We all **procrastinate,** or voluntarily delay doing some task despite expecting to be worse off for the delay. These delays can result in academic difficulties, financial problems, relationship problems, and a multitude of stress-related ailments.

How can you avoid the procrastination bug? According to psychologist Peter Gollwitzer and colleagues, a key is setting clear "implementation intentions," a series of goals to be accomplished toward a specific end.[58] For example, set a goal of spending at least 2 hours per day for the next week focusing on the review of literature for your next big term paper. Having a plan that includes deadlines and rewarding yourself for meeting

sympathomimetics Food substances that can produce stresslike physiological responses.

procrastinate Intentionally put off doing something.

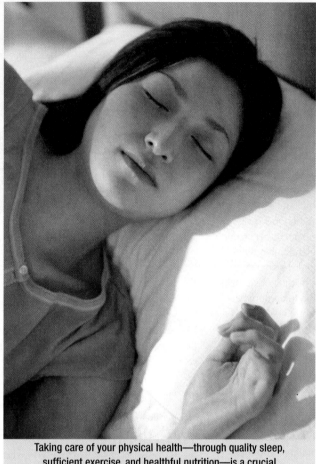

Taking care of your physical health—through quality sleep, sufficient exercise, and healthful nutrition—is a crucial component of stress management.

you must do, but not immediately; and the things that it would be nice to do. Consider the nice-to-do items only if you finish the others or if they include something fun.

● **Find a clean, comfortable place to work, and avoid interruptions.** When you have a project that requires total concentration, schedule uninterrupted time. Don't answer the phone; close your door and post a "Do Not Disturb" sign; or go to a quiet room in the library or student union where you can hide and work.

● **Reward yourself for work completed.** When you finish a task, do something nice for yourself. Rest breaks give you time to recharge and refresh your energy levels.

● **Work when you're at your best.** If you're a morning person, study and write papers in the morning, and take breaks when you start to slow down.

● **Break overwhelming tasks into small pieces, and allocate a certain amount of time to each.** If you are floundering in a task, move on and come back to it when you're refreshed.

● **Remember that time is precious.** If you have trouble saying no to people and projects that steal your time, see the **Skills for Behavior Change** box on page 89 for some suggestions.

34.4%
of college students report that their finances have been very difficult to handle during the past 12 months.

Consider Downshifting

Today's lifestyles are hectic and pressure packed, and stress often comes from trying to keep up. Many people are questioning whether "having it all" is worth it, and they are taking a step back and simplifying their lives. This trend has been labeled **downshifting,** or *voluntary simplicity.* Moving from a large urban area to a smaller town, leaving a high-paying and high-stress job for one that makes you happy, decluttering your life, and making a host of other changes in lifestyle typify downshifting.

Downshifting involves a fundamental alteration in values and honest introspection about what is important in life. It means cutting down on shopping habits, buying only what you need to get by, and living within modest means. When you contemplate any form of downshift or perhaps even start your career this way, it's important to move slowly and consider the following:

● **Complete a financial inventory.** How much money will you need to do the things you want to do? Will you live alone or share costs with roommates? Do you need a car, or can you rely on public transportation? (See **Focus On: Improving Your Financial Health** on page 26 for more on assessing your finances.)

downshifting Taking a step back and simplifying a lifestyle that has become focused on trying to keep up, hectic, and packed with pressure and stress; also known as *voluntary simplicity.*

those deadlines can motivate you to stay on task. Like most plans, it is important to be realistic in the number of goals you set. Start with a simple plan and be flexible. Another strategy is to get started early and set a personal end date that is well ahead of the class due date.

Learning to manage your time better overall is key to reducing stress. Keep a journal for 2 days to note how you spend your time. Write down your activities every day—everything from going to class to doing your laundry to texting your friends—and the amount of time you spend doing each. Are you completing the tasks you need to do on a daily basis? Are there any activities you can stop doing or that you would like to do more frequently? Use the following time-management tips in your stress-management program:

● **Do one thing at a time.** Don't try to watch television, wash clothes, and write your term paper all at once. Stay focused.

● **Clean off your desk.** Go through the things on your desk, toss unnecessary papers, and put into folders the papers for tasks that you must do. Read your mail, recycle what you don't need, and file what you will need later.

● **Prioritize your tasks.** Make a daily "to do" list and stick to it. Categorize the things you must do today; the things that

Learn to Say No and Mean It!

Is your calendar so full you barely have time to breathe? Are you unable to say no to other people? When you are asked to do something you don't really want to do or are overextended, practice the following tips to avoid overcommitment:

❯ **Be sympathetic, but firm.** Explain that although you think it's a great cause or idea, you can't participate right now. Don't waver if they persist or pressure you.

❯ **Don't say you want to think about it and will get back to them.** This only leads to more forceful requests later.

❯ **Don't give in to guilt.** Stick to your guns. Remember you don't owe anyone your time.

❯ **Even if something sounds good, avoid spontaneous "yes" responses.** Make a rule that you will take at least a day to think about committing your time.

❯ **Schedule time for yourself first.** If you don't have time for the things you love to do, stop and prioritize your activities. Don't let your time be sucked up by things that you really don't want to do.

● **Develop an Expense Plan.** Manage your budget and plan ahead for college tuition and book costs, as well as for rent, food, and entertainment expenses. It's also extremely important to understand your health insurance plan so that you know what services are covered (and what you have to pay for) if you go to an urgent care clinic or doctor.

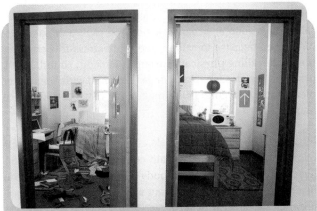

Can reducing clutter help me de-stress in college?

When a dorm room for two is only about 226 sq. ft., reducing clutter can head off stress from a disorganized environment. Less stuff and good organization can help you avoid the stress of playing hide-and-seek with your cell phone or your car keys. Which of these two rooms appears to be a less stressful environment?

● **Determine your ultimate goal.** What is most important to you, and what will you need to reach that goal? What can you do without?

● **Make both short-term and long-term plans for simplifying your life.** Set up your plans in doable steps, and work slowly toward each step.

● **Select the right career.** Look for work that you enjoy and that isn't necessarily driven by salary. Can you be happy taking a lower-paying job if it is less stressful?

● **Consider options for saving money.** Downshifting doesn't mean you renounce money; it means you choose not to let money rule your life. Saving is still important, and you need to prepare for emergencies and for future plans.

Relaxation Techniques for Stress Management

Relaxation is the body's natural antidote to stress. Some common relaxation techniques have been practiced for centuries, including yoga, qigong, tai chi, deep breathing, meditation, visualization, and massage therapy; other techniques include progressive muscle relaxation, biofeedback, and hypnosis. These techniques work because they trigger the relaxation response, a constellation of effects that are the opposite of the stress response: heart rate decreases, blood pressure decreases, blood flow increases, respiration rate decreases, metabolic rate slows, oxygen consumption decreases, muscle tension decreases, and so on.[59]

Yoga Yoga is an ancient practice that combines meditation, stretching, and breathing exercises designed to relax, refresh, and rejuvenate. It began about 5,000 years ago in India and has been evolving ever since. Some 15 million adults practice many versions in the United States today.[60]

Classical yoga is the ancestor of nearly all modern forms of yoga. Breathing, poses, and verbal mantras are often part of classical yoga. Of the many branches of classical yoga, *hatha yoga* is the most well-known because it is the most body focused. This style of yoga involves the practice of breath control and *asanas*—held postures and choreographed movements that enhance strength and flexibility. (Several other, more athletic, forms of yoga are discussed in **Chapter 11.**) Recent research has provided increased evidence of the benefits of hatha yoga in reducing inflammation, boosting mood, and reducing stress among those who practice it regularly.[61] (See **Focus on: Cultivating Your Spiritual Health,** starting on page 60, for additional information on yoga.)

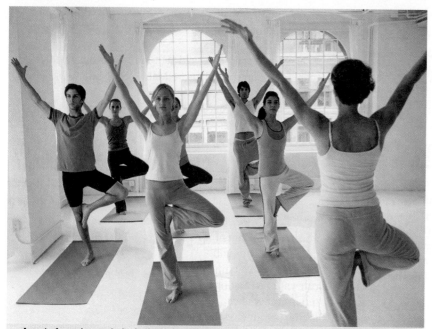

A part of yoga's popularity in the United States comes from the positive effect it can have on physical, spiritual, and emotional health.

than involving the abdominal region. Simply stated, diaphragmatic breathing is deep breathing that maximally fills the lungs by involving the movement of the diaphragm and lower abdomen. This technique is commonly used in yoga exercises and in other meditative practices. Try the diaphragmatic breathing exercise in **Figure 3.5** (page 91) right now and see whether you feel more relaxed!

Meditation There are many different forms of **meditation.** Most involve sitting quietly for 15 to 20 minutes, focusing on a particular word or symbol, and controlling breathing. Practiced by Eastern religions for centuries, meditation is believed to be an important form of introspection and personal renewal. In stress management, it can calm the body and quiet the mind, creating a sense of peace. A recent review of accumulated research found that one form of meditation, *transcendental meditation (TM)*, helped adults reduce their blood pressure and significantly reduce their need for blood pressure medications. Importantly, TM reduced symptoms of angina, CVD risks, and overall CVD mortality.[62] (Meditation and other aspects of spiritual health are discussed in detail in **Focus On: Cultivating Your Spiritual Health** beginning on page 60.) Meditation can be performed alone or in a group. Many colleges and universities offer classes on how to meditate. Check with your campus wellness center.

Visualization Often our thoughts and imagination provoke distress by conjuring up worst-case scenarios. Our imagination, however, can also be tapped to reduce stress. In **visualization,** you use your imagination to create mental scenes. The choice of mental images is unlimited, but natural settings such as ocean beaches and mountain lakes are often used because they often represent stress-free environments. Recalling physical sensations of sight, sound, smell, taste, and touch can replace stressful stimuli with peaceful or pleasurable thoughts. Try to make your visualization as real and detailed as possible.

Progressive Muscle Relaxation Progressive muscle relaxation involves systematically contracting and relaxing different muscle groups in your body. The standard pattern is to begin with the feet and work your way up your body, contracting and releasing as you go (**Figure 3.6,** page 91). The process is designed to teach awareness of the different feelings of muscle tension and muscle release. With practice, you can quickly identify tension in your body when you are facing stressful situations and consciously release that tension to calm yourself.

Massage Therapy If you have ever had someone massage your stiff neck, aching feet, or hands, you know that massage

Qigong *Qigong* (pronounced "chee-kong"), one of the fastest-growing, most widely accepted forms of mind–body health exercise, is used by some of the country's largest health care organizations, such as Kaiser Permanente, particularly for people suffering from chronic pain or stress. Qigong is an ancient Chinese practice that involves becoming aware of and learning to control *qi* (or *chi,* pronounced "chee"), or vital energy in your body. According to Chinese medicine, a complex system of internal pathways called *meridians* carry *qi* throughout your body. If *qi* becomes stagnant or blocked, you'll feel sluggish or powerless. Qigong incorporates a series of flowing movements, breath techniques, mental visualization exercises, and vocalizations of healing sounds that are designed to restore balance and integrate and refresh the mind and body.

Tai Chi *Tai chi* (pronounced "ty-chee") is sometimes described as "meditation in motion." Originally developed in China as a form of self-defense, this graceful form of exercise has existed for about 2,000 years. Tai chi is noncompetitive and self-paced. To do tai chi, you perform a defined series of postures or movements in a slow, graceful manner. Each movement or posture flows into the next without pause. Tai chi has been widely practiced in China for centuries and is now becoming increasingly popular around the world, both as a basic exercise program and as a complement to other health care methods. Health benefits include stress reduction, greater balance, and increased flexibility.

meditation A relaxation technique that involves deep breathing and concentration.

visualization The creation of mental images to promote relaxation.

Diaphragmatic or Deep Breathing Typically, we breathe using only the upper chest and thoracic region rather

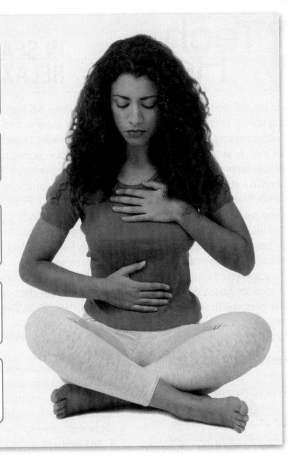

1. Assume a natural, comfortable position either sitting up straight with your head, neck, and shoulders relaxed, or lying on your back with your knees bent and your head supported. Close your eyes and loosen binding clothes.

2. In order to feel your abdomen moving as you breathe, place one hand on your upper chest and the other just below your rib cage.

3. Breathe in slowly and deeply through your nose. Feel your stomach expanding into your hand. The hand on your chest should move as little as possible.

4. Exhale slowly through your mouth. Feel the fall of your stomach away from your hand. Again, the hand on your chest should move as little as possible.

5. Concentrate on the act of breathing. Shut out external noise. Focus on inhaling and exhaling, the route the air is following, and the rise and fall of your stomach.

FIGURE 3.5 **Diaphragmatic Breathing**
This exercise will help you learn to breathe deeply as a way to relieve stress. Practice this for 5 to 10 minutes several times a day, and soon diaphragmatic breathing will become natural for you.

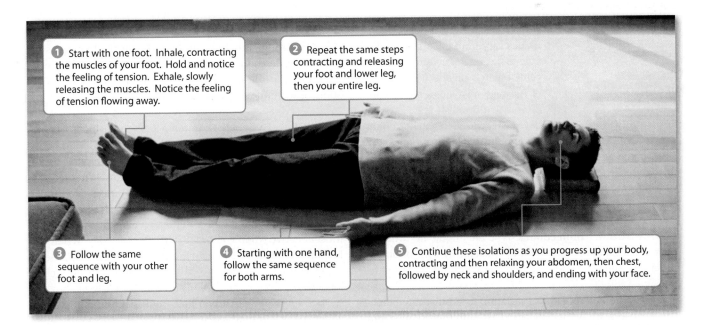

1. Start with one foot. Inhale, contracting the muscles of your foot. Hold and notice the feeling of tension. Exhale, slowly releasing the muscles. Notice the feeling of tension flowing away.

2. Repeat the same steps contracting and releasing your foot and lower leg, then your entire leg.

3. Follow the same sequence with your other foot and leg.

4. Starting with one hand, follow the same sequence for both arms.

5. Continue these isolations as you progress up your body, contracting and then relaxing your abdomen, then chest, followed by neck and shoulders, and ending with your face.

FIGURE 3.6 **Progressive Muscle Relaxation**
Sit or lie down in a comfortable position and follow the steps described to increase your awareness of tension in your body and your ability to release it.

IN SEARCH OF APPS FOR THE RELAXATION RESPONSE

One of the wonderful things about being human is that when we're hit with stressors, we have many more options than fight or flight. With practice, you can learn to make the relaxation response just as automatic as the stress response. That practice—whether it is yoga, deep breathing, meditation, or one of many other relaxation techniques—has an immediate benefit: You get to relax! There are many apps that can help guide you through a meditation or yoga session, gauge your stress, and otherwise help you fit stress management and relaxation practice into your life. Here are a few of the available apps:

* **Stress Check** (Free: Android, iPhone, iPod), www.azumio.com/apps/stress-check

This nifty app has a stress gauge and heart monitor onboard. Just put your finger over your phone's camera hole, and using the app's software, it will pick up your heart rate and give you readouts.

* **Pocket Yoga** (Modest cost: iPhone), http://pocket-sports.com

With three different practices designed by experienced instructors, three different levels of difficulty, and three different session durations, you can tailor the app to your needs. Both visual and voice-over instructions are included.

* **Breathe2Relax** (Free: Android, iPhone, iPod, iPad), http://t2health.org/apps/breathe2relax

This relaxation tool uses guided information to help you learn and practice diaphragmatic breathing.

* **Ambiance** (Modest cost: Android, iPhone, iPod, iPad, Desktop), http://ambianceapp.com

This app is marketed as an "environmental enhancer" and includes over 2,500 downloadable sounds, from natural soundscapes like ocean waves to electronic sounds and music. You can use the sounds as background when studying or just "chilling."

* **GPS for the Soul** (Free: iPhone), www.heartmath.org/free-services/solutions-for-stress/gps-for-the-soul.html

This app uses your device's camera to gauge stress levels by measuring your heart rate. It contains guided meditation, poetry, visuals, sound or music, and a breathing pacer to help you relax.

* **Insight Timer** (Modest cost: Android, iPhone, iPod, iPad), www.spotlightsix.com

This app uses the sound of Tibetan singing bowls to signal the start and end of a meditation session. You can set the timer for sessions of different lengths, choose from seven different bowls (each with a unique sound), adjust the number of times the bell rings, log your meditation sessions, and create journal entries. You can also connect with a community for meditation support.

This is just a sample of the broad array of stress management and relaxation apps. And remember, technology cuts both ways. It can be a stressor if you let it. But you can also use it to help yourself deal with hassles, stressors, and beat stress.

Source: GPS for the Soul Link reprinted by permission of Institute of HeartMath.

---

biofeedback A technique that involves self-monitoring, usually with the aid of a device, and learning to control physical responses to stress.

hypnosis A trancelike state in which people are unusually responsive to suggestion.

is an excellent way to relax. Techniques vary from deep-tissue massage to the gentler acupressure. Recent research on the effectiveness of massage as a stress-reducer indicates that Swedish massage may have beneficial effects on hormones that regulate blood pressure and reduce inflammation, as well as invoke a general relaxation response in the body.[63] (Focus On: Complementary and Alternative Medicine, starting on page 000, provides more information about the benefits of massage and other body-based methods such as acupressure and shiatsu.)

Biofeedback **Biofeedback** is a technique in which a person learns to use the mind to consciously control bodily functions, such as heart rate, body temperature, and breathing rate. Using devices as simple as stress dots that change color with body temperature variation to sophisticated electrical sensors, individuals learn to listen to their bodies and make necessary adjustments, such as relaxing certain muscles. Or, through breathing and mind control, they may slow the heart rate and relax. Eventually practitioners of biofeedback develop the ability to recognize and lower stress responses without using any devices.

Hypnosis **Hypnosis** requires a person to focus on one thought, object, or voice, thereby freeing the right hemisphere of the brain to become more active. The person then becomes unusually responsive to suggestion. Whether self-induced or induced by someone else, hypnosis can reduce certain types of stress.

Relaxation techniques, whether ancient or modern, are most effective when you practice them every day. When you become experienced at evoking the relaxation response in quiet settings, you can use it to help cope with life's challenges and stresses as they occur. The **Tech & Health** box describes some apps that can help you start and maintain an effective relaxation practice.

How Stressed Are You?

Let's face it: Some periods in life, including your college years, can be especially stressful! Learning to "chill" starts with an honest examination of your life experiences and your reactions to stressful situations. Respond to each section, assigning points as directed. Total the points from each section, then add them and compare to the life-stressor scale.

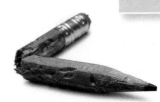

1 Recent History

In the last year, how many of the following major life events have you experienced? (Give yourself **five points** for each event you experienced; if you experienced an event more than once, give yourself **ten points,** etc.)

1. Death of a close family member of friend _____
2. Ending a relationship (whether by choice or not) _____
3. Major financial upset jeopardizing your ability to stay in college _____
4. Major move, leaving friends, family, and/or your past life behind _____
5. Serious illness (you) _____
6. Serious illness (of someone you're close with) _____
7. Marriage or entering a new relationship _____
8. Loss of a beloved pet _____
9. Involved in a legal dispute or issue _____
10. Involved in a hostile, violent, or threatening relationship _____

Total _____

2 Self-Reflection

For each of the following, indicate where you are on the scale of 0 to 5.

	Strongly Disagree					Strongly Agree

1. I have a lot of worries at home and at school. — 0 1 2 3 4 5

2. My friends and/or family put too much pressure on me. — 0 1 2 3 4 5

3. I am often distracted and have trouble focusing on schoolwork. — 0 1 2 3 4 5

4. I am highly disorganized and tend to do my schoolwork at the last minute. — 0 1 2 3 4 5

5. My life seems to have far too many crisis situations. — 0 1 2 3 4 5

6. Most of my time is spent sitting; I don't get much exercise. — 0 1 2 3 4 5

7. I don't have enough control in decisions that affect my life. — 0 1 2 3 4 5

8. I wake up most days feeling tired/like I need a lot more sleep. — 0 1 2 3 4 5

9. I often have feelings that I am alone and that I don't fit in very well. — 0 1 2 3 4 5

10. I don't have many friends or people I can share my feelings or thoughts with. — 0 1 2 3 4 5

11. I am uncomfortable in my body, and I wish I could change how I look. — 0 1 2 3 4 5

12. I am very anxious about my major and whether I will get a good job after I graduate. — 0 1 2 3 4 5

13. If I have to wait in a restaurant or in lines, I quickly become irritated and upset. — 0 1 2 3 4 5

14. I have to win or be the best in activities or in classes or I get upset with myself. — 0 1 2 3 4 5

15. I am bothered by world events and am cynical and angry about how people behave. — 0 1 2 3 4 5

16. I have too much to do, and there are never enough hours in the day. — 0 1 2 3 4 5

17. I feel uneasy when I am caught up on my work and am relaxing or doing nothing. — 0 1 2 3 4 5

18. I sleep with my cell phone near my bed and often check messages/tweets/texts during the night. — 0 1 2 3 4 5

19. I enjoy time alone but find that I seldom get enough alone time each day. — 0 1 2 3 4 5

20. I worry about whether or not others like me. — 0 1 2 3 4 5

21. I am struggling in my classes and worry about failing. — 0 1 2 3 4 5

22. My relationship with my family is not very loving and supportive. — 0 1 2 3 4 5

23. When I watch people, I tend to be critical and think negatively about them. — 0 1 2 3 4 5

24. I believe that people are inherently selfish and untrustworthy, and I am careful around them. — 0 1 2 3 4 5

25. Life is basically unfair, and most of the time there is little I can do to change it. — 0 1 2 3 4 5

26. I give more than I get in relationships with people. — 0 1 2 3 4 5

27. I tend to believe that what I do is often not good enough or that I should do better. — 0 1 2 3 4 5

28.	My friends would describe me as highly stressed and quick to react with anger and/or frustration.	O	1	2	3	4	5
29.	My friends are always telling me I "need a vacation to relax."	O	1	2	3	4	5
30.	Overall, the quality of my life right now isn't all that great.	O	1	2	3	4	5

Total _____

Scoring
Total your points from Sections 1 and 2. _____

Although the following scores are not meant to be diagnostic, they do serve as an indicator of potential problem areas. If your scores are:

0–50, your stress levels are low, but it is worth examining areas where you did score points and taking action to reduce your stress levels.

51–100, you may need to reduce certain stresses in your life. Long-term stress and pressure from your stresses can be counterproductive. Consider what you can do to change your perceptions of things, your behaviors, or your environment.

100–150, you are probably pretty stressed. Examine what your major stressors are and come up with a plan for reducing your stress levels right now. Don't delay or blow this off because it could lead to significant stress-related problems, affecting your grades, your social life, and your future!

151–200, you are carrying high stress, and if you don't make changes, you could be heading for some serious difficulties. Find a counselor on campus to talk with about some of the major issues you identified above as causing stress. Try to get more sleep and exercise, and find time to relax. Surround yourself with people who are supportive of you and make you feel safe and competent.

YOUR PLAN FOR CHANGE

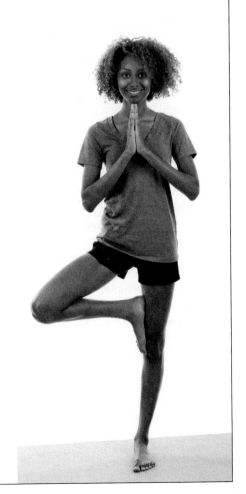

The **Assessyourself** activity gave you the chance to look at your sources of chronic stress, identify major stressors that you experienced in the last year, and see how you typically respond to stress. Now that you are aware of these patterns, you can focus on developing behaviors that lead to reduced stress.

Today, you can:

○ Practice one new stress-management technique. For example, you could spend 10 minutes doing a deep-breathing exercise or find a good spot on campus to meditate.

○ In a journal, write down stressful events or symptoms of stress that you experience.

Within the next 2 weeks, you can:

○ Attend a class or workshop in yoga, tai chi, qigong, meditation, or some other stress-relieving activity. Look for beginner classes offered on campus or in your community.

○ Make a list of the papers, projects, and tests that you have over the coming semester and create a schedule for them. Break projects and term papers into small, manageable tasks, and be realistic about how much time you'll need to get these tasks done.

○ Chart your day. Keep track of how much time you spend on Facebook, Twitter, or chatting on line and how much you spend on schoolwork, exercise, and watching TV. Set time aside for you, but limit your nonproductive time each day.

By the end of the semester, you can:

○ Keep track of the money you spend and where it goes. Establish a budget and follow it for at least a month.

○ Find some form of exercise you can do regularly. You may consider joining a gym or just arranging regular "walk dates" or pickup basketball games with your friends. Try to exercise at least 30 minutes every day. (See **Chapter 11** for more information about physical fitness.)

MasteringHealth™

Build your knowledge—and health!—in the Study Area of MasteringHealth with a variety of study tools.

Summary

* Stress is an inevitable part of our lives. *Eustress* refers to stress associated with positive events; *distress* refers to stress associated with negative events.

* The alarm, resistance, and exhaustion phases of the general adaptation syndrome (GAS) involve physiological responses to both real and imagined stressors and cause a complex cascade of hormones to rush through the body.

* Undue stress for extended periods of time can compromise the immune system and result in serious health consequences. Stress has been linked to numerous health problems, including cardiovascular disease (CVD), weight gain, hair loss, diabetes, digestive problems, and increased susceptibility to infectious diseases. Psychoneuroimmunology is the science that analyzes the relationship between the mind's reaction to stress and the function of the immune system.

* Stress can have negative impacts on your intellectual and psychological health, including impairing memory and concentration and contributing to depression, anxiety, and other mental health disorders.

* Psychosocial factors that impact stress include change, hassles, relationships, academic and financial pressure, frustrations and conflict, overload, and environmental stressors. Persons subjected to discrimination or bias may face unusually high levels of stress. Some sources of stress are internal and are related to appraisal, self-esteem, self-efficacy, personality, and psychological hardiness.

* College can be especially stressful. Recognizing the signs of stress is the first step toward better health. Managing stress begins with learning coping skills. Finding out what works best for you—probably some combination of managing emotional responses, taking mental or physical action, developing a support network, cultivating spirituality, downshifting, learning time management, managing finances, or learning relaxation techniques—will help you better cope with stress in the long run.

Pop Quiz

1. Even though Andre experienced stress when he graduated from college and moved to a new city, he viewed these changes as an opportunity for growth. What is Andre's stress called?
   a. Strain
   b. Distress
   c. Eustress
   d. Adaptive response

2. Which of the following is an example of a chronic stressor?
   a. Giving a talk in public
   b. Meeting a deadline for a big project
   c. Dealing with a permanent disability
   d. Preparing for a job interview

3. In which stage of the general adaptation syndrome does the fight-or-flight response occur?
   a. Exhaustion stage
   b. Alarm stage
   c. Resistance stage
   d. Response stage

4. The branch of the autonomic nervous system that is responsible for energizing the body for either fight or flight and for triggering many other stress responses is the
   a. central nervous system.
   b. parasympathetic nervous system.
   c. sympathetic nervous system.
   d. endocrine system.

5. During what phase of the general adaptation syndrome has the physical and psychological energy used to fight the stressor been depleted?
   a. Alarm phase
   b. Resistance phase
   c. Endurance phase
   d. Exhaustion phase

6. Losing your keys is an example of what psychosocial source of stress?
   a. Pressure
   b. Inconsistent behaviors
   c. Hassles
   d. Conflict

7. A state of physical and mental exhaustion caused by excessive stress is called
   a. conflict.
   b. overload.
   c. hassles.
   d. burnout.

8. Which of the following test-taking techniques is *not* recommended to reduce test-taking stress?
   a. Plan ahead and study over a period of time for the test.
   b. Eat a balanced meal before the exam.
   c. Do all your studying the night before the exam so it is fresh in your mind.
   d. Manage your time during the test.

9. Which of the following is *not* an example of a time-management technique?
   a. Doing one thing at a time
   b. Prioritizing your tasks
   c. Practicing procrastination in completing homework assignments
   d. Developing a plan of action

10. After 5 years of 70-hour workweeks, Tom decided to leave his high-paying, high-stress law firm and lead a simpler lifestyle. What is this trend called?
    a. Adaptation
    b. Conflict resolution
    c. Burnout reduction
    d. Downshifting

Answers to these questions can be found on page A-1.

Think about It!

1. Describe the alarm, resistance, and exhaustion phases of the general adaptation syndrome and the body's physiological response to stress. Does stress lead to more irritability or emotionality, or does irritability or emotionality lead to stress? Provide examples.

2. What are some of the health risks that result from chronic stress? How does the study of psychoneuroimmunology link stress and illness?

3. Why are the college years often high-stress for many? What factors increase stress risks? What actions can you take to manage your stressors?

4. How does anger affect the body? Discuss the steps you can take to manage your own anger and help your friends control theirs.

5. How much of a procrastinator are you? What can you do to reduce procrastination?

Accessing Your Health on the Internet

The following websites explore further topics and issues related to personal health. For links to the websites below, visit the Study Area in MasteringHealth.

1. *American College Counseling Association.* The website of the professional organization for college counselors offers useful links and articles.
   www.collegecounseling.org

2. *American Psychological Association.* Here you can find current information and research on stress and stress-related conditions as well as an annual survey.
   www.apa.org/topics/stress/index.aspx

3. *National Institute of Mental Health.* A resource for information on all aspects of mental health, including the effects of stress.
   www.nimh.nih.gov

Improving Your Sleep

LEARNING OUTCOMES

✱ Describe the problem of sleep deprivation in the United States and globally.

✱ Identify the groups that are most likely to be sleep deprived and indicate why they are at higher risk than others.

✱ Explain why we need sleep and what happens if we don't get enough, including potential physical, emotional, social, and safety threats to health.

✱ Explain circadian rhythms and why they are important to daily functioning.

✱ Explain sleep needs and factors that contribute to sleep deficits.

✱ Explore what you can do to make sure you get enough sleep.

✱ Describe the common sleep-related disorders insomnia, sleep apnea, and restless legs syndrome.

100 How does sleep deprivation threaten your health?

105 Why do caffeinated drinks keep me awake?

105 What sleep disorders are common among college students?

108 What should I do if I can't fall asleep?

Josh knew he wasn't ready for tomorrow's physics exam, but he went to his roommate's basketball game anyway. By the time it was over and he hit the books, it was nearly midnight. To keep himself awake, he drank a can of Mountain Dew, an energy drink, and then a cup of instant coffee as he plowed through the text, his notes, and the online study guide. Just before 4:00 AM, he fell into bed exhausted. But instead of drifting into sleep, his mind kept racing. *Dynamics, inertia, action,* and *reaction* tumbled around with disjointed memories of all the stressful situations he'd been through in the past few days . . . losing his cell phone, the fight with his girlfriend, his empty bank account and looming credit card due date . . . . He glanced at the clock: It was 5:30 AM. The exam was in 3 hours.

You can probably predict what happened to Josh: He failed the test.

All people need **sleep,** which is a readily reversible state of reduced responsiveness to and interaction with the environment.[1] The importance of sleep is highlighted by new evidence that links inadequate sleep with a variety of health problems, including weight

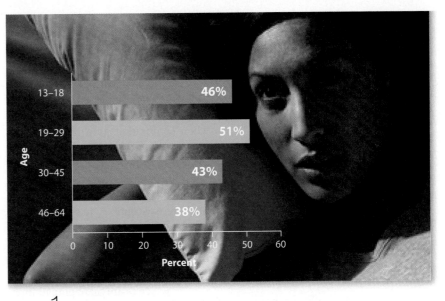

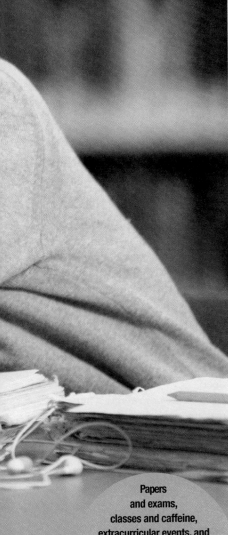

FIGURE 1 Percentage of the U.S. Population Who Rarely/Never Get a Good Night's Sleep on Weekdays

Source: Data from National Sleep Foundation, "2011 Sleep in America Poll: Communications Technology in the Bedroom, Summary of Findings," (Washington, DC: National Sleep Foundation, 2011). Available at www.nationalsleepfoundation.org

Papers and exams, classes and caffeine, extracurricular events, and on- and off-line social lives all help make today's college students a largely sleep-deprived bunch—and their health may be in jeopardy as a result.

gain, high blood pressure, depression, lowered immunity, and other ailments. Inadequate sleep isn't just an American problem: Globally, nearly 45 percent of the world's population report not getting enough sleep, largely due to excess stress.[2]

Sleepless in America

In a recent survey from the American College Health Association (ACHA), only 10.8 percent of students reported getting enough sleep to feel well rested in the morning 6 or more days per week. Over 62 percent of students said they felt tired or sleepy for 3 or more days in the past week, and 10.4 percent of students say they were tired, dragged out, or sleepy during the last 7 days.[3] It's widely acknowledged that college students are among the most sleep-deprived age group in the United States, with nearly 60 percent of those in the 18- to 29-year-old age group describing themselves as night owls who are still awake in the wee hours of the morning yet must get up early—resulting in regular sleep deficiency.[4] In general, the sleepiest members of the population are people aged 13 to 29, with people aged 30 to 64 reporting they are less sleepy **(Figure 1)**.[5]

These sleep deficiencies have been linked to a host of problems, including poor academic performance, increased alcohol abuse, accidents, daytime drowsiness, relationship issues, depression, and other problems.[6]

Several major studies indicate that younger Americans, particularly those between the ages of 18 and 24 and those over the age of 65, are most likely to fall asleep unintentionally during the day, suffering from a condition known as **excessive daytime sleepiness.**[7]

Wired and Tired: Technology's Toll on Our Sleep

Why are younger Americans so tired? Technology. If you can't live without your interactive device or are constantly wondering who might be texting you, you may be among the growing number of *wired and tired* Americans. Whether awake or sleeping, the urge to check in costs us many hours each day. In fact, according to a recent poll, technology invades the bedrooms of millions, with over 95 percent of respondents reporting using electronic devices in the hours right before going to bed and over two thirds of these people saying they seldom get enough sleep. Sleep experts indicate that it isn't just the time you spend using technology that cuts into your sleep time. Increased exposure to interactive technology may increase alertness compared to just watching television. Artificial light exposure

sleep A readily reversible state of reduced responsiveness to, and interaction with, the environment.

excessive daytime sleepiness Disorder characterized by unusual patterns of falling asleep during normal waking hours.

melatonin: A hormone that affects sleep cycles, increasing drowsiness.

from multiple devices in the hours before we go to bed may suppress the release of **melatonin,** a hormone that helps regulate biological rhythms and promotes sleep, while increasing alertness and shifting circadian rhythms to a later hour, making it harder to fall asleep. Some experts believe that as children develop into their teenage years, their bodies may be biologically predisposed toward later bedtimes and shorter sleep times, causing morning wake-up problems.[8]

54.6%
of college students have difficulty falling asleep one or more days of the week.

Sleepy Workers

Adult workers also suffer from sleepiness, and the costs are high. Drowsiness may contribute to poor work performance, off-task thinking, difficulties in concentrating, and irritability or edginess on the job. Drowsy workers are also more likely to have on-the-job accidents, be depressed, miss more work, and have motor vehicle accidents when commuting. In a recent survey, over 30 percent of workers reported falling asleep or being barely awake in the past month while at work, driving while drowsy, or both. Shift workers are particularly susceptible to sleep-related problems.[9]

When there aren't enough hours in the day, sleep typically gets short-changed. Because Americans are managing to function on campus and on the job, even though they report sleeping less, you might conclude that sufficient sleep isn't all that necessary. In fact, the evidence grows daily for the importance of adequate sleep to overall health and daily functioning. Let's look at the benefits of sleep and find out what happens when you don't get enough.

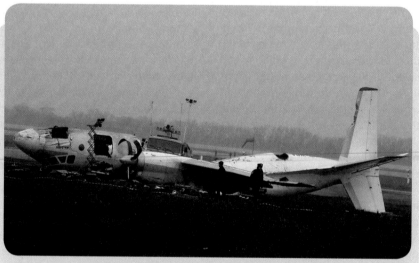

How does sleep deprivation threaten your health?

People we trust for transportation suffer from on-the-job sleepiness at alarming rates. Over 26 percent of train operators and 23 percent of pilots admit to sleepiness on the job in the last week. Twenty percent of pilots, 18 percent of train operators, and 14 percent of truck drivers report making a serious error or having a "near miss" while at work.

Source: Data from National Sleep Foundation, "Sleepy Pilots, Train Operators and Drivers," March 2012, www.sleepfoundation.org

Why Do You Need to Sleep?

You need to sleep because it maintains your physical health, affects your ability to function, and promotes your psychological health. It achieves these results by serving at least two biological purposes:

● *It restores you both physically and mentally.* For example, certain reparative chemicals are released while you sleep. And there is some evidence, discussed shortly, that during sleep the brain is cleared of daily minutiae, learning is synthesized, and memories are consolidated. Also, supplies of neurotransmitters that are used up during waking hours are restored during sleep.

● *It conserves body energy.* When you sleep, your core body temperature and the rate at which you burn calories drop. This leaves you with more energy to perform activities throughout your waking hours.

Sleep Maintains Your Physical Health

Sleep has beneficial effects on most body systems. That's why, when you consistently don't get a good night's rest, your body doesn't function as well, and you become more vulnerable to a wide variety of health problems.[10] The following is a brief summary of the physical benefits of sleep.

● **Sleep helps maintain your immune system.** The common cold, strep throat, the flu, mononucleosis, cold sores, and a variety of other ailments are more common when your immune system is depressed. And that's more likely to happen if you're not getting enough sleep. For instance, one recent study found that poor sleep quality and shorter sleep duration increased susceptibility to the common cold.[11] Another key study reports that sleep disruption, particularly when circadian rhythms are disrupted repeatedly, results in an overall disruption of immune functioning.[12]

● **Sleep helps reduce your risk for cardiovascular disease.** Several studies have indicated that high blood pressure is more common in people who get fewer than 7 hours of sleep a night.[13] Newer research points to a strong association between short-duration sleep and cardiovascular disease.[14]

● **Sleep contributes to a healthy metabolism and helps regulate hunger.** Chemical reactions in your cells break down food and synthesize compounds that the body needs. The sum of all these reactions is called *metabolism*. Several recent studies suggest that sleep contributes to healthy metabolism and possibly a healthy body weight. Those who sleep less tend to eat more, particularly high-fat, high-protein foods, and exercise less than those who get adequate amounts of sleep, and thus they may be more prone to obesity.

Some experts have theorized that when you don't get enough sleep, two hormones that regulate appetite may get knocked out of whack. *Ghrelin*, a "hungry hormone," may increase in the body and stimulate your appetite. Another hormone, *leptin*, tells you that you are full. But when you're sleep deprived, your body may not create as much of it, allowing you to eat more than you otherwise would. Several early studies showed to varying degrees that people who slept less than 8 hours per night had lower levels of leptin, higher levels of ghrelin, and higher body mass indexes (a measure of overweight and obesity). A newer controlled clinical trial provides compelling evidence that going short on sleep increases total ghrelin levels in men, but not in women, and reduces the satiety hormone GLP-1 levels of women, but not of men. Men who sleep 4 hours or less (short sleep) are likely to experience an increase in appetite, and after a short sleep, women are less likely to feel full after eating.[15] There is also evidence that sleep deficiencies, and particularly sleep disorders such as sleep apnea, can increase the risk of *type 2 diabetes*, a disorder of glucose metabolism.[16]

Sleep Affects Your Ability to Function

It's easy to see how not getting enough sleep can be detrimental. But sleep does more for you than simply maintain your health. Let's take a look at what the research says about the benefits of enough sleep.

● **Sleep contributes to neurological functioning.** Restricting sleep can cause a wide range of neurological problems, including lapses of attention, slowed or poor memory, reduced cognitive ability, and a tendency for your thinking to get "stuck in a rut."[17] Your ability not only to remember facts but also to integrate them, make meaningful generalizations about them, and consolidate what you've learned into lasting memories requires adequate sleep time.[18] College students who pull all-nighters, as well as students who are short sleepers, have significantly lower overall grade-point averages compared with classmates who get adequate sleep.[19]

● **Sleep improves motor tasks.** Sleep also has a restorative effect on motor function, that is, the ability to perform tasks such as shooting a basket, playing a musical instrument, or driving a car. Motor function is affected by sleep throughout the life span.[20] Some sleep researchers contend that a night without sleep impairs your motor skills and reaction time as much as if you were driving drunk.[21] As Americans have become more and more sleep-deprived, the incidence of *drowsy driving* and so-called *fall-asleep crashes* has become a national concern. Nearly one third of people report that they have driven when they couldn't keep their eyes open in the last 30 days. Drivers 16 to 24 are the most likely of any age group to report falling asleep at the wheel within the last year, and men of all ages are more likely to fall asleep than are women. Data from the National Highway Traffic Safety Administration (NHTSA) indicate that sleepy drivers are involved in 2 percent of all fatal crashes; however, other sources estimate these figures may be considerably higher, ranging from 15 to 33 percent.[22]

Sleep Promotes Your Psychosocial Health

Research suggests that certain brain regions, including the cerebral cortex (your "master mind"), can achieve some form of essential rest only during sleep.[23]

In addition, you're more likely to feel stressed-out, worried, or sad when you're sleep deprived. The relationship between sleep and stress is highly complex: Stress can cause or contribute to sleep problems, and sleep problems can cause or increase your level of stress! The same is true of depression and anxiety disorders: Reduced or poor quality sleep can trigger these disorders, but it's also a common symptom resulting from them. Individuals who

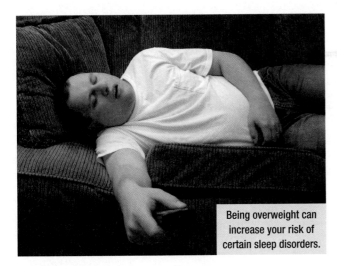

Being overweight can increase your risk of certain sleep disorders.

See It! Videos
How you can avoid nodding off behind the wheel? Watch **Dozing and Driving** in the Study Area of MasteringHealth™

suffer from chronic insomnia have over twice the risk of developing depression compared to people who experience no problems sleeping.[24]

What Goes on When You Sleep?

If you've ever taken a flight that crossed two or more time zones, then you've probably experienced *jet lag,* a feeling that your body's "internal clock" is out of sync with the hours of daylight and darkness at your destination. Jet lag happens because the new day/night pattern disrupts the 24-hour biological clock by which you are accustomed to going to sleep, waking up, and performing habitual behaviors throughout

---

circadian rhythm The 24-hour cycle by which you are accustomed to going to sleep, waking up, and performing habitual behaviors.

non-REM (NREM) sleep A period of restful sleep dominated by slow brain waves; during non-REM sleep, rapid eye movement is rare.

REM sleep A period of sleep characterized by brain-wave activity similar to that seen in wakefulness; rapid eye movement and dreaming occur during REM sleep.

---

your day. This cycle, known as your **circadian rhythm,** is regulated by a master clock that coordinates the activity of nerve cells, protein, and genes. The hypothalamus and a tiny gland in your brain called the *pineal body,* which is responsible for the drowsiness-inducing hormone called melatonin, are key to these cyclical rhythms.[25]

You can fight the effects of melatonin for hours—even days!—especially if, like Josh in our opening story, you load up on caffeine. But like all human beings—in fact, all mammals—you will eventually crash and succumb to sleep. Sleep researchers generally distinguish between two primary sleep stages: a stage of deeper sleep that is not characterized by rapid eye movement, called **non-REM (NREM) sleep,** and a stage of lighter sleep in which rapid eye movement and dreaming occur, called **REM sleep.** During the night, you slide through the stages of NREM sleep, then into REM sleep, then back through NREM again, repeating one full cycle about once every 90 minutes.[26] Overall, you spend about 75 percent of each night in NREM sleep, and 25 percent in REM (Figure 2). As you age, you may sleep more lightly and spend even less time in REM sleep.

Non-REM Sleep Is Restorative

During non-REM (NREM), or quiet sleep, the body rests. Movement can occur, for instance, to shift your position in bed, but muscle tension is reduced. Both your body temperature and your energy use drop; sensation is dulled; and your brain waves, heart rate, and breathing slow. In contrast, digestive processes speed up, and your body stores nutrients. During NREM sleep, you do not typically dream. Four distinct stages of NREM sleep have been distinguished by their characteristic progressive slowing of brain-wave patterns.

Stage 1. Your eyes may be open or closed. Stage 1 lasts only a few minutes, and it is the lightest stage of sleep from which you are most easily awakened. This is the transition period between wakefulness and sleep in which the brain produces *theta waves,* which are slow brain waves. Many experience a sudden feeling of falling in this stage that may cause them to have a quick, jerky muscular reaction.

Stage 2. This stage is slightly deeper than stage 1 and lasts from 5 to 15 minutes with even slower brain waves than in stage 1. Your eyes are closed, eye and body movements gradually cease, and you disengage from your environment.

Stage 3. NREM sleep is also called *slow-wave sleep,* because during stages 3 and 4, a sleeper's brain generates slow brain waves known as *delta waves.* Your blood pressure drops, your heart rate and respiration slow considerably, and you enter deep sleep.

Stage 4. This is the deepest stage of sleep. Speech and movement are rare during this stage, but can and do sometimes occur. For example,

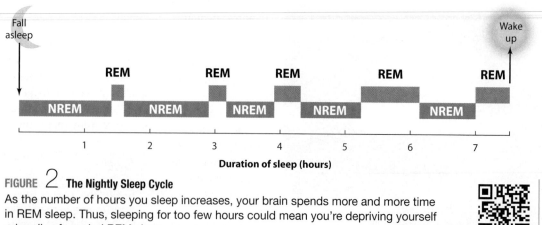

FIGURE 2 **The Nightly Sleep Cycle**
As the number of hours you sleep increases, your brain spends more and more time in REM sleep. Thus, sleeping for too few hours could mean you're depriving yourself primarily of needed REM sleep.

Video Tutor: Improving Your Sleep

sleepwalking typically occurs during the first stage 4 period of the night. You've probably heard that it's difficult to awaken a sleepwalker, and that's true of anyone in stage 4 sleep.

During the deep phases of NREM sleep, human growth hormone is released, and your body repairs and regenerates tissue, builds bone and muscle, and promotes immune system health. If you don't reach or stay in deep NREM sleep for long periods, you may find that you tire more readily and have less resistance to disease.

REM Sleep Is Energizing

Dreaming takes place primarily during REM sleep. A REM sleeper's brain-wave activity increases to be almost indistinguishable from that of someone who is wide awake, and the brain's energy use is higher than that of a person who is performing a difficult math problem![27] Your muscles are paralyzed during REM sleep: You may dream that you're rock climbing, but your body is incapable of movement. Almost the only exceptions are the heart, your respiratory muscles, which allow you to breathe,

and the tiny muscles of your eyes, which move your eyes rapidly as if you were following the scenario of your dream. This rapid eye movement gives REM sleep its name.

During REM sleep, your brain processes the experiences you've had and consolidates the information you've learned during the day. A growing chorus of researchers have theorized that if you are deprived of REM sleep, you may have declines in cognitive function, particularly short-term memory.[28] As the night progresses, the duration of NREM sleep declines and you spend more and more time in REM. That's why a full night's sleep is important for getting as much REM sleep as you need.

How Much Sleep Do You Need?

Researchers find most people need between 7 and 8 hours of sleep per day, on average.[29] But sleep needs vary from person to person, and your gender, health, and lifestyle also affect how much rest your body demands. For example, women need more sleep than men overall.

It is worth noting that sleep patterns change over the life span. Infants need the most sleep, and teens and younger adults need 8 to 9 hours per night, slightly more than the adult average. It is a myth that people need less sleep as they grow older, though older adults may experience sleep difficulties that result in fewer hours of rest per night owing to health conditions

such as sleep apnea, pain, and the need to use the bathroom more frequently.[30]

Research has consistently shown that sleep really is the "great elixir" and that sleep deprivation and disorders contribute significantly to premature death and disability from a variety of conditions, including cardiovascular disease, cancer, and diabetes, in particular. In fact, many scientists believe that diabetes, obesity, and other metabolic disorders may be linked with biological clock activity.[31] In general, those who get adequate amounts of sleep live longer and enjoy more quality days than those who don't.[32]

Sleep Need Includes Baseline plus Debt

Pay attention to how you feel after different amounts of sleep, and aim for the duration that feels best for you.[33] In addition to your body's physiological need, consider your **sleep debt.** That's the total number of hours of missed sleep you're carrying around with you, either because you got up before your body was fully rested or because your sleep was interrupted. Let's say that last week you managed just 5 hours of sleep a night Monday through Thursday. Even if you get 7 to 8 hours a night Friday through Sunday, your unresolved sleep debt of 8 to 12 hours will leave you feeling tired and groggy when you start the week again. That means you need *more than* 8 hours a night for the next several nights to "catch up."

The good news is that you *can* catch up if you go about it sensibly. Getting 5 hours of sleep a night all semester long, then sleeping 48 hours the first weekend you're home on break won't restore your functioning, and it's likely to disrupt your circadian rhythm. Instead, whittle away at that sleep debt by sleeping 9 hours a night throughout your break—then start the new term resolved to sleep 7 to 8 hours a night.

sleep debt The difference between the number of hours of sleep an individual needed in a given time period and the number of hours he or she actually slept.

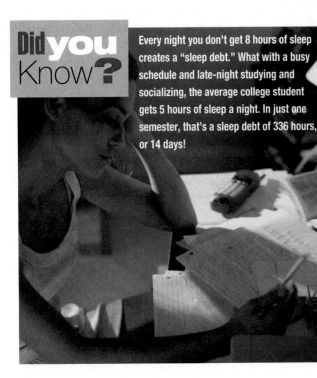

Did you Know?

Every night you don't get 8 hours of sleep creates a "sleep debt." What with a busy schedule and late-night studying and socializing, the average college student gets 5 hours of sleep a night. In just one semester, that's a sleep debt of 336 hours, or 14 days!

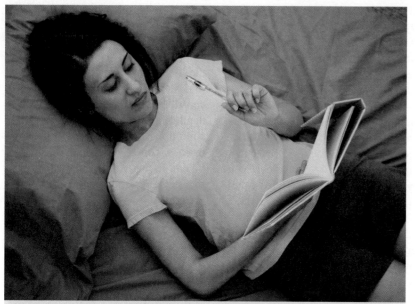

If a worry keeps you awake, jot it down in a journal. You'll be better prepared to handle it in the morning after a good night's sleep.

Do Naps Count?

Speaking of catching up, do naps count? Although naps can't entirely cancel out a significant sleep debt, they can help improve your mood, alertness, and performance. Regular naps may also improve immune function and help ward off infections.[34] It's best to nap in the early to mid-afternoon, when the pineal body in your brain releases a small amount of melatonin and your body experiences a natural dip in its circadian rhythm. Never nap in the late afternoon, because it could interfere with your ability to fall asleep that night. Keep your naps short, because a long nap of more than 30 minutes can leave you in a state of **sleep inertia,** which is characterized by cognitive impairment, grogginess, and a disoriented feeling.

what do you think?

Do you find it difficult to get 7 or 8 hours of sleep each night?
● Do you think you are able to catch up on sleep you miss?
● Have you noticed any negative consequences in your life when you get too little sleep?

How to Get a Good Night's Sleep

Do you need a jolt of caffeine to get you jump-started in the morning? Do you find it hard to stay awake in class? Have you ever nodded off behind the wheel? These are all signs of inadequate or poor quality sleep. To find out whether you're sleep-deprived, take the **Assess Yourself** questionnaire on page 109.

Do's and Don'ts for Restful Sleep

The following tips can help you get a longer and more restful night's sleep.

● **Let there be light.** Throughout the day, stay in sync with your circadian rhythm by spending time in the sunlight. If you live in an area where the sun seldom shines for weeks at a time, invest in special light-emitting diode (LED) lighting designed to mimic the sun's rays.

sleep inertia A state characterized by cognitive impairment, grogginess, and disorientation that is experienced upon rising from short sleep or an overly long nap.

Exposure to natural light outdoors is most beneficial, but opening the shades indoors and, on overcast days, turning on room lights can also help keep you alert.
● **Stay active, but avoid exercise before bed.** Make sure you get plenty of physical activity during the day. Activity speeds up your metabolism and makes it harder to fall asleep, so make sure you don't exercise for several hours before you want to sleep.
● **Sleep tight.** Don't let a pancake pillow, scratchy or pilled sheets, or a threadbare blanket keep you from sleeping soundly. If your mattress is uncomfortable and you can't replace it, try putting a foam mattress topper on it. And make your bed in the morning; neat sheets and covers are inviting for sleep.
● **Create a sleep "cave."** As bedtime approaches, keep your bedroom quiet, cool, and dark. If you live in an apartment or dorm where there's noise outside or in the halls, wear ear plugs or get an electronic device that produces "white noise," such as the sound of gentle rain. Turn down the thermostat or, on hot nights, run a quiet electric fan. Install room-darkening shades or curtains, or wear an eye mask if necessary, to block out any light from the street.

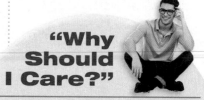

"Why Should I Care?"

It probably won't surprise you to find out that students cite sleep problems as the second largest negative impact on their academic performance, right after stress. But did you know that sleepy people are more likely to be grumpy and confrontational, wreaking havoc with their social life? Lack of sleep reduces libido and makes people less interested in having sex, zapping their love life, too.

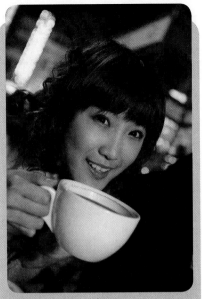

Why do caffeinated drinks keep me awake?

After-dinner coffee? Not unless it's decaf. Caffeine promotes alertness by blocking the neurotransmitter adenosine in your brain—a useful thing when you are studying, but a potential problem when you are trying to sleep. Your body needs 6 hours to process half of the caffeine you drink (and another 6 to process half of what remains, and so on). So coffee at 8:00 PM means you won't be sleeping soundly until well after midnight.

● **Condition yourself into better sleep.** Go to bed and get up at the same time each day. Establish a bedtime ritual that signals to your body that it's time for sleep. For instance, sit by your bed and listen to a quiet song, meditate, write in a journal, take a warm bath or shower, or read something that lets you quietly wind down.

● **Make your bedroom a mental escape.** Don't stew about things you can't fix right now. Clear your mind of worries and frustrations. Focus on listening to your body unwind.

● **Avoid foods and drinks that keep you awake.** Large meals, nicotine, energy drinks, caffeine, and alcohol close to bedtime can affect your ability to get to sleep and stay asleep. Your body takes about 6 hours to clear *half* the caffeine you consume from your system.[35]

● **Don't toss and turn.** If you're not asleep after 20 minutes, get up. Turn on a low light, and read something relaxing, not stimulating, or listen to some gentle music. Once you feel sleepy, go back to bed.

● **Get rid of technology in the bedroom.** Make a rule: No TV, texting, or tweeting your time away in bed. If you can't sleep, don't surf the net or check your Facebook page. Sit quietly, focus on deep breathing and relaxation, block your worries, and try to capture that drowsy, sleepy feeling.

● **Don't drink large amounts of any liquid before bed.** Drinking liquids may contribute to **nocturia,** or overactive bladder, meaning you have to get up several times during the night. A variety of conditions, besides too much fluid intake, including urinary tract infection or other ailments, can cause nocturia. See your doctor if bathroom trips have begun to be a regular thing at night.

● **Don't take nonprescribed sleeping pills or nighttime pain medications.** Casual use of over-the-counter sleeping

nocturia Frequent urination at night due to an overactive bladder.

aids can interfere with your brain's natural progression through the healthy stages of sleep.

● **Don't get revved by emotional upheavals.** Stop all incoming messages 1 hour before bed. One reason is to avoid late-night phone calls, texts, or e-mails that can end up in arguments, disappointments, and other emotional stressors. If something—or someone—does jazz you up shortly before bed, journal about it briefly, then promise yourself that you'll make time the next day to explore your feelings more deeply.

What If You Still Can't Sleep?

As many as 70 million U.S. adults suffer from sleep-related disorders.[36] Ironically, fewer than 5 percent of college students are diagnosed and in

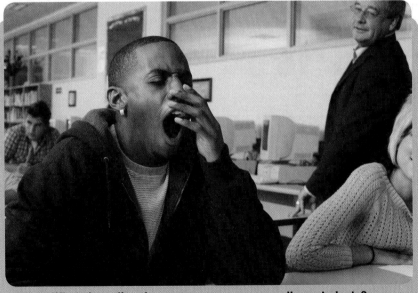

What sleep disorders are common among college students?

From insomnia to sleepwalking to narcolepsy, sleep disorders are more common than you might think. There are more than 80 different clinical sleep disorders, and it is estimated that 70 million adult Americans—and millions of children—suffer from one. At least some of the college students short-changed on sleep—27 percent, the same as the general adult population—may be suffering from a sleep disorder.

treatment for sleep disorders, although nearly 25 percent of students say that they have had sleep difficulties in the last year that were difficult to handle.[37] Millions of sleep-deprived people have difficulty performing everyday activities (Table 1). However, if you're following the advice in this chapter and you still aren't sleeping well, then it's time to see your health care provider. To aid in diagnosis, you will probably be asked to keep a sleep diary like the one in Figure 3, and you may be referred to a sleep disorders center for an overnight stay. This type of evaluation is known as a clinical **sleep study**. While you are asleep in the sleep center, sensors and electrodes record data that will be reviewed by a sleep specialist who will work with your doctor to diagnose and treat your sleep problem.

sleep study A clinical assessment of sleep in which the patient is monitored while spending the night in a sleep disorders center.

TABLE 1

Self-Reported Sleep-Related Difficulties Among Adults 20 Years Old and Older

Difficulty	Percentage of Adults
Concentrating on things	23.2%
Remembering things	18.2%
Working on hobbies	13.3%
Driving or taking public transportation	11.3%
Taking care of financial affairs	10.5%
Performing employed or volunteer work	8.6%

Source: Centers for Disease Control and Prevention, "Insufficient Sleep is a Public Health Epidemic," 2013, www.cdc.gov

	Day 1	Day 2	Day 3
Fill out in morning			
Bedtime	11 pm	11:30 pm	
Wake time	7:30 am	8:30 am	
Time to fall asleep	45 min	30 min	
Awakenings (how many and how long?)	2 times 1 hour	1 time 45 min	
Total sleep time	6.75 hrs	7.75 hrs	
Feeling at waking (refreshed, groggy, etc.)	Still tired	Energized	
Fill out at bedtime			
Exercise (what, when, how long?)	Jog at 2 pm 30 min	Soccer practice at 4 pm; 2 hrs	
Naps (when, where, how long?)	4 pm, my bed 30 min	2 pm, library 1 hour	
Caffeine (what, when, how much?)	2 cups coffee at 8 am	1 latte at 10 am; 1 soda at 9 pm	
Alcohol (what, when, how much?)	1 beer at 8 pm	None	
Evening snacks (what, when, how much?)	Bag of popcorn at 10 pm	Chips and soda at 9 pm	
Medications (what, when, how much?)	None	None	
Feelings (happiness, anxiety, major cause, etc.)	Stressed about paper	Worried about sister	
Activities 1 hour before bed (what and how long?)	Wrote paper	Watched TV	

FIGURE 3 Sample Sleep Diary
Using a sleep diary such as this one can help you and your health care provider discover any behavioral factors that might be contributing to your sleep problem.

Maybe you're already practicing ways to get a better night's sleep. Which of the following sleep-promoting behaviors are you already incorporating into your life?

- ☐ I exercise regularly, but not before going to bed.
- ☐ My bedroom is my sleep cave, designed to help me sleep comfortably.
- ☐ I have a text/e-mail-free zone in my bedroom at night.
- ☐ I make sure not to nap late in the day.

The American Academy of Sleep Medicine identifies more than 80 specific sleep disorders. The most common disorders in adults are *insomnia, sleep apnea,* and *restless legs syndrome.* Other common sleep disorders include narcolepsy and a group of disorders called parasomnias.

Insomnia

Insomnia—difficulty in falling asleep, frequent arousals during sleep, or early morning awakening—is the most common sleep complaint. Recent research indicates that at some point every year, between 30 and 40 percent of adults report some insomnia symptoms, and 10 to 15 percent of adults have *chronic insomnia* that lasts longer than a month.[38] About 4 percent of college students are being treated for insomnia.[39] Insomnia is more common among women than men, and its prevalence increases with age.

Insomnia Symptoms and Causes
Symptoms of insomnia include difficulty falling asleep, waking up frequently during the night, difficulty returning to sleep, waking up too early in the morning, unrefreshing sleep, daytime sleepiness, and irritability. Sometimes insomnia is related to stress and worry. In other cases it may be related to disrupted circadian rhythms, which may occur with travel across time zones, shift work, and other major schedule changes. Insomnia can also occur as a side effect from taking certain medications. Left untreated, insomnia can be associated with increased illness or morbidity.

Treatment for Insomnia
Because of the close connection between behavior and insomnia, cognitive behavioral therapy is often part of any treatment for insomnia. A cognitive behavioral therapist assists a patient in identifying thought and behavioral patterns that contribute to the inability to fall asleep. Once these patterns are recognized, the patient practices new habits that produce positive change.

In some cases of insomnia, *hypnotic* or *sedative* medications may be prescribed. These drugs induce sleep, and some may help relieve anxiety. However, some have undesirable side effects ranging from daytime sleepiness and hallucinations to sleepwalking and other strange nighttime behaviors. Some drugs can actually promote anxiety or depression. Many sedatives are also addictive and can lead to tolerance and dependence. Antidepressants are also commonly prescribed for insomnia.

Relaxation techniques, including yoga and meditation, can be especially helpful in preparing the body to sleep. Exercise, done early in the day, can also help reduce stress and promote deeper sleep. The **Skills for Behavior Change** box presents some specific tips for preventing insomnia related to jet lag and other schedule disruptions.

insomnia A disorder characterized by difficulty in falling asleep quickly, frequent arousals during sleep, or early morning awakening.

sleep apnea A disorder in which breathing is briefly and repeatedly interrupted during sleep.

Sleep Apnea

Sleep apnea is a disorder in which breathing is briefly and repeatedly interrupted during sleep.[40] *Apnea* refers to a breathing pause that lasts at least 10 seconds. Sleep apnea affects more than 18 million Americans, or 1 in every 15 people; it affects all age groups and both sexes.[41]

Symptoms and Causes of Sleep Apnea
There are two major types of sleep apnea: *central* and *obstructive. Central sleep apnea* occurs when the brain fails to tell the respiratory muscles to initiate breathing. Consumption of alcohol, certain illegal drugs, and certain medications can contribute to central sleep apnea.

Beat Jet Lag

Insomnia, fatigue, stomachache, and headache: These are symptoms of jet lag and not a great way to spend a spring break vacation. In general, the more time zones you cross, the worse the jet lag will be. There are ways to avoid or reduce jet lag. Here's how:

- ❭ Begin the trip rested (preexisting sleep deprivation intensifies jet lag).
- ❭ Schedule a daytime flight.
- ❭ Reset your watch as soon as you depart.
- ❭ Avoid alcohol, caffeine, and nicotine.
- ❭ Eat small meals at the appropriate mealtime for your destination.
- ❭ Several days before going west, go to bed and wake up 1 hour later each day.
- ❭ Once in the west, seek morning light and avoid afternoon light.
- ❭ Several days before going east, go to bed and wake up 1 hour earlier each day.
- ❭ Once in the east, seek evening light and avoid morning light.
- ❭ If you take an overnight flight, avoid sleeping too much on the day of your arrival. You'll find it hard to fight the fatigue, but sleeping during the day will make it harder for you to adjust to your new time zone's schedule.

Skills for Behavior Change

Obstructive sleep apnea (OSA) is more common and occurs when air cannot move in and out of a person's nose or mouth, even though the body tries to breathe. Typically, OSA occurs when a person's throat muscles and tongue relax during sleep and block the airways, causing snorting, snoring, and gagging. These sounds occur because falling oxygen saturation levels in the blood stimulate the body's autonomic nervous system to trigger inhalation, often via a sudden gasp of breath. This response may wake the person (and anyone else in the bed!), preventing deep sleep and causing the person to wake in the morning feeling like they haven't slept.

People who are overweight often have sagging throat tissue, which puts them at higher risk for OSA; in these cases, weight loss can reduce apnea. In addition to being overweight, other risk factors include smoking and alcohol use, being age 40 or older, and ethnicity (African Americans, Pacific Islanders, and Hispanics). Anatomical risk factors for OSA can include: a small upper airway (or large tongue, tonsils or uvula), a recessed chin, small jaw or a large overbite, and a large neck size (17 inches or greater in a man, or 16 inches or greater in a woman). Because OSA runs in some families, genetics may also play a role.[42]

More serious risks of OSA include chronic high blood pressure, irregular heartbeats, heart attack, and stroke. Apnea-associated sleeplessness may also increase the risk of type 2 diabetes, immune system deficiencies, and a host of other problems.[43]

Treatment for Sleep Apnea The most commonly prescribed therapy for OSA is *continuous positive airway*

restless legs syndrome (RLS) A neurological disorder characterized by an overwhelming urge to move the legs when they are at rest.

narcolepsy A lifelong condition that causes people (and animals!) to fall asleep involuntarily during the day.

pressure (CPAP), which consists of an airflow device, long tube, and mask. People with sleep apnea wear this mask during sleep, and air is forced into the nose to keep the airway open.

Other methods for treating OSA include dental appliances, which reposition the lower jaw and tongue, and surgery to remove tissue in the upper airway. In general, these approaches are most helpful for mild disease or heavy snoring. Lifestyle changes, which may include losing weight, avoiding alcohol, and quitting smoking, are often effective ways of reducing symptoms of OSA.

Restless Legs Syndrome

Restless legs syndrome (RLS) is a neurological disorder characterized by unpleasant sensations in the legs when at rest combined with an uncontrollable urge to move in an effort to relieve these feelings. These sensations range in severity from uncomfortable to irritating to painful. In general, the symptoms are more pronounced in the evening or at night. Lying down or trying to relax activates the symptoms, so people with RLS often have difficulty falling and staying asleep. Some researchers estimate that RLS affects as many as 12 million Americans. Others think it may be even more common, but is underdiagnosed or misdiagnosed, because of the wide range in severity of symptoms.[44]

The cause of RLS is unknown. However, there is growing support for some form of genetic predisposition to the disorder. In other cases, RLS appears to be related to other conditions such as kidney failure, diabetes, and peripheral neuropathy. Pregnancy or hormonal changes can worsen symptoms.[45] If there is an underlying condition, treatment of that condition may provide relief. Other treatment options include use of prescribed

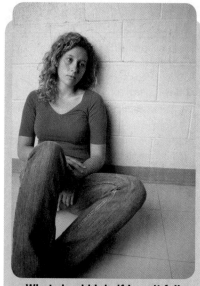

What should I do if I can't fall asleep?

If you have difficulty falling asleep, it may be that noises, lights, interruptions, or persistent worries are keeping you awake. Use ear plugs or a white noise machine to block out noise, wear an eye shade to block out light, and turn off your phone and computer to prevent interruptions.

medication, decreasing tobacco and alcohol use, and applying heat to the legs. For some people practicing relaxation techniques or performing stretching exercises can help alleviate symptoms.

Narcolepsy

Narcolepsy is a lifelong condition that causes people to fall asleep involuntarily during the day, while in class, at work, driving, or in the middle of a sentence. It often starts during the teen years or young adulthood, but it may occur in preteen youth or in people in their 50s. Narcolepsy affects as many as 200,000 Americans, with men and women affected in equal numbers. There appears to be a genetic basis for the disorder.[46]

Assess yourself

Are You Sleeping Well?

Read each statement below, then circle True or False according to whether or not it applies to you in the current school term.

1. I sometimes doze off in my morning classes. — True / False
2. I sometimes doze off in my last class of the day. — True / False
3. I go through most of the day feeling tired. — True / False
4. I feel drowsy when I'm a passenger in a bus or car. — True / False
5. I often fall asleep while reading or studying. — True / False
6. I often fall asleep at the computer or watching TV. — True / False
7. It usually takes me a long time to fall asleep. — True / False
8. My roommate tells me I snore. — True / False
9. I wake up frequently throughout the night. — True / False
10. I have fallen asleep while driving. — True / False

If you answer True more than once, you may be sleep deprived. Try the strategies in this chapter for getting more or better quality sleep, but if you still experience sleepiness, see your health care provider.

YOUR PLAN FOR CHANGE

The **Assess yourself** activity gave you the chance to determine whether you are sleep-deprived. Now that you have considered your answers, you can take steps to improve your sleep, starting tonight.

Today, you can:

○ Evaluate your behaviors and identify things you're doing that get in the way of a good night's sleep. Develop a plan. What can you do differently starting today?

○ Write a list of personal Do's and Don'ts. For instance: Do turn off your cell phone after 11:00 PM. Don't drink anything with caffeine after 3:00 PM. No strenuous exercise after dinner.

Within the next 2 weeks, you can:

○ Keep a sleep diary, noting not only how many hours of sleep you get each night, but also how you feel and how you function the next day.

○ Arrange your room to promote restful sleep. Remember the "cave": Keep it quiet, cool, and dark, and replace any uncomfortable bedding.

○ Visit your campus health center and ask for more information about getting a good night's sleep.

By the end of the semester, you can:

○ Establish a regular sleep schedule. Get in the habit of going to bed and waking up at the same time, even on weekends.

○ Create a ritual, such as stretching, meditation, reading something light, or listening to music, that you follow each night to help your body ease from the activity of the day into restful sleep.

○ If you are still having difficulty sleeping and feel you may have a sleep disorder or an underlying health problem disrupting your sleep, contact your health care provider.

Preventing Violence and Injury

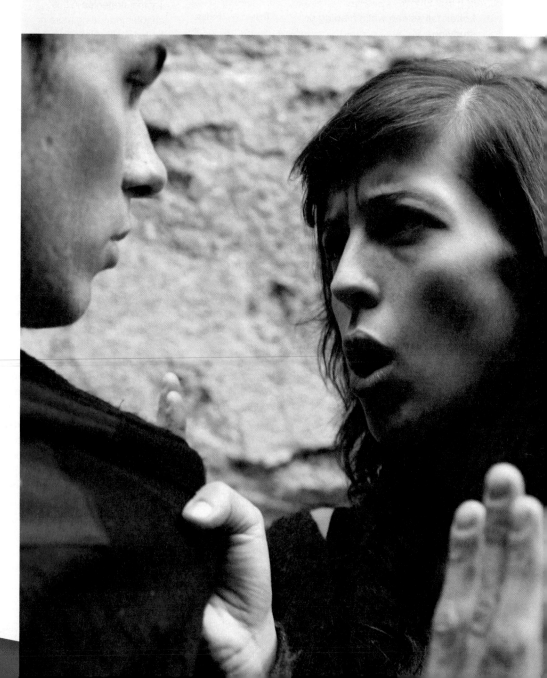

LEARNING OUTCOMES

* Differentiate between intentional and unintentional injuries.

* Identify societal and personal factors that contribute to violence in American society.

* Discuss the prevalence and common causes of homicide, gang violence, terrorism, and other intentional acts of violence.

* Describe types of and social contributors to sexual victimization.

* Articulate personal and community strategies for preventing violence.

* Describe precautions to take to minimize the risk and effect of unintentional injuries.

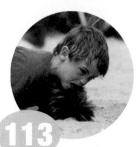

113

What makes some people act out their anger with violence?

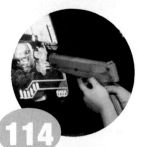

114

Does violence in the media cause violence in real life?

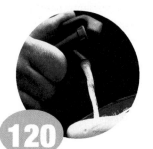

120

What is meant by *acquaintance rape*?

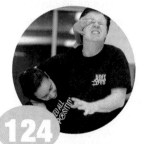

124

How can I protect myself from becoming a victim of violence?

"Fear follows crime, and is its punishment."
—Voltaire, 1694–1778[1]

Acts of hatred and brutality have always played a major role in our history as humans struggle to dominate one another. Today, violence is pervasive and takes many forms. With the news media reporting on a seemingly endless barrage of shootings, kidnappings, hate crimes, rapes, domestic violence, and other crimes, many people learn to live in fear even though they may not have experienced violence personally. Is violence in the United States out of control? Based on the evidence, are those fears justified? And to which kinds of violence are college students particularly vulnerable?

Before we can discuss the nature and extent of violence, it's important that we have an understanding of what the word *violence* means. The World Health Organization (WHO) defines **violence** as "the intentional use of physical force or power, threatened or actual, against oneself, another person, or against a group or community, that either results in or has a high likelihood of resulting in injury, death, psychological harm, maldevelopment, or deprivation."[2] Today, most experts realize that emotional and psychological forms of violence can be as devastating as physical blows to the body.

The U.S. Public Health Service has categorized violence resulting in injuries into two categories: intentional injuries or unintentional injuries. **Intentional injuries** are those committed with intent to harm and typically include assaults, homicides, self-inflected injuries, and suicides. **Unintentional injuries,** on the other hand, are those committed without intent to harm, such as motor vehicle crashes, fires, and drownings.

So, why devote an entire chapter to violence and injury in an introductory health text for college and university students? The answer is simple: Young adults are disproportionately affected by violence and injury. Unintentional injuries, particularly from motor vehicle crashes, are the number one cause of death among 15- to 24-year-olds in the United States today, whereas the second and third leading causes of death in young adults are homicide and suicide.[3]

Violence in the United States

Violence has been a part of the American landscape since colonial times; however, it wasn't until the 1980s that the U.S. Public Health Service identified *violence* as a leading cause of death and disability and gave it chronic disease status, indicating that it was a pervasive threat to society. Statistics from the Federal Bureau of Investigation (FBI) have shown that, after steadily increasing from 1973 to 2006, the rates of overall crime and certain types of violent crime have been slowly decreasing in recent years.[4] However, in October 2012, the news media caused confusion by running conflicting headlines about violence. Some outlets reported a 4 percent decline in violent crime,[5] whereas others claimed there had been a huge jump in violent crime—*up 18 to 22 percent in 1 year!*[6]

Which report was right? Actually, both of them! Historically, we use two methods: the FBI's *Uniform Crime Reporting (UCR) Program* and the Bureau of Justice Statistics *National Crime Victimization Survey (NCVS)*. These two systems are meant to be complementary, with overlapping, but not identical methods for collecting violent crime data. Usually, the two of them come to fairly similar conclusions, but not always, as in 2012.

So, why the differences in reports? While the FBI's UCR collects data on violent crimes involving force or threat *reported* to law enforcement agencies—crimes like murder and nonnegligent manslaughter, forcible rape, robbery, aggravated assault, and more than 20 other categories of crime—the Bureau of Justice statistics collects detailed information on the frequency and nature of the crimes of rape, sexual assault, personal robbery, aggravated and simple assault, home burglary, theft, and motor vehicle theft twice a year through *surveys* of over 100,000 people.[7] In addition to using a method that differs from the FBI, the Bureau of Justice also does not keep track of homicides or crimes against businesses. See **Figure 4.1** for the percent change of violent crimes in 2012 and **Figure 4.2** for the frequency of different types of crimes.

Violence trends are difficult to assess, but whether total rates of crime are up or down, there are huge disparities in crime rates based on race, sex, age, socioeconomic status, geography, and other factors. Finally, there were still an estimated 6 million violent crimes against U.S. residents aged 12 and older in 2011.[8] Even if we have never been victims ourselves, we all are victimized by violent acts that cause us to be fearful; impinge on our liberty; and damage the reputation of our campus, city, or nation. If you don't go out for a walk or run at night because you are worried about being attacked, you are a victim of societal violence.

Violence on U.S. Campuses

Campus gun violence has made headline news far too many times in recent years. Whether at Virginia Tech University, where 32 people died in the deadliest mass shooting in U.S. history; at Oikos University, where 7 were killed by a former student; or at Sandy Hook Elementary, where 26 elementary school students and teachers were gunned down by a 20-year-old, campus shootings tragically persist, and no age group seems immune. Tragedies like these have sparked dialogue and action across the nation, prompting increases in campus security and student and faculty safety measures. Today it would be hard to find a campus without a safety plan in place to prevent and respond to violent crime.

Campuses have stepped up to protect their students and the students' sense of safety, but gun violence is not the only

violence A set of behaviors that produces injuries, as well as the outcomes of these behaviors (the injuries themselves).

intentional injuries Injury, death, or psychological harm caused by violence with the intent to harm.

unintentional injuries Injury, death, or psychological harm caused unintentionally, often as a result of circumstances.

culprit. Relationship violence is one of the most prevalent problems on college campuses. In the most recent American College Health Association's survey, 10.3 percent of women and 6.7 percent of men reported being emotionally abused in the past 12 months by a significant other. Almost 7 percent of women and 3.5 percent of men reported being stalked, and 1.9 percent of men and 2.1 percent of women reported being involved in a physically abusive relationship. Nearly 1 percent of men and 2 percent of women reported being in a sexually abusive relationship.[9]

How many of the actual relationship crimes committed are reported? It is believed that fewer than 25 percent of campus relationship crimes are reported to *any* authority.[10] Even though as many as 20 to 25 percent of college women will be raped or sexually assaulted before

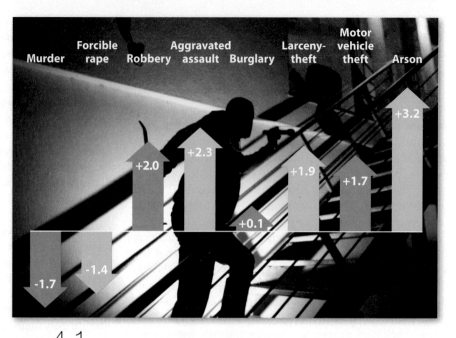

FIGURE 4.1 First Increases in Crime Rates in Decades?
According to the FBI's preliminary semiannual uniform crime report, some types of violent crime increased for the first time in years during the first 6 months of 2012.
Source: Federal Bureau of Investigation, "Early 2012 Crime Stats," January 2013, www.fbi.gov

they graduate, 95 percent of these women never report these crimes.[11]

Why would students fail to report crimes? Typical reasons include concerns over privacy, fear of retaliation, embarrassment or shame, lack of support, perception that the crime was too minor or they were somehow at fault, or uncertainty that it was a crime. This is particularly true in the situations where a victim knew her rapist or where drinking was involved and crime details were fuzzy.[12]

79% of crimes against college students occur at off-campus locations.

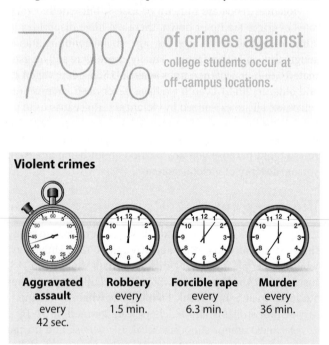

FIGURE 4.2 Crime Clock
The crime clock represents the annual ratio of crime to fixed time intervals. The crime clock should not be taken to imply a regularity in the commission of crime.
Source: Adapted from Federal Bureau of Investigation, "Crime in the United States, 2011," 2012, www.fbi.gov

Factors Contributing to Violence

Several social, community, relationship, and individual factors increase the likelihood of violent acts, as discussed in the following list:[13]

● **Poverty.** Low socioeconomic status can create a hopeless environment in which some people view violence as the only way to obtain what they want.[14]

● **Unemployment.** Financial strain, losing or fear of losing a job, economic downturns, and living in economically depressed areas can increase rates and severity of violence.[15]

● **Parental and peer influence.** Children raised in environments where shouting, hitting, emotional abuse, antisocial behavior, and other forms of violence are commonplace are more apt to act out these behaviors as adults. Lack of social connections and having peers with high delinquency rates increase risks.[16]

- **Cultural beliefs.** Cultures that objectify women, believe men are in charge, and empower men to be tough and aggressive show higher rates of violence in the home.[17]
- **Discrimination or oppression.** Whenever one group is oppressed or perceives that its members are oppressed by those of another group, violence against others is more likely.
- **Religious beliefs and differences.** Strong religious beliefs can lead some people to think that violence against others is justified.
- **Political differences.** Civil unrest and differences in political party affiliations and beliefs have historically been triggers for violent acts.
- **Breakdowns in the criminal justice system.** Overcrowded prisons, lenient sentences, early releases, and inadequate treatment/training all encourage future violence.
- **Stress.** People who are in crisis or under stress are more apt to be highly reactive, striking out at others or acting irrationally.[18]

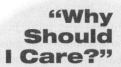

what do you think?

Why do you think rates of violence in the United States are so much higher than those of other nations, such as Great Britain and Japan?
- Which of the factors listed here do you think is the single greatest cause of violence, and why?
- What could be done to reduce risk from this factor?

may also be prone to react with violence in future situations.[23]

Aggressive behavior is often a key aspect of violent interactions. **Primary aggression** is goal-directed, hostile self-assertion that is destructive in nature. **Reactive aggression** is more often part of an emotional reaction brought about by frustrating life experiences. Whether aggression is reactive or primary, it is most likely to flare up in times of acute stress.

Substance Abuse
Alcohol and drug abuse are often catalysts for violence at all levels of society, both nationally and internationally.[24] Consumption of alcohol precedes over half of all violent

"Why Should I Care?"

The amount you drink tonight can directly affect your chances of becoming a victim of injury or assault. College students are particularly at risk for crimes committed under the influence of alcohol, including assault, rape, and intimate partner violence, but understanding the impact of alcohol in escalating potentially violent situations can help you stay out of harm's way.

primary aggression Goal-directed, hostile self-assertion that is destructive in character.

reactive aggression Hostile emotional reaction brought about by frustrating life experiences.

What Makes Some People Prone to Violence?

In addition to the broad, societal-based factors that contribute to crime, personal factors also can increase risks for violence. Emerging evidence suggests that one's family and home environment may be the greatest contributor to eventual violent behavior among family members.[19] The following are several other predictors of aggressive behavior.[20]

Anger People who anger quickly often have a low tolerance for frustration. The cause may be genetic or physiological; there is evidence that some people are born with strong tendencies toward being angry. Family background may be the most important factor. Typically, anger-prone people come from families that are disruptive, chaotic, and unskilled in emotional expression.[21] Also, people who are taught not to express anger in public do not know how to handle it when it reaches a level they can no longer hide.[22] Those who have been bullied in school

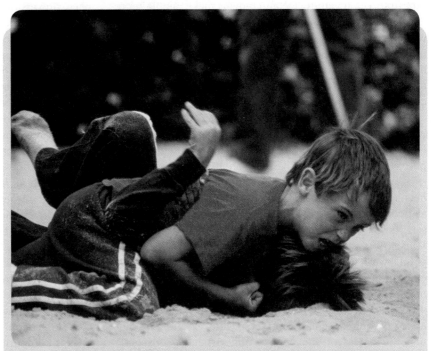

What makes some people act out their anger with violence?

If you are like most people, you probably acted out your anger more as a child than you do today. With age and maturity, most people learn to control outbursts of anger in a socially acceptable and rational manner. However, some people go through life acting out their aggressive tendencies in much the same way they did as children—with anger and violence that are a form of self-assertion or a response to frustration.

crimes and is a major factor in domestic violence at all levels.[25] Men who are heavier drinkers and more frequently drink to intoxication are the most likely to be violent perpetrators, and alcohol abuse, particularly binge drinking, is associated with physical victimization among males and sexual victimization (particularly rape) among females on campuses.[26] The social and emotional consequences of substance abuse takes a tool on the perpetrators as well: Numbers of suicide attempts and completions are also highly correlated to drug and alcohol intake.[27]

How Much Impact Do the Media Have?

After the massacre at Sandy Hook elementary, the media again focused its attention squarely on what are widely perceived as causes of violence: (1) too many high-capacity assault rifles, (2) something of a crisis in mental health, and last, but not least, (3) a daily dose of media violence. Does a regular diet of heinous crimes and bloody massacres from video games, TV, and movies make people more likely to engage in murder and mayhem? Are those who witnessed the type of media attention given to the perpetrators of mass shootings more likely to try to grab the spotlight in the same way? Is there such a thing as becoming so desensitized to violence that life and death scenarios feel commonplace?

Although the media are blamed for playing a major role in the escalation of violence, this association has been challenged continuously. While early studies seemed to support a link between excessive exposure to violent media and subsequent violent behavior, much of this research has now been called into question for methodological problems such as poor measures of violence, biased subject selection, and sample size issues.[28] More recent studies of a possible relationship between media violence and violent acts seem to point a weak finger toward a connection between media violence and short-term aggression, but there is no strong link to subsequent violent acts. Although there appears to be an association between celebrity suicide depicted in the media and subsequent increases in fan suicides, it is no stronger than the increase in suicides that occur when a peer suicide occurs.[29]

While some continue to believe that viewing violent media somehow numbs people to humanity, allows people to commit violence without empathy or regret, or even triggers violent events, several studies have disputed this premise.[30] Even so, several potential restrictions have been proposed to ban violent media for youth. The Supreme Court has steadfastly

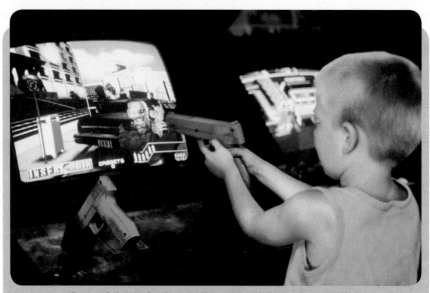

Does violence in the media cause violence in real life?

Evidence of the real-world effects of violence in the media is inconclusive. Arguably, Americans today—especially children—are exposed to more depictions of violence in the news, movies, music, and games than ever before. To date, however, research has not shown a clear link between exposure to violent media and a person's propensity to be violent.

rejected them, echoing the claims that a relationship between violent acts and the consumption of violent media has not been proven through consistent, rigorous research. President Obama and several professional groups have called for more research to better understand the complex factors that prompt violence and what might be done to reduce risks.

Critics of theories blaming media violence point out that today's young people are exposed to more media violence—on the Internet and TV and in movies and video games—than any previous generation, yet rates of violent crime among youth have fallen to 40-year lows.[31] But just because a connection between the media and violence has not been established does not mean it's healthy to consume an excessive amount of it. Debate continues over whether a person who regularly sees violence enacted in the media becomes *desensitized* to violence, and concerns have been raised about those who spend a disproportionate amount of time online or watching TV instead of interacting in real-time, face-to-face communication. Will they miss the important lessons that come from talking with people in person and learning to get along with others? What will be the result of a generation that opts out of significant "live" interactions with their peers?

what do you think?

Do you think the media influence your behavior? If so, in what ways?

● Could that influence lead to your becoming violent? Why or why not?

● Are there instances in which curtailing violent viewing or restricting the nature and extent of violence and sex in the media is warranted? If so, under what circumstances?

Intentional Injuries

Intentional injury can be categorized into three major types—*interpersonal violence*, *collective violence*, and *self-directed violence*—although there is some degree of overlap among these groups.[32] Interpersonal violence and collective violence are discussed below. (Self-directed violence, including suicide, is discussed in **Chapter 2.**) **Collective violence** refers to violence committed by groups of individuals.[33] **Interpersonal violence** includes intentionally using physical force or power, whether threatened or actual, to inflict violence against one individual by another (or by a group of others) that results in injury, death, or psychological harm.[34] Homicide, hate crimes, domestic violence, child abuse, elder abuse, and sexual victimization all fit into this category.

Homicide

Homicide, defined as murder or nonnegligent manslaughter (killing of another human), is the fifteenth leading cause of death in the United States overall, but the second leading cause of death for persons aged 15 to 24 and is among the top five leading causes of death for ages 1 to 44.[35] Today, homicide accounts for nearly 15,000 premature deaths in the United States annually, the majority of which are caused by firearms.[36] Over half of all homicides occur among people who know one another; in two thirds of these cases, the perpetrator and victim are friends or acquaintances, and in one third of those cases, they are family members.[37]

Homicide rates reveal particularly clear disparities among races. Whereas overall homicide rates in the United States have fluctuated minimally and have even decreased in some populations, those involving young victims and perpetrators, particularly young black males, have surged. In 2011, homicide rates were nearly 52 per 100,000 for African American males aged 10 to 24, compared with almost 14 per 100,000 for Hispanic males and only 3 per 10,000 for white males. Additionally, homicide was the leading cause of death for 10- to 24-year-old African Americans in 2011, the second leading cause of death for Hispanics, and the third leading cause of death for American Indians and Alaska Natives.[38] See the **Health Headlines** box on the following page for a discussion of the role guns play in the high rates of homicide in the United States.

Hate and Bias-Motivated Crimes

A **hate crime** is a crime committed against a person, property, or group of people that is motivated by the offender's bias against a race, religion, disability, sexual orientation, or ethnicity. As a result of national efforts to promote understanding and appreciation of diversity, reports of hate crimes declined to an all-time low of 6,222 incidents in 2011, according to the FBI's recent hate crime statistics report **(Figure 4.3)**.[39] Of these hate crimes, nearly 47 percent were a result of bias toward a particular race, 21 percent were motivated by bias based on sexual orientation, 20 percent reflected bias toward religion, just over 11 percent were motivated by ethnicity/national origin bias, and nearly 1 percent reflected bias toward disabilities. In 2012, *gender* and *gender identity* were added to the hate/bias crimes to be included in hate crime statistics.[40] Fear of retaliation keeps many hate crimes hidden; it is estimated that fewer than 44 percent of hate crimes are reported, and only about one fourth of those are reported by victims themselves.[41]

Bias-motivated crime, sometimes referred to as **ethnoviolence,** describes violence based on prejudice and discrimination among ethnic groups in the larger society. **Prejudice** is an irrational attitude of hostility directed against an individual; a group; a race; or the supposed characteristics of an individual, group, or race. **Discrimination** constitutes actions that deny equal treatment or opportunities to a group of people, often based on prejudice.

See It! Videos
What would you do if you saw someone being bullied for being gay? Watch **Teen Bullied for Being Gay** in the Study Area of MasteringHealth™

collective violence Violence committed by groups of individuals.

interpersonal violence The intentional use of physical force or power, threatened or actual, against another person or against a group or community that results in or has a high likelihood of resulting in injury, death, psychological harm, maldevelopment, or deprivation.

homicide Death that results from intent to injure or kill.

hate crime A crime targeted against a particular societal group and motivated by bias against that group.

ethnoviolence Violence directed at persons affiliated with a particular ethnic group.

prejudice A negative evaluation of an entire group of people that is typically based on unfavorable and often wrong ideas about the group.

discrimination Actions that deny equal treatment or opportunities to a group, often based on prejudice.

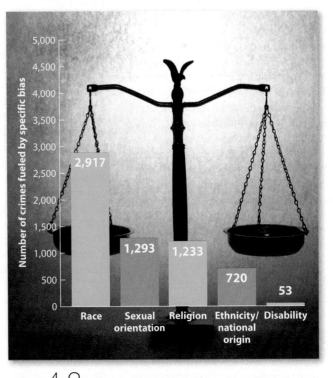

FIGURE 4.3 Bias-Motivated Crimes, Single-Bias Incidence, 2011
Source: Data from Federal Bureau of Investigation, "Hate Crime Statistics, 2011," Table 1, 2011, www.fbi.gov

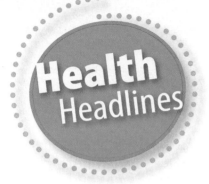

Health Headlines

BRINGING THE GUN DEBATE TO CAMPUS

On average, each year in the United States 100,000 people are shot. Over 31,000 of them die, and of those who survive, many experience significant physical and emotional repercussions. Some facts about guns and gun violence include the following:

* Firearm homicide is a leading cause of death for people aged 15 to 24, second only to motor vehicle crashes. The rate of firearm deaths for this age group is 42.7 times higher in the United States than it is in 22 other high-income countries with stricter gun laws and fewer guns.
* Handguns are consistently responsible for more murders than any other single type of weapon (see the figure to the right).
* Today, 35 percent of American homes have a gun on the premises, with nearly 300 million privately owned guns registered—and millions more that are unregistered and/or illegal.
* Firearms are the weapons most often used in attacks on American campuses, followed by knives/bladed weapons, a combination of weapons, and strangulation. The most common reason for an incident is "related to an intimate relationship" followed by "retaliation for a specific action." The presence of a gun in the home triples the risk of a homicide in that location and increases suicide risk more than five times.

What factors contribute to gun deaths in the United States? Gun critics argue that large numbers of guns in the United States as well as relatively lax gun-control laws are the culprits. However, gun-rights advocates say that the problem lies not with guns, but with the people who own them; as evidence, they point to countries

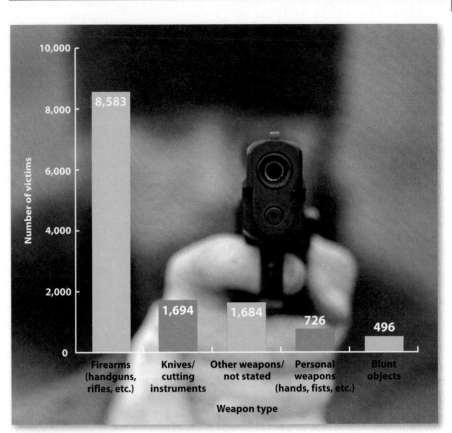

Homicide in the United States by Weapon Type, 2011
Sixty-seven percent of murders in the United States are committed using firearms, far outweighing all other weapons combined.

Source: Data from U.S. Department of Justice, Federal Bureau of Investigation, *Crime in the United States, 2011, Expanded Homicide Data,* Table 11, 2012, www.fbi.gov

like Canada that have similar numbers of guns as the United States but much lower gun-related crime rates.

High-profile shootings at schools and in other public places have brought the gun debate into sharp focus, particularly on college and university campuses. The National Conference on State Legislatures reported that 22 states ban carrying a concealed weapon on a college campus. But in 25 other states, the decision to ban or allow concealed weapons on campuses is made by each institution. Mississippi and Wisconsin passed some form of concealed weapon bills in 2011, and in 2012, so did 16 other states, even though most bills failed to secure enough votes for passage in earlier attempts. Proponents argue that there is no evidence that legally allowing guns on campus would increase the risk of campus violence. What do you think?

* How would you feel about students or instructors in your classes having guns? Would it make you feel more or less safe? What about bringing a gun to a sporting event, party on campus, or other venue?
* Do you think making guns illegal on campus would prevent students from bringing guns to school? Why or why not?
* What factors should be taken into consideration as states vote on guns on campus?

Sources: D. Drysdale, W. Modzeleski, and A. Simons, "Campus Attacks: Targeted Violence Affecting Institutions of Higher Learning," Washington DC: United States Secret Service, United States Department of Education, and the Federal Bureau of Investigation, 2010; National Conference of State Legislatures, "Guns on Campus: Overview," 2013; Brady Campaign to Prevent Gun Violence, "Facts: Gun Violence," Revised 2010, www.bradycampaign.org; S. Lewis, "Concealed Carry on Campus—Guns on Campus—College Campus Carry," CNN Report, 2011, www.campuscarry.com

Prejudice and discrimination can stem from a fear of change and a desire to blame others when forces such as the economy and crime seem to be out of control. Teaching tolerance, understanding, and respect for people from different backgrounds can reduce bias-related crimes. Interacting with those from different backgrounds and recognizing the shared humanity in each of us can break down barriers that may appear to exist.

Common reasons given to explain hate and bias-motivated crimes include (1) *thrill seeking* by multiple offenders through a group or peer attack; (2) *feeling threatened* that others will take their jobs or property or beset them in some way; (3) *retaliating* for some real or perceived insult or slight; and (4) *fearing the unknown or differences*. For other people, hate crimes are a part of their mission in life, either due to religious or political zeal or distorted moral beliefs.

Nearly 10 percent of reported hate crimes occur on campuses, and schools and colleges have the fastest growing risks for such crimes.[42] Campuses have responded to reports of hate crimes by offering courses that emphasize diversity, *zero tolerance* for violations, training faculty to recognize possible offenses and act appropriately, and developing policies that strictly enforce punishment for hate crimes.

Gang Violence

Gangs are continuing to expand and evolve, accounting for nearly 50 percent of violent crime in some U.S. jurisdictions and over 90 percent in others.[43] Increasingly, gangs are linked to alien smuggling, human trafficking, and prostitution, as well as drug trafficking, sex trafficking, shootings, beatings, thefts, carjackings, and the killing of innocent victims caught in the crossfire of gang shootouts. They are well-organized, well-armed, and well-connected in many regions of the world.[44]

Why do young people join gangs? Although the reasons are complex, gangs seem to meet many of the personal needs of young people. Often, gangs give members a sense of self-worth, companionship, security, and excitement. In other cases, gangs provide economic incentives that far exceed options available through legal endeavors. Once young people become involved in gang subculture, it is difficult for them to leave.

Who is at risk for joining a gang? The age range of gang members is typically 12 to 22. Risk factors include low self-esteem, academic problems, low socioeconomic status, alienation from family and society, recent immigration to the United States, a history of family violence, and living in gang-controlled neighborhoods.[45] Programs that attempt to combat the problems that lead to gang membership can also reduce the strength of gangs.

1 in 3 women and 1 in 10 men
have been victims of intimate partner violence in the form of rape, stalking, or physical violence in their lifetimes.

Numerous terrorist attacks around the world reveal the vulnerability of all nations to domestic and international threats. Today, threats against our airlines, mass transportation systems, cities, national monuments, and population fuel our fears of looming terrorist attacks. Effects on our economy, costs of food and fuel, travel restrictions, additional security measures, and military buildups are but a few of the examples of how terrorist threats have affected our lives.

Over the past decade the Centers for Disease Control and Prevention (CDC) created the *Emergency Preparedness and Response Division* to monitor potential public health risks, such as bioterrorism, chemical emergencies, radiation emergencies, mass casualties, national disaster and severe weather; develop plans for mobilizing communities in the case of emergency; and provide information about terrorist threats. In addition, the Department of Homeland Security works to prevent future attacks, and the FBI and other government agencies aim to ensure citizens' health and safety.

Terrorism

As defined in the U.S. Code of Federal Regulations, **terrorism** is the "unlawful use of force or violence against persons or property to intimidate or coerce a government, the civilian population, or any segment thereof in furtherance of political or social objectives."[46]

terrorism The unlawful use of force or violence against persons or property to intimidate or coerce a government, the civilian population, or any segment thereof, in furtherance of political or social objectives.

domestic violence The use of force to control and maintain power over another person in the home environment, involving both actual harm and the threat of harm.

intimate partner violence (IPV) Describes physical, sexual, or psychological harm by a current or former partner or spouse. This type of violence can occur among heterosexual or same-sex couples and does not require sexual intimacy.

Domestic Violence

Domestic violence refers to the use of force to control and maintain power over another person in the home environment. It can occur between parent and child, between spouses or intimate partners, or between siblings or other family members. The violence may involve emotional abuse; verbal abuse; threats of physical harm; and physical violence ranging from slapping and shoving to beatings, rape, and homicide.

Intimate Partner Violence

The term **intimate partner violence (IPV)** describes physical, sexual, or psychological harm done by a current or former partner or spouse. This type of violence can occur among heterosexual or same-sex couples and does not require sexual intimacy. On average, 24 people per minute are victims of rape, physical violence, or stalking by an intimate partner in the United States. Over the

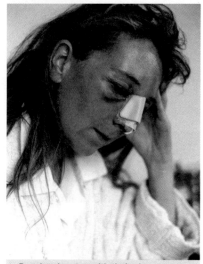

People who stay with their abusers may do so because they are dependent on the abuser, because they fear the abuser, or even because they love the abuser. In some cultures, women may not be free to leave an abusive relationship because of restrictive laws, religious beliefs, or social mores. Such women sometimes turn to drastic measures in order to escape.

child maltreatment Any act or series of acts of commission or omission by a parent or caregiver that results in harm, potential for harm, or threat of harm to a child.

stant criticism, verbal attacks, displays of explosive anger meant to intimidate, and controlling behavior. Psychological abusers seek to intimidate and debase their partners, thereby gaining control over the partner and the relationship. Those who have experienced this violence are more likely to report depression, difficulty in intimate relationships, frequent headaches, chronic pain, difficulty with sleeping, activity limitations, poor physical health, irritable bowel syndrome, and other health problems.[49]

The Cycle of IPV

Have you ever heard of a woman who is repeatedly beaten by her partner and wondered, "Why doesn't she just leave him?" There are many reasons some women find it difficult to break ties with their abusers. Some women, particularly those with small children, are financially dependent on their partners. Others fear retaliation against themselves or their children. Some hope the situation will change with time, and others stay because cultural or religious beliefs forbid divorce. Finally, some women still love the abusive partner and are concerned about what will happen to him if they leave.

course of a year, that equals more than 12 million women and men. Homicide committed by a current or former intimate partner is the leading cause of death of pregnant women in the United States.[47] In addition, 74 percent of all murder-suicides in the United States involve an intimate partner.[48]

Nearly half of all women and men in the United States have experienced psychological aggression by an intimate partner in their lifetime. This abuse can take the form of con-

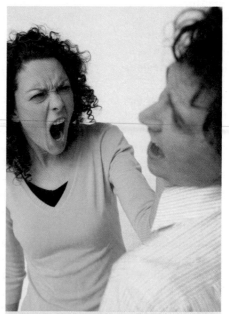

Both men and women are subject to violence and abuse from their intimate partners.

In the 1970s, psychologist Lenore Walker developed a theory called the *cycle of violence* that explained predictable, repetitive patterns of psychological and/or physical abuse that seemed to occur in abusive relationships.[50] Over the years, Walker's initial work has been criticized for its lack of scientific rigor, anecdotal approach, and seeming overstatement of selected patterns as universal truths. In her most recent book, *The Battered Woman Syndrome*, Walker responds to many of her early critics with improved quantitative analysis, reviews of recent research, and an extensive list of experts in the field of violence.[51]

Today, the cycle of violence continues to be important to understanding why people stay in otherwise unhealthy relationships. The cycle consists of three major phases:

1. **Tension building.** This phase typically occurs prior to the overtly abusive act and includes breakdowns in communication, anger, psychological aggression and violent language, growing tension, and fear.

2. **Incident of acute battering.** At this stage, the batterer usually is trying to "teach her a lesson," and when he feels he has inflicted enough pain, he'll stop. When the acute attack is over, he may respond with shock and denial about his own behavior or blame her for making him do it.

3. **Remorse/reconciliation.** During this "honeymoon" period, the batterer may be kind, loving, and apologetic, swearing that he will work to change his behavior. However, when the same things that triggered past abuse begin to resurface, the cycle starts over again.

For a woman who gets caught in this cycle, it is often very hard to summon the resolve to extricate herself. Most need effective outside intervention.

Causes of Domestic Violence and IPV

There is no single reason to explain abuse in relationships. Alcohol abuse is often associated with such violence, as are having a history of family violence and marital dissatisfaction. Numerous studies also point to differences in the communication patterns between abusive and nonabusive relationships. Stress, mental health issues, economic uncertainty/frustration, issues of power/control, and issues with self-esteem are among common rationale given for IPV, as well as modeling learned from the perpetrator's family while growing up.[58]

Child Maltreatment: Child Abuse and Neglect

Child maltreatment is defined as any act or series of acts of commission or omission by a parent or caregiver that results in harm, potential for harm, or threat of harm to a child.[53] **Child abuse** refers to *acts of commission*, or deliberate or intentional words or actions that cause harm, potential harm, or threat of harm to a child. The abuse may be sexual, psychological, physical, or any combination of these. **Neglect** is an *act of omission*, meaning a failure to provide for a child's basic physical, emotional, or education needs or to protect a child from harm or potential harm. Failure to provide food, shelter, clothing, medical care, or supervision or exposing a child to unnecessary environmental violence or threats are examples of neglect. Although exact figures for child abuse are difficult to obtain, in 2011 an estimated 3.4 million cases of child abuse were reported, involving the alleged maltreatment of approximately 6.2 million children (Figure 4.4).[54]

There is no single profile of a child abuser, but the most common perpetrators in general child maltreatment cases are biological parents. Frequently, the perpetrator is a young adult in his or her mid-twenties without a high school diploma; lives at or below the poverty level; is depressed, socially isolated, with a poor self-image; and has difficulty coping with stressful situations. In many instances, the perpetrator has experienced violence and is frustrated by life.

Not all violence against children is physical. Health can be severely affected by psychological violence. The negative consequences of this kind of victimization can include depression, low self-esteem, and a pervasive fear of offending the abuser.

Elder Abuse By 2030, the number of people in the United States over the age of 65 will exceed 71 million—nearly double their number in 2000. As people live longer, the chances they will become vulnerable and need family and community support will increase. Each year, hundreds of thousands of adults over the age of 60 are abused, neglected, or financially exploited as they enter the later years of life, and these statistics are likely an underestimate.[55] Many victims are unable or afraid to report abuse because of embarrassment; fears that the abuser will get in trouble, retaliate by putting them in a nursing home, or the abuse will get worse; or guilt because someone has to take care of them. Others suffer from dementia and may not be aware of the abuse. Today, a variety of social services focus on protecting our seniors in much the same way that we endeavor to protect other vulnerable populations.

Sexual Victimization

The term *sexual victimization* refers to any situation in which an individual is coerced or forced to comply with or endure another's sexual acts or overtures. It can run the gamut from harassment and stalking to assault and rape by perpetrators known or unknown to the victim. It can even include sexual coercion and rape by spouses within the confines of marriage. Sexual victimization and violence can have devastating and far-reaching effects on people of any age.

Sexual Assault and Rape

Sexual assault is any act in which one person is sexually intimate with another person without that person's consent. This may range from simple touching to forceful penetration and may include, for example, ignoring indications that intimacy is not wanted, threatening force or other negative consequences, and actually using force.

Considered to be the most extreme form of sexual assault, **rape** is defined as "penetration without the victim's consent." Incidents of rape generally fall into one of two types—aggravated or simple. An **aggravated rape** is any rape involving one or multiple attackers, strangers, weapons, or physical beatings. A **simple rape** is a rape perpetrated by one person, whom the victim knows, and does not involve a physical beating or use of a weapon. Most rapes are classified as simple rape, but that terminology should not be taken to mean that a simple rape is any less violent or criminal. The FBI ranks rape as the second ranked type of violent crime, trailing only murder.[56] Nearly 1 in 5 women and 1 in 71 men in the United States have been raped at some time in their lives, with nearly 80 percent of female rape victims experiencing their first rape before the age of 25. More than one fourth of male rape victims were raped before they were 10 years old.[57]

By most indicators, reported cases of rape appear to have declined in the United States since the early 1990s, even as reports of

child abuse Deliberate or intentional words or actions that cause harm, potential harm, or threat of harm to a child.

neglect Failure to provide for a child's basic needs such as food, shelter, medical care, and clothing.

sexual assault Any act in which one person is sexually intimate with another person without that person's consent.

rape Sexual penetration without the victim's consent.

aggravated rape Rape that involves one or multiple attackers, strangers, weapons, or physical beating.

simple rape Rape by one person, usually known to the victim, that does not involve a physical beating or use of a weapon.

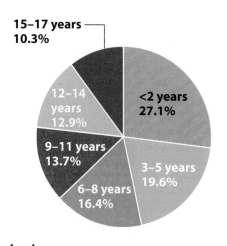

15–17 years 10.3%

12–14 years 12.9%

<2 years 27.1%

9–11 years 13.7%

6–8 years 16.4%

3–5 years 19.6%

FIGURE 4.4 **Child Abuse and Neglect Victims, by Age, 2011**
Source: U.S. Department of Health and Human Services, Administration on Children, Youth and Families, "Child Maltreatment 2011," 2012, www.acf.hhs.gov

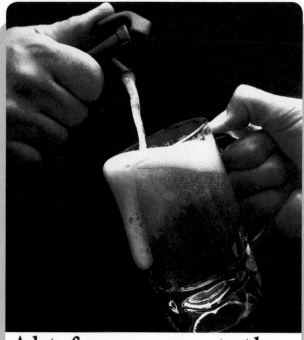

A lot of campus rapes start here.

Whenever there's drinking or drugs, things can get out of hand. So it's no surprise that many campus rapes involve alcohol.

But you should know that under any circumstances, sex without the other person's consent is considered rape. A felony, punishable by prison. And drinking is no excuse.

That's why, when you party, it's good to know what your limits are. You see, a little sobering thought now can save you from a big problem later.

What is meant by *acquaintance* rape?

The term *date rape* used to be applied to sexual assault (coercive, nonconsensual sexual activity) occurring in the context of a dating relationship. However, the term has fallen out of favor because the word *date* implies something reciprocal or arranged, thus minimizing the crime. The term *acquaintance rape* is now more commonly used, referring to any rape in which the rapist is known to the victim, even if only minimally. Acquaintance rape is particularly common on college campuses, where alcohol and drug use can impair young people's judgment and self-control.

acquaintance rape Any rape in which the rapist is known to the victim. A term that replaces the term *date rape*.

other forms of sexual assault have increased. This decline is thought to be due to shifts in public awareness and attitudes about rape, combined with tougher crime policies, major educational campaigns, and media attention. These changes enforce the idea that rape is a violent crime and should be treated as such. However, numerous sources indicate that rape is among one of the most underreported crimes.[58]

Acquaintance Rape

The terms *date rape* and *acquaintance rape* have been used interchangeably in the past. However, most experts now believe that the term *date rape* is inappropriate because it implies a consensual interaction in an arranged setting and may, in fact, minimize the crime of rape when it occurs. Today, **acquaintance rape** refers to

any rape in which the rapist is known to the victim. Acquaintance rape is more common when drugs or alcohol have been consumed by the offender or victim; this makes the campus party environment a high-risk venue for young college women and men.[59]

78% of sexual violence

involves an offender who was a family member, intimate partner, friend, or acquaintance of the victim.

Rape on U.S. Campuses Although rape is a notoriously "underreported" crime, 18 percent of all reported campus crimes were forcible rape.[60] By some estimates, between 20 and 25 percent of college women have experienced an attempted or completed rape in college.[61] The vast majority of rape victims know their attacker and alcohol is frequently involved, as are a growing number of rape-facilitating drugs such as Rohypnol and gamma-hydroxybutyrate (GHB). See the **Skills for Behavior Change** box for more on how to avoid rape-facilitating drugs.

In previous decades, the accuracy of campus reports of sexual assault and rape were highly questionable, with many campuses reporting zero assaults or rapes in a given year. In 1992, Congress passed the Campus Sexual Assault Victim's Bill of Rights, known as the *Ramstad Act,* which allows assault victims to call in nonuniversity authorities

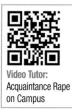

Video Tutor: Acquaintance Rape on Campus

Avoiding Rape-Facilitating Drugs

❯ Do not accept beverages or open-container drinks from anyone you do not know well and trust. At a bar or a club, accept drinks only from the bartender or wait staff.

❯ Never leave a drink or food unattended. If you get up to dance, have someone you trust watch your drink or take it with you.

❯ Go with friends and leave with friends. Never leave a bar or a party with someone you don't know well.

❯ If you think someone slipped something into your drink, tell a friend and have him or her get you to an emergency room.

❯ If a friend seems disproportionately intoxicated in relation to what he or she has had to drink, stay with your friend and watch him or her carefully. Call 9-1-1 if anyone experiences seizures, vomits, passes out, has difficulty breathing, or experiences other complications.

to investigate crime and mandates the reporting of all such crimes; it also requires universities to provide counseling and educational programs to increase student awareness. More recently, this act provides options for victims and notification procedures for accused perpetrators.

Marital Rape Although its legal definition varies within the United States, marital rape can be any unwanted intercourse or penetration (vaginal, anal, or oral) obtained by force, threat of force, or when the spouse is unable to consent. Effectively, if a spouse says "no" to sex, "no" should mean "no," and it is a crime to force sexual acts. This problem has undoubtedly existed since the origin of marriage as a social institution, and it is noteworthy that marital rape did not become a crime in all 50 states until 1993. Even more noteworthy is the fact that many states still allow exemptions from marital rape prosecution, meaning that the judicial system may treat it as a lesser crime.[62]

In general, women under the age of 25 and those from lower socioeconomic groups are at highest risk of marital rape. Internationally, women raised in cultures where male dominance is the norm tend to have higher rates of forced sex within the confines of marriage. Likewise, women from homes where other forms of domestic violence are common and where there is a high rate of alcoholism or substance abuse also tend to be victimized at greater rates.

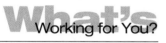
Working for You?

Maybe you already practice some strategies to stay safe in social situations. Which of these are you already incorporating into your life?

☐ When I go to parties, I go with a friend and we look out for each other.

☐ I decide before I go out how much I am going to drink.

☐ I don't leave bars alone with people I've just met.

Child Sexual Abuse

Sexual abuse of children by adults or older children includes sexually suggestive conversations; inappropriate kissing; touching; petting; oral, anal, or vaginal intercourse; and other kinds of sexual interaction. Recent studies indicate that the rates of sexual abuse in children range from 3 to 32 percent of all children, with girls being at greater risk than boys, even though young boys are abused in significant numbers.[63]

Most experts believe that as high as these numbers are, the shroud of secrecy surrounding child sexual abuse makes it very likely the number of actual cases is grossly underestimated. Unfortunately, the programs taught in schools today may give children the false impression that they are more likely to be assaulted by a stranger. In reality, 90 percent of child sexual abuse victims know their perpetrator in some ways, with nearly 70 percent of children abused by family members, usually an adult male.[64]

People who were abused as children bear spiritual, psychological, or physical scars. Studies have shown that child sexual abuse has an impact on later life: Children who experience sexual abuse are at increased risk for anxiety disorders, depression, eating disorders, post-traumatic stress disorder (PTSD), and suicide attempts.[65] Youth who have been sexually abused are 25 percent more likely to experience teen pregnancy, 30 percent more likely to abuse their own children, and they are much more likely to have problems with alcohol abuse or drug addiction.[66]

Sexual Harassment

Sexual harassment is defined as unwelcome sexual conduct that is related to any condition of employment or evaluation of student performance. The victim or harasser may be a woman or a man, and the victim does not have to be of the opposite sex. Unwelcome sexual advances, requests for sexual favors, and other verbal or physical conduct of a sexual nature constitute sexual harassment when:[67]

● Submission to such conduct is made either explicitly or implicitly a term or condition of an individual's employment or education;

● Submission to or rejection of such conduct by an individual is

sexual harassment Any form of unwanted sexual attention related to any condition of employment or performance evaluation.

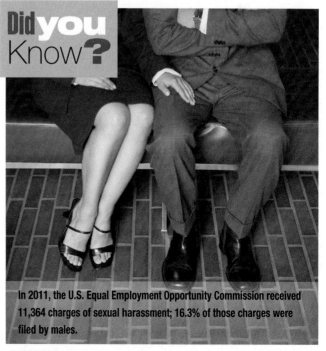

In 2011, the U.S. Equal Employment Opportunity Commission received 11,364 charges of sexual harassment; 16.3% of those charges were filed by males.

Source: Data from The U.S. Equal Employment Opportunity Commission, "Sexual Harassment," February 2013, www.eeoc.gov

used as the basis for employment or education-related decisions affecting such an individual; or

- Such conduct is sufficiently severe or pervasive that it has the effect, intended or unintended, of unreasonably interfering with an individual's work or academic performance because it has created an intimidating, hostile, or offensive environment and would have such an effect on a reasonable person of that individual's status.

Commonly, people think of harassment as involving only faculty members or persons in power, where sex is used to exhibit control of a situation. However, peers can harass one another, too. Sexual harassment may include unwanted touching; unwarranted sex-related comments or subtle pressure for sexual favors; deliberate or repeated humiliation or intimidation based on sex; and gratuitous comments, jokes, questions, photos, or remarks about clothing or bodies, sexuality, or past sexual relationships.

Most schools and companies have sexual harassment policies in place, as well as procedures for dealing with harassment problems. If you feel you are being harassed, the most important thing you can do is to be assertive:

- **Tell the harasser to stop.** Be clear and direct. Tell the person if it continues that you will report it. If harassing is via phone or Internet, block the person.
- **Document the harassment.** If the harassment becomes intolerable, a record of exactly what occurred (and when and where) will help make your case. Save copies of all communication that the harasser sends you.
- **Try to make sure you aren't alone in the harasser's presence.** Witnesses to harassment can ensure appropriate validation of the event.
- **Complain to a higher authority.** Talk to legal authorities or your instructor, adviser, or counseling center psychologist about what happened.
- **Remember that you have not done anything wrong.** You will likely feel awful after being harassed (especially if you have to complain to superiors). However, feel proud that you are standing up for yourself.

what do you think?

What policies does your school have regarding consensual relationships between faculty members and students?

- Should consenting adults have the right to become intimate or interact socially, regardless of their positions within a school system or workplace?
- What are the potential dangers of such interactions? Are there ever situations in which such interactions are okay?

stalking The willful, repeated, and malicious following, harassing, or threatening of another person.

Stalking

The crime of **stalking** can be defined as a course of conduct directed at a specific person that would cause a reasonable person to feel fear. This may include repeated visual or physical proximity, nonconsensual written or verbal communication, and implied or explicit threats.[68] Stalking can even occur online (see the **Tech & Health** box on page 123 about staying safe when using social networking sites). Over 1 in 4 victims report being stalked through the use of some form of technology, such as cell phones, e-mail, instant messaging, electronic monitoring, websites, Global Positioning Systems (GPS), listening devices, and video cameras. The most common stalking behaviors include unwanted phone calls and messages, spreading rumors, spying on the victim, and showing up at the same places as the victim without having a reason to be there.[69] Millions of women and men are stalked annually in the United States, and the vast majority of stalkers are persons involved in relationship breakups or other dating acquaintances; fewer than 10 percent of stalkers are strangers to their victims.[70] Adults between the ages of 18 and 24 experience the highest rates of stalking. Like sexual harassment, stalking is an underreported crime. Often students do not think a stalking incident is serious enough to report, or they worry that the police will not take it seriously.

Social Contributors to Sexual Violence

Sexual violence and intimate partner violence share common factors that increase the likelihood of their occurrence. Certain societal assumptions and traditions can promote sexual violence, including the following:

- **Trivialization.** Many consider rape by a husband or intimate partner not to count or not to be serious.
- **Blaming the victim.** In spite of efforts to combat this type of thinking, there is still the belief that a scantily clad woman "asks" for sexual advances.
- **Pressure to be macho.** Males are taught from a young age that showing emotions is a sign of weakness. This portrayal often depicts men as aggressive and predatory and females as passive targets.
- **Male socialization.** Many still believe that ideas like "sowing wild oats" and "boys will be boys" are merely normal parts of development to adulthood in males. Women are often *objectified*, or treated as sexual objects in the media, which contributes to the idea that it's only natural for men to be predatory.
- **Male misperceptions.** With media implying that sex is the focus of life, it's not surprising that some men believe that when a woman says no, she is really asking to be seduced. Later, these same men may be surprised when the woman says she was raped.
- **Situational factors.** Dates in which the male makes all the decisions, pays for everything, and generally controls the entire situation are more likely to end in an aggressive sexual scenario. Alcohol and other drugs also increase the risk and severity of assaults.

Tech & Health

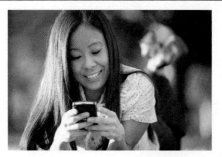

IDENTITY THEFT, INTERNET VICTIMIZATION, AND SOCIAL NETWORKING SAFETY

At any given time, millions of people are chatting away on social networking sites with friends, family, and strangers, posting photos and personal information that may be available to people they barely know. Others have outdated or inadequate anti-malware and security software that leaves them vulnerable to a wide range of intrusions. Even those who secure their home computer systems may face major invasions of privacy as they bank, use credit or debit cards, or use unprotected cell phones and other devices. As we use our latest devices, predators lie in wait, ready to steal our identity and engage in crimes. Consider the following:

✳ A first-year student at Virginia Commonwealth University was murdered by someone she met on MySpace.
✳ A student at the University of Kansas learned the consequences of revealing too much information on Facebook when she was stalked by a man who accessed her class schedule online.
✳ More than 11.5 million Americans became victims of identity fraud in 2011, a disappointing 12.6 percent increase after a dramatic decline in 2010.
✳ The highest identify fraud rate was among LinkedIn users, 10.1 percent of whom had their identities stolen. Google+ users came in second, with a fraud rate of 7 percent, followed by Twitter and Facebook users, who suffered higher average rates of fraud than the 4.9 percent experienced by all consumers nationally.
✳ Identity fraud was also significantly higher among people who checked into

To stay safe online, think before you tweet.

social media sites using the GPS function on their mobile devices and people who clicked on new applications.
✳ The largest groups of identity theft victims were aged 20 to 29, followed by those 30 to 39.

Although very real threats to health, reputation, financial security, and future employment lie in wait for those who post indiscriminately and unwisely to the Web, social networking sites can be used safely. To reduce your risks of *identity theft* (unauthorized access to personal information without explicit permission) or *identity fraud* (misuse of personal information for illicit financial or material gain) and safely enjoy the benefits of social networking sites, personal devices, and other activities, practice a little caution and use some common sense. The following tips will help you to remain safe, protect your identity, and feel free to express yourself without fear of repercussions:

✳ Don't post anything on the Web that you wouldn't want someone to pick out of your trash can and read. Your address,

phone numbers, banking information, calendar, family secrets, and other information should be kept off the sites. Invest in high-quality security software, make sure it is up to date, and run scans regularly.
✳ Don't post compromising pictures, videos, or other things that you wouldn't want your mother or coworkers to see.
✳ Never meet a stranger in person whom you've met only online without bringing a trusted friend along, or at the very least, notifying a close friend of where you will be and when you will return. Choose a well-established, public place to meet during daylight hours, and arrange a ride home with a friend in advance. Don't give your address or traceable phone numbers to the person you are meeting.
✳ Shred personal information with a micro-shredder. Protect your social security or student identification number. Don't write your ID numbers on checks or other places where others could get them.
✳ Change your passwords and security questions often, and don't give them to your friends.
✳ Avoid doing banking or accessing sensitive personal financial documents when using public WiFi servers. Make sure your cell phone is not posting your location publicly. Knowing that you are somewhere other than your home at night or during the day can be an open invitation for others to enter your home.

Sources: 2012 NCVRW Resource Guide, "Internet Victimization," February 2013, Available at www.ncjrs.gov; Javelin Strategy and Research, "2011 Identity Fraud Survey Report: Identity Fraud Decreases But Remaining Frauds Cost Consumers More Time & Money," 2012, www.javelinstrategy .com

Minimize Your Risk of Becoming a Victim of Violence

It is far better to prevent a violent act than to recover from it. Both individuals and communities can play important roles in the prevention of violence and intentional injuries.

Self-Defense against Personal Assault and Rape

Assault can occur no matter what preventive actions you take, but commonsense self-defense tactics can lower the risk. Self-defense is a process that includes increasing your awareness, developing self-defense skills, taking reasonable precautions, and having the judgment necessary to respond to different situations. It is important to know ways to avoid

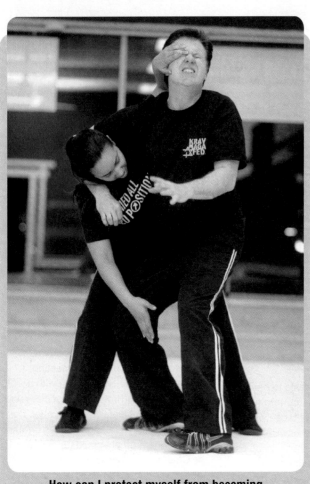

How can I protect myself from becoming a victim of violence?

Safety workshops and self-defense classes can arm students with physical and mental skills that may help them repel or deter an assailant.

Skills for Behavior Change

Reducing Your Risk of Dating Violence

Remember that if a romantic partner truly cares for you and respects you, that person will respect your wishes and feelings. Here are some tips for dealing with sexual pressure or unwanted advances when dating and socializing:

❭ Prior to your date, think about your values, and set personal boundaries before you walk out the door.
❭ Set limits. Practice what you will say to your date if things go in an uncomfortable direction. If the situation feels like it is getting out of control, stop and talk, say no directly, and don't be coy or worry about hurting feelings. Be firm.
❭ Watch your alcohol consumption. Drinking might get you into situations you could otherwise avoid.
❭ Pay attention to your date's actions. If there is too much teasing, if there is a tendency to keep you from doing things with friends, and if all the decisions are made for you, it may mean trouble. Trust your intuition.
❭ Go out in groups when dating someone new.
❭ Stick with your friends. Agree to keep an eye out for one another at parties, and have a plan for leaving together and checking in with each other. Never leave a bar or party alone with a stranger.

and extract yourself from potentially dangerous situations. The **Skills for Behavior Change** box identifies practical tips for preventing dating violence.

Most attacks by unknown assailants are planned in advance. Many rapists use certain ploys to initiate their attacks. Examples include asking for help, offering help, staging a deliberate "accident" such as bumping into you, or posing as a police officer or other authority figure. Sexual assault frequently begins with a casual, friendly conversation.

Trust your intuition. Be assertive and direct to someone who is getting out of line or threatening—this may convince the would-be rapist or attacker to back off. Don't try to be nice, and don't fear making a scene. Use the following tips to let a potential assailant know that you are prepared to defend yourself:

● **Speak in a strong voice.** State, "Leave me alone" rather than, "Will you please leave me alone?" Avoid apologies and excuses. Sound like you mean it.

● **Maintain eye contact.** This keeps you aware of the person's movements and conveys an aura of strength and confidence.
● **Stand up straight, act confident, and remain alert.** Walk as though you own the sidewalk.

If you are attacked, act immediately. Draw attention to yourself and your assailant. Scream, "Fire!" loudly. Research has shown that passersby are much more likely to help if they hear the word *fire* rather than just a scream.

What to Do if Rape Occurs

If you are a rape victim, report the attack. This can give you a sense of control. Follow these steps:

● Call 9-1-1.
● Do not bathe, shower, douche, clean up, or touch anything the attacker may have touched.
● Save the clothes you were wearing, and do not launder them. They will be needed as evidence. Bring a clean change of clothes to the clinic or hospital.
● Contact the rape assistance hotline in your area, and ask for advice on therapists or counseling if you need additional help.

If a friend is raped, here's how you can help:

- Believe her, and don't ask questions that may appear to implicate her in the assault.
- Recognize that rape is a violent act and that the victim was not looking for this to happen.
- Encourage your friend to see a doctor immediately because she may have medical needs but feel too embarrassed to seek help on her own. Offer to go with her.
- Encourage her to report the crime.
- Be understanding, and let her know you will be there for her.
- Recognize that this is an emotional recovery, and it may take time for her to bounce back.
- Encourage your friend to seek counseling.

Campuswide Responses to Violence

Increasingly, campuses have become microcosms of the greater society, complete with the risks, hazards, and dangers that people face in the world. Many college administrators have been proactive in establishing violence-prevention policies, programs, and services. They have also begun to examine the aspects of campus culture that promote and tolerate violent acts.[71]

Prevention and Early Response Efforts

Campuses are conducting emergency response drills and reviewing the effectiveness of emergency messaging systems via e-mail, text message, and other mobile alerts. The REVERSE 9-1-1 system uses database and mapping technologies to notify campus police and community members in the event of problems, and other systems allow campus administrators to send out alerts in text, voice, e-mail, or instant message format. Some schools program the phone numbers, photographs, and basic student information for all incoming first-year students into a university security system so that in the event of a threat students need only hit a button on their phones, whereupon campus police will be notified and tracking devices will pinpoint their location.

Changes in the Campus Environment There are many changes to the campus environment that can improve safety. Campus lighting, parking lot security, call boxes for emergencies, removal of overgrown shrubbery along bike paths and walking trails, and stepped-up security are increasingly on the radar of campus safety personnel. Buildings can be designed with better lighting and more security provisions, and security cameras can be installed in hallways, in classrooms, and in public places throughout campus. Safe rides are often provided for students who have consumed too much alcohol; and health promotion

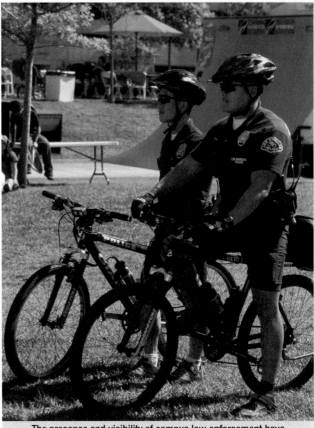

The presence and visibility of campus law enforcement have increased in recent years.

programs can step up their violence prevention efforts through seminars on acquaintance rape, sexual assault, harassment, and other topics.

Campus Law Enforcement Campus law enforcement has changed over the years by increasing both numbers of its members and its authority to prosecute student offenders. Campus police are responsible for emergency responses, and they have the power to enforce laws with students in the same way they are handled in the general community. In fact, many campuses now hire state troopers or local law enforcement officers to deal with campus issues rather than maintain a separate police staff.

Coping in the Event of Campus Violence Although schools have worked tirelessly to implement plans for preventing violence, it can and does still occur. In its aftermath, some may find it difficult to remain on campus because it represents a place of violation and lack of safety; others may experience problems with concentration, studying, and other essential activities. Although there is no easy "fix," several strategies can be helpful for coping with traumatic events. First, members of the campus community should be allowed to mourn. Memorial services and acknowledgment of grief, fear, anger, and other emotions are critical to healing. Secondly, students, faculty, and staff should be involved in planning for prevention of future problems—it can help them feel

what do you think?

What types of safety and violence response resources are available to you on your campus?

● Does your school have a system for sending campus alerts to all students?

● Does it have an emergency plan in the event of a threat to students?

like they have some control. Once a prevention plan is in place, the school should be sure to educate all members of the campus community on what it is. Third, students should seek out support groups, therapists who specialize in PTSD, and trusted family or friends if they need to talk and work through their feelings. Journaling or writing about feelings can also help.

Community Strategies for Preventing Violence

There are many steps you can take to ensure your own personal safety (see the **Skills for Behavior Change** box). However, it is also necessary to address the issues of violence and safety on a community level. Because the factors that contribute to violence are complex and interrelated, community strategies for prevention must also be multidimensional, focusing on individuals, schools, families, communities, policies, programs, and services designed to reduce risk. Violence-prevention strategies recommended by the CDC's Injury Response initiatives are as follows:

● Inoculate children against violence in the home. Youth exposed to physical and emotional abuse in their families are much more likely to victimize others. Teaching youth principles of respect and responsibility are fundamental to the health and well-being of future generations.

● Develop policies and laws that prevent violence.

● Develop skills-based educational programs teaching basics of interpersonal communication, parenting skills, dating behavior, elements of healthy relationships, anger management, conflict resolution, peaceful negotiation, appropriate assertiveness, healthy coping, stress management, and other health-based behaviors.

● Begin early and through families, schools, community programs, athletics, music, faith-based groups, or wherever feasible, provide experiences that help youth develop self-esteem and confidence (self-efficacy).

● Promote tolerance and acceptance, and establish and enforce policies that forbid discrimination.

● Improve community services focused on family planning, mental health services, day care and respite care, alcohol, and substance abuse prevention.

● Improve community-based support and treatment for victims. Ensure that support services are available and that individuals have choices available when trying to stop the violence in their lives.

Stay Safe on All Fronts

Follow these tips to protect yourself from assault.

OUTSIDE ALONE

❱ Carry a cell phone, but stay off it. Be aware of what is happening around you.

❱ If you are being followed, don't go home. Head for a location where there are other people. If you decide to run, run fast and scream loudly to attract attention.

❱ Vary your routes. Stay close to others.

❱ Park near lights; avoid dark areas where people could hide.

❱ Carry pepper spray or other deterrents. Consider using your campus escort service.

❱ Tell others where you are going and when you expect to be back.

IN YOUR CAR

❱ Lock your doors. Do not open your doors or windows to strangers.

❱ If someone hits you while you are driving, drive to the nearest gas station or other public place. Call the police or road service for help, and stay in your car until help comes.

IN YOUR HOME

❱ Install dead bolts on all doors and locks on all windows. Make sure the locks work, and don't leave a spare key outside.

❱ Lock doors when at home, even during the day. Close blinds and drapes whenever you are away and in the evening when you are home.

❱ Rent apartments that require a security code or clearance to gain entry, and avoid easily accessible apartments, such as first-floor units.

❱ Don't let repair people in without asking for their identification, and have someone else with you when repairs are being made in your home or apartment.

❱ Keep a cell phone near your bed and program it to dial 9-1-1.

❱ If you return home to find your residence has been broken into, don't enter. Call the police. If you encounter an intruder, it is better to give up your money than to fight.

Unintentional Injuries

As stated at the beginning of the chapter, unintentional injuries occur without planning or intention to harm. How big of a problem is unintentional injury? For Americans aged 15 to 44, unintentional injuries are the leading cause of death, killing approximately 40,000 people in the prime of life.[72] In fact, unintentional injuries are responsible for about 28 percent of

TRAUMATIC BRAIN INJURY: YOUNG ADULTS AT HIGH RISK

Lately you can't miss it in the news: Another story of a former NFL player suffering the effects of repeated bashings to the head in the crushing tackles that make up football. What those players are experiencing are the cumulative effects of traumatic brain injuries (TBIs). But don't think TBIs are solely the concern of professional athletes. The most common source of TBIs is falling, but motor vehicle accidents, skiing, and skateboarding are responsible for many as well. Approximately 1.7 million people sustain a TBI each year, and 52,000 of them die. TBIs contribute to a third of all injury deaths in the United States, and young adults are at particularly high risk for them.

TBIs are caused by bumps or blows to the head or by a penetrating head injury. Injuries of this type cause the brain to move or twist in the skull, damaging brain cells, causing unhealthy chemical changes, and disrupting the normal function of the brain. TBIs can range from mild to severe, and fortunately about 75 percent of TBIs are considered mild. One common example of a mild TBI is a concussion. Males aged 0 to 4 years have the highest rates of TBI-related emergency department visits, hospitalizations, and deaths.

TBIs can affect a variety of brain functions. Memory, reasoning, perception of sensations like taste and smell, communication, language comprehension, and emotional responses and regulation can all be compromised. The risks for Alzheimer's and Parkinson's diseases, as well as epilepsy and other brain disorders, can be increased in someone who has suffered a TBI. Once someone has sustained a TBI, they are at an increased risk of suffering another one. Repeated mild TBIs can be especially damaging or even fatal if they occur in a short amount of time.

It's important that TBIs be treated by a doctor, but prevention is the best medicine. How can you protect yourself?

✳ Always wear your seat belt, even for short trips.
✳ Wear bike and motorcycle helmets whenever riding, even if your state does not require them.

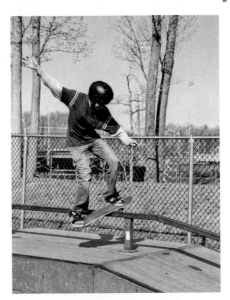

Skateboarding without a helmet? You're at prime risk for a TBI.

✳ Drink in moderation. Injuries are less likely when you have full control of your body.
✳ Use common sense in all contact and recreational sports. Follow rules for head contact. Wear a helmet whenever a fall is a possibility. Never wear head protection devices that are cracked, brittle, or don't fit your head correctly.
✳ Avoid falls at home by using stepladders, handrails, nonslip mats in the bathtub, and removing tripping hazards like loose electrical cords.

Source: Centers for Disease Control and Prevention, "Traumatic Brain Injury," Updated March 2013. www.cdc.gov

---

all deaths in this age group.[73] Most efforts to prevent unintentional injuries focus on changing personal behaviors, the environment, or the circumstances (policies, procedures) that put people in harm's way.

Two types of accidents that cause numerous deaths and unintentional injuries every year are motor vehicle crashes and cycling incidents. Motor vehicles account for most unintentional injury deaths; in 2010 alone, they caused nearly 33,000 deaths and 2.4 million serious injuries.[74] (See the **Health Headlines: Traumatic Brain Injury** box for more on head injuries.) Bicycle injuries account for more than 500,000 emergency room visits every year, most of them in younger adults. If you drive a car or ride a bicycle, you must be aware of what causes accidents and how to ensure your safety.

Vehicle Safety

According to the National Safety Council, the most common contributing factors to motor vehicle accidents are *impaired driving, distracted driving, speeding, driver age,* and *vehicle safety issues.* Being a new, younger driver or an older driver increases risk of accidents. While we cannot change our age, the rest of the factors are mostly within personal control.

Impaired Driving Nearly 32 percent of all motor vehicle accident (MVA) fatalities are due to alcohol impairment, and over 60 percent of those deaths involve drivers aged 21–34.[75] Alcohol is not the only cause of **impaired driving;** drugs and even severe sleep deprivation claim many lives each year, too.

impaired driving Driving under the influence of alcohol or other drugs.

Distracted Driving **Distracted driving** includes using a cell phone, texting, sending e-mails, searching for songs on your iPod or radio, eating your lunch, putting on makeup, fixing your hair, studying, using navigation systems, chatting with passengers, or any other type of distracting activity while simultaneously operating a vehicle. The best way to prevent crashes is to avoid distracted or impaired driving, practice risk-management driving, and learn accident-avoidance techniques. See the **Points of View** box on page 129 for more on the debate surrounding distracted driving.

Risk-Management Driving
Risk-management driving techniques reduce the chances of being involved in a collision:

- Don't use electronic devices while driving, even a hands-free cell phone.
- Don't drink and drive. Take a taxi or arrange for someone to be the "designated driver."
- Pay attention to prescription and OTC medication labels that caution against drinking when using them because they may cause drowsiness.
- Don't drive when tired, highly emotional, or highly stressed.
- Never tailgate. The rear bumper of the car ahead of you should be at least 3 seconds worth of distance away, making stopping safely possible.
- Scan the road ahead of you and to both sides.
- Drive with your low-beam headlights on *day and night* to make your car more visible.
- Drive defensively. Be on the alert for unsignaled lane changes, sudden braking, or other unexpected maneuvers.
- Obey all traffic laws.
- Secure your pet in a safe kennel or safety seat to avoid distractions.
- Preplan your navigation so you don't have to deal with GPS or maps while driving.
- If you get a call or text, pull over, respond later, or ask a passenger to handle it for you.
- Whether you are the driver or a passenger, always wear a seat belt.

Accident-Avoidance Techniques
To avoid a serious accident, you may need to steer into another, less severe collision. Here are the Automobile Association of America's (AAA) rules for accident avoidance:

- Generally, veer to the right.
- Steer, don't skid, off the road to avoid rolling your vehicle.
- If you have to hit a vehicle, hit one moving in the same direction as your own.
- If you have to hit a stationary object, try to hit a soft one (bushes, small trees) rather than a hard one (boulders, brick walls, giant trees).
- If you have to hit a hard object, hit it with a glancing blow.
- Avoid hitting pedestrians, motorcyclists, and bicyclists at all costs.

Cycling Safety

The National Highway Traffic Safety Administration (NHTSA) reports over 620 cyclist fatalities per year and over 52,000 injuries.[76] Most fatal collisions are caused by cyclists' errors, usually failure to yield at intersections. However, alcohol also plays a significant role in bicycle deaths and injuries: In 2010 more than one third of cyclist fatalities involved alcohol, either in the cyclist or the driver of the vehicle that hit them.[77] To avoid accidents, cyclists should avoid alcohol, follow the rules of the road, ride with the flow of traffic, wear reflective clothing, know proper hand signals, avoid using a cell phone or listening to music while riding, and most importantly, wear a bike helmet.

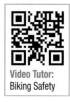

Video Tutor:
Biking Safety

Bike Helmets There are very good reasons why you should wear a helmet every time you ride: Even a low-speed fall on a bicycle path can cause a serious injury, and wearing a helmet is the single most effective way to prevent a head injury in a bike crash, according to the NHTSA. Seventy percent of bicyclists killed in 2010 reportedly were not wearing helmets.[78]

You can buy an effective helmet by doing the following:

- Buy a helmet that has the Consumer Product Safety Commission (CPSC) safety sticker and reflective decals.
- Forego wild or unusually shaped helmets, dark-colored helmets, or helmets with straps that are flimsy or have limited adjustments.
- Buy a helmet that fits snugly on your head, doesn't rock side-to-side, and sits low on your forehead (1–2 finger widths above eyebrows).
- Read "Buyer's Guide to Bicycle Helmets," updated regularly at www.helmets.org for the latest information on helmet ratings.

Banning Phone Use While Driving:
GOOD IDEA OR GOING TOO FAR?

Okay, 'fess up: How often in recent history have you chatted on the phone while driving, tried to read a text message, or switched the music on your iPod? For many of us, that answer is more than once. In fact, texting drivers make up 31 percent of drivers aged 16–24, 41 percent of drivers aged 25–39, and 5 percent of drivers 55 and older. In addition, 70 percent of all drivers report talking on their cell phones regularly while driving. So, what's the problem? The fact is that driving while distracted by cell phones is deadly. In 2011, 3,331 people were killed and an estimated 387,000 were injured in crashes that were reported to involve distracted driving.

Recognizing that increased reliance on cell phones could be contributing to motor vehicle accidents, state and federal officials are beginning to enact laws that restrict their use. Thirty-nine states ban texting while driving, 10 states ban the use of handheld phones completely but allow hands-free phone calls, and 33 states ban all phone use for novice drivers. All laws are primary enforcement, meaning that an officer may cite a driver for handheld use without any other traffic offenses. Are these laws worth the effort, or are they going too far?

Arguments Favoring Banning Cell Phone Use While Driving:

○ Other laws to improve public safety while driving, such as laws against drunk driving or mandating seat belt use, have saved millions of lives. Cell phone bans could do the same.

○ Statistics have shown that texting while driving is about six times more likely to result in an accident than driving while intoxicated, and drivers who use handheld devices are four times as likely to get into crashes resulting in injury than those who do not use them. Headset cell phone use is not substantially safer than handheld use.

Arguments Opposing Banning Cell Phone Use While Driving:

○ Although distracted driving from phone calls and texting is a problem, there are many other distractions that are just as serious: talking with passengers, eating, working a GPS device, putting on makeup, changing the radio station, and more. Why ban cell phones without banning the others?

○ These laws will be difficult to enforce and will spend tax dollars that might be better spent improving traffic safety in other ways.

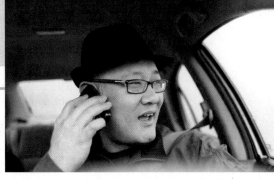

Where Do You Stand?

○ Do you currently use a cell phone while driving? Do you text/tweet while driving? If so, would a law make you stop? Even if it wasn't made illegal, would you or could you stop?

○ Do you think cell phone use while driving should be banned? If so, all forms or only certain things like texting? Why?

○ Do you agree with the states that have banned cell phone use for novice drivers but allow it for more experienced ones? Do you think you can become experienced enough to use a cell phone safely while driving?

○ What about other distractions? Do you personally think they are as dangerous as cell phone use? Why or why not? How could you avoid getting distracted while driving?

Sources: Governors Highway Safety Association, "Cell Phone and Texting Laws," February 2013, www.ghsa.org; U.S. Department of Transportation, "Statistics and Facts about Distracted Driving," February 2013, www.distraction.gov; M. Reardon, "Study: Distractions, Not Phones, Cause Car Crashes" in CNET.com Signal Strength, January 29, 2010, http://news.cnet.com

Are You at Risk for Violence or Injury?

How often are you at risk for sustaining an intentional or unintentional injury? Answer the questions below to find out.

1 Relationship Risk

How often does your partner:

	Never	Sometimes	Often
1. Criticize you for your appearance (weight, dress, hair, etc.)?	○	○	○
2. Embarrass you in front of others by putting you down?	○	○	○
3. Blame you or others for his or her mistakes?	○	○	○
4. Curse at you, shout at you, say mean things, insult, or mock you?	○	○	○
5. Demonstrate uncontrollable anger?	○	○	○
6. Criticize your friends, family, or others who are close to you?	○	○	○
7. Threaten to leave you if you don't behave in a certain way?	○	○	○
8. Manipulate you to prevent you from spending time with friends or family?	○	○	○
9. Express jealousy, distrust, and anger when you spend time with other people?	○	○	○
10. Make all the significant decisions in your relationship?	○	○	○
11. Intimidate or threaten you, making you fearful or anxious?	○	○	○
12. Make threats to harm others you care about, including pets?	○	○	○
13. Control your telephone calls, monitor your messages, or read your e-mail without permission?	○	○	○
14. Punch, hit, slap, or kick you?	○	○	○
15. Make you feel guilty about something?	○	○	○
16. Use money or possessions to control you?	○	○	○
17. Force you to perform sexual acts that make you uncomfortable or embarrassed?	○	○	○
18. Threaten to kill himself or herself if you leave?	○	○	○
19. Follow you, call to check on you, or demonstrate a constant obsession with what you are doing?	○	○	○

2 Risk for Assault or Rape

How often do you:

	Never	Sometimes	Often
1. Drink more than one or two drinks while out with friends or at a party?	○	○	○
2. Leave your drink unattended while you get up to dance or go to the bathroom?	○	○	○
3. Accept drinks from strangers while out at a bar or party?	○	○	○
4. Leave parties with people you barely know or just met?	○	○	○
5. Walk alone in poorly lit or unfamiliar places?	○	○	○
6. Open the door to strangers?	○	○	○
7. Leave your car or home door unlocked?	○	○	○
8. Talk on your cell phone, oblivious to your surroundings?	○	○	○

3 Risk for Vehicular Injuries

How often do you:

	Never	Sometimes	Often
1. Drive after you have had one or two drinks?	○	○	○
2. Drive after you have had three or more drinks?	○	○	○
3. Drive when you are tired?	○	○	○
4. Drive while you are extremely upset?	○	○	○
5. Drive while using your cell phone?	○	○	○
6. Drive or ride in a car while not wearing a seat belt?	○	○	○
7. Drive faster than the speed limit?	○	○	○
8. Accept rides from friends who have been drinking?	○	○	○

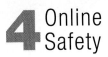

Online Safety

How often do you:

	Never	Sometimes	Often
1. Give out your name or address on the Internet?	○	○	○
2. Put personal identifying information on your blog, Facebook, or other websites?	○	○	○
3. Post personal pictures, travel/vacation plans, and other private material on social networking sites?	○	○	○
4. Date people you meet online?	○	○	○
5. Use a shared or public computer to check e-mail without clearing the browser cache?	○	○	○
6. Make financial transactions online without confirming security measures?	○	○	○

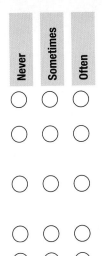

Analyzing Your Responses

Look at your responses to the list of questions in each of these sections. Part 1 focused on relationships—if you answered "sometimes" or "often" to several of these questions, you may need to evaluate your situation. In Parts 2 through 4, if you answered "often" to any question, you may need to take action to ensure that you stay safe.

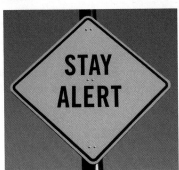

YOUR PLAN FOR CHANGE

The **Assessyourself** activity gave you a chance to consider symptoms of abuse in your relationships and signs of unsafe behavior in other realms of your life. Now that you are aware of these signs and symptoms, you can work on changing behaviors to reduce your risk.

Today, you can:

○ Pay attention as you walk your normal route around campus, and think about whether you are taking the safest route. Is it well lit? Do you walk in areas that receive little foot traffic? Are there any emergency phone boxes along your route? Does campus security patrol the area? If part of your route seems unsafe, look around for alternate routes. Vary your route when possible.

○ Look at your residence's safety features. Is there a secure lock, dead bolt, or keycard entry system on all outer doors? Can

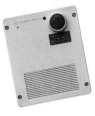

windows be shut and locked? Is there a working smoke alarm in every room and hallway? Are the outside areas well lit? If you live in a dorm or apartment building, is there a security guard at the main entrance? If you notice any potential safety hazards, report them to your landlord or campus residential life administrator right away.

Within the next 2 weeks, you can:

○ If you are worried about potentially abusive behavior in a partner or in a friend's partner, visit the campus counseling center and ask about resources on campus or in your community to help you deal with potential relationship abuse. Consider talking to a counselor

about your concerns or sitting in on a support group.

○ Next time you go out to a bar or a party, set limits for yourself in order to avoid putting yourself in a dangerous or compromising position. Decide ahead of time on the number of drinks you will have, arrange with a friend to look out for each other during the party, and be sure you have a reliable, safe way of getting home.

By the end of the semester, you can:

○ Learn ways to protect yourself by signing up for a self-defense workshop or violence prevention class.

○ Get involved in an on-campus or community group dedicated to promoting safety. You might want to attend a meeting of an antiviolence group, join in a Take Back the Night rally, or volunteer at a local rape crisis center or battered women's shelter.

MasteringHealth™

Build your knowledge—and health!—in the Study Area of MasteringHealth with a variety of study tools.

Summary

* Violence in the form of intentional and unintentional injuries continues to be a major problem in the United States today. Intentional injuries result from actions committed with the intent to do harm.

* Violence affects everyone in society—from direct victims, to children and families who witness it, to those who modify their behaviors because they are fearful. Shootings and acts of violence on campuses have resulted in a groundswell of activities designed to protect students.

* Factors that lead to violence include poverty, unemployment, parental influences, cultural beliefs, discrimination or oppression, religious or political differences, breakdowns in the criminal justice system, stress, and heavy substance use. Anger and substance abuse can contribute to patterns of violence and aggression in individuals.

* Hate crimes divide people, but examining personal biases and taking time to get to know other groups of people will help foster tolerance, understanding, and respect. Gang violence continues to rise, nationally and internationally, but efforts to reduce gang membership, improve enforcement, and increase penalties for gang activities can help reduce risks.

* Most sexual victimization crimes are committed by someone the victim already knows and includes unwanted touching, stalking, harassment, rape, and child sexual abuse. Recognizing how to protect yourself and your loved ones; knowing where to turn for help; and having honest, straightforward dialogue about sexual matters in dating situations are sound strategies to reduce risk.

* Preventing violence is a public health priority. It means community activism, prioritizing mental and emotional health, providing services to people in trouble, alcohol and drug abuse prevention, and providing behavioral skills training.

* Unintentional injuries, particularly motor vehicle injuries, continue to be a leading cause of death for people aged 15–44. Impaired driving and distracted driving are key contributors to vehicular deaths and injuries.

* To avoid unintentional injuries, focus on personal protection (wear seat belts, bike helmets, and pay attention to threats).

Pop Quiz

1. _____ is an example of an *intentional injury*.
   a. A car accident
   b. Murder
   c. Accidental drowning
   d. A traumatic brain injury from not wearing a bicycle helmet

2. Which of the following is not an underlying contributor or cause of violence?
   a. Cultural, religious, or political differences
   b. Poverty and unemployment
   c. Lack of education
   d. Alcohol or drug abuse

3. Domestic violence includes all of the following except:
   a. marital rape.
   b. threats.
   c. physical violence.
   d. infidelity.

4. Psychologist Lenore Walker developed a theory known as the
   a. aggression cycle.
   b. sexual harassment cycle.
   c. cycle of child abuse.
   d. cycle of violence.

5. Jack beats his wife Melissa "to teach her a lesson." Afterward, he denies attacking her. The phase of the cycle of violence that this illustrates is
   a. acute battering.
   b. chronic battering.
   c. remorse/reconciliation.
   d. tension building.

6. Rape by a person known to the victim that does not involve a physical beating or use of a weapon is called
   a. simple rape.
   b. sexual assault.
   c. simple assault.
   d. aggravated rape.

7. Jane rejected a sexual advance by her supervisor. Three weeks later he gave her a negative performance evaluation and told her if she went on a date with him he would change it. His actions constitute:
   a. no problematic behavior.
   b. sexual assault.
   c. sexual harassment.
   d. sexual battering.

8. Which of the following is an example of stalking?
   a. Making intimate and personal sexually charged comments to another person
   b. Repeated visual or physical seeking out of another person
   c. An unwelcome sexual conduct by the perpetrator
   d. Sexual abuse upon a child

9. In a sociology class, a group of students was discussing sexual assault. One student commented that some women dress too provocatively. The social assumption this student made is
   a. minimization.
   b. trivialization.
   c. blaming the victim.
   d. male socialization.

10. What is the leading cause of death for persons aged 15–44 in the United States?
    a. Homicide
    b. Heart disease/CVD
    c. Motor vehicle accidents
    d. Suicide

Answers to these questions can be found on page A-1.

Think about It!

1. What forms of violence do you think are most significant or prevalent in the United States today? Why?
2. What type of violence is most common on your campus? How do you think campus violence affects students at your school? Are there differences in how men and women respond to news that there has been a rape or violent assault on campus? If so, why?
3. Why do some people develop into violent or abusive adults and others become pacifists or peaceful adults? What key factors influence violent offenders to be violent?
4. What actions need to be taken to stem the tide of violence in the United States at the individual level? At the community level? In schools? On college campuses? Nationally?
5. Think about an unintentional injury that affected you. What led up to it? What could have been done to prevent it? How much control did you have over the situation and how much was it affected by others?

Accessing Your Health on the Internet

The following websites explore further topics and issues related to personal health. For links to the websites below, visit the Study Area in MasteringHealth.

1. *Centers for Disease Control and Prevention: National Center for Injury Prevention and Control (NCIPC).* Key national resource for a wide range of topics and resources about violence. Also includes the latest information from the National Intimate Partner and Sexual Violence Survey. www.cdc.gov/violenceprevention

2. *United Nations, "Ending Violence against Women and Girls."* International website for information about global violence against women and girls. Includes resources for speakers and videos focused on issues surrounding global violence. www.un.org/en/globalissues/briefingpapers/endviol/index.shtml

3. *Men Can Stop Rape.* Practical suggestions and training for men interested in helping to protect women from sexual predators and assault. www.mencanstoprape.org

4. *National Center for Victims of Crime.* Provides information and resources to help victims of violence rebuild their lives and cope with the aftermath of crime. www.victimsofcrime.org

5. *National Sexual Violence Resource Center.* An excellent resource for victims of sexual violence, including e-learning opportunities for those interested in prevention. www.nsvrc.org

5 Building Healthy Relationships and Understanding Sexuality

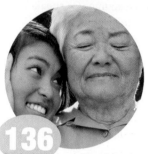

136

Do intimate relationships have to be sexual?

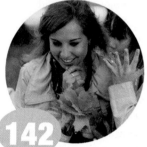

142

To what extent do people communicate without words?

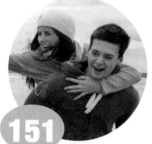

151

What influences sexual identity besides biology?

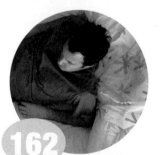

162

Are sexual disorders more physical or more psychological?

LEARNING OUTCOMES

✻ Identify characteristics of successful relationships, including how to maintain them and overcome common barriers.

✻ Discuss ways to improve communication skills and interpersonal interactions.

✻ Compare and contrast the different types of committed relationships.

✻ Describe the demographic trends related to remaining single.

✻ Examine the factors that affect the decision of when or whether to have children.

✻ Discuss issues that influence the success of an intimate relationship, reasons why relationships end, and how to cope when they do.

✻ Define *sexual identity,* and discuss its major components, including biology, gender identity, gender roles, and sexual orientation.

✻ Identify major features and functions of sexual anatomy and physiology and explain the nature of the human sexual response.

✻ Describe the varieties of sexual expression.

✻ Classify sexual dysfunctions, and describe major disorders.

✻ Discuss the impact of drugs on sexual behavior.

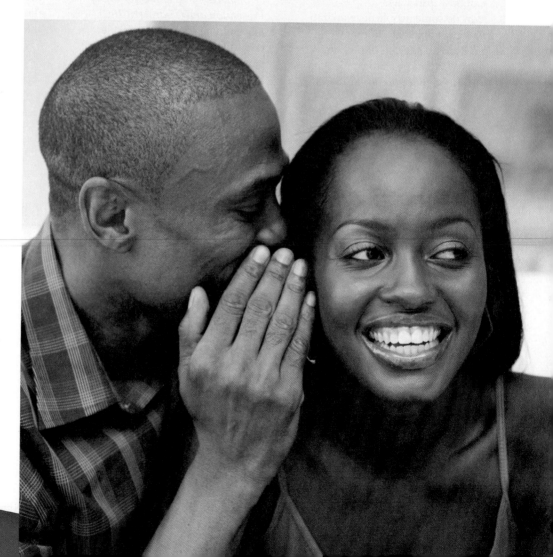

Humans are social beings—we have a basic need to belong and to feel loved, accepted, and wanted. We can't thrive without relating to and interacting with others in some way. In fact, numerous studies have shown that having supportive interpersonal relationships is beneficial to health.[1]

All relationships involve a degree of risk. However, only by taking these risks can we grow and truly experience all that life has to offer. In this chapter, we examine healthy relationships and the communication skills necessary to maintain them. We also explore sexual identity, gender roles, and sexual orientation—key aspects of our identity—which help us better understand who we are.

Intimate Relationships

We can define **intimate relationships** in terms of four characteristics: behavioral interdependence, need fulfillment, emotional attachment, and emotional availability. Each of these characteristics may be related to interactions with family, close friends, and romantic partners.

Behavioral interdependence refers to the mutual impact that people have on each other as their lives and daily activities intertwine. What one person does influences what the other person wants to do and can do. Behavioral interdependence may become stronger over time to the point that each person would feel a great void if the other were gone.

Intimate relationships also fulfill psychological needs and so are a means of *need fulfillment.* Through relationships with others, we fulfill our needs for the following:

- **Intimacy**—someone with whom we can share our feelings freely
- **Social integration**—someone with whom we can share worries and concerns
- **Nurturance**—someone we can take care of and who will take care of us
- **Assistance**—someone to help us in times of need
- **Affirmation**—someone who will reassure us of our own worth and tell us that we matter

In mutually rewarding intimate relationships, partners and friends meet each other's needs. They disclose feelings, share confidences, and provide support and reassurance. Each person comes away feeling better for the interaction and validated by the other person.

In addition to behavioral interdependence and need fulfillment, intimate relationships involve strong bonds of *emotional attachment,* or feelings of love. When we hear the word *intimacy,* we often think of a sexual relationship. Although sex can play an important role in emotional attachment, a relationship can be very intimate and yet not sexual. Two people can be emotionally intimate (share feelings) or spiritually intimate (share spiritual beliefs and meanings), or they can be intimate friends. With such a range of possibilities, the intimacy level that two people experience cannot be judged easily by those outside the relationship **(Figure 5.1)**.

Emotional availability, the ability to give to and receive from others emotionally without fear of being hurt or rejected, is the fourth characteristic of intimate relationships. At times, all of us may limit our emotional availability. For example, after a painful breakup we may decide not to jump into another relationship immediately, or we may decide to talk about it with only one or two close friends. Holding back can offer time for introspection and healing, as well as for considering the lessons learned. However, some people who have experienced intense trauma find it difficult to ever be fully available emotionally. This limits their ability to experience intimate relationships.

Healthy intimate relationships can benefit all parties involved. Historically, research examining the benefits of intimate relationships has focused on marriage. More recently, studies examining other forms of intimate relationships have reported that all types of close relationships are good for our health.[2] People with positive, fulfilling relationships with spouses, family members, friends, and coworkers are 50 percent more likely to survive over time than are people with

intimate relationships Relationships with family members, friends, and romantic partners, characterized by behavioral interdependence, need fulfillment, emotional attachment, and emotional availability.

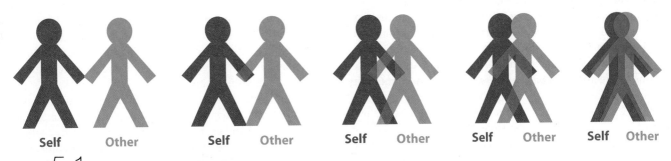

| Self | Other | Self | Other | Self | Other | Self | Other | Self | Other |

FIGURE 5.1 **How Intimate Is a Relationship?**
Relationships exist on a continuum of closeness and inclusion. Asking people to choose the diagram that best portrays a particular relationship does a remarkably good job of assessing the closeness they feel.

Source: Adapted from A. Aron, E. N. Aron and D. Smollan, "Inclusion of Other in the Self Scale and the Structure of Interpersonal Closeness," *Journal of Personality & Social Psychology* 63, no. 4 (1992): 596–612. Copyright © 1992. American Psychological Association. Adapted with permission.

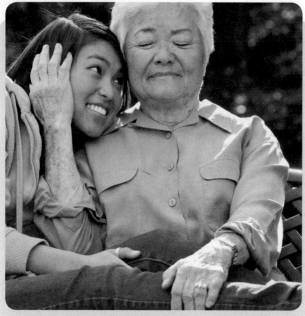

Do intimate relationships have to be sexual?

We may be accustomed to hearing "intimacy" used to describe romantic or sexual relationships, but intimate relationships can take many forms. The emotional bonds that characterize intimate relationships often span the generations and help individuals gain insight and understanding into each other's worlds.

poor relationships.[3] People with very few positive, trusting relationships have decreased immune system functioning, hormone regulation, and ability to handle stress and anxiety. A study looking at the physical and mental health of college students in committed relationships found that those in committed relationships reported fewer mental health problems and were less likely to be overweight or obese.[4]

Relating to Yourself

You have probably heard the notion that you must love yourself before you can love someone else. What does this mean? Learning how you function emotionally and how to nurture yourself through all life's situations is a lifelong task. You should certainly not postpone intimate connections with others until you achieve this state. However, a certain level of individual maturity will help you maintain relationships.

Two concepts that are especially important to any good relationship are *accountability* and *self-nurturance*. **Accountability** means that both partners see themselves as responsible for their own decisions, choices, and actions. They don't hold the other person responsible for positive or negative experiences. **Self-nurturance,** which goes hand in hand with accountability, means developing individual potential through a

accountability Accepting responsibility for personal decisions, choices, and actions.

self-nurturance Developing individual potential through a balanced and realistic appreciation of self-worth and ability.

family of origin People present in the household during a child's first years of life—usually parents and siblings.

balanced and realistic appreciation of self-worth and ability. To make good choices in life, a person must balance many physical and emotional needs, including sleeping, eating, exercising, working, relaxing, and socializing. When the balance is disrupted, as inevitably it will be at times, self-nurturing people are patient with themselves and try to put things back on course. Learning to live in a balanced and healthy way is a lifelong process. Individuals who are on a path of accountability and self-nurturance have a much better chance of maintaining a satisfying relationship with others.

Self-Esteem and Self-Acceptance Important factors that affect your ability to nurture yourself and maintain healthy relationships with others include the way you define yourself (*self-concept*) and the way you evaluate yourself (*self-esteem*). Your self-concept is like a mental mirror that reflects how you view your physical features, emotional states, talents, likes and dislikes, values, and roles. A person might define herself as an activist, a mother, an honor student, an athlete, or a pianist. In contrast, how you feel about yourself or evaluate yourself constitutes your self-esteem. You might consider yourself an excellent student, a horrible singer, a great lover, or a "10" in terms of appearance—such judgments indicate your level of self-esteem or self-evaluation.

Your perception and acceptance of yourself influences your relationship choices. If you feel unattractive, uncomfortable, or inferior to others, you may choose not to interact with other people or to avoid social events. Or you may unconsciously seek out individuals who confirm your negative view of yourself by treating you poorly. Conversely, if you are secure about your unique characteristics and talents, that positive self-concept will make it easier to form relationships with people who support and nurture you, and to interact with a variety of people in a healthy, balanced way.

Family Relationships

A family is a recognizable group of people with roles, tasks, boundaries, and personalities whose central focus is to protect, care for, love, and socialize with one another. Because the family is a dynamic institution that changes as society changes, the definition of *family,* and those individuals believed to constitute family membership, changes over time as well. Who are members of today's families? Historically, most families have been made up of people related by blood, marriage or long-term committed relationships, or adoption. Yet today, many other groups of people are being recognized and are functioning as family units.

Although there is no "best" family type, we do know that a healthy family's key roles and tasks are to nurture and support. Healthy families foster a sense of security and feelings of belonging that are central to growth and development. In the early years of people's lives, families provide the most significant relationships. Gradually, the circle widens to include friends, coworkers, and acquaintances. However, it is from our **family of origin,** the people present in our household during our first years of life, that we initially learn about feelings, problem solving, love, intimacy, and gender roles. We learn to negotiate relationships and have opportunities to communicate effectively, develop attitudes and values, and explore spiritual belief systems. It is not uncommon when we establish relationships outside the family to rely on these initial experiences and on skills modeled by our family of origin.

Friendships

Friendships are often the first relationships we form outside our immediate families, and they can be some of life's most stable and enduring relationships. Establishing and maintaining strong friendships may be a good predictor of your success in establishing love relationships, because each requires shared interests and values, mutual acceptance, trust, understanding, respect, and levels of confiding. Healthy friendships involve the following:[5]

● Understanding the roles and boundaries within the friendship.
● Communicating understandings, needs, expectations, limitations, and affections.
● Having a sense of equity in which both participants share confidences and contribute fairly and equally to maintaining the friendship.
● Consistently trying to give as much as one gets from the relationship.

Developing meaningful friendships is more than merely "friending" someone on Facebook. Getting to know someone well requires time, effort, and commitment. A recent study reported that Americans have, on average, four close social contacts, yet only half of those contacts are solely friends and not also linked through kinship or romantic relationship.[6] Take a few minutes to examine one of your current friendships. What characteristics in that relationship benefit you? How can you make that friendship stronger?

Romantic Relationships

Most people choose at some point to enter into an intimate romantic and sexual relationship with another person. Romantic relationships typically include all the characteristics of friendship as well as the following characteristics related to passion and caring:

● **Fascination.** Lovers tend to pay attention to the other person even when they should be involved in other activities. They are preoccupied with the other and want to think about, talk to, or be with the other.
● **Exclusiveness.** Lovers have a special relationship that usually precludes having the same relationship with a third party. The love relationship often takes priority over all others.
● **Sexual desire.** Lovers desire physical intimacy and want to touch, hold, and engage in sexual activities with the other.
● **Giving the utmost.** Lovers care enough to give the utmost when the other is in need, sometimes to the point of extreme sacrifice.
● **Being a champion or advocate.** Lovers actively champion each other's interests and attempt to ensure that the other succeeds.

Theories of Love What is love? This four-letter word has been written about and engraved on walls; it has been the theme of countless novels, movies, and plays. There is no single definition of *love,* and the word may mean different things to different people, depending on cultural values, age, gender, and situation. Although we may not know how to put our feelings into words, we all know it when the "lightning bolt" of love strikes.

Several theories related to how and why love develops have been proposed. In his classic Triangular Theory of Love, psychologist Robert Sternberg posits the following three key components to loving relationships (Figure 5.2):[7]

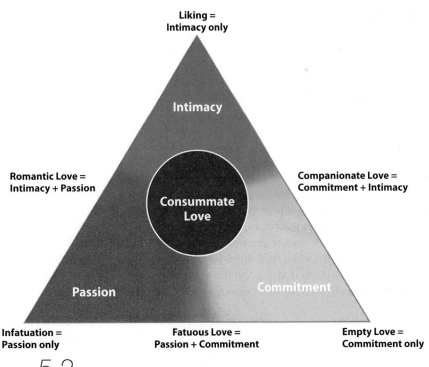

FIGURE 5.2 **Sternberg's Triangular Theory of Love**
According to Sternberg's model, three elements—intimacy, passion, and commitment—existing alone or in combination form different types of love. The most complete, ideal type of love in the model is consummate love, which combines balanced amounts of all three elements.

- **Intimacy.** The emotional component, which involves closeness, sharing, and mutual support.
- **Passion.** The motivational component, which includes lust, attraction, sexual arousal, and sharing.
- **Commitment.** The cognitive component, which includes the decision to be open to love in the short term and the commitment to the relationship in the long term.

The quality of love relationships is reflected by the level of intimacy, passion, and commitment each person brings to the relationship over time. Sternberg believes that relationships that include two or more of the above are more likely to endure than those that include only one. He uses the term **consummate love** to describe a combination of intimacy, passion, and commitment—an ideal and deep form of love that is, unfortunately, all too rare.

consummate love A relationship that combines intimacy, passion, and commitment.

Quite different from Sternberg's approach are theories of love and attraction based on brain chemistry and circuitry. Anthropologist Helen Fisher, among others, has hypothesized that attraction and falling in love follow a fairly predictable pattern based on the following: (1) *imprinting,* in which our evolutionary patterns, genetic predispositions, and past experiences trigger a romantic reaction; (2) *attraction,* in which neurochemicals produce feelings of euphoria and elation; (3) *attachment,* in which endorphins—natural opiates—cause lovers to feel peaceful, secure, and calm; and (4) *production of a cuddle chemical;* that is, the brain secretes the hormone oxytocin, which stimulates sensations during lovemaking and elicits feelings of satisfaction and attachment.[8]

According to Fisher's theory, lovers who claim that they are swept away by passion may not be far from the truth. Why? The love-smitten person's endocrine system secretes chemical substances such as dopamine, norepinephrine, and phenylethylamine (PEA), which are chemical cousins of amphetamines.[9] Although attraction may in fact be a "natural high," this passion loses effectiveness over time as the body builds up a tolerance. Fisher speculates that some people become attraction junkies, seeking the intoxication of new love much as the drug user seeks a chemical high. Fisher also speculates that PEA levels drop significantly over a 3- to 4-year period, leading to the "4-year itch" that manifests in the peaking fourth-year divorce rates present in over 60 cultures. Romances that last beyond the 4-year mark are then influenced by endorphins that give lovers a sense of security, peace, and calm.

Choosing a Romantic Partner

Choosing a relationship partner is influenced by more than just chemical and psychological processes. One important factor is proximity, or being in the same place at the same time. The more often that you see a person in your hometown, at social gatherings, or at work, the more likely it is that interaction will occur. Thus, if you live in New York, you'll probably end up with another New Yorker. However, the advent of the Internet has made geographic proximity less important. (See the **Tech & Health** box on the following page for guidelines on meeting people online.)

You also choose a partner based on *similarities* (in attitudes, values, intellect, interests, education, and socioeconomic status); the old adage that "opposites attract" usually isn't true. If your potential partner expresses interest or liking, you may react with mutual regard known as *reciprocity*. The more you express interest, the safer it is for someone else to return the regard, and the cycle spirals onward.

A final factor that plays a significant role in selecting a partner is *physical attraction.* Whether such attraction is caused by a chemical reaction or a socially learned behavior, men and women appear to have different attraction criteria. When selecting mates, men tend to be attracted primarily to youth and beauty, while women tend to be attracted to older mates and to place higher emphasis on partners who have good financial prospects and who appear to be dependable and industrious.[10]

Communicating: A Key to Good Relationships

From the moment of birth, we strive to be understood. We flail our arms, cry, scream, smile, frown, and make sounds and gestures to attract attention or to communicate what we want or need. By adulthood, each of us has developed a unique way of communicating with others via gestures, words, expressions, and body language. No two of us communicate exactly the same way or have the same need for connecting with others.

Different cultures have different ways of expressing feelings and using body language. Some cultures gesture broadly; others maintain a closed and rigid means of speaking. Some are offended by direct eye contact; others welcome a steady look in the eyes. Men and women also tend to have different styles of communication that are largely dictated by culture and socialization (see the **Health in a Diverse World** box on page 140).

Although people differ in the way they communicate, this doesn't mean that one sex, culture, or group is better at it than another. We have to be willing to accept differences and work to keep communication lines open and fluid. Remaining interested, actively engaged in the interaction, and open and willing to exchange ideas and thoughts is something that we typically learn with practice and hard work.

Technology has revolutionized our access to information and the ways we communicate. Couples can meet on a site like Match.com, keep in constant contact via texting, and inform the world of their relationship highs and lows via Facebook and Twitter. With all these tools available, it can be easy to share TMI (too much information). Ilana Gershon, author of *The Breakup 2.0: Disconnecting over New Media,* suggests we lack standard etiquette for the use of new media in relationships. At its best, social media can bring people closer together; at its worst, it can be used intentionally or unintentionally to embarrass or hurt. Consider the following suggestions to safeguard yourself:

WHEN MEETING

✳ If you join a dating site, be honest about yourself; state your interests and characteristics fairly, including things that you think might be less attractive than stereotypes and cultural norms dictate.

✳ If you meet someone online, and want to meet in person, put safety first! Plan something brief, preferably during daylight hours. Meet in a public place, like

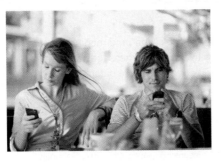

a coffee shop. Do not meet with anyone who wants to keep the time and location a secret. Tell a friend or family member the details of when and where you are meeting and any information you have about the person you are meeting.

WHILE DATING

✳ Discuss limits with your partner on the type of info you each want shared online. Agree to share only within those limits.

✳ Recognize that constant electronic updates throughout the day can leave little to share when you are together. Save some information for face-to-face talks!

✳ Sober up before you click "submit." Things that seem funny under the influence may not seem funny the next morning.

✳ Remember that the Internet is forever. Once a picture or a post is sent, it can never be completely erased. Never post anything that would embarrass someone if it was seen by a family member or potential employer.

✳ Respect your partner's privacy. Logging in to his/her e-mail or Facebook account to look at private messages is a breach of trust.

✳ Know that the GPS in a phone can be used to track your location, and cell phone spyware can be installed that allows e-mail and texts to be read from another device. If you think you may be a victim of "cyberstalking" by a current or former partner, get a new phone or ask the phone company to reinstall the phone's operating system to wipe out the software.

IF BREAKING UP

✳ Do not break up with someone via text/e-mail/Tweet/Facebook/chat. People deserve the respect of a more personal break up.

✳ Upon breaking up, be sure to change any passwords you may have confided in your partner. The temptation to use those for ill may be too strong to resist.

Learning Appropriate Self-Disclosure

Sharing personal information with others is called **self-disclosure.** If you are willing to share personal information with others, they will likely share personal information with you. Likewise, if you want to learn more about someone, you have to be willing to share parts of your personal self with that person. Self-disclosure is not only storytelling or sharing secrets, it is also revealing how you are reacting to the present situation and giving any information about the past that is relevant to the other person's understanding of your current reactions.

Self-disclosure can be a double-edged sword, as there is risk in divulging personal insights and feelings. If you sense that sharing feelings and personal thoughts will result in a closer relationship, you will likely take such a risk. But if you believe that the disclosure may result in rejection or alienation, you may not open up so easily. If the confidentiality of previously shared information has been violated, you may hesitate to disclose yourself in the future.

However, the risk in not disclosing yourself to others is that you will lack intimacy in relationships. Psychologist Carl Rogers stressed the importance of understanding yourself and others through self-disclosure. He believed that weak relationships were characterized by inhibited self-disclosure.[11]

If self-disclosure is a key element in creating healthy communication, but fear is a barrier to that process, what can we do? The following suggestions can help:

● **Get to know yourself.** Remember that your "self" includes your feelings, beliefs, thoughts, and concerns. The more you know about yourself, the more likely you will be able to communicate with others about yourself.

self-disclosure Sharing feelings or personal information with others.

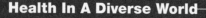

HE SAYS/SHE SAYS

There are some gender-specific communication patterns and behaviors that are obvious to the casual observer (see graphic). However, according to Dr. Cynthia Burggraf Torppa at Ohio State University, the bigger difference is the way in which men and women interpret or process the same message. She indicates that that women are more sensitive to interpersonal meanings "between the lines" and men are more sensitive to subtle messages about status. Recognizing these differences and how they make us unique is a good first step in avoiding unnecessary frustrations and miscommunications.

Sources: C. Burggraf Torppa, Family and Consumer Sciences, Ohio State University Extension, "Gender Issues: Communication Differences in Interpersonal Relationships," 2010, http://ohioline.osu.edu; J. Wood, *Gendered Lives: Communication, Gender, and Culture,* 10th ed. (Belmont, CA: Cengage, 2013); M. L. Knapp and A. L. Vangelisti, *Interpersonal Communication and Human Relationships,* 6th ed. (Boston: Allyn & Bacon, 2009).

Video Tutor:
Gender Differences in Communication

Women

FACIAL EXPRESSIONS
- Smile and nod more often
- Maintain better eye contact

SPEECH PATTERNS
- Higher pitched, softer voices
- Use approximately 5 speech tones
- May sound more emotional
- Make more tentative statements
- Interrupt less often

BODY LANGUAGE
- Take up less space
- Gesture toward the body
- Lean forward when listening
- More gentle when touching others
- More feedback via body language

BEHAVIORAL DIFFERENCES
- Express intimate feelings more readily
- More likely to ask for help
- Apologize more frequently
- Talk is primarily a means of rapport, establishing connections, and negotiating relationships

Men

FACIAL EXPRESSIONS
- Frown more often
- Often avoid eye contact

SPEECH PATTERNS
- Lower pitched, louder voices
- Use approximately 3 speech tones
- May sound more abrupt
- Make more direct statements
- More likely to interrupt

BODY LANGUAGE
- Occupy more space
- Gesture away from the body
- Lean back when listening
- More forceful gestures
- Less feedback via body language

BEHAVIORAL DIFFERENCES
- Have more difficulty in expressing intimate feelings
- Less likely to ask for help
- Apologize less often
- Talk is primarily a means of preserving independence and negotiating and maintaining status

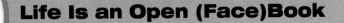

STUDENT HEALTH Today

Life Is an Open (Face)Book

Headlines such as "*Prince Harry parties naked in Las Vegas*" and "*Gay students accidentally outed to parents via Facebook*" remind us that we cannot expect privacy in a world where nearly everyone has a camera and an Internet connection. We are all one photo tag away from a family member or potential employer seeing us in less than flattering circumstances or knowing information we'd prefer kept secret.

"Social Media Screening," the practice of searching out all possible information on a prospective employee (sometimes to the point of asking for a Facebook password at an interview) is practiced by nearly half of employers. Their biggest concerns: Inappropriate photos, evidence of drug or alcohol use or abuse, and poor writing skills.

If you are concerned about your privacy, make sure your publicly available information is what you want prospective employers, family, and other people to see. Then tighten your privacy settings and untag yourself in photos you don't want people to see. Due to cached sites and reposts, you can't erase everything, so you may need to prepare an explanation for past posts, photos, and other information. As our "private" lives get more public all the time, we may have to accept Mark Zuckerberg's philosophy, that "privacy is no longer a social norm."

Sources: N. Messieh, "Survey: 37% of Your Prospective Employers Are Looking You up on Facebook," News: Social Media, Blog, *The Next Web*, April 18, 2012, http://thenextweb.com; B. Johnson, "Privacy No Longer a Social Norm,

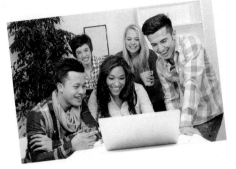

Says Facebook Founder," *The Guardian*, January 10, 2010, www.guardian.co.uk; N. Evans, "Back to Face the Music? Prince Harry Flies Home After Las Vegas Naked Photos Scandal," *Mirror News* Online, August 22, 2012, www.mirror.co.uk; G. Fowler, "When the Most Personal Secrets Get Outed on Facebook," *The Wall Street Journal*, October 13, 2012, http://online.wsj.com

---

● **Become more accepting of yourself.** No one is perfect or has to be.

● **Be willing to discuss your sexual history.** In a culture that puts many taboos on discussions of sex in everyday conversation, it's no wonder we find it hard to disclose our sexual feelings to those with whom we are intimate. However, with the soaring rate of sexually transmitted infections and the ever-looming threat of AIDS, there has never been a more important time to discuss sexual history with a partner.

● **Choose a safe context for self-disclosure.** When and where you make such disclosures and to whom may greatly influence the response. Choose a setting in which you feel safe to let yourself be known.

● **Be thoughtful about self-disclosure via social media.** Self-disclosure can be an effective method of building intimacy with another person, but not with large groups. Sharing information that is too personal on Facebook or Twitter may leave you embarrassed or vulnerable later. See the **Student Health Today** box for more on online privacy.

Becoming a Better Listener

Listening is a vital part of interpersonal communication; it allows us to share feelings, express concerns, communicate wants and needs, and let our thoughts and opinions be known. Improving listening skills will enhance our relationships, improve our grasp of information, and allow us to interpret more effectively what others say. We listen best when (1) we believe that the message is somehow important and relevant to us; (2) the speaker holds our attention through humor, dramatic effect, or other techniques; and (3) we are in the mood to listen (free of distractions and worries).

How many times have you been caught pretending to listen when you were not? Sometimes this tuned-out behavior is due to lack of sleep, stress overload, being preoccupied, having had too much to drink, or being under the influence of drugs. Other times the reason is that the speaker is a motormouth who talks for the sake of talking, or that you find the speaker or topic of conversation boring. Some of the most common listening difficulties are things that we can work to improve. See the **Skills for Behavior Change** box on page 142 for suggestions to improve your listening.

Using Nonverbal Communication

Understanding what someone is saying often involves much more than listening and speaking. Often, what is not actually said may speak louder than any words can say. Rolling the eyes, looking at the floor or ceiling rather than maintaining eye contact, body movements and hand gestures—all these nonverbal clues influence the way we interpret messages. **Nonverbal communication** includes all unwritten and unspoken messages, both intentional and unintentional. Ideally, our nonverbal communication matches and supports our verbal communication. This is not always the case. Research shows that when verbal and nonverbal communications don't match, we are more likely to believe the nonverbal cues.[12] This is one reason why it is important to be aware of all the nonverbal cues we use regularly and to understand how others might interpret them.

Nonverbal communication can include the following:[13]

- **Touch.** This can be a handshake, a warm hug, a hand on the shoulder, or a kiss on the cheek.

Are You Really Listening?

To become an excellent listener, practice the following skills and consciously use them on a daily basis:

❱ Pay attention. Good listeners participate and acknowledge what the other person is saying. Nodding, smiling, saying "yes" or "uh-huh," and asking questions at appropriate times all convey that you are attentive. Use positive body language and voice tone.

❱ Make sure to shut off the TV and put away your cell phone.

❱ Show empathy and sympathy. Watch for verbal and nonverbal clues to the other person's feelings and try to relate.

❱ Ask for clarification. If you aren't sure what the speaker means, indicate that you're not sure you understand, or paraphrase what you think you heard.

❱ Control the desire to interrupt. Try taking a deep breath for 2 seconds, then hold your breath for another second and really listen to what is being said as you slowly exhale.

❱ Avoid snap judgments based on what other people look like or are saying.

❱ Resist the temptation to "set the other person straight."

❱ Try to focus on the speaker. Hold back the temptation to launch into your own rendition of a similar situation.

❱ Be tenacious. Stick with the speaker and try to stay on topic. If the person seems to wander, gently bring the topic back by saying, "You were just saying. . . ."

❱ Offer your thoughts and suggestions, but remember that you should advise only up to a certain point. Clarify statements with "This is my opinion" as a reminder that it is only a viewpoint rather than a fact.

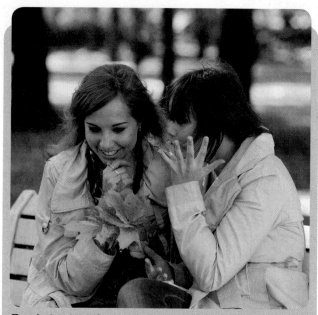

To what extent do people communicate without words?

Researchers have found that 93 percent of communication effectiveness is determined by nonverbal cues. Positive communication means using positive body language. Laughing, smiling, and gesturing all help convey meaning and assure your partner you are engaged.

- **Gestures.** These can include physical mannerisms that replace words, such as a thumbs-up or a wave hello or good-bye, or movements that augment verbal communication, such as indicating with your hands the size of the fish that got away. Gestures can also be rude, such as glancing at one's watch to indicate a wish to leave or rolling one's eyes to show contempt for what has been said.
- **Interpersonal space.** This is the amount of physical space that separates two people.
- **Facial expressions.** These can signal moods and emotions and often have universal meaning.
- **Body language.** This includes things like folding your arms across your chest, crossing your legs, or leaning forward in your chair.
- **Tone of voice.** This refers not to what you say, but how you say it—the elements of speaking that color the use of words, such as pitch, volume, and speed.

While facial expressions are believed to have near universal meaning, most other body language is culturally specific. A gesture of agreement in one culture can be offensive in another. To communicate as effectively as possible, it is important to recognize and use nonverbal cues that support and help clarify your verbal messages. Awareness and practice of your verbal and nonverbal communication will also enhance your skills in interpreting messages others send to you.

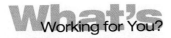
Managing Conflict through Communication

A **conflict** is an emotional state that arises when the behavior of one person interferes with that of another. Conflict is inevitable whenever people live or work together. Not all conflict is bad; in fact, airing feelings and coming to some form of resolution over differences can sometimes strengthen relationships. **Conflict resolution** and successful conflict management form a systematic approach to resolving differences fairly and constructively, rather than allowing them to fester. The goal of conflict resolution is to solve differences peacefully and creatively.

Here are some strategies for conflict resolution.

1. Identify the problem or issues. Talk with each other to clarify exactly what the conflict or problem is. Try to understand both sides of the problem. In this first stage, you must say what you want and listen to what the other person wants. Focus on using "I" messages and avoid using any blaming "you" messages. Be an active listener—repeat what the other person has said and ask questions for clarification or additional information.

2. Generate several possible solutions. Base your search for solutions on the goals and interests identified in the first step. Come up with several different alternatives, and avoid evaluating any of them until you have finished brainstorming.

3. Evaluate the alternative solutions. Discard any that are unacceptable to either of you, and keep narrowing down the solutions to one or two that seem to work for both parties. Be honest with each other about a solution that you feel is unsatisfactory, but also be open to compromise.

4. Decide on the best solution. Choose an alternative that is acceptable to both parties. You both need to be committed to the decision for this solution to be effective.

5. Implement the solution. Discuss how the decision will be carried out. Establish who is responsible to do what and when. The solution stands a better chance of working if you agree on the plans for implementing it.

6. Follow up. Evaluate whether the solution is working. Check in with the other person to see how he or she feels about it. Are you both satisfied with the way the solution is working? If something is not working as planned, or if circumstances have changed, discuss revising the plan. Remember that both parties must agree to any changes to the plan, as they did with the original.

"Why Should I Care?"

Learning to communicate effectively, especially about emotions, is essential to all healthy relationships. Time spent developing listening skills, understanding nonverbal communication patterns, and learning to have difficult conversations will serve you well through the rest of your life.

Committed Relationships

Commitment in a relationship means that one intends to act over time in a way that perpetuates the well-being of the other person, oneself, and the relationship. Polls show that the majority of Americans strive to develop a committed relationship.[14] These relationships can take several forms, including marriage, cohabitation, and gay and lesbian partnerships.

Marriage

In many societies around the world, traditional committed relationships take the form of marriage. In the United States, marriage means entering into a legal agreement that includes shared financial plans, property, and responsibility for raising children. Many Americans also view marriage as a religious bond that emphasizes certain rights and obligations for each spouse. Marriage is socially sanctioned and highly celebrated in our culture, so there are numerous incentives for couples to formalize their relationship with a wedding ceremony.

conflict An emotional state that arises when the behavior of one person interferes with the behavior of another.

conflict resolution A concerted effort by all parties to constructively resolve differences or points of contention.

Historically, close to 90 percent of Americans married at least once during their lifetime, and at any given time, more than 50 percent of U.S. adults are married (see **Figure 5.3** on page 144). However, in recent years Americans have become less likely to marry; since 1960, annual marriages of adult men and women have steadily declined.[15] This decrease may be due to several factors, including delay of first marriages, increase in cohabitation, and a small decrease in the number of divorced persons who remarry. In 1960, the median age for first marriage was 23 years for men and 20 years for women; now, the median age of first marriage has risen to 28.6 years for men and 26.6 years for women.[16]

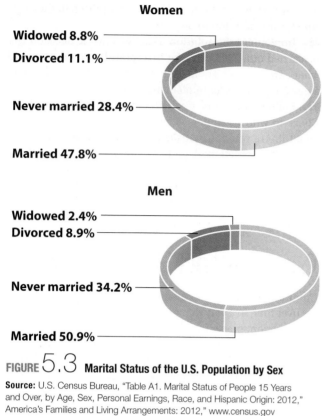

Women

Widowed 8.8%
Divorced 11.1%
Never married 28.4%
Married 47.8%

Men

Widowed 2.4%
Divorced 8.9%
Never married 34.2%
Married 50.9%

FIGURE 5.3 **Marital Status of the U.S. Population by Sex**

Source: U.S. Census Bureau, "Table A1. Marital Status of People 15 Years and Over, by Age, Sex, Personal Earnings, Race, and Hispanic Origin: 2012," America's Families and Living Arrangements: 2012," www.census.gov

Note that the figure does not list the percentages for married men and women with a spouse absent and separated.

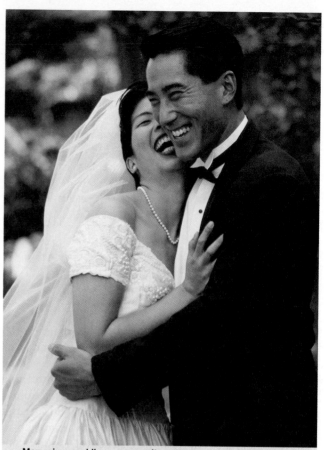

Many view weddings or commitment ceremonies as the ultimate symbol of commitment between two people and a validation of their love for each other.

monogamy Exclusive sexual involvement with one partner.

serial monogamy A series of monogamous sexual relationships.

open relationship A relationship in which partners agree that sexual involvement can occur outside the relationship.

cohabitation Living together without being married.

common-law marriage Cohabitation lasting a designated period of time (usually 7 years) that is considered legally binding in some states.

Many Americans believe that marriage involves **monogamy,** or exclusive sexual involvement with one partner. In fact, the lifetime pattern for many Americans appears to be **serial monogamy,** which means that a person has a monogamous sexual relationship with one partner before moving on to another monogamous relationship. However, some people prefer to have an **open relationship,** or open marriage, in which the partners agree that there may be sexual involvement for each person outside their relationship.

A healthy marriage combines the benefits of friendship and a loving committed relationship and thereby provides emotional support. It also provides stability for both the couple and those involved in the couple's life. Considerable

research indicates that married people live longer, feel happier, remain mentally alert longer, and suffer fewer physical and mental health problems.[17] Couples in healthy marriages have less stress, which in turn contributes to better overall health. Healthy marriage contributes to lower levels of stress in three important ways: financial stability, expanded support networks, and improved personal behaviors. Married adults are about half as likely to be smokers as are cohabitating, divorced, or separated adults. They are also less likely to be heavy drinkers. The one negative health indicator for married people is body weight in men. Married men are far more likely than never-married men to be overweight, but no more likely than divorced or widowed men.[18]

Despite its benefits, traditional marriage is not for everyone, and it is not the only path to a happy and successful committed relationship.

Cohabitation

Cohabitation is a relationship in which two unmarried people with an intimate connection live together in the same household. In some states, cohabitation that lasts a designated number of years (usually 7) legally constitutes a **common-law marriage** for purposes of purchasing real

66% of women who marry between ages 24 to 26 report very happy marriages, more than women who marry at younger or older ages.

estate and sharing other financial obligations. For a variety of reasons, more Americans are choosing cohabitation. In fact, cohabitation is increasingly the first coresidential partnership formed by young adults.[19]

Cohabitation before marriage has been a controversial issue for decades. While some voiced moral objections, other concerns were related to higher divorce rates among couples that cohabited before marriage. However, according to a recent report from the National Center for Health Statistics, cohabitation is no longer a clear predictor of marriage success or failure. In a group of 13,000 men and women aged 15 to 44, 71 percent of men who were engaged when they moved in with their fiancé were still married to the same woman after 10 years. For men who didn't cohabit before getting married, the success rate dropped slightly to 69 percent. Sixty-five percent of cohabiting engaged women were still married after 10 years, compared to 66 percent of women who waited until after marriage to move in with their husband.[20] In other words, for today's couples, what seems to matter is the level of commitment when moving in. Couples who move in together with plans to marry have about the same chances of divorcing as couples who never cohabit before marriage, but those who move in together without specific plans to marry have an increased risk of divorce.

Although cohabitation has advantages, it also has drawbacks. Perhaps the greatest disadvantage is the lack of societal validation for the relationship, especially if the couple then has children. Many cohabitors must deal with pressures from parents and friends, difficulties in obtaining insurance and tax benefits, and legal issues over property.

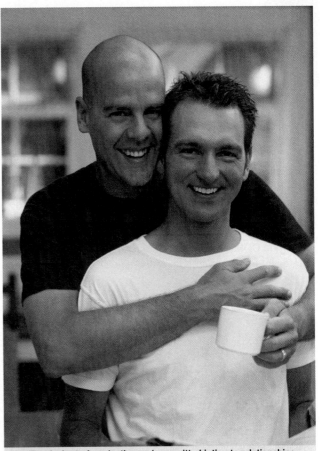

The desire to form lasting and committed intimate relationships is shared by most adults, regardless of sexual orientation.

Gay and Lesbian Marriage/Partnerships

Whether they are gay or straight, most adults want intimate, committed relationships. Lesbians and gay men seek the same things in primary relationships that heterosexual partners do: love, friendship, communication, validation, companionship, and a sense of stability. The American Community Survey identified an estimated 646,000 same-sex couples in the United States, 20 percent of whom are legally married.[21]

Challenges to successful lesbian and gay relationships often stem from discrimination and difficulties dealing with social, legal, and religious doctrines. For lesbian and gay couples, obtaining the same level of "marriage benefits," such as tax deductions, power-of-attorney rights, partner health insurance, child custody rights, and other rights, continues to be a challenge. In 2013, the U.S. Supreme Court overturned a portion of the Defense of Marriage Act (DOMA) that prevented married homosexual couples from being legally recognized by the federal government. Due to this recent change, married homosexual couples are now eligible for federal benefit programs. DOMA was originally established in 1996 to normalize heterosexual marriage on a federal level and to permit each state to decide whether or not to recognize

same-sex unions. See the **Points of View** box on the following page for more on the two sides to this issue.

As of 2013, New York, Massachusetts, Connecticut, Iowa, New Hampshire, Vermont, Maine, Washington, Maryland, Rhode Island, Minnesota, Delaware, California, and the District of Columbia are the only states or districts to grant same-sex couples marriage equality. Six other states currently have broad relationship-recognition laws that extend to same-sex couples all, or nearly all, the state rights and responsibilities of married heterosexual couples, whether labeled "civil unions" or "domestic partnerships." More limited rights and protections for same-sex couples and/or the recognition of same-sex marriages performed in other states are legislated in three additional states.[22] Worldwide, the number of countries that have legalized same-sex marriages or who approve civil unions or registered domestic partnerships for same-sex couples continues to grow. As of 2013, sixteen countries allow same-sex marriage.[23]

Staying Single

Increasing numbers of adults of all ages are electing to marry later or to remain single altogether. According to data from the most recent U.S. Census, 54 percent of women aged 20 to

The Defense of Marriage Act:
FOR BETTER OR FOR WORSE?

The federal Defense of Marriage Act (DOMA), enacted in 1996, is a law defining marriage as a legal union exclusively between one man and one woman and establishing that no state must recognize the relationship between persons of the same sex as a marriage, even if the relationship is considered a marriage in another state. Before DOMA was partially repealed by the Supreme Court in 2013, it denied gay couples the federal protections and benefits that apply to heterosexual couples.

When DOMA was enacted, federal law deferred to states in defining marriage. At the time DOMA was enacted, same-sex couples were not allowed to marry in any U.S. state. Since then, thirteen states and the District of Columbia have recognized equal marriage rights for same-sex couples, and thousands of couples have married. As of 2013, the portion of DOMA still in effect does not require states to recognize or legalize same-sex marriages carried out in other states. However, the Supreme Court rulings carried out in 2013 appear to pave the way for greater acceptance of same-sex couple marriages. Should DOMA be entirely repealed? Here are some of the arguments for and against the law.

Arguments to Keep DOMA

○ Marriage is largely a religious institution, and many religious groups are opposed to the idea of same-sex marriage.

○ Civil unions and domestic partnerships offer same-sex couples many of the same protections and rights as marriage, so allowing same-sex couples to marry is unnecessary.

○ Allowing same-sex couples to marry would undermine the institution of marriage itself.

Arguments to Repeal DOMA

○ The U.S. Constitution is supposed to guarantee equal rights for all U.S. citizens. Having unequal marriage rights is a form of discrimination.

○ Civil unions and domestic partnerships do not offer all of the benefits of marriage, and they vary greatly from state to state.

○ The U.S. Constitution requires each state to give "full faith and credit" to the laws of other states, including states' obligations to honor marriages validated in other states and districts.

Where Do You Stand?

○ Do you think all legally married couples should be treated equally under the law? Do you think states should be able to make their own determinations about who can legally marry?

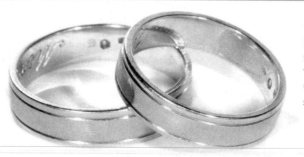

○ Are you aware of the rights, responsibilities, and protections granted to married couples by the federal government?

○ What person(s) or institution(s) should define marriage?

---

34 have never been married. Likewise, men in this age group postponed marriage in increasing numbers, with 64 percent remaining unmarried.[24]

Singles clubs, social outings arranged by communities and religious groups, extended family environments, and many social services support the single lifestyle. Many singles live rich, rewarding lives and maintain a large network of close friends and family. Although sexual intimacy may or may not be present, the intimacy achieved through other interactions with loved ones is a key aspect of the single lifestyle.

Choosing Whether to Have Children

If you decide to raise children, your relationship with your partner will change. Resources of time, energy, and money are split many ways, and you will no longer be able to give each other undivided attention. Babies and young children do not time their requests for food, sleep, and care for the convenience of adults. Therefore, if your own basic needs for security, love, and purpose are already met, you will be better parents. Any stresses existing in your relationship will be further accentuated when parenting is added to your responsibilities. Having a child does not save a bad relationship—in fact, it seems only to compound the problems that already exist. A child cannot and should not be expected to provide the parents with self-esteem and security.

Changing patterns in family life affect the way children are raised. For instance, in modern society, it is not always clear which partner will adjust his or her work schedule to provide the primary care of children. And today, the "blended family" is the most common family unit; creating instant families for stepparents and stepchildren.

You could also be among the increasing numbers of individuals choosing to have children in a family structure other than a heterosexual marriage. Single women or lesbian couples can choose adoption or alternative insemination as a way to create a family. Single men or gay couples can choose to adopt or obtain the services of a surrogate mother.

According to the U.S. Census Bureau, in 2012, over 28 percent of all children under age 18 were living in families headed by a man or woman raising a child alone, reflecting a growing trend in America.[25]

Regardless of the structure of the family, certain factors remain important to the well-being of the unit: consistency, communication, affection, and mutual respect. Good parenting does not necessarily come naturally. Many people parent as they were parented (see Table 5.1). This strategy may or may not lead to sound child-rearing principles. Establishing a positive, respectful parenting style sets the stage for healthy family growth and development.

Finally, as a potential parent you must consider the financial implications of deciding to have a child. It is estimated that a middle-income family that had a child in 2012 will spend, on average, about $241,080 for food, clothing, shelter, education, and other necessities for the child over

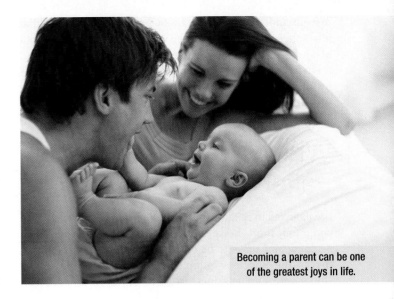

Becoming a parent can be one of the greatest joys in life.

the next 17 years. Keep in mind that these numbers do not include the cost of childbearing or the costs of a college education.[26] Compared to 1975, when only 39 percent of women with preschool-aged children worked outside the home, today about 64 percent of mothers with young children juggle a job along with parenting.[27] Most families rely on a network of day care workers, family members, friends, grandparents, neighbors, and nannies to care for children during work hours. The price of day care centers can be shocking to those who don't have children. In 2011, the average annual cost of full-time infant care ranged from about $4,600 in Mississippi to nearly $15,000 in Massachusetts. Put another way, it can cost as much to send a baby to full-time day care as it does to send a child to college.[28]

Given that roughly half of all pregnancies in the United States are unintended, it's safe to say that many people become parents without a lot of forethought.[29] Some children are born into a relationship that doesn't last. This does not mean it is impossible to do a good job of parenting. Children are amazingly resilient and forgiving if parents show

TABLE 5.1	Common Parenting Styles
Authoritarian "giving orders"	Parents use a set of rules that are clear and unbending. Obedience is highly valued and rewarded. Misbehavior is punished. Children may behave for a reward or out of fear of punishment. Children are not encouraged to think for themselves or to question those in authority.
Permissive "giving in"	Parents take a hands-off approach. Children are allowed great freedom with few boundaries, minimal guidance, and little discipline. Without limits and expectations, children often struggle with impulse control, poor choices, and insecurity, and have trouble taking responsibility for their actions.
Assertive-Democratic "giving choices"	Parents have clear expectations for children, clarify issues, and give reasons for limits. Children are given lots of practice in making choices and are guided to see the consequences of their decisions. Encouragement and acknowledgment of good behavior form the focal point of this style. Misbehavior is handled with an appropriate consequence or by problem solving with the child.

Source: Adapted from S. Dinwiddie, "Effective Parenting Styles: Why Yesterday's Models Won't Work Today," June 21, 2013, www.kidsource.com. Copyright © 2009 Sue Dinwiddie. Reprinted by permission of the author.

respect and communicate about household activities that affect their lives. Even children who grew up in a household of conflict can feel loved and respected if their parents treat them fairly. This means that parents must take responsibility for their own emotions and make it clear to children that they are not the reason for the conflict.

When Relationships Falter

Breakdowns in relationships usually begin with a change in communication, however subtle. Either partner may stop listening and cease to be emotionally present for the other. In turn, the other feels ignored, unappreciated, or unwanted. Unresolved conflicts increase, and unresolved anger can cause problems in sexual relations.

When a couple who previously enjoyed spending time together find themselves continually in the company of others, spending time apart, or preferring to stay home alone, it may be a sign that the relationship is in trouble. Of course, the need for individual privacy is not a cause for worry—it's essential to health. If, however, a partner decides to change the amount and quality of time spent together without the input or understanding of the other, it may be a sign of hidden problems. Figure 5.4 on page 149 illustrates some of the factors that signal a healthy or unhealthy relationship.

College students, particularly those who are socially isolated and far from family and hometown friends, may be particularly vulnerable to staying in unhealthy relationships. They may become emotionally dependent on a partner for everything from eating meals to recreation and study time. Mutual obligations, such as shared rental arrangements, transportation, and child care, can make it tough to leave. It's also easy to mistake sexual advances for physical attraction or love. Without a network of friends and supporters to talk with, to obtain validation for feelings, or to share concerns, a student may feel stuck in a relationship that is headed nowhere.

jealousy An aversive reaction evoked by a real or imagined relationship involving a person's partner and a third person.

power The ability to make and implement decisions.

Honesty and verbal affection are usually positive aspects of a relationship. In a troubled relationship, however, they can be used to cover up irresponsible or hurtful behavior. "At least I was honest" is not an acceptable substitute for acting in a trustworthy way, and claiming "But I really do love you" is not a license for being inconsiderate or rude.

Confronting Couples Issues

Couples seeking a long-term relationship must confront several issues that can either enhance or diminish their chances of success. Some of these issues involve jealousy, gender roles, power sharing, and open communication about unmet expectations.

Jealousy in Relationships **Jealousy** has been described as an aversive reaction evoked by a real or imagined relationship involving one's partner and a third person. Jealousy often indicates underlying problems, such as insecurity, low self-esteem, or possessiveness, which are barriers to a healthy relationship. In some cases, there may be a valid reason for jealousy, such as the violation of relationship boundaries. In both men and women, jealousy is related to believing it would be difficult to find another relationship if the current one ends. For men, jealousy is positively correlated with the degree to which the man's self-esteem is affected by his partner's judgments. Although a certain amount of jealousy can be expected in any loving relationship, it doesn't have to threaten the relationship as long as partners communicate openly about it.[30]

Changing Gender Roles Throughout history, women and men have taken on various roles in their relationships. In agricultural America, gender roles were determined by tradition, and each task within a family unit held equal importance. Our modern society has fewer gender-specific roles. Rather than taking on traditional female and male roles, many couples find it makes more sense to divide tasks on the basis of schedule, convenience, and preference. However, it rarely works out that the division is equal between men and women. The U.S. Bureau of Labor Statistics estimates that 19 percent of men did housework on an average day in 2011, compared to 48 percent of women. Sixty-six percent of women prepared meals compared to 40 percent of men.[31] It is important in contemporary relationships that couples are able to communicate how they feel about the multiple roles and tasks they will share in a dual-earner household or the relationship is likely to suffer.

Sharing Power **Power** can be defined as the ability to make and implement decisions. There are many ways to exercise power, but powerful people are those who know what they want and have the ability to attain it. In traditional relationships, men were the wage earners and consequently had decision-making power. Women exerted much influence, but often they needed a man's income for survival. That pattern has evolved. In recent years women have outpaced men in education, and their earnings have grown at faster rates than men's have. However, women still trail men in earnings in almost every field. According to the Bureau of Labor Statistics, only 28 percent of wives have incomes that top their husbands', even though 81 percent of wives have an education level that is equal to or greater than their husbands'.[32] As women's earning potential continues to increase and they can be financially

what do you think?

Have you ever experienced jealousy in a relationship?
● Can you identify what actions or events caused you to feel this way?
● Did you have actual facts to support your feelings, or was your response based on suspicions?

In an unhealthy relationship...	In a healthy relationship...
You care for and focus on another person only and neglect yourself or you focus only on yourself and neglect the other person.	You both love and take care of yourselves before and while in a relationship.
One of you feels pressure to change to meet the other person's standards and is afraid to disagree or voice ideas.	You respect each other's individuality, embrace your differences, and allow each other to "be yourselves."
One of you has to justify what you do, where you go, and people you see.	You both do things with friends and family and have activities independent of each other.
One of you makes all the decisions and controls everything without listening to the other's input.	You discuss things with each other, allow for differences of opinion, and compromise equally.
One of you feels unheard and is unable to communicate what you want.	You express and listen to each other's feelings, needs, and desires.
You lie to each other and find yourself making excuses for the other person.	You both trust and are honest with yourselves and with each other.
You don't have any personal space and have to share everything with the other person.	You respect each other's need for privacy.
Your partner keeps his or her sexual history a secret or hides a sexually transmitted infection from you, or you do not disclose your history to your partner.	You share sexual histories and information about sexual health with each other.
One of you is scared of asking the other to use protection or has refused the other's requests for safer sex.	You both practice safer sex methods.
One of you has forced or coerced the other to have sex.	You both respect sexual boundaries and are able to say no to sex.
One of you yells and hits, shoves, or throws things at the other in an argument.	You resolve conflicts in a rational, peaceful, and mutually agreed upon way.
You feel stifled, trapped, and stagnant. You are unable to escape the pressures of the relationship.	You both have room for positive growth, and you both learn more about each other as you develop and mature.

FIGURE 5.4 **Healthy versus Unhealthy Relationships**

Source: Reprinted with permission from Advocates for Youth, www.advocatesforyouth.org. Copyright © 2000, Washington, D.C. 20036.

independent, the power dynamics between women and men will continue to shift.

Unmet Expectations We all have expectations of ourselves and our partners—how we will spend our time, how we will spend our money, how and how often we will express love and intimacy, and how we will grow together as a couple. Expectations are an extension of our values, beliefs, hopes, and dreams for the future. When communicated and agreed upon, they help relationships thrive. If we are unable to communicate our expectations, we set ourselves up for disappointment and hurt. Partners in healthy relationships can communicate wants and needs and have honest discussions when things aren't going as expected or as planned.

When and Why Relationships End

Often we hear in the news that 50 percent of American marriages end in divorce. This number is based on comparing the annual marriage rate with the annual divorce rate. This comparison is misleading because in any given year, the people who are divorcing are mostly not the same people who just got married. It is more accurate to look at the total number of married people and calculate how many of them eventually divorce. By this calculation, the divorce rate in the United States has never exceeded 40 percent.[33] Although this number is still high, it should be noted that the divorce rate in the United States shot up in the 1970s, peaked in the early 1980s, and has since declined to about 30 percent.

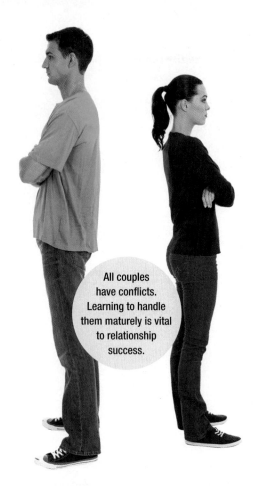

All couples have conflicts. Learning to handle them maturely is vital to relationship success.

The divorce rate, however, represents only a portion of the actual number of failed relationships. Couples who stop living together but never go through a legal divorce process are not counted in these statistics. Similarly, cohabitants and unmarried partners who raise children, own homes together, and exhibit all the outward appearances of marriage but without the license, are also not included.

Why do relationships end? There are many reasons, including illness, financial concerns, career problems, and personality conflicts. Many people enter a relationship with certain expectations about how they and their partner will behave. Failure to communicate or live up to these beliefs can lead to resentment and disappointment. Differences in sexual needs may also contribute to the demise of a relationship. Under stress, communication and cooperation between partners can break down. Conflict, negative interactions, and a general lack of respect between partners can erode even the most loving relationship.

Coping with Failed Relationships

No relationship comes with a guarantee. Losing love is as much a part of life as falling in love. That being said, uncoupling can be very painful (see the **Skills for Behavior Change** box for advice on approaching this difficult process). Whenever we get close to another, we also risk being hurt if things don't work out. Remember that knowing, understanding, and feeling good about oneself before entering the relationship is very important. Consider these tips for coping with a failed relationship.[34]

● Acknowledge that you've gone through a rough spot. You may feel grief, loneliness, rejection, anger, guilt, relief, sadness, or all of these. Remember, it's good to reach out to others to deal with these feelings. Seek out trusted friends and, if needed, professional help.

● Let go of negative thought patterns and habits. Engage in activities that make you happy. Walk, read, listen to music, go to the movies, the theater, concerts, spend time with fun friends, volunteer with a community organization, or write in a journal. Find your joy!

● Explore the new person you want to be while reconnecting with your old self. Take time to evaluate who you are at this point in your life. Think about what makes you happy and spend time with people who you enjoy and who are nurturing.

● Make a promise to yourself: no new relationships until you have moved past the last one. You need time to resolve your past experience rather than escape from it. It can be difficult to be trusting and intimate in a new relationship if you are still working on getting over a past one. Heal first, before looking for love again.

How Do You End It?

Relationship endings are just as important as their beginnings. Healthy closure affords both parties the opportunity to move on without wondering or worrying about what went wrong and whose fault it was. If you need to end a relationship, do so in a manner that preserves and respects the dignity of both partners. If you are the person "breaking up," you probably have had time to think about the process and may be at a different stage than your partner.

Here are some tips for ending a relationship in a respectful and caring way:

❱ Arrange a time and quiet place where you can talk without interruption.

❱ Say in advance that there is something important you want to discuss.

❱ Accept that your partner may express strong feelings and be prepared to listen quietly.

❱ Consider in advance if you might also become upset and what support you might need.

❱ Communicate honestly using "I" messages and without personal attacks. Explain your reasons as much as you can without being cruel or insensitive.

❱ Don't let things escalate into a fight, even if you have very strong feelings.

❱ Provide another opportunity to talk about the end of the relationship when you both have had time to reflect.

Your Sexual Identity: More Than Biology

Sexual identity, the recognition and acknowledgment of oneself as a sexual being, is determined by a complex interaction of genetic, physiological, environmental, and social factors. The beginning of sexual identity occurs at conception with the combining of chromosomes that determine sex. All eggs carry an X sex chromosome; sperm may carry either an X or a Y chromosome. If a sperm carrying an X chromosome fertilizes an egg, the resulting combination of sex chromosomes (XX) provides the blueprint to produce a female. If a sperm carrying a Y chromosome fertilizes an egg, the XY combination produces a male.

Sometimes chromosomes are added, lost, or rearranged in this process and the sex of the offspring is not clear, a condition known as **intersexuality.** *Disorders of sexual development* (*DSDs*) is a less confusing term that has been recommended to refer to intersex conditions, which may occur as often as 1 in 1,500 live births.[35]

The genetic instructions included in the sex chromosomes lead to the differential development of male and female **gonads** (reproductive organs) at about the eighth week of fetal life. Once the male gonads (testes) and the female gonads (ovaries) develop, they play a key role in all future sexual development because the gonads are responsible for the production of sex hormones. The primary female sex hormones are estrogen and progesterone. The primary male sex hormone is testosterone. The release of testosterone in a maturing fetus stimulates the development of a penis and other male genitals. If no testosterone is produced, female genitals form.

At the time of **puberty,** sex hormones again play major roles in development. Hormones released by the **pituitary gland,** called *gonadotropins,* stimulate the testes and ovaries to make appropriate sex hormones. The increase of estrogen production in females and testosterone production in males leads to the development of **secondary sex characteristics.** Male secondary sex characteristics include deepening of the voice, development of facial and body hair, and growth of the skeleton and musculature. Female secondary sex characteristics include growth of the breasts, widening of the hips, and the development of pubic and underarm hair.

In addition to a person's biological status as a male or female, another important component of sexual identity is gender. **Gender** refers to characteristics and actions typically associated with men or women (masculine or feminine) as defined by the culture in which one lives. Our sense of masculine and feminine traits is largely a result of **socialization** during our childhood. **Gender roles** are the behaviors and activities we use to express our maleness or femaleness in ways that conform to society's expectations. For example, you may have learned to play with dolls or trucks, based on how your parents influenced your actions.

For some, gender roles can be very confining when they lead to stereotyping. Bounds established by **gender-role stereotypes** can make it difficult to express one's true sexual identity. In the United States, men are traditionally expected to be independent, aggressive, logical, and always in control of their emotions, whereas women are traditionally expected to be passive, nurturing, intuitive, sensitive, and emotional. **Androgyny** refers to the combination

sexual identity Recognition of oneself as a sexual being; a composite of biological sex characteristics, gender identity, gender roles, and sexual orientation.

intersexuality Not exhibiting exclusively male or female sex characteristics; also known as disorders of sexual development (DSD).

gonads The reproductive organs that produce germ cells and sex hormones in a man (testes) or woman (ovaries).

puberty The period of sexual maturation.

pituitary gland The endocrine gland in the brain controlling the release of hormones from the gonads.

secondary sex characteristics Characteristics associated with sex but not directly related to reproduction, such as vocal pitch, amount of body hair, breasts, and location of fat deposits.

gender The characteristics and actions associated with being feminine or masculine as defined by the society or culture in which one lives.

socialization Process by which a society communicates behavioral expectations to its individual members.

gender roles Expression of maleness or femaleness in everyday life that conform to society's expectations.

gender-role stereotypes Generalizations concerning how men and women should express themselves and the characteristics each possesses.

androgyny Combination of traditional masculine and feminine traits in a single person.

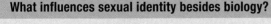

What influences sexual identity besides biology?

How you perceive yourself as a sexual being is influenced by socialization and personal experience. Your understanding of gender roles, your contact with people of various gender identities or sexual orientations, and your own degree of emotional maturity can all affect your sense of sexual identity.

gender identity *Personal sense or awareness of being masculine or feminine, a male or a female.*

transgendered *When one's gender identity does not match one's biological sex.*

transsexual *A person who is psychologically of one sex but physically of the other.*

sexual orientation *A person's enduring emotional, romantic, sexual, or affectionate attraction to other persons.*

heterosexual *Experiencing primary attraction to and preference for sexual activity with people of the other sex.*

homosexual *Experiencing primary attraction to and preference for sexual activity with people of the same sex.*

bisexual *Experiencing attraction to and preference for sexual activity with people of both sexes.*

gay *Sexual orientation involving primary attraction to people of the same sex; usually but not always applies to men attracted to men.*

lesbian *Sexual orientation involving attraction of women to other women.*

sexual prejudice *Negative attitudes and hostile actions directed at those with a different sexual orientation.*

See It! Videos

Is being gay in the spotlight no big deal? Watch **Celebrities Coming Out, Casually** in the Study Area of MasteringHealth™

of traditional masculine and feminine traits in a single person. Androgynous people do not always follow traditional sex roles but instead choose behaviors based on the given situation.

Whereas gender roles are an expression of cultural expectations for behavior, **gender identity** is the personal sense or awareness of being masculine or feminine, a male or a female. A person's gender identity does not always match his or her biological sex; this is called being **transgendered.** There is a broad spectrum of expression among transgendered persons that reflects the degree of dissatisfaction they have with their sexual anatomy. Some transgendered persons are very comfortable with their bodies and are content simply to dress and live as the other gender. At the other end of the spectrum are **transsexuals,** who feel trapped in their bodies and may opt for therapeutic interventions, such as sex reassignment surgery.

Sexual Orientation

Sexual orientation refers to a person's enduring emotional, romantic, sexual, or affectionate attraction to others. You may be primarily attracted to members of the other sex (**heterosexual**), your same sex (**homosexual**), or both sexes (**bisexual**). Many homosexuals prefer the terms **gay,** queer, or **lesbian** to describe their sexual orientation. *Gay* and *queer* can apply to both men and women, but *lesbian* refers specifically to women.

Most researchers today agree that sexual orientation is best understood using a model that incorporates biological, psychological, and socioenvironmental factors. Biological explanations focus on research into genetics, hormones, and differences in brain anatomy, whereas psychological and socioenvironmental explanations examine parent–child interactions, sex roles, and early sexual and interpersonal interactions. Collectively, this growing body of research suggests that the origins of homosexuality, like heterosexuality, are complex.[36] To diminish the complexity of sexual orientation to "a choice" is a clear misrepresentation of current research. Homosexuals do not "choose" their sexual orientation any more than heterosexuals do.

Sexual orientation is often viewed as a concept based entirely on whom one has sex with, but this is an inaccurate and overly simplistic idea. It depends not only on whom you are

sexually attracted to, fantasize about, and actually have sex with, but also factors such as who you feel close to emotionally and in which "community" you feel most comfortable. In reality there are a whole range of complex, interacting, and fluid factors that influence your sexuality over time.

Gay, lesbian, and bisexual persons are repeatedly the targets of **sexual prejudice.** Sexual prejudice refers to negative attitudes and hostile actions directed at a social group and its members.[37] Hate crimes, discrimination, and hostility targeting sexual minorities are evidence of ongoing sexual prejudice. Recent data from the Department of Justice indicate that bias regarding sexual orientation is the motivation for approximately 21 percent of all hate crimes reported in the United States.[38]

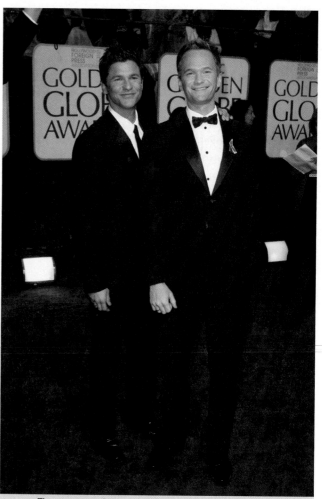

The presence of gay and lesbian celebrities in the media contributes to the increasing acceptance of gay relationships in everyday life. Actor Neil Patrick Harris and his partner David Burtka are an openly gay couple who plan to marry now that New York state has legalized gay marriage.

Sexual Anatomy and Physiology

An understanding of the functions of the female and male reproductive systems will help you derive pleasure and satisfaction from your sexual relationships, be sensitive to your partner's wants and needs, and make responsible choices regarding your own sexual health.

Female Sexual Anatomy and Physiology

The female reproductive system includes two major groups of structures, the external genitals and the internal organs (Figure 5.5). The external female genitals are collectively known as the **vulva** and include all structures that are outwardly visible: the mons pubis, the labia minora and majora, the clitoris, the urethral and vaginal openings, and the vestibule of the vagina and its glands. The **mons pubis** is a pad of fatty tissue covering and protecting the pubic bone; after the onset of puberty, it becomes covered with coarse hair. The **labia majora** are folds of skin and erectile tissue that enclose the urethral and vaginal openings; the **labia minora,** or inner lips, are folds of mucous membrane found just inside the labia majora.

The **clitoris** is located at the upper end of the labia minora and beneath the mons pubis, and its only known function is to provide sexual pleasure. Directly below the clitoris is the urethral opening through which urine is expelled from the body. Below the urethral opening is the vaginal opening. In some women, the vaginal opening is covered by a thin membrane called the **hymen**. It is a myth that an intact hymen is proof of virginity, as the hymen can be stretched or torn by physical activity and is not present in all women to begin with.

The **perineum** is the area of smooth tissue found between the vulva and the anus. Although not technically part of the external genitalia, the tissue in this area has many nerve endings and is sensitive to touch; it can play a part in sexual excitement.

The internal female genitals include the vagina, uterus, fallopian tubes, and ovaries. The **vagina** is a tubular organ that serves as a passageway from the uterus to the outside of the body. This passage allows menstrual flow to exit from the uterus during a woman's monthly cycle, receives the penis during intercourse, and serves as the birth canal during childbirth. The **uterus (womb)** is a hollow, muscular, pear-shaped organ. Hormones acting on the inner lining of the uterus (the **endometrium**), either prepare the uterus for implantation and development of a fertilized egg or signal that no fertilization has taken place, in which case the endometrium deteriorates and becomes menstrual flow.

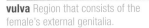

vulva Region that consists of the female's external genitalia.

mons pubis Fatty tissue covering the pubic bone in females; in physically mature women, the mons is covered with coarse hair.

labia majora "Outer lips," or folds of tissue covering the female sexual organs.

labia minora "Inner lips," or folds of tissue just inside the labia majora.

clitoris A pea-sized nodule of tissue located at the top of the labia minora; central to sexual arousal and pleasure in women.

hymen Thin tissue covering the vaginal opening in some women.

perineum Tissue that forms the "floor" of the pelvic region, found between the vulva and the anus.

vagina The passage in females leading from the vulva into the uterus.

uterus (womb) Hollow, muscular, pear-shaped organ whose function is to contain the developing fetus.

endometrium Soft, spongy matter that makes up the uterine lining.

External Anatomy

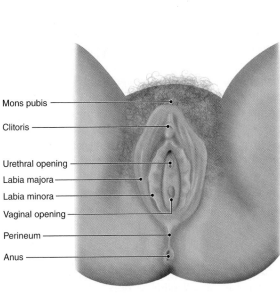

Mons pubis
Clitoris
Urethral opening
Labia majora
Labia minora
Vaginal opening
Perineum
Anus

Internal Organs

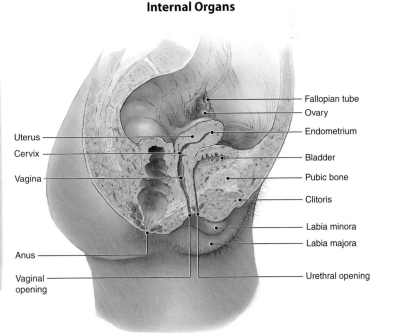

Uterus
Cervix
Vagina
Anus
Vaginal opening

Fallopian tube
Ovary
Endometrium
Bladder
Pubic bone
Clitoris
Labia minora
Labia majora
Urethral opening

FIGURE 5.5 **Female Reproductive System**

The lower end of the uterus, the **cervix,** extends down into the vagina. The **ovaries,** almond-sized organs suspended on either side of the uterus, produce the hormones estrogen and progesterone and are the reservoir for immature eggs. All the eggs a woman will ever have are present in her ovaries at birth. Eggs mature and are released from the ovaries in response to hormone levels. Extending from the upper end of the uterus are two thin, flexible tubes called the **fallopian tubes.** The fallopian tubes, which do not actually touch the ovaries, capture eggs as they are released from the ovaries during ovulation, and they are the site where sperm and egg meet and fertilization takes place. The fallopian tubes then serve as the passageway to the uterus, where the fertilized egg becomes implanted and development continues.

The Onset of Puberty and the Menstrual Cycle

With the onset of puberty, the female reproductive system matures, and the development of secondary sex characteristics transforms young girls into young women. The first sign of puberty is the beginning of breast development, which generally occurs around age 11. The pituitary gland, the **hypothalamus,** and the ovaries all secrete hormones that act as chemical messengers among them. Working in a feedback system, hormonal levels in the bloodstream act as the trigger mechanism for release of more or different hormones.

Around age $9^1/_2$ to $11^1/_2$, the hypothalamus receives the message to begin secreting *gonadotropin-releasing hormone (GnRH)*. The release of GnRH in turn signals the pituitary gland to release hormones called *gonadotropins*. Two gonadotropins, *follicle-stimulating hormone (FSH)* and *luteinizing hormone (LH)*, signal the ovaries to start producing **estrogens** and **progesterone.** Estrogens regulate the menstrual cycle, and increased estrogen levels assist in the development of female secondary sex characteristics. Progesterone helps the endometrium to develop in preparation to nourish a fertilized egg and helps maintain pregnancy.

The normal age range for the onset of the first menstrual period, termed **menarche,** is 9 to 17 years, with the average age being $11^1/_2$ to $13^1/_2$ years. Body fat heavily influences the onset of puberty, and increasing rates of obesity in children may account for the fact that girls in the United States and other countries are reaching puberty earlier than they used to.[39] Other theories on early menarche include family disruption, high stress levels, and endocrine disruptors in the food supply.

The average menstrual cycle lasts 28 days and consists of three phases: the proliferative phase, the secretory phase, and the menstrual phase. The *proliferative phase* begins with the end of menstruation. During this time, the endometrium develops, or "proliferates." How does this process work? By the end of menstruation, the hypothalamus senses very low levels of estrogen and progesterone in the blood. In response, it increases its secretions of GnRH, which in turn triggers the pituitary gland to release FSH. When FSH reaches the ovaries, it signals several **ovarian follicles** to begin maturing (Figure 5.6 on page 155) . Normally, only one of the follicles, the **graafian follicle,** reaches full maturity in the days preceding ovulation. While the follicles mature, they begin producing estrogen, which in turn signals the endometrium to proliferate. If fertilization occurs, the endometrium will become a nesting place for the developing embryo. High estrogen levels signal the pituitary gland to slow down FSH production and increase release of LH. Under the influence of LH, the ovarian follicle ruptures and releases a mature **ovum** (plural: *ova*), a single mature egg cell, near a fallopian tube (around day 14). This is the process of **ovulation.** The other ripening follicles degenerate and are reabsorbed by the body. Occasionally, two ova mature and are released during ovulation. If both are fertilized, fraternal (nonidentical) twins develop. Identical twins develop when one fertilized ovum (called a *zygote*) divides into two separate zygotes.

The phase following ovulation is called the *secretory phase*. The ruptured graafian follicle, which has remained in the ovary, is transformed into the **corpus luteum** and begins secreting large amounts of estrogen and progesterone. These hormone secretions peak around the twentieth or twenty-first day of the average cycle and cause the endometrium to thicken and continue preparing for a potential fertilized ovum. If fertilization and implantation take place, cells surrounding the developing embryo release a hormone called *human chorionic gonadotropin (HCG)*, increasing estrogen and progesterone secretions that maintain the endometrium and signal the pituitary not to start a new menstrual cycle.

If no implantation occurs, the hypothalamus responds by signaling the pituitary gland to stop producing FSH and LH, thus causing the levels of progesterone in the blood to peak. The corpus luteum begins to decompose, leading to rapid declines in estrogen and progesterone levels. These hormones are needed to sustain the lining of the uterus. Without them, the endometrium is sloughed off in the menstrual flow, and this begins the *menstrual phase*. The low estrogen levels of the menstrual phase signal the hypothalamus to release GnRH, which acts on the pituitary gland to secrete FSH, and the cycle begins again.

Menstrual Problems

Premenstrual syndrome (PMS) is a term used for a collection of physical, emotional, and behavioral symptoms that many women experience 7 to 14 days prior to their menstrual period. The most common symptoms are tender breasts, food cravings, fatigue,

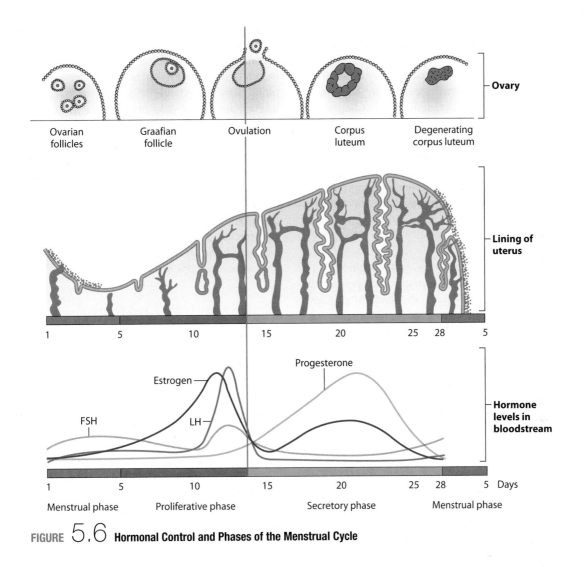

Ovary

Ovarian follicles | Graafian follicle | Ovulation | Corpus luteum | Degenerating corpus luteum

Lining of uterus

1   5   10   15   20   25   28   5

Hormone levels in bloodstream

Estrogen
Progesterone
FSH
LH

1   5   10   15   20   25   28   5   Days

Menstrual phase | Proliferative phase | Secretory phase | Menstrual phase

FIGURE 5.6 **Hormonal Control and Phases of the Menstrual Cycle**

irritability, and depression. It is estimated that 75 percent of menstruating women experience some signs and symptoms of PMS each month.[40] For the majority of women, these disappear as their period begins, but for a small subset of women (3 to 5 percent), symptoms are severe enough to affect their daily routines and activities to the point of being disabling. This severe form of PMS has its own diagnostic category in the *DSM-5*, **premenstrual dysphoric disorder (PMDD),** with symptoms that include severe depression, hopelessness, anger, anxiety, low self-esteem, difficulty concentrating, irritability, and tension.[41]

There are several natural approaches to managing PMS that can also help PMDD. These strategies include eating more carbohydrates (grains, fruits, and vegetables), reducing caffeine and salt intake, exercising regularly, and taking measures to reduce stress. Recent investigation into methods of controlling the severe emotional swings has led to the use of antidepressants for treating PMDD, primarily selective serotonin reuptake inhibitors (SSRIs; e.g., Prozac, Paxil, and Zoloft).

Dysmenorrhea is a medical term for menstrual cramps, the pain or discomfort in the lower abdomen that many women experience just before or during menstruation. Along with cramps, some women can experience nausea and vomiting, loose stools, sweating, and dizziness. Menstrual cramps can be classified as primary or secondary dysmenorrhea. Primary dysmenorrhea doesn't involve any physical abnormality and usually begins 6 months to a year after a woman's first period, while secondary dysmenorrhea has an underlying physical cause such as endometriosis or uterine fibroids.[42] You can reduce the discomfort of primary dysmenorrhea by using over-the-counter nonsteroidal anti-inflammatory drugs (NSAIDS) such as aspirin, ibuprofen (Advil or Motrin), or naproxen (Aleve). Other self-care strategies such as soaking in a hot bath or using a heating pad on your abdomen may also ease your cramps. For severe cramping, your health care provider may recommend a low-dose oral contraceptive to prevent ovulation, which in turn may reduce the production of **prostaglandins** and therefore the severity of your cramps. Managing secondary dysmenorrhea involves treating the underlying cause.

premenstrual dysphoric disorder (PMDD) Collective name for a group of negative symptoms similar to but more severe than PMS, including severe mood disturbances.

dysmenorrhea Condition of pain or discomfort in the lower abdomen just before or during menstruation.

prostaglandin A hormone-like substance associated with muscle contraction and inflammation.

Toxic shock syndrome (TSS), although rare today, is still something women should be aware of. TSS is caused by a bacterial infection facilitated by tampon or diaphragm use (see **Chapter 6**). Symptoms, which occur during one's period or a few days after, are sometimes hard to recognize because they mimic the flu and include sudden high fever, vomiting, diarrhea, dizziness, fainting, or a rash that looks like sunburn. Proper treatment usually ensures recovery in 2 to 3 weeks.

Menopause Just as menarche signals the beginning of a woman's reproductive years, **menopause**—the permanent cessation of menstruation—signals the end. Menopause generally occurs between the ages of 40 and 60; the average age is 51 in the United States. It results in decreased estrogen levels, which may produce troublesome symptoms in some women. Decreased vaginal lubrication, hot flashes, headaches, dizziness, and joint pain have all been associated with the onset of menopause.

Hormones, such as estrogen and progesterone, have long been prescribed as **hormone replacement therapy** to relieve menopausal symptoms and reduce the risk of heart disease and osteoporosis. (The National Institutes of Health prefers the term **menopausal hormone therapy,** because this hormone treatment is not a replacement and does not restore the physiology of youth.) However, recent studies, including results from the Women's Health Initiative (WHI),

suggest that hormone therapy may actually do more harm than good. In fact, the WHI terminated research on this therapy ahead of schedule because of concerns about participants' increased risk of breast cancer, heart attack, stroke, blood clots, and other health problems.[43] New data, however, indicate that these risks may be related to the age at which women begin HRT and the form (pill or patch) utilized.[44] Conflicting research such as this highlights the need for all women to discuss the risks and benefits of menopausal hormone therapy with their health care provider and come to an informed decision. It is crucial to find a doctor who specializes in women's health and keeps up-to-date with the latest research findings. Certainly a healthy lifestyle, such as regular exercise, a balanced diet, and adequate calcium intake, can also help protect postmenopausal women from heart disease and osteoporosis.

Male Sexual Anatomy and Physiology

The structures of the male reproductive system are divided into external and internal genitals (Figure 5.7). The external genitals are the penis and the scrotum. The internal male genitals include the testes, epididymides, vasa deferentia, ejaculatory ducts, urethra, and three other structures—the seminal vesicles, the prostate gland, and the Cowper's glands—that secrete components that, with sperm, make up semen. These three structures are sometimes referred to as the *accessory glands.*

The **penis** is the organ that deposits sperm in the vagina during intercourse. The urethra, which passes through the center of the penis, acts as the passageway for both semen

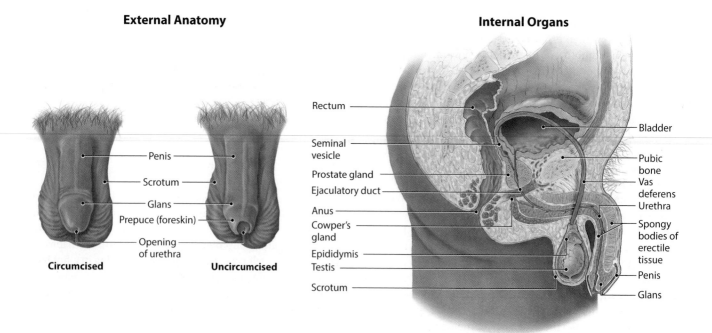

External Anatomy

Penis
Scrotum
Glans
Prepuce (foreskin)
Opening of urethra

Circumcised   **Uncircumcised**

Internal Organs

Rectum

Seminal vesicle
Prostate gland
Ejaculatory duct
Anus
Cowper's gland
Epididymis
Testis
Scrotum

Bladder
Pubic bone
Vas deferens
Urethra
Spongy bodies of erectile tissue
Penis
Glans

FIGURE 5.7 **Male Reproductive System**

and urine to exit the body. During sexual arousal, the spongy tissue in the penis becomes filled with blood, making the organ stiff (erect). Further sexual excitement leads to **ejaculation,** a series of rapid, spasmodic contractions that propel semen out of the penis.

Situated behind the penis and also outside the body is a sac called the **scrotum.** The scrotum protects the testes and helps control the temperature within the testes, which is vital to proper sperm production. The **testes** (singular: *testis*) manufacture sperm and **testosterone,** the hormone responsible for the development of male secondary sex characteristics.

The development of sperm is referred to as **spermatogenesis.** Like the maturation of eggs in the female, this process is governed by the pituitary gland. Follicle-stimulating hormone (FSH) is secreted into the bloodstream to stimulate the testes to manufacture sperm. Immature sperm are released into a comma-shaped structure on the back of each testis called the **epididymis** (plural: *epididymides*), where they ripen and reach full maturity.

Each epididymis contains coiled tubules that gradually "unwind" and straighten out to become the **vas deferens.** The two vasa deferentia, as they are called in the plural, make up the tubular transportation system whose sole function is to store and move sperm. Along the way, the **seminal vesicles** provide sperm with nutrients and other fluids that comprise **semen.**

The vasa deferentia eventually connect each epididymis to the ejaculatory ducts, which pass through the prostate gland and empty into the urethra. The **prostate gland** contributes more fluids to the semen, including chemicals that help the sperm fertilize an ovum and neutralize the acidic environment of the vagina to make it more conducive to sperm motility (ability to move) and potency (potential for fertilizing an ovum). Just below the prostate gland are two pea-shaped nodules called the **Cowper's glands.** The Cowper's glands secrete a fluid that lubricates the urethra and neutralizes any acid that may remain in the urethra after urination. Urine and semen do not come into contact with each other. During ejaculation of semen, a small valve closes off the tube to the urinary bladder.

Debate continues over the practice of *circumcision,* the surgical removal of a fold of skin, known as the *foreskin,* covering the end of the penis. While nearly universal in the United States a few decades ago, only about 55 percent of baby boys are now circumcised, mostly for religious or cultural reasons or because of hygiene concerns. However, recent research supports the claim that circumcision yields medical benefits, including decreased risk of urinary tract infections in the first year, decreased risk of penile cancer (although cancer of the penis is very rare), and decreased risk of sexual transmission of human papillomavirus (HPV) and human immunodeficiency virus (HIV). Strong arguments that can be made against circumcision include a lack of medical necessity, a possible reduction in sexual sensitivity, and the possibility of bleeding, infection, and surgical complications. The American Academy of Pediatrics

recently took a stand on the issue stating that scientific evidence shows potential medical benefits of newborn male circumcision but that the evidence is not currently strong enough to recommend routine circumcision.[45]

Human Sexual Response

Video Tutor: Male and Female Sexual Response

Psychological factors greatly influence sexual response and sexual desire. Thus, you may find a sexual relationship with one partner vastly different from experiences with another.

Sexual response is a physiological process that generally follows a pattern. Sexual responses in both men and women are somewhat arbitrarily divided into four stages: excitement/arousal, plateau, orgasm, and resolution. Researchers agree that each individual has a personal response pattern that may or may not conform to these phases. Regardless of the type of sexual activity (stimulation by a partner or self-stimulation), the response stages for an individual are the same.

During the first stage, *excitement/arousal,* **vasocongestion** (increased blood flow that causes swelling in the genitals) stimulates male and female genital responses. The vagina begins to lubricate in preparation for penile penetration, and the penis becomes partially erect. Both sexes may exhibit a "sex flush," or light blush all over their bodies. Excitement/arousal can be generated through fantasy or by touching parts of the body, kissing, viewing images or videos, or reading erotic literature.

During the *plateau phase,* the initial responses intensify. Voluntary and involuntary muscle tensions increase. The woman's nipples and the man's penis become erect. The penis secretes a few drops of preejaculatory fluid, which may contain sperm.

During the *orgasmic phase,* vasocongestion and muscle tensions reach their peak, and rhythmic contractions occur through the genital regions. In women, these contractions are centered in the uterus, outer vagina, and anal sphincter. In men, the contractions occur in two stages. First, contractions within the prostate gland begin propelling semen through the urethra. In the second stage, the muscles of the pelvic floor, urethra, and anal sphincter contract. Semen usually, but not always, is ejaculated from the penis. In both

ejaculation The propulsion of semen from the penis.

scrotum External sac of tissue that encloses the testes.

testes Male sex organs that manufacture sperm and produce hormones.

testosterone The male sex hormone manufactured in the testes.

spermatogenesis The development of sperm.

epididymis The duct system atop each testis where sperm mature.

vas deferens A tube that transports sperm from the epididymis to the ejaculatory duct.

seminal vesicles Glandular ducts that secrete nutrients for the semen.

semen Fluid containing sperm and nutrients that increase sperm viability and neutralize vaginal acid.

prostate gland Gland that secretes chemicals that help sperm fertilize an ovum and provides neutralizing fluids into the semen.

Cowper's glands Glands that secrete a fluid that lubricates the urethra and neutralizes any acid remaining in the urethra after urination.

vasocongestion The engorgement of the genital organs with blood.

sexes, spasms in other major muscle groups also occur, particularly in the buttocks and abdomen. In both men and women, feet and hands may also contract, and facial features often contort.

Muscle tension and congested blood subside in the *resolution phase,* as the genital organs return to their pre-arousal states. Both sexes usually experience deep feelings of well-being and profound relaxation. Following orgasm and resolution, many women can become aroused again and experience additional orgasms. However, some men experience a refractory period, during which their systems are incapable of subsequent arousal. This refractory period may last from a few minutes to several hours and tends to lengthen with age.

Men and women experience the same stages in the sexual response cycle; however, the length of time spent in any one stage varies. Thus, one partner may be in the plateau phase while the other is in the excitement or orgasmic phase. Such variations in response rates are entirely normal. Some couples believe that simultaneous orgasm is desirable for sexual satisfaction. Although simultaneous orgasm is pleasant, so are orgasms achieved at different times.

Sexual pleasure and satisfaction are also possible without orgasm or intercourse. Expressing sexual feelings for another person involves many pleasurable activities, of which intercourse and orgasm are only a part.

what do you think?

Why do we place so much importance on orgasm?
● Can sexual pleasure and satisfaction be achieved without orgasm?
● What is the role of desire in sexual response?

Expressing Your Sexuality

Finding healthy ways to express your sexuality is an important part of developing sexual maturity. Many avenues of sexual expression are available.

Sexual Behavior: What Is "Normal"?

How do we know which sexual behaviors are considered normal? What or whose criteria should we use? These are not easy questions.

Every society sets standards and attempts to regulate sexual behavior. Boundaries arise that distinguish good from bad, acceptable from unacceptable, and they result in criteria used to establish what is viewed as normal or abnormal. Some of the common sociocultural standards for sexual behavior commonly held in Western culture today include the following:[46]

celibacy State of not engaging in sexual activities or a sexual relationship.

● **The coital standard.** Penile-vaginal intercourse (coitus) is viewed as the ultimate sex act.
● **The orgasmic standard.** Sexual interaction should lead to orgasm.
● **The two-person standard.** Sex is an activity to be experienced by two.
● **The romantic standard.** Sex should be related to love.
● **The safer sex standard.** If we choose to be sexually active, we should act to prevent unintended pregnancy or disease transmission.

These are not laws or rules, but rather social scripts that have been adopted over time. Sexual standards often shift through the years, and many people choose not to follow them. Rather than making blanket judgments about normal versus abnormal, we might ask the following questions:[47]

● Is a sexual behavior healthy and fulfilling for a particular person?
● Is it safe?
● Does it lead to the exploitation of others?
● Does it take place between responsible, consenting adults?

In this way, we can view behavior along a continuum that takes into account many individual factors. As you read about the options for sexual expression in the pages ahead, use these questions to explore your feelings about what is normal for you.

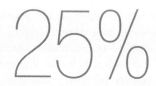

25%
of college students report having had more than one sex partner in the past 12 months.

Options for Sexual Expression

The range of human sexual expression is virtually infinite. What you find enjoyable may not be an option for someone else. The ways you choose to meet your sexual needs today may be very different from what they were 2 weeks ago, or will be 2 years from now. Accepting yourself as a sexual person with individual desires and preferences is the first step in achieving sexual satisfaction.

Celibacy Celibacy is avoidance of or abstention from sexual activities. Some individuals choose celibacy for religious or moral reasons. Others may be celibate for a period of time because of illness, the breakup of a long-term relationship, or lack of an acceptable partner. For some, celibacy is a lonely, agonizing state, but others find it an opportunity for introspection, values assessment, and personal growth. While abstinence and celibacy are related terms, abstinence usually refers to the avoidance of intercourse, and celibacy usually refers to abstention from all sexual behaviors with another person or all sexual activities whatsoever.

Autoerotic Behaviors

Autoerotic behaviors involve sexual self-stimulation. The two most common are sexual fantasy and masturbation.

Sexual fantasies are sexually arousing thoughts and dreams. Fantasies may reflect real-life experiences, forbidden desires, or the opportunity to practice new or anticipated sexual experiences. The fact that you may fantasize about a particular sexual experience does not mean that you want to, or have to, act out that experience. Sexual fantasies are just that—fantasy.

Masturbation is self-stimulation of the genitals. Although many people feel uncomfortable discussing masturbation, it is a common sexual practice across the life span. Masturbation is a natural pleasure-seeking behavior in infants and children. It is a valuable and important means for adolescents, as well as adults, to explore sexual feelings and responsiveness. In one survey of college students, 48 percent of women and 92 percent of men reported that they have masturbated.[48]

Kissing and Erotic Touching

Kissing and erotic touching are two very common forms of nonverbal sexual communication. Both men and women have **erogenous zones**, areas of the body that when touched lead to sexual arousal. Erogenous zones may include genital as well as nongenital areas, such as the earlobes, mouth, breasts, and inner thighs. Almost any area of the body can be conditioned to respond erotically to touch. Spending time with your partner to explore and learn about his or her erogenous areas is another pleasurable, safe, and satisfying means of sexual expression.

Manual Stimulation

Both men and women can be sexually aroused and achieve orgasm through manual stimulation of the genitals by a partner. For many women, orgasm is more likely to be achieved through manual stimulation than through intercourse. *Sex toys* include a wide variety of objects that can be used for sexual stimulation alone or with a partner. Vibrators and dildos are two common types of toys and can be found in a variety of shapes, styles, and sizes. Sex toys can add zest to sexual experiences and, for women who may not reach orgasm by intercourse, may provide another option for satisfaction. (Note that toys must be cleaned after each use.)

Oral-Genital Stimulation

Cunnilingus refers to oral stimulation of a woman's genitals and **fellatio** to oral stimulation of a man's genitals. Many partners find oral-genital stimulation intensely pleasurable. In the most recent National College Health Assessment (NCHA), 42 percent of college students reported having oral sex in the past month.[49] For some people, oral sex is not an option because of moral or religious beliefs. Remember, HIV (human immunodeficiency virus) and other sexually transmitted infections (STIs) can be transmitted via unprotected oral-genital sex, just as

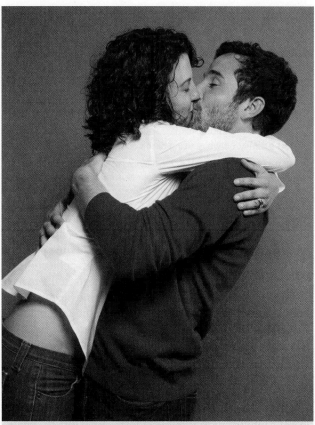

As with any other human behavior, the idea of "normal" sexual activity varies from person to person and from society to society.

they can through intercourse. Use of an appropriate barrier device is strongly recommended if a partner's disease status is unknown.

Vaginal Intercourse

The term *intercourse* generally refers to **vaginal intercourse** (*coitus,* or insertion of the penis into the vagina), which is the most often practiced form of sexual expression. In the latest NCHA survey, 46 percent of college students reported having vaginal intercourse in the past month.[50] Coitus can involve a variety of positions, including the missionary position (man on top facing the woman), woman on top, side by side, or man behind (rear entry). Many partners enjoy experimenting with different positions. Knowledge of yourself and your body, along with your ability to communicate effectively, will play a large part in determining the enjoyment and meaningfulness of intercourse for you and your partner. Also, it is easier to relax and enjoy sex when you know that you are protected from disease and unintended pregnancy. (See **Chapter 13** for more about safer sex.)

autoerotic behaviors Sexual self-stimulation.

sexual fantasies Sexually arousing thoughts and dreams.

masturbation Self-stimulation of genitals.

erogenous zones Areas of the body of both men and women that, when touched, lead to sexual arousal.

cunnilingus Oral stimulation of a woman's genitals.

fellatio Oral stimulation of a man's genitals.

vaginal intercourse The insertion of the penis into the vagina.

Maybe you already make healthy, responsible, and satisfying decisions about your sex life. Which of these behaviors are you already practicing?

☐ I've chosen to be celibate—with so many other obligations and pressures in my life, this choice makes sense to me right now.

☐ I'm in a monogamous sexual relationship. We're not ready to start a family, so we're using birth control.

☐ My partner doesn't want to have sex—he says he's not ready. We still manage to show each other our love by kissing and touching.

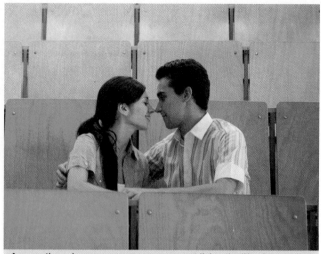

Are you the only person on your campus not living the life of the typical reality TV hottie? Probably not. You may think everyone else is having more sex with more partners than you are, but generally speaking, the actual numbers don't measure up to college students' perceptions.

Anal Intercourse The anal area is highly sensitive to touch, and some couples find pleasure in the stimulation of this area. **Anal intercourse** is the insertion of the penis into the anus. Research indicates that 5 percent of college students have had anal sex in the past month.[51] Stimulation of the anus by mouth or with the fingers is also practiced. As with all forms of sexual expression, anal stimulation or intercourse is not for everyone. If you enjoy this form of sexual expression, note that condom usage is especially important, as the delicate tissues of the anus are more likely to tear than are vaginal tissues, significantly increasing the risk of transmission of HIV and other STIs. Also, anything inserted into the anus should not be inserted into the vagina without cleaning because bacteria commonly found in the anus can cause vaginal infections.

anal intercourse The insertion of the penis into the anus.

Responsible and Satisfying Sexual Behavior

Sexuality is a fascinating, complex, contradictory, and sometimes frustrating aspect of our lives. Healthy sexuality doesn't happen by chance. It is a product of assimilating information and skills, of exploring values and beliefs, and of making responsible and informed choices. Healthy and responsible sexuality includes the following:

● **Good communication as the foundation.** Open and honest communication with your partner is the basis for establishing respect, trust, and intimacy. Do you communicate with your partner in caring and respectful ways? Can you share your thoughts and emotions freely with your partner? Do you talk about being sexually active and what that means? Can you share your sexual history with your partner? Do you discuss contraception and disease prevention? Are you able to communicate what you like and don't like? All of these are components of open communication that accompany healthy, responsible sexuality.

● **Acknowledging that you are a sexual person.** People who can see and accept themselves as sexual beings are more likely to make informed decisions and take responsible actions. If you see yourself as a potentially sexual person, you will plan ahead for contraception and disease prevention. If

you are comfortable being a sexually active person, you will not need or want your sexual experiences clouded by alcohol or other drug use. If you choose not to be sexually active, you do so consciously, as a personal decision based on your convictions. Even if you are not sexually active, it is important to acknowledge that sex is a natural aspect of life and to recognize that you are in charge of your own decisions about your sexuality.

● **Understanding sexual structures and their functions.** If you understand how your body works, sexual pleasure and response will not be mysterious events. You will be able to pleasure yourself as well as communicate to your partner how best to pleasure you. You will understand how pregnancy and sexually transmitted infections can be prevented. You will be able to recognize sexual dysfunction and take responsible actions to address the problem.

● **Accepting and embracing your gender identity and your sexual orientation.** "Being comfortable in your own skin" is an old saying that is particularly relevant when it comes to sexuality. It is difficult to feel sexually satisfied if you are

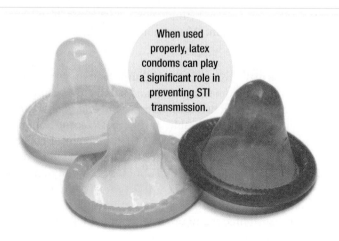

When used properly, latex condoms can play a significant role in preventing STI transmission.

conflicted about your gender identity or sexual orientation. You should explore and address questions and feelings you may have. Good communication skills, acknowledging that you are a sexual person, and understanding your sexual anatomy and its functions will allow you to complete this task.

Variant Sexual Behavior

Although attitudes toward sexuality have changed radically over time, some behaviors are still considered to be outside the norm. People who study sexuality prefer the neutral term **variant sexual behavior** to describe sexual activities that most people do not engage in, such as the following:

- **Group sex**—sexual activity involving more than two people. Participants in group sex run a higher risk of exposure to HIV and other STIs.
- **Transvestism**—wearing the clothing of the opposite sex. Most transvestites are male, heterosexual, and married.
- **Fetishism**—sexual arousal achieved by looking at or touching inanimate objects, such as underclothing or shoes.

Some variant sexual behaviors can be harmful to the individual, to others, or to both. Many of the following activities are illegal in at least some states:

- **Exhibitionism**—exposing one's genitals to strangers in public places. Most exhibitionists are seeking a reaction of shock or fear from their victims. Exhibitionism is a minor felony in most states.
- **Voyeurism**—observing other people for sexual gratification. Most voyeurs are men who attempt to watch women undressing or bathing. Voyeurism is an invasion of privacy and is illegal in most states.
- **Sadomasochism**—sexual activities in which gratification is achieved by inflicting pain (verbal or physical abuse) on a partner or by being the object of such infliction. A sadist is a person who enjoys inflicting pain, and a masochist is a person who enjoys experiencing it.
- **Pedophilia**—sexual activity or attraction between an adult and a child. Any sexual activity involving a minor, including possession of child pornography, is illegal in all states.
- **Autoerotic asphyxiation**—practice of reducing or eliminating oxygen to the brain, usually by tying a cord around one's neck, to increase pleasure while masturbating to orgasm. Tragically, some individuals accidentally strangle themselves.

Sexual Dysfunction

Research indicates that *sexual dysfunction,* the term used to describe problems that can hinder sexual functioning, is quite common. Sexual dysfunction can be divided into four major categories: desire disorders, arousal disorders,

TABLE 5.2	Types of Sexual Dysfunction	
	Description
Desire Disorders	
Inhibited sexual desire	Lack of interest in sexual activity
Sexual aversion disorder	Phobias (fears) or anxiety about sexual contact
Arousal Disorders	
Erectile dysfunction	Inability to achieve or maintain an erection
Female sexual arousal disorder	Inability to remain sexually aroused
Orgasmic Disorders	
Premature ejaculation	Reaching orgasm rapidly or prematurely
Retarded ejaculation	Inability to ejaculate once an erection is achieved
Female orgasmic disorder	Inability to have an orgasm or difficulty/delay in reaching orgasm
Pain Disorders	
Dyspareunia	Pain during or after sex
Vaginismus	Forceful contraction of the vaginal muscles that prevents penetration from occurring

orgasmic disorders, and pain disorders (see **Table 5.2**). All of them can be treated successfully.

People should not feel embarrassed about sexual dysfunction. The reproductive system can malfunction just as any other body system can. If you experience a problem with sexual function, an important first step is to seek out a qualified health care provider to investigate the possible causes. Causes can be varied and overlapping and commonly include biological/medical factors; substance-induced factors (recreational, over-the-counter, or prescription drug use); psychological factors (stress, performance pressure); and factors related to social context (relationship tensions, poor communication).[52]

variant sexual behavior A sexual behavior that most people do not engage in.

what do you think?

Why do we find it so difficult to discuss sexual dysfunction?
- Do you think it is more difficult for men or for women to talk about dysfunction? Why?

Sexual dysfunctions are most common in the early adult years, with the majority of people seeking care for these conditions during their late twenties and into their thirties. The incidence of dysfunction increases again during perimenopause and postmenopause years in women and in older age for both men and women.[53]

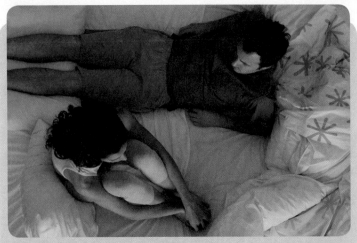

Are sexual disorders more physical or more psychological?

Sexual disorders can have both physical and psychological roots. Sexual desire disorders, orgasmic disorders, and sexual performance disorders often arise as a result of stress, fatigue, depression, or anxiety, but they frequently have physiological bases, such as medication or substance use, as well. Sexual arousal disorders and sexual pain disorders, on the other hand, often are strongly related to physical conditions and risk factors, but they may be exacerbated by stress and mental health problems. Interpersonal problems, including lack of trust and communication between partners, are also significant contributors to the development of sexual dysfunctions.

of alcohol or other drugs. However, these drugs probably have only a placebo effect in men with normal erections, and combining them with other drugs, such as ketamine, amyl nitrate, or methamphetamine, can lead to potentially fatal drug interactions. In particular, when combined with amyl nitrate, these drugs can lead to a sudden drop in blood pressure and possible cardiac arrest.[54]

"Date rape" drugs have been a growing concern in recent decades. They have become prevalent on college campuses, where they are often used in combination with alcohol. (The dangers of these drugs are discussed in more detail in **Chapters 4** and **7**.)

Perhaps the most common danger associated with use of drugs during sex is the tendency to blame the drug for negative behavior or unsafe sexual activities. "I can't help what I did last night because I was drunk" is a statement that demonstrates sexual immaturity. A sexually mature person carefully examines risks and benefits and makes decisions accordingly. If drugs are necessary to increase erotic feelings or reduce inhibitions, it is likely that the partners are being dishonest about their feelings for each other. Good sex should not depend on chemical substances.

Drugs and Sex

Because psychoactive drugs affect the body's entire physiological functioning, it is only logical that they also affect sexual behavior. Promises of increased pleasure make drugs very tempting to people seeking greater sexual satisfaction. Too often, however, drugs become central to sexual activities and damage the relationship. Drug use can also lead to undesired or unplanned (and thus unprotected) sexual activity.

Alcohol is notorious for reducing inhibitions and promoting feelings of well-being and desirability. At the same time, alcohol inhibits sexual response; thus, the mind may be willing, but not the body. An increasing number of young men have begun experimenting with the recreational use of drugs intended to treat erectile dysfunction, including Viagra, Cialis, and Levitra. These drugs work by relaxing the smooth muscle cells in the penis, allowing for increased blood flow to the erectile tissues. Young men who take this type of medication are hoping to increase their sexual stamina or counteract sexual performance anxiety or the effects

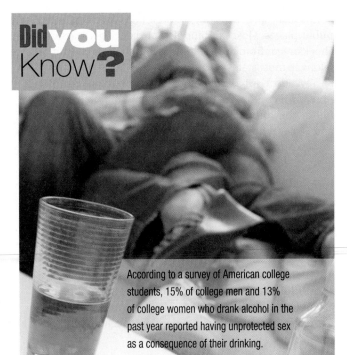

Did you Know?

According to a survey of American college students, 15% of college men and 13% of college women who drank alcohol in the past year reported having unprotected sex as a consequence of their drinking.

Source: Data from American College Health Association, *American College Health Association–National College Health Assessment II: Undergraduate Students Reference Group Data Report, Fall 2012* (Hanover, MD: American College Health Association, 2013), Available at www.acha-ncha.org

How Well Do You Communicate?

How do you think you rate as a communicator? How do you think others might rate you? Are you generally someone who expresses his or her thoughts easily, or are you more apt to say nothing for fear of saying the wrong thing? Read the following scenarios and indicate how each describes you, based on the following rating scale.

5 = Would describe me *all* or *nearly all* of the time
3 = Would describe me *sometimes*, but it would be a struggle for me
1 = Would describe me *never* or *almost never*

1. In a roomful of mostly strangers, you would find it easy to mingle and strike up conversations with just about anyone in the room.

2. Someone you respect is very critical/hateful about someone that you like a lot. You would be comfortable speaking up and saying you disagree and why you feel this way.

3. Someone in your class is not doing her part on a group project and her work is substandard. You would be direct and tell her the work isn't acceptable.

4. One of your friends asks you to let him look at your class assignment because he hasn't had time to do his. You know that he skips class regularly and seems to never do his own work, so you politely tell him no.

5. You realize that the person you are dating is not right for you and you are probably not right for him or her. When he or she blurts out, "I love you," you say, "I'm sorry, but I don't have those same feelings for you."

6. Your instructor asks you to give a speech at a state conference, discussing health problems faced by students on campus. You tell the instructor that you'd love to do it and begin planning what you will say.

7. You don't want to go out drinking at a party on Friday night, even though all of your good friends are going to go. When asked what time they should pick you up, you tell them you appreciate the offer, but you really don't want to go.

8. Your best friend, Bill, is in an abusive relationship with his girlfriend, Molly. You tell him that you think he might benefit by visiting the campus counseling center.

9. Students in your class have done poorly on a recent exam and believe that the test was unfair. You volunteer to be the spokesperson and talk with the instructor, telling her what the class thinks of the exam.

10. You see someone you are really attracted to. You walk up to him or her at a party and strike up a conversation, with the intention of asking him or her out on a date.

How Did You Do?

The higher your score on the above scenarios (the more 5s you have), the more likely it is that you are a direct and clear communicator. Are there areas that you rated as 3s or as 1s? Why do you think you have difficulties in these situations? How might you best communicate in these situations to achieve the results you want? Any time you have to communicate with others about difficult topics, it is best to speak and listen carefully, keep the other person's feelings in mind, and show respect for the individual. Try to think about what you might say ahead of time so that you are prepared to speak.

YOUR PLAN FOR CHANGE

The Assess**yourself** activity gave you the chance to look at how you communicate. Now that you have considered your responses, you can take steps toward becoming a better communicator and improving your relationships.

Today, you can:

○ Call a friend you haven't talked to in a while or arrange a coffee date with a new acquaintance you'd like to get to know better.

○ Start a journal in which you keep track of communication and relationship issues that arise. Look for trends and think about ways you can change your behavior to address them.

Within the next 2 weeks, you can:

○ Sit down with the person with whom you are having a sexual relationship and have an honest and open discussion about sex. Before the discussion, think about what you would like to talk about and how you will bring it up.

○ If there is someone with whom you have a conflict, arrange a time to sit down with that person in a neutral setting away from distractions to talk about the issues.

By the end of the semester, you can:

○ Practice being an active listener and notice when your mind wanders while you are listening to someone.

○ Think about the ways you communicate with a sexual partner. Consider removing yourself from an unhappy relationship or improving communication with a partner to reach a satisfying relationship.

MasteringHealth™

Summary

* Characteristics of intimate relationships include behavioral interdependence, need fulfillment, emotional attachment, and emotional availability. Intimate relationships help us fulfill our needs for intimacy, social integration, nurturance, assistance, and affirmation. Family, friends, and partners or lovers provide the most common opportunities for intimacy. Each relationship may include healthy and unhealthy characteristics that affect daily functioning.

* To improve our ability to communicate with others, we need to develop our skills in using self-disclosure, listening effectively, conveying and interpreting nonverbal communication, and managing and resolving conflicts.

* For most people, commitment is an important ingredient in successful relationships. The major types of committed relationships include marriage and cohabitation. Gays and lesbians seek love, friendship, communication, validation, companionship, and a sense of stability, just as heterosexuals do.

* Remaining single is more common than ever. Most single people lead healthy, happy, and well-adjusted lives.

* Those who decide to have or not to have children can lead rewarding, productive lives as long as they have given this decision the utmost thought.

* Factors that can strain a relationship are breakdowns in communication and mutual respect, jealousy, changing gender roles, power sharing, and unmet expectations. Before relationships fail, often many warning signs appear. By recognizing these signs and taking action to change behaviors, partners may save and enhance their relationships.

* Sexual identity is determined by a complex interaction of genetic, physiological, environmental, and social factors. Biological sex, gender identity, gender roles, and sexual orientation all are blended into our sexual identity.

* Sexual orientation refers to a person's enduring emotional, romantic, sexual, or affectionate attraction to other persons. Gay, lesbian, and bisexual persons are often the targets of sexual prejudice. Sexual prejudice refers to negative attitudes and hostile actions directed at a social group and its members.

* The major components of the female sexual anatomy include the mons pubis, labia minora and majora, clitoris, urethral and vaginal openings, vagina, cervix, fallopian tubes, uterus, and ovaries. The major components of the male sexual anatomy are the penis, scrotum, testes, epididymides, vasa deferentia, and seminal vesicles.

* Physiologically, men and women experience the same four phases of sexual response: excitement/arousal, plateau, orgasm, and resolution.

* Responsible and satisfying sexuality involves good communication, recognition of yourself as a sexual being, an understanding of sexual structures and functions, and acceptance of your gender identity and sexual orientation.

* Sexual dysfunctions can be classified into disorders of sexual desire, sexual arousal, orgasm, and sexual pain, and can be caused by biological factors, substance use, psychological factors, or social factors. All are treatable.

* Alcohol and other psychoactive drugs can affect sexual behavior. Drug use can decrease inhibitions and lead people to engage in undesired or unsafe sexual activity.

Pop Quiz

1. Terms such as *behavioral interdependence, need fulfillment,* and *emotional availability* describe which type of relationship?
   a. Dysfunctional relationship
   b. Sexual relationship
   c. Intimate relationship
   d. Behavioral relationship

2. Intimate relationships fulfill our psychological need for someone to listen to our worries and concerns. This is known as our need for
   a. dependence.
   b. social integration.
   c. enjoyment.
   d. spontaneity.

3. Lovers tend to pay attention to the other person even when they should be involved in other activities. This is called
   a. inclusion.
   b. exclusivity.
   c. fascination.
   d. authentic intimacy.

4. Intense feelings of elation, sexual desire, and ecstasy toward a partner are characteristic of
   a. companionate love.
   b. mature love.
   c. passionate love.
   d. intimacy.

5. According to anthropologist Helen Fisher, attraction and falling in love follow a pattern based on
   a. lust, attraction, and attachment.
   b. intimacy, passion, and commitment.
   c. imprinting, attraction, attachment, and the production of specific brain chemicals.

d. fascination, exclusiveness, sexual desire, giving the utmost, and being a champion.

6. Which of the following is *not* a good way to resolve a conflict?
   a. Express anger and resentment so the other person feels your heartache.
   b. Clarify exactly what the conflict or problem is.
   c. Come up with several possible solutions.
   d. Be honest about what you find unsatisfactory.

7. One factor in choosing a partner is *proximity,* which refers to
   a. mutual regard.
   b. attitudes and values.
   c. physical attraction.
   d. being in the same place at the same time.

8. Your personal inner sense of maleness or femaleness is known as your
   a. sexual identity.
   b. sexual orientation.
   c. gender identity.
   d. gender.

9. Individuals who are sexually attracted to both sexes are identified as
   a. heterosexual.
   b. bisexual.
   c. homosexual.
   d. intersexual.

10. The most sensitive or erotic spot in the female genital region is the
   a. mons pubis.
   b. vagina.
   c. clitoris.
   d. labia.

Answers to these questions can be found on page A-1.

Think about It!

1. Why are relationships with family important? Explain how your family unit was similar to or different from a historically traditional family unit. What people made up your family of origin?
2. What problems can form barriers to intimacy? What actions can you take to reduce or remove these barriers?
3. How have gender roles changed over your lifetime? Do you view the changes as positive for both men and women?
4. What is "normal" sexual behavior? What criteria should we use to determine healthy sexual practices?
5. If scientists ever established a genetic basis for homosexual, heterosexual, or bisexual orientation, would that put an end to antigay prejudice? Why or why not?

Accessing Your Health on the Internet

The following websites explore further topics and issues related to personal health. For links to the websites below, visit the Study Area in MasteringHealth.

1. *American Association of Sexuality Educators, Counselors, and Therapists (AASECT).* Professional organization providing standards of practice for treating sexual issues and disorders. www.aasect.org
2. *The BACCHUS Network.* Student-friendly source of information about sexual and other health issues. www.bacchusnetwork.org
3. *Go Ask Alice!* An interactive question-and-answer resource from the Columbia University Health Services. "Alice" is available to answer questions about any health-related issues, including relationships, nutrition and diet, exercise, drugs, sex, alcohol, and stress. www.goaskalice.columbia.edu
4. *Sexuality Information and Education Council of the United States (SIECUS).* Information, guidelines, and materials for advancement of healthy and proper sex education. www.siecus.org
5. *The Human Rights Campaign.* Advocacy and resources about LGBT issues by the largest civil rights organization for lesbian, gay, bisexual and transgender Americans. www.hrc.org
6. *Advocates for Youth.* Current news, policy updates, research, and other resources about the sexual health of and choices particular to high-school and college-aged students. www.advocatesforyouth.org

Considering Your Reproductive Choices

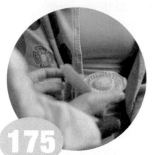

175

How can I learn more about my birth control options?

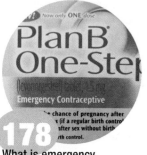

178

What is emergency contraception?

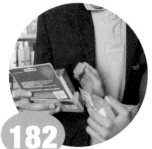

182

How do I choose a method of birth control?

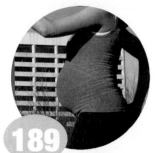

189

What should I consider before becoming a parent?

LEARNING OUTCOMES

✱ Explain how each of the main categories of contraception affects the process of conception and understand how the effectiveness of contraception is measured.

✱ Compare and contrast the advantages, disadvantages, and effectiveness of different barrier methods in preventing pregnancy and sexually transmitted infections.

✱ Compare the advantages, risks, and effectiveness of different hormonal methods in preventing pregnancy.

✱ Describe intrauterine contraceptives, their effectiveness, and their advantages and disadvantages.

✱ Describe emergency contraception and how it is used.

✱ Explain how behavioral methods of contraception work and compare their effectiveness to other methods of birth control.

✱ Describe surgical methods of birth control and discuss their advantages and disadvantages.

✱ List the questions you should consider when choosing a method of contraception.

✱ Summarize the legal decisions surrounding abortion and the various types of abortion procedures.

✱ Discuss key issues to consider when thinking about pregnancy and parenthood.

✱ Describe fetal development and explain the importance of prenatal care.

✱ Describe the process of labor and delivery, discuss complications of pregnancy and childbirth, and identify key features of the postpartum period.

✱ Review primary causes of and possible solutions to infertility.

✱ Describe the advantages and disadvantages of adoption.

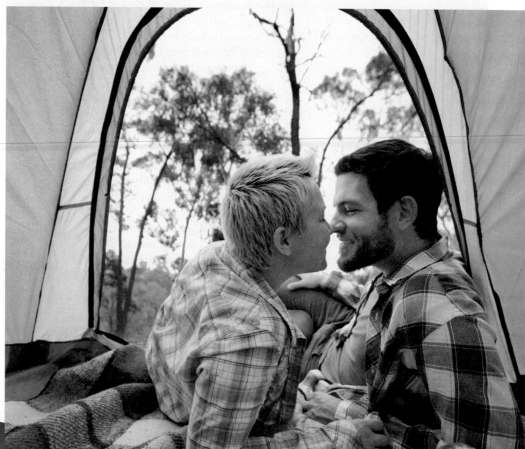

Today, we not only understand the intimate details of reproduction, but we also possess technologies that can control or enhance our **fertility.** Along with information and technological advances comes choice, which goes hand in hand with responsibility. Choosing whether and when to have children is a great responsibility. Children transform people's lives. They require a lifelong personal commitment of love and nurturing. Before having children, a person should ask: Am I mature enough physically, emotionally, and financially to care for another human being?

One measure of maturity is the ability to discuss reproduction and birth control with one's sexual partner before engaging in sexual activity. Men often assume that their partners are taking care of birth control. Women sometimes feel that broaching the topic implies that they are promiscuous. Both may feel that bringing up the subject might interfere with romance and spontaneity.

Too often, neither partner brings up the topic, resulting in unprotected sex. In a recent survey, only 54 percent of college women and 50 percent of college men reported having used a method of contraception the last time they had vaginal intercourse.[1] This ambivalence toward contraceptives has serious consequences. Each year, there are 20 million new cases of sexually transmitted infections—half of which are in ages 15 to 24 (see **Chapter 13** for more information).[2] Half of all pregnancies in the United States—more than 3 million a year—are unintended, meaning they are mistimed or unwanted.[3]

Discussing the topic with your health care provider or your sexual partner will be easier if you understand human reproduction and contraception and have taken the time to honestly consider your attitudes toward these matters. This chapter provides important information for you to think about as you contemplate your own sexual and reproductive choices.

Birth control methods prevent conception by interfering with one of these three conditions.

Without birth control, 85 percent of sexually active women would become pregnant within 1 year.[4] Society has searched for a simple, infallible, and risk-free way to prevent pregnancy since people first associated sexual activity with pregnancy. Outside of abstinence, we have not yet found one.

To evaluate the effectiveness of a particular contraceptive method, you must be familiar with two concepts: perfect-use failure rate and typical-use failure rate. **Perfect-use failure rate** refers to the number of pregnancies that are likely to occur in the first year of use (per 100 users of the method) if the method is used without any error. The **typical-use failure rate** refers to the number of pregnancies that are likely to occur in the first year of use with the normal number of errors, memory lapses, and incorrect or incomplete use. The typical-use information is much more practical in helping people make informed decisions about contraceptive methods.

Hear It! Podcasts

Want a study podcast for this chapter? Download the podcast **Birth Control, Pregnancy, and Childbirth: Managing Your Fertility** in the Study Area of MasteringHealth™

fertility A person's ability to reproduce.

birth control (contraception) Methods of preventing pregnancy.

conception The fertilization of an ovum by a sperm.

perfect-use failure rate The number of pregnancies (per 100 users) that are likely to occur in the first year of use of a particular birth control method if the method is used consistently and correctly.

typical-use failure rate The number of pregnancies (per 100 users) that are likely to occur in the first year of use of a particular birth control method if the method's use is not consistent or always correct.

Basic Principles of Birth Control

The term **birth control** (also called **contraception**) refers to methods of preventing conception. **Conception** occurs when a sperm fertilizes an egg. This usually takes place in a woman's fallopian tube. The following conditions are necessary for conception:

1. **A viable egg.** A sexually mature woman will release one egg (sometimes more) from one of her two ovaries once every 28 days, on average. Eggs remain viable for 24 to 36 hours after their release from the ovary into the fallopian tube.

2. **A viable sperm.** Each ejaculation contains between 200 and 500 million sperm cells. Once sperm reach the fallopian tubes they survive an average of 48 to 72 hours—and can survive up to a week.

3. **Access to the egg by the sperm.** To reach the egg, sperm must travel up the vagina, through the cervical opening into the uterus, and from there to the fallopian tubes.

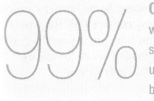

99% of U.S. women who have ever been sexually active report having used at least one form of birth control.

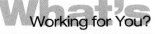

What's Working for You?

Maybe you are already sexually active and practicing safer sex. Which of the following behaviors are you already incorporating into your life?

☐ I keep a package of condoms handy—I don't want to get caught unprepared.

☐ I made an appointment with my doctor to discuss birth control options.

☐ I've decided I'm not ready to have sex, so I'm choosing to abstain at this point in my life.

☐ My partner and I have started talking about what birth control we want to use. Even though it can be embarrassing, it's a relief to talk it over!

barrier methods Contraceptive methods that block the meeting of egg and sperm by means of a physical barrier (such as condom, diaphragm, or cervical cap); a chemical barrier (such as spermicide); or both.

hormonal methods Contraceptive methods that introduce synthetic hormones into the woman's system to prevent ovulation, thicken cervical mucus, or prevent a fertilized egg from implanting.

surgical methods Surgically altering a man's or woman's reproductive system to permanently prevent pregnancy.

behavioral methods Temporary or permanent abstinence or planning intercourse in accordance with fertility patterns.

sexually transmitted infections (STIs) Infectious diseases caused by pathogens transmitted through some form of intimate, usually sexual, contact.

male condom A single-use sheath of thin latex or other material designed to fit over an erect penis and catch semen upon ejaculation.

spermicides Substances designed to kill sperm.

Present methods of contraception fall into several categories. **Barrier methods** block the egg and sperm from joining. **Hormonal methods** introduce synthetic hormones into the woman's system that prevent ovulation, thicken cervical mucus, or prevent a fertilized egg from implanting. **Surgical methods** prevent pregnancy permanently. **Behavioral methods** involve temporary or permanent abstinence or planning intercourse in accordance with fertility patterns. Table 6.1 lists the most popular forms of contraception among sexually active college students today.

Some contraceptive methods can also protect, to some degree, against **sexually transmitted infections (STIs).** This is an important factor to consider when choosing a contraceptive. Table 6.2 on the following page summarizes the effectiveness, STI protection, frequency of use, and costs of various methods.

TABLE 6.1	Top Reported Contraceptive Methods Sexually Active College Students or Their Partners Used the Last Time They Had Intercourse		
Method	Male	Female	Total
Male condom	70%	61%	64%
Birth control pills (monthly or extended cycle)	64%	60%	62%
Withdrawal	28%	31%	30%
Fertility awareness (calendar, mucus, basal body temperature)	5%	7%	6%
Intrauterine device	5%	6%	6%
Cervical ring	4%	4%	4%
Spermicide (foam, jelly, cream)	7%	3%	4%

Note: Survey respondents could select more than one method.

Source: Data from American College Health Association, *American College Health Association—National College Health Assessment II: Undergraduate Students Reference Group Data Report, Fall 2012* (Hanover, MD: American College Health Association, 2013), www.acha-ncha.org

Male Condom

The **male condom** is a thin sheath designed to cover the erect penis and catch semen, preventing it from entering the vagina. Most male condoms are made of latex, although condoms made of polyurethane or lambskin also are available. Condoms come in a wide variety of styles. They can be purchased in pharmacies, supermarkets, public bathrooms, and many health clinics. A new condom must be used for each act of vaginal, oral, or anal intercourse.

A condom must be rolled onto the penis before the penis touches the vagina, and it must be held in place when removing the penis from the vagina after ejaculation to prevent slippage (see Figure 6.1). Condoms come with or without **spermicide** and with or without lubrication. If desired, users

Barrier Methods

Barrier methods work on the simple principle of preventing sperm from ever reaching the egg by use of a physical or chemical barrier during intercourse. Some barrier methods prevent semen from having any contact with the woman's body, and others prevent sperm from going past the cervix. In addition, many barrier methods contain or are used in combination with a substance that kills sperm.

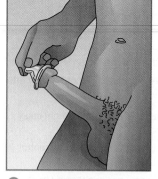 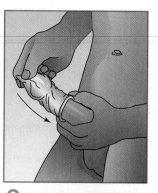 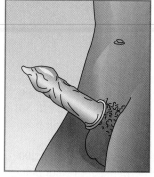 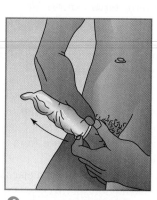

① Pinch the air out of the top half-inch of the condom to allow room for semen.

② Holding the tip of the condom with one hand, use the other hand to unroll it onto the penis.

③ Unroll the condom all the way to the base of the penis, smoothing out any air bubbles.

④ After ejaculation, hold the condom around the base until the penis is totally withdrawn to avoid spilling any semen.

FIGURE 6.1 How to Use a Male Condom

Contraceptive Effectiveness, STI Protection, Frequency of Use, and Costs

Method	Failure Rate Typical Use	Failure Rate Perfect Use	STI Protection	Frequency of Use	Cost
Continuous abstinence	0	0	Yes	N/A	None
Implanon	0.05	0.05	No	Inserted every 3 years	$400–$800/exam, device, and insertion; $100–$300 for removal
Male sterilization	0.15	0.1	No	Done once	$350–$1,000/interview, counseling, examination, operation, and follow-up sperm count
Female sterilization	0.5	0.5	No	Done once	$1,500–$6,000/interview, counseling, examination, operation, and follow-up visit
IUD (intrauterine device)					
ParaGard (copper T)	0.8	0.6	No	Inserted every 10 years	$500–$1,000/exam, insertion, and follow-up visit
Mirena	0.2	0.2	No	Inserted every 5 years	$500–$1,000/exam, insertion, and follow-up visit
Depo-Provera	6	0.2	No	Injected every 12 weeks	$30–$100/3-month injection; $35–$175 for initial exam; $20–$40 for further visits to clinician for shots
Oral contraceptives (combined pill and progestin-only pill)	9	0.3	No	Take daily	$15–$50 monthly pill pack at drugstores, often less at clinics; check for family planning programs in your student health center, $35–$250 for initial exam
Ortho Evra patch	9	0.3	No	Applied weekly	$15–$80/month at drugstores; often less at clinics, $35–$250 for initial exam
NuvaRing	9	0.3	No	Inserted every 4 weeks	$15–$80/month at drugstores, often less at clinics; $35–$250 for initial exam
Diaphragm (with spermicidal cream or jelly)	12	6	Some	Used every time	$15–$75 for diaphragm; $50–$200 for initial exam; $8–$17/supplies of spermicide jelly or cream
Cervical cap (FemCap) (with spermicidal cream or jelly)					
Women who have never given birth	14	4	Some	Used every time	$60–$75 for cap; $50–$200 for initial exam; $8–$17/supplies of spermicide jelly or cream
Women who have given birth	32	No data	Some	Used every time	
Male condom (without spermicides)	18	2	Some	Used every time	$1 and up/condom—some family planning or student health centers give them away or charge very little. Available in drugstores, family planning clinics, some supermarkets, and from vending machines
Today sponge					
Women who have never given birth	12	9	No	Used every time	$9–$15/package of three sponges. Available at family planning centers, drugstores, online, and in some supermarkets
Women who have given birth	24	20	No	Used every time	
Female condom (without spermicides)	21	5	Some	Used every time	$2-4/condom. Available at family planning centers, drugstores, and in some supermarkets
Withdrawal	22	4	No	Used every time	None
Fertility awareness-based methods	24	0.04–5.0	No	Followed every month	$10–$12 for temperature kits. Charts and classes often free in health centers and churches
Spermicides (foams, creams, gels, vaginal suppositories, and vaginal film)	28	18	No	Used every time	$8/applicator kits of foam and gel ($4–$8 refills). Film and suppositories are priced similarly. Available at family planning clinics, drugstores, and some supermarkets
No method	85	85	No	N/A	None
Emergency contraceptive pill					Treatment initiated within 72–120 hours after unprotected intercourse reduces the risk of pregnancy by 75%–89% (with no protection against STIs). Costs depend on what services are needed: $39–$60/Plan B-One Step; $20–$50/one pack of combination pills; $50–$70/two packs of progestin-only pills; $35–$150/visit with health care provider; $10–$20/pregnancy test; ella $77–$97/in addition to visit with health care provider

Notes: "Failure Rate" refers to the number of unintended pregnancies per 100 women during the first year of use. "Typical Use" refers to failure rates for men and women whose use is not consistent or always correct. "Perfect Use" refers to failure rates for those whose use is consistent and always correct.

Some family planning clinics charge for services and supplies on a sliding scale according to income.

Sources: Adapted from R. Hatcher et al., *Contraceptive Technology*, 20th rev. ed. (New York: Ardent Media, 2011); R. Hatcher et al., *Contraceptive Technology*, 19th rev. ed. Copyright © 2007 Contraceptive Technology Communications, Inc. Reprinted by permission of Ardent Media, Inc.

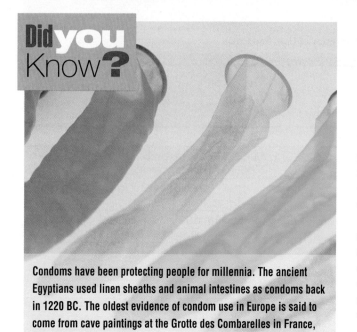
Condoms have been protecting people for millennia. The ancient Egyptians used linen sheaths and animal intestines as condoms back in 1220 BC. The oldest evidence of condom use in Europe is said to come from cave paintings at the Grotte des Combarelles in France, dating from AD 100–200!

can lubricate their own condoms with contraceptive foams, creams, and jellies or other water-based lubricants. Never use products such as baby oil, cold cream, petroleum jelly, vaginal yeast infection medications, or body lotion with a condom. These products contain substances that will cause the latex to disintegrate.

Condoms are less effective and more likely to break during intercourse if they are old or improperly stored. To maintain effectiveness, store them in a cool place (not in a wallet or glove compartment) and inspect them for small tears before use. Lightly squeeze the package before opening to feel that air is trapped inside and the package has not been punctured. Discard all condoms that have passed their expiration date.

female condom (FC2) A single-use nitrile sheath for internal use during intercourse to catch semen upon ejaculation.

Advantages When used consistently and correctly, condoms can be up to 98 percent effective.[5] The condom is the only temporary means of birth control available for men, and latex and polyurethane condoms are the only barriers that effectively prevent the spread of HIV and some STIs. (Skin condoms, made from lamb intestines, are not effective against STIs.) Many people choose condoms as their form of birth control because they are inexpensive and readily available without a prescription and because their use is limited to times of sexual activity, with no negative health effects. Some men find that condoms help them stay erect longer or help prevent premature ejaculation.

Disadvantages There is considerable potential for user error; as a result, the typical-use effectiveness of condoms in preventing pregnancy is around 82 percent.[6] Improper use of a condom can lead to breakage, leakage, or slippage, potentially exposing the users to STI transmission or an unintended pregnancy. Even when used perfectly, a condom doesn't protect against transmission of STIs that may have external areas of infection (e.g., herpes).

For some people, a condom interrupts the spontaneity of sex because stopping to put it on may break the mood. Others report that the condom decreases sensation. These inconveniences and perceptions contribute to improper use or avoidance of condoms altogether. Partners who put on a condom as part of foreplay are generally more successful with this form of birth control.

Female Condom

The **female condom (FC2)** is a single-use, soft, lubricated, loose-fitting sheath meant for internal vaginal use. The newest, improved versions are made from nitrile, rather than polyurethane. The sheath has a flexible ring at each end. One ring lies inside the sheath to serve as an insertion mechanism and hold the condom in place behind the cervix. The other ring remains outside the vagina once the condom is inserted and protects the labia and the base of the penis from exposure to STIs. Figure 6.2 on page 171 shows the proper use of the female condom.

Advantages Used consistently and correctly, female condoms are 95 percent effective at preventing pregnancy.[7] They also can prevent the spread of HIV and other STIs, including those that can be transmitted by external genital contact. The female condom can be inserted in advance, so its use doesn't have to interrupt lovemaking. Some women choose to use the female condom because it gives them more personal control over pregnancy prevention and STI protection, or because they cannot rely on their partner to use a male condom. Because the nitrile material is thin and pliable, there is less loss of sensation with the female condom than there is with the latex male condom. The female condom is relatively inexpensive, readily available without a prescription, and causes no negative health effects.

Disadvantages As with the male condom, there is potential for user error with the female condom, including possible slipping or leaking, which could lead to STI transmission or unintended pregnancy. Because of the potential problems, the typical-use effectiveness of the female condom is 79 percent.[8] Some people dislike using the female condom

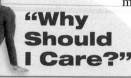

"Why Should I Care?"

Even if you use another method for contraception, it's a good idea to use a condom as well for protection against STIs. You don't want to get an STI—not only can they be unpleasant right now, but some of them can stay with you for life and cause lasting harm to your health and your fertility, not to mention wreaking havoc on your love life!

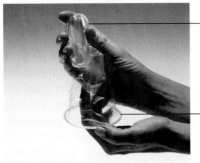

Inner ring is used for insertion and to help hold the sheath in place during intercourse.

Outer ring covers the area around the opening of the vagina.

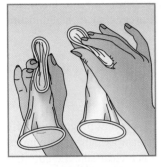

1 Grasp the flexible inner ring at the closed end of the condom, and squeeze it between your thumb and second or middle finger so it becomes long and narrow.

2 Choose a comfortable position for insertion: squatting, with one leg raised, or sitting or lying down. While squeezing the ring, insert the closed end of the condom into your vagina.

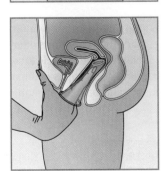

3 Placing your index finger inside of the condom, gently push the inner ring up as far as it will go. Be sure the sheath is not twisted. The outer ring should remain outside of the vagina.

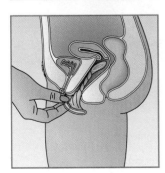

4 During intercourse, be sure that the penis is not entering on the side, between the sheath and the vaginal wall. When removing the condom, twist the outer ring so that no semen leaks out.

FIGURE 6.2 **How to Use a Female Condom**

because they feel it is disruptive, noisy, odd looking, or difficult to use. Some women have reported external or vaginal irritation from using the female condom. As with the male condom, a new condom is required for each act of intercourse. Male and female condoms should never be used simultaneously.

Jellies, Creams, Foams, Suppositories, and Film

Like condoms, some other barrier methods—jellies, creams, foams, suppositories, and film—do not require a prescription. They are referred to as spermicides—substances designed to kill sperm. The active ingredient in most of them is nonoxynol-9 (N-9).

jellies and creams Spermicide packaged in tubes and inserted into the vagina with an applicator.

suppositories Waxy capsules that are inserted deep into the vagina, where they melt and release a spermicide.

vaginal contraceptive film A thin film infused with spermicidal gel that is inserted into the vagina so that it covers the cervix.

Jellies and creams are packaged in tubes, and foams are available in aerosol cans. All have applicators designed for insertion into the vagina. They must be inserted far enough to cover the cervix, thus providing both a chemical barrier that kills sperm and a physical barrier that stops sperm from continuing toward an egg. Jellies and creams usually need to be inserted 10 minutes before intercourse and remain effective for about 1 hour after insertion.

Suppositories are waxy capsules that are inserted deep into the vagina, where they melt. They must be inserted 10 to 20 minutes before intercourse to have time to melt, but no longer than 1 hour prior to intercourse, or they lose their effectiveness. An additional suppository must be inserted for each subsequent act of intercourse.

Vaginal contraceptive film is another method of spermicide delivery. A thin film infused with spermicidal gel is inserted into the vagina so that it covers the cervix. The film dissolves into a spermicidal gel that is effective for up to 3 hours. As with other spermicides, a new film must be inserted for each act of intercourse.

Advantages Spermicides are most effective when used in conjunction with another barrier method (condom, diaphragm, etc.); used alone they offer only 72 percent (typical use) to 82 percent (perfect use) effectiveness at preventing pregnancy.[9] Like condoms, spermicides are inexpensive, do not require a prescription or pelvic examination, and are readily available over the counter. They are simple to use and their use is limited to the time of sexual activity.

Disadvantages Spermicides can be messy and must be reapplied for each act of intercourse. Some people experience irritation or allergic reactions to spermicides, and recent studies indicate that while spermicides containing N-9 are effective at preventing pregnancy, they are not effective in preventing transmission of HIV, chlamydia, or gonorrhea. In fact, frequent (more than once a day) use of N-9 spermicides has been shown to cause irritation and breaks in the mucous layer or skin of the genital tract, creating a point of entry for viruses and bacteria that cause disease. Spermicides containing N-9 have also been associated with increased risk of urinary tract infection. New spermicides without N-9 are being tested to enter the market.

Diaphragm with Spermicidal Jelly or Cream

Invented in the mid-nineteenth century, the **diaphragm** was the first widely used birth control method for women. The device is a soft, shallow cup made of thin latex rubber. Its flexible, rubber-coated ring is designed to fit snugly behind the pubic bone in front of the cervix and over the back of the cervix on the other side so it blocks access to the uterus. Diaphragms must be used with spermicidal cream or jelly, which is applied to the inside of the diaphragm before it is inserted, up to 6 hours before intercourse. The diaphragm holds the spermicide in place, creating a physical and chemical barrier against sperm **(Figure 6.3)**. Diaphragms are manufactured in different sizes and must be fitted to the woman by a trained health care provider, who should make sure the user knows how to insert her diaphragm correctly before she leaves the provider's office.

> **diaphragm** A latex, cup-shaped device designed to cover the cervix and block access to the uterus; should always be used with spermicide.
>
> **cervical cap** A small cup made of latex or silicone that is designed to fit snugly over the entire cervix; should always be used with spermicide.

Advantages If used consistently and correctly, diaphragms can be 94 percent effective in preventing pregnancy.[10] Due to its shape, when used with spermicidal jelly or cream, the diaphragm also offers some protection against gonorrhea and possibly chlamydia and human papillomavirus (HPV). After the initial prescription and fitting, the only ongoing expense involved with diaphragm use is spermicide. Because the diaphragm can be inserted up to 6 hours in advance and used for multiple acts of intercourse, some users find it less disruptive than other barrier methods.

Disadvantages Although the diaphragm can be left in place for multiple acts of intercourse, additional spermicide must be applied before each act. The diaphragm must then stay in place for 6 to 8 hours after intercourse to allow the chemical to kill any sperm remaining in the vagina. Some women find inserting the device awkward, especially if the woman is rushed. When inserted incorrectly, diaphragms are much less effective. It is also possible for a diaphragm to slip out of place, be difficult to remove, or require refitting by a physician (e.g., following a pregnancy or a significant weight gain or loss).

Cervical Cap with Spermicidal Jelly or Cream

One of the oldest methods used to prevent pregnancy, early **cervical caps** were made from beeswax, silver, or copper. The currently available FemCap is a clear silicone cup that fits snugly over the entire cervix. It comes in three sizes and must be fitted by a health care provider. The FemCap is designed for use with spermicidal jelly or cream. It is held in place by suction created during application and works by blocking sperm from the uterus.

Advantages Cervical caps can be reasonably effective (86%) with typical use.[11] They may offer some protection against transmission of gonorrhea, and possibly HPV and chlamydia. They are relatively inexpensive because the only ongoing cost is for the spermicide.

The FemCap can be inserted up to 6 hours prior to intercourse. The device must be left in place for 6 to 8 hours afterward, but after that time period, it can be removed, cleaned, and reinserted immediately. Because the FemCap is made of surgical-grade silicon, it is a suitable alternative for people who are allergic to latex.

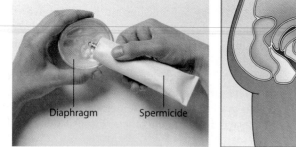

❶ Place spermicidal jelly or cream inside the diaphragm and all around the rim.

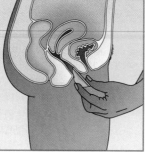

❷ Fold the diaphragm in half and insert dome-side down (spermicide-side up) into the vagina, pushing it along the back wall as far as it will go.

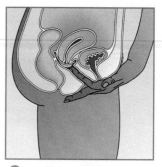

❸ Position the diaphragm with the cervix completely covered and the front rim tucked up against your pubic bone; you should be able to feel your cervix through the rubber dome.

FIGURE 6.3 **The Proper Use and Placement of a Diaphragm**

troublesome at first; but within a year, most women are amenorrheic (have no menstrual periods). Weight gain is commonly reported. Prolonged use is linked with loss of bone density.[28] Other possible side effects include dizziness, nervousness, and headache. Unlike other methods of contraception, this method cannot be stopped immediately if problems arise, and the drug and its side effects may linger for up to 6 months after the last shot. Also, after the final injection, it may take women who wish to get pregnant up to a year to conceive.

Contraceptive Implants

A single-rod implantable contraceptive, **Implanon** (now named **Nexplanon**) is a small soft plastic capsule (about the size of a matchstick) that is inserted just beneath the skin on the inner side of a woman's upper underarm by a health care provider. Implanon/Nexplanon continually releases a low, steady dose of progestin for up to 3 years, suppressing ovulation during that time.

Advantages After insertion, Implanon/Nexplanon is generally not visible, making it a discreet method of birth control. Its main advantages are that it is highly effective (99.95%), not subject to user error, and need only be replaced every 3 years.[29] It has similar benefits as other progestin-only forms of contraception, including the lightening or cessation of menstrual periods, the lack of estrogen-related side effects, and safety for use by breast-feeding women. Fertility usually returns immediately after removal of the implant.

Disadvantages Insertion and removal of Implanon/Nexplanon must be performed by a clinician. There is a higher initial cost for this method, and it may not be covered by all health plans. Potential minor side effects include irritation, allergic reaction, swelling, or scarring around the area of insertion, and there is also a possibility of infection or complications with removal. Implanon/Nexplanon may be less effective in women who are overweight.[30] As with other progestin-only contraceptives, users can experience irregular bleeding. Implanon/Nexplanon offers no protection against transmission of STIs, and it may require a backup method during the first week of use.

Intrauterine Contraceptives

The **intrauterine device (IUD)** is a small, plastic, flexible device, with a nylon string attached. It is placed in the uterus through the cervix and provides protection from pregnancy for 5 to 10 years. The exact mechanism by which it works is not clearly understood, but researchers believe IUDs affect the way sperm and eggs move, thereby preventing fertilization, and/or affect the lining of the uterus to prevent a fertilized ovum from implanting.

See It! Videos

Why are IUDs gaining popularity? Watch **New Support for IUDs** in the Study Area of MasteringHealth™

The IUD was once extremely popular in the United States; however, most brands were removed from the market because of serious complications such as pelvic inflammatory disease and infertility. Redesigned for safe use, the IUD is again very popular with women around the world and is experiencing a resurgence of popularity among U.S. women.[31]

ParaGard and Mirena IUDs

Two IUDs are currently available in the United States. **ParaGard** is a T-shaped plastic device with copper around the shaft. It does not contain any hormones and can be left in place for 10 years. A newer IUD, **Mirena,** is effective for 5 years and releases small amounts of progestin.

A clinician must insert an IUD. One or two strings extend from the IUD into the vagina so the user can periodically check to make sure that the device is in place. While IUDs were initially not recommended for women who had never had a baby, the American Congress of Obstetricians and Gynecologists now supports their use for most women.[32]

Advantages The IUD is a safe, discreet, and highly effective method of birth control (more than 99% effective).[33] It is effective immediately and needs to be replaced only every 5 years (Mirena) or every 10 years (ParaGard). ParaGard has the benefit of containing no hormones at all and thus has none of the potential negative health impacts of hormonal contraceptives.

Implanon (Nexplanon) A small soft plastic capsule inserted just beneath the skin on the inner side of a woman's upper underarm that continually releases a low, steady dose of progestin for up to 3 years, suppressing ovulation during that time.

intrauterine device (IUD) A device, often T-shaped, that is implanted in the uterus to prevent pregnancy.

ParaGard An IUD with a copper-wound shaft and containing no hormones, which can be left in place for up to 10 years.

Mirena An IUD that releases small amount of progestin and is effective for up to 5 years.

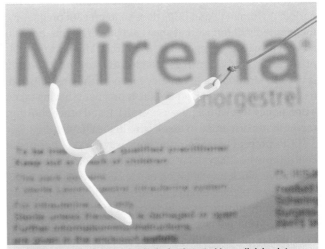

Mirena IUD is a flexible plastic device inserted by a clinician into a woman's uterus, where it releases progestin for up to 5 years.

Mirena, on the other hand, likely offers some of the potential health benefits of other progestin-only methods. Both IUDs can be used by breast-feeding women. With Mirena, periods become lighter or stop altogether. The IUDs are fully reversible; after removal, there is usually no delay in return of fertility. Both of these methods offer sexual spontaneity, as there is no need to keep supplies on hand or to interrupt lovemaking. The IUD can be removed at any time by a clinician if a woman wants to discontinue use.

Disadvantages Disadvantages of IUDs include possible discomfort, the cost of insertion, and potential complications. Also, the IUD does not protect against STIs. In some women, the device can cause heavy menstrual flow and severe cramps for the first few months. Other negative side effects include acne, headaches, nausea, breast tenderness, mood changes, uterine cramps, and backache, which seem to occur most often in women who have never been pregnant. Women using IUDs also have a higher risk of benign ovarian cysts.

Emergency Contraception

Emergency contraception is the use of a contraceptive to prevent pregnancy after unprotected intercourse, a sexual assault, or the failure of another birth control method. Combination estrogen-progestin pills and progestin-only pills are two common types of **emergency contraceptive pills (ECPs),** sometimes referred to as "morning-after pills."

Morning-after pills are not the same as the "abortion pill," although the two are often confused. ECPs contain the same type of hormones as regular birth control pills and are used after unprotected intercourse but before a woman misses her period. A woman taking ECPs does so to prevent pregnancy; the method will not work if she is already pregnant, nor will it harm an existing pregnancy. In contrast, Mifeprex or mifepristone (formerly known as RU-486), the *early abortion pill,* is used to terminate a pregnancy that is already established; it is taken after a woman is sure she is pregnant (having taken a pregnancy test with a positive result). It and other abortion methods are discussed in detail later in the chapter.

ECPs prevent pregnancy the same way as other hormonal contraceptives—they delay or inhibit ovulation, inhibit fertilization, or block implantation of a fertilized egg, depending on the phase of the woman's menstrual cycle. Although ECPs use the same hormones as birth control pills, not all brands of birth control pills can be used for emergency contraception. When taken within 24 hours, ECPs reduce the risk of pregnancy by up to 95 percent; when taken 2 to 5 days later, ECPs reduce the risk of pregnancy by 88 percent.[34]

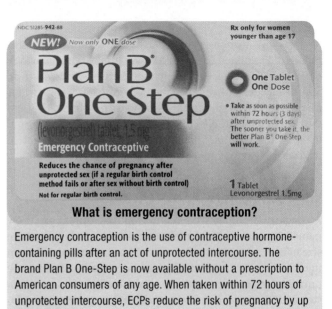

What is emergency contraception?

Emergency contraception is the use of contraceptive hormone-containing pills after an act of unprotected intercourse. The brand Plan B One-Step is now available without a prescription to American consumers of any age. When taken within 72 hours of unprotected intercourse, ECPs reduce the risk of pregnancy by up to 95 percent.

New FDA regulations now allow Plan B One-Step to be sold on the shelf with no age restrictions. The generic versions, Next Choice One Dose and My Way, will soon be on the shelf as well, but consumers will need to be 17 to purchase them. Generic two-pill versions will remain behind the pharmacy counter but available to anyone 17 and older without a prescription. Plan B One-Step is a progestin-only pill that should be taken as soon as possible (but no later than 72 hours, or 3 days) after unprotected intercourse. My Way, Next Choice, One Dose, and levonorgestrel tablets are generic equivalents of Plan B.[35]

The FDA has more recently approved **ella.** Unlike other ECPs, ella is only available by prescription. A progesterone receptor modulator, ella works by inhibiting or preventing ovulation. It can prevent pregnancy when taken up to 120 hours (5 days) following unprotected intercourse.

According to a recent national survey, 10 percent of sexually active college students reported using emergency contraception within the past year (or reported their partner had used it.)[36]

ECPs are no substitute for taking proper precautions before having sex (such as using latex condoms with a spermicide). However, their potential for preventing pregnancy resulting from sexual assault and for reducing the rate of unintended pregnancy, and ultimately abortion, is an exciting advance in reproductive health care.

Behavioral Methods

Some methods of contraception rely on one or both partners altering their sexual behavior. In general, these methods require more self-control, diligence, and commitment, making them more prone to user error than hormonal and barrier methods.

Withdrawal

Withdrawal, also called *coitus interruptus,* involves removing the penis from the vagina just prior to ejaculation. In the 2012 American Health College Association's National College Heath Assessment (ACHA-NCHA), approximately 30 percent of respondents reported that withdrawal was used as a method of birth control the last time they had sexual intercourse.[37] This statistic is startlingly high, considering the high risk of pregnancy (78%, typical use)[38] or contracting an STI associated with this method of birth control.

Advantages and Disadvantages Although withdrawal can be practiced when absolutely no other contraceptive is available, and it is better than using no contraceptive at all, it is unreliable, even with "perfect" use, because there can be up to half a million sperm in the drop of fluid at the tip of the penis *before* ejaculation. Timing withdrawal is also difficult, and males concentrating on accurate timing may not be able to relax and enjoy intercourse. Withdrawal offers no protection against the transmission of STIs and requires a high degree of self-control, experience, and trust.

Abstinence and "Outercourse"

Strictly defined, *abstinence* means "deliberately avoiding intercourse." This definition would allow one to engage in such forms of sexual intimacy as massage, kissing, and solitary masturbation. Couples who go beyond massage and kissing and engage in activities such as oral–genital sex and mutual masturbation, but not vaginal or anal sex, are sometimes said to be engaging in "outercourse."

Advantages and Disadvantages Abstinence is the only method of avoiding pregnancy that is 100 percent effective. It is also the only method that is 100 percent effective against transmitting disease. Like abstinence, outercourse can be 100 percent effective for birth control as long as the male does not ejaculate near the vaginal opening. Unlike abstinence, however, outercourse is not 100 percent effective against STIs. Oral–genital contact can transmit disease, although the practice can be made safer by using a condom on the penis or a latex barrier, such as a dental dam, on the vaginal opening. Both abstinence and outercourse can be difficult for couples to sustain over long periods of time.

Fertility Awareness Methods

Fertility awareness methods (FAMs) of birth control rely on altering sexual behavior during certain times of the month (Figure 6.4).

Fertility awareness methods are rooted in an understanding of basic physiology. A released ovum can survive about 36 hours after ovulation, and sperm can live for as long as 7 days in the reproductive tract. These techniques require observing female fertile periods and abstaining from sexual intercourse (or any penis–vagina contact) during the times

when a sperm and egg could meet. Some of the more common forms include the following:

- **Cervical mucus method.** The cervical mucus method requires women to examine the consistency and color of their normal vaginal secretions. Prior to ovulation, vaginal mucus becomes gelatinous and stretchy, and normal vaginal secretions may increase. To prevent pregnancy, partners must avoid sexual activity involving penis–vagina contact while this mucus is present and for several days afterward.
- **Body temperature method.** The body temperature method relies on the fact that the woman's basal (resting) body temperature rises between 0.4 and 0.8 degrees after ovulation has occurred. For this method to be effective, the woman must chart her temperature for several months to learn to recognize her body's temperature fluctuations. To prevent

> **withdrawal** A method of contraception that involves withdrawing the penis from the vagina before ejaculation; also called *coitus interruptus.*
>
> **fertility awareness methods (FAMs)** Several types of birth control that require alteration of sexual behavior rather than chemical or physical intervention in the reproductive process.

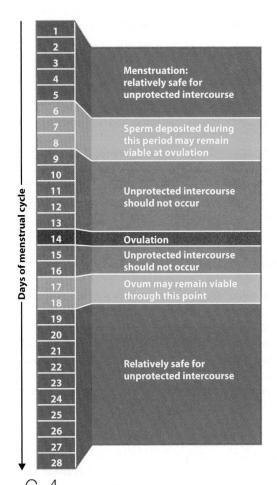

FIGURE 6.4 The Fertility Cycle
Fertility awareness methods (FAMs) can combine the use of a calendar, the cervical mucus method, and body temperature measurements to identify the fertile period. It is important to remember that most women do not have a consistent 28-day cycle.

Days of menstrual cycle

1
2
3
4
5
6
7
8
9
10
11
12
13
14
15
16
17
18
19
20
21
22
23
24
25
26
27
28

Menstruation: relatively safe for unprotected intercourse

Sperm deposited during this period may remain viable at ovulation

Unprotected intercourse should not occur

Ovulation

Unprotected intercourse should not occur

Ovum may remain viable through this point

Relatively safe for unprotected intercourse

pregnancy, partners must abstain from penis–vagina contact before the temperature rise until several days after the temperature rise is observed.

● **Calendar method.** The calendar method requires the woman to record the exact number of days in her menstrual cycle. Because few women menstruate with complete regularity, this method involves keeping a record of the menstrual cycle for 12 months, during which time some other method of birth control must be used. This method assumes that ovulation occurs during the midpoint of the cycle. To prevent pregnancy, the couple must abstain from penis–vagina contact during the fertile time.

Advantages and Disadvantages Fertility awareness methods are the only forms of birth control that comply with certain religious teachings, including those of the Roman Catholic Church. They don't require a medical visit or prescription, and there are no negative health effects. The effectiveness of fertility awareness methods depends on diligence, commitment, and self-discipline; they are 76 percent effective with typical use.[39] Women who attempt to use these methods without proper training run a high risk of unintended pregnancy; anyone interested in using them is advised to take a class. Classes are often offered free by health centers and churches, and there is only minimal expense for supplies. These methods offer no STI protection, and they may not work for women with irregular menstrual cycles.

sterilization Permanent fertility control achieved through surgical procedures.

tubal ligation Sterilization of the woman that involves cutting and tying off or cauterizing of the fallopian tubes.

Essure A minimally invasive sterilization procedure that places microcoils into the fallopian tubes via the vagina.

Adiana A minimally invasive sterilization procedure in which a soft insert is placed in each fallopian tube in order to induce scarring and blockage.

hysterectomy Surgical removal of the uterus.

Surgical Methods

In the United States, **sterilization** has become the second leading method of contraception for women of all ages and the leading method of contraception among married women and women over the age of 30.[40] Because sterilization is permanent, anyone considering it should think through possibilities such as divorce and remarriage or a future improvement in financial status that might make a pregnancy realistic or desirable.

Female Sterilization

One method of sterilization for women is **tubal ligation,** a surgical procedure in which the fallopian tubes are sealed shut to block sperm's access to released eggs (see **Figure 6.5**). The operation is usually done laparoscopically in a hospital on an outpatient basis. The procedure usually takes less than an hour, and the patient is generally allowed to return home within a short time.

A tubal ligation does not affect ovarian and uterine function. The woman's menstrual cycle continues, and released eggs simply disintegrate and are absorbed by the lymphatic system. As soon as her incision heals, the woman may resume sexual intercourse with no fear of pregnancy.

A newer sterilization procedure, **Essure,** involves the placement of small microcoils into the fallopian tubes via the vagina. The entire procedure takes about 35 minutes and can be performed in a physician's office. Once in place, the microcoils expand to the shape of the fallopian tubes. The coils promote the growth of scar tissue around the device and lead to the fallopian tubes becoming blocked. Like traditional forms of tubal ligation, Essure is permanent.

Adiana is another new, minimally invasive method of blocking a woman's fallopian tubes. A soft insert about the size of a grain of rice is placed in each fallopian tube. Scar tissue grows around the insert and eventually blocks the fallopian tubes. The insertion can be performed in a physician's office in about 15 minutes.

A **hysterectomy,** or removal of the uterus, is a method of sterilization requiring major surgery. It is usually done only when a woman's uterus is diseased or damaged, not as a primary means of female sterilization.

Advantages The main advantage to female sterilization is that it is highly effective (99.5%) and permanent.[41] After the one-time expense and operation or procedure, no other cost or ongoing action is required. Sterilization has no negative effect on a woman's sex drive. A potential advantage of the Essure and Adiana methods is that they do not require an incision.

Disadvantages As with any surgery, there are risks involved with a tubal ligation. Although rare, possible complications include infection, pulmonary embolism, hemorrhage, anesthesia complications, and ectopic pregnancy. Essure and Adiana do not require an incision, so the immediate risks are lower. However, because there are relatively new techniques, the long-term risks are unknown. Sterilization

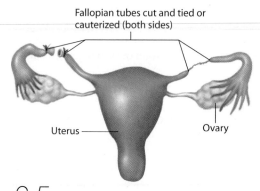

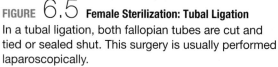

FIGURE 6.5 **Female Sterilization: Tubal Ligation** In a tubal ligation, both fallopian tubes are cut and tied or sealed shut. This surgery is usually performed laparoscopically.

offers no protection against STI transmission and is initially expensive, if not covered by your insurance plan. The procedure is permanent and should be used only if both partners are certain they do not want more children.

Male Sterilization

Sterilization in men is less complicated than it is in women. A **vasectomy** is frequently done on an outpatient basis, using a local anesthetic (see **Figure 6.6**). This procedure involves making a small incision in the side of the scrotum to expose a vas deferens, cutting the vas deferens and either tying off or cauterizing the ends, then repeating this on the other side.

Many men are reluctant to consider sterilization because they fear the operation will affect their sexual performance or sex drive. However, a vasectomy in no way affects sexual response. Because sperm constitute only a small part of the semen (about 2%), the amount of ejaculate is not changed significantly. The testes continue to produce sperm, but the sperm can no longer enter the ejaculatory duct. Any sperm that are manufactured disintegrate and are absorbed into the lymphatic system.

Advantages A vasectomy is a highly effective and permanent means of preventing pregnancy. After 1 year, the pregnancy rate in women whose partners have had vasectomies is 0.15 percent (or about 1 in 1,500).[42] A vasectomy is a fairly simple outpatient procedure requiring minimal recovery time, and after the one-time expense and operation, no other cost or ongoing action is required.

Disadvantages Male sterilization offers no protection against STI transmission. Also, a vasectomy is not immediately effective in preventing pregnancy. Because sperm are stored in other areas of the reproductive system besides the vasa deferentia, couples must use alternative methods of birth control for at least 1 month after the vasectomy. A physician must perform a semen analysis to determine when unprotected intercourse can take place. As with any surgery,

there are some risks involved with a vasectomy. In a small percentage of cases, serious complications occur, such as formation of a blood clot in the scrotum, infection, or inflammatory reactions. Very infrequently the vasa deferentia may create a new path, negating the procedure. Sterilization is initially expensive if not covered by your insurance plan.

vasectomy Sterilization of the man that involves cutting and tying off or cauterizing both vasa deferentia.

Choosing a Method of Contraception

With all the options available, how does a person or a couple decide what method of contraception is best? You must research the various methods, ask questions of your health care provider, and be honest with yourself and your partner about your preferences. Questions to ask yourself are included below.

Video Tutor: Choosing Contraception

- **How comfortable would I be using a particular method?** If you aren't at ease with a method, you may not use it consistently, and it probably will not be a reliable choice for you. Think about whether the method may cause discomfort for you or your partner, and consider your own comfort level with touching your body. For women, some methods, such as the diaphragm, sponge, or NuvaRing, require inserting a device into the vagina and taking it out. For men, using a condom requires rolling it onto the penis.
- **Will this method be convenient for me and my partner?** Some methods require more effort than do others. Be honest with yourself about how likely you are to use the method consistently. Are you willing to interrupt lovemaking, to abstain from sex during certain times of the month, or to take a pill every day? You may feel condoms are easy and convenient to use, or you may prefer something that requires little ongoing thought, such as injections or an IUD.
- **Am I at risk for the transmission of STIs?** If you have multiple sex partners or are uncertain about the sexual history or disease status of your current sex partner, then you are at risk for transmission of STIs and HIV (the virus that causes AIDS). Condoms (both male and female) are the *only* birth control method that protects against STIs and HIV (although some other barrier methods offer limited protection).
- **Do I want to have a biological child in the future?** If you are unsure about your plans for future childbearing, you should use a temporary birth control method rather than a permanent one such as sterilization. Keep in mind that you may regret choosing a permanent method if you are young, if you have few or no children, or if you are choosing this method because you feel pressured by your partner. If you know you

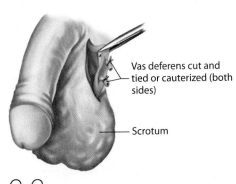

FIGURE 6.6 **Male Sterilization: Vasectomy**
In a vasectomy, the surgeon makes an incision in the scrotum, then locates and cuts the vasa deferentia, either sealing or tying both sides shut.

Vas deferens cut and tied or cauterized (both sides)

Scrotum

want to have children in the future, consider how soon that will be, as some methods, such as Depo-Provera, will cause a delay in return to fertility.

● **How would an unplanned pregnancy affect my life?** If an unplanned pregnancy would be a potentially devastating event for you, or would have a serious impact on your plans for the future, then you should choose a highly effective birth control method, such as abstinence, the pill, patch, ring, implant, shot, or IUD. If, however, you are in a stable relationship, have a reliable source of income, are planning to have children in the future, and would embrace a pregnancy should it occur now, then you may be comfortable with a less reliable method such as condoms, fertility awareness, the diaphragm, or spermicides.

● **What are my religious and moral values?** Fertility awareness methods are a good option if your beliefs prevent you from considering other birth control methods. When both partners are motivated to use these methods, they can be successful at preventing unintended pregnancy. If you are considering this option, sign up for a class to get training to use the method effectively.

● **How much will the birth control method cost?** Some contraceptive methods involve an initial outlay of money and few continuing costs (e.g., sterilization, IUD), whereas others are fairly inexpensive but must be purchased repeatedly (e.g., condoms, spermicides, monthly pill prescriptions). You should consider whether a method will be cost-effective for you in the long run. Remember that any prescription method requires routine checkups, which may involve some cost to you. Be sure to check your health insurance to determine if the Affordable Care

abortion The termination of a pregnancy by expulsion or removal of an embryo or fetus from the uterus.

Act's requirement to cover "preventive services" now makes hormonal contraceptives available to you at no cost.

● **Do I have any health factors that could limit my choice?** Hormonal birth control methods can pose potential health risks to women with certain preexisting conditions, such as high blood pressure, a history of stroke or blood clots, liver disease, migraines, or diabetes. You should discuss this issue with your health care provider when considering birth control methods. In addition, women who smoke or are over the age of 35 are at risk from complications of combination hormonal contraceptives. Breast-feeding women can use progestin-only methods, but should avoid methods containing estrogen. Men and women with latex allergies may need to use barrier methods made of polyurethane, silicone, or other materials.

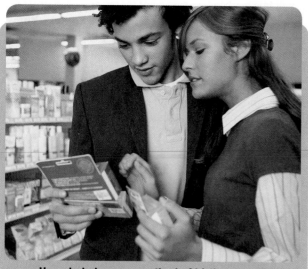

How do I choose a method of birth control?

There are many different methods of birth control on the market. When you choose a method, you'll need to consider several factors, including effectiveness, cost, comfort level, convenience, and health risks.

Abortion

Women obtain abortions for a variety of reasons. The vast majority of abortions occur because of unintended pregnancies.[43] As we know, even the best birth control methods can fail. In addition, some pregnancies are terminated because they are a consequence of rape or incest. Other reasons commonly cited are not being ready financially or emotionally to care for a child at that time.[44] When an unwanted pregnancy does occur, a woman must decide whether to terminate the pregnancy, carry it to term and keep the baby, or carry it to term and give the baby up for adoption. This is a personal decision that each woman must make, based on her personal beliefs, values, and resources, and after carefully considering all alternatives.

In 1973, the landmark U.S. Supreme Court decision in *Roe v. Wade* stated that the "right to privacy . . . founded on the Fourteenth Amendment's concept of personal liberty . . . is broad enough to encompass a woman's decision whether or not to terminate her pregnancy."[45] The decision maintained that during the first trimester of pregnancy, a woman and her practitioner have the right to terminate the pregnancy through **abortion** without legal restrictions. It allowed individual states to set conditions for second-trimester abortions. Third-trimester abortions were ruled illegal unless the mother's life or health was in danger. Prior to the legalization of abortions, women wishing to terminate a pregnancy had to travel to a country where the procedure was legal, consult an illegal abortionist, or perform their own abortions. These procedures sometimes led to infertility from internal scarring or death from hemorrhage or infection.

50% **of pregnancies**
that occur each year
are unintended.

The Debate over Abortion

Abortion is a highly charged and politically thorny issue in American society, and it is highly intertwined with unintended pregnancy, as 40 percent of unintended pregnancies end in abortion.[46] Pro-choice individuals feel that it is a woman's right to make decisions about her own body and health, including the decision to continue or terminate a pregnancy. On the other side of the issue, pro-life individuals believe that the embryo or fetus is a human being with rights that must be protected. In a recent national poll, 53 percent of people feel that *Roe v. Wade* should be kept in place, 29 percent felt it should be overturned, and 18 percent had no opinion.[47] The political debate continues as pro-life groups lobby for laws prohibiting the use of public funds for abortion and abortion counseling at the same time that pro-choice groups lobby for laws that make abortions more widely available. At times, violence has arisen as a result of this controversy in the form of attacks on clinics or on individual physicians who perform abortions.

In the 40 years since *Roe v. Wade* legalized abortion nationwide, hundreds of laws have been passed at the state and federal level to narrow or expand its limits. For example, a 2012 Mississippi law requiring physicians in abortion clinics (but not other clinics) to have admitting privileges at a local hospital threatened to close the state's only abortion clinic; and in 2013, North Dakota passed a law that would ban most abortions after approximately 6 weeks gestation (before many women know they are pregnant). Thus, while abortion remains legal in all 50 states, for many women its availability is limited.

Emotional Aspects of Abortion

The best scientific evidence available indicates that among adult women who have an unplanned pregnancy, the risk of mental health problems is no greater if they have an abortion than if they deliver a baby. Although a variety of feelings such as regret, guilt, sadness, relief, and happiness are normal, no evidence has shown that an abortion causes long-term negative mental health outcomes.[48] Researchers report that the best predictor of a woman's emotional well-being following an abortion is her emotional well-being prior to the procedure.[49] The factors that place a woman at higher risk for negative psychological responses following an abortion include the following: perception of stigma, need for secrecy, low levels of social support for the abortion decision, prior

history of mental health issues, low self-esteem, and avoidance and denial coping strategies.[50] The majority of women who have an abortion are able to view an abortion as one of life's events. Certainly the presence of a support network and the assistance of mental health professionals are helpful to any woman who is struggling with the emotional aspects of her abortion decision.

Methods of Abortion

The choice of abortion procedure is determined by how many weeks the woman has been pregnant. Length of pregnancy is calculated from the first day of her last menstrual period.

Surgical Abortions The majority of abortions performed in the United States today are surgical. If performed during the first trimester of pregnancy, abortion presents a relatively low health risk to the mother. About 88 percent of abortions occur during the first 12 weeks of pregnancy (see **Figure 6.7**).[51] The most commonly used method of first-trimester abortion is **suction curettage**, also called vacuum aspiration or dilation and curettage (D&C) (see **Figure 6.8** on page 184). The vast majority of abortions in the United States are done using this procedure, which is usually performed under a local anesthetic. The cervix is dilated with instruments or by placing laminaria, a sterile seaweed product, in the cervical canal. The laminaria is left in place for a few hours or overnight and slowly dilates the cervix. After it is removed, a long tube is inserted into the uterus through the cervix, and gentle suction removes fetal tissue from the uterine walls.

> **suction curettage** An abortion technique that uses gentle suction to remove fetal tissue from the uterus; also called vacuum aspiration or dilation and curettage (D&C).

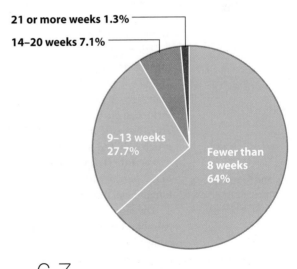

21 or more weeks 1.3%
14–20 weeks 7.1%
9–13 weeks 27.7%
Fewer than 8 weeks 64%

FIGURE 6.7 When Women Have Abortions (in weeks from the last menstrual period)
Source: K. Pazol et al., "Abortion Surveillance—United States 2009," *Surveillance Summaries* 61, no. SS08 (2012): 1–44, www.cdc.gov

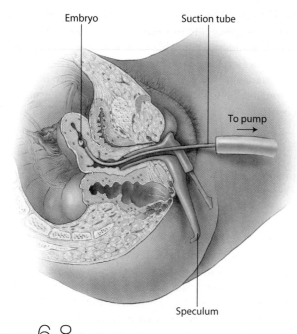

Embryo   Suction tube

To pump →

Speculum

FIGURE 6.8 **Suction Curettage Abortion**
This procedure, in which a long tube with gentle suction is used to remove fetal tissue from the uterine walls, can be performed up to the twelfth week of pregnancy.

Pregnancies that progress into the second trimester (after week 12) are usually terminated through **dilation and evacuation (D&E).** For this procedure, the cervix is dilated for 1 to 2 days, and a combination of instruments and vacuum aspiration is used to empty the uterus. Second-trimester abortions may be done under general anesthetic. The D&E can be performed on an outpatient basis (usually in the physician's office), with or without pain medication. Generally, however, the woman is given a mild tranquilizer to help her relax. This procedure may cause moderate to severe uterine cramping and blood loss. After a D&E, a return visit to the clinician is an important follow-up.

Abortions during the third trimester are very rare (less than 2% of abortions in the United States).[52] When they are performed, a D&E or saline **induction abortion** can be performed. The much debated **intact dilation and extraction (D&X),** often referred to as "partial birth abortion," is no longer legal in the United States.

The risks associated with surgical abortion include infection, incomplete abortion (when parts of the placenta remain in the uterus), excessive bleeding, and cervical and uterine trauma. Follow-up and attention to danger signs decrease the chances of long-term problems.

dilation and evacuation (D&E) An abortion technique that uses a combination of instruments and vacuum aspiration; fetal tissue is both sucked and scraped out of the uterus.

induction abortion An abortion technique in which chemicals are injected into the uterus through the uterine wall; labor begins, and the woman delivers a dead fetus.

intact dilation and extraction (D&X) A late-term abortion procedure in which the body of the fetus is extracted up to the head and then the contents of the cranium are aspirated; no longer legal in the United States.

medication abortion The termination of a pregnancy during its first 9 weeks using hormonal medications that cause the embryo to be expelled from the uterus.

The mortality rate for women undergoing first-trimester abortions in the United States averages 1 death per every 1,000,000 procedures at 8 or fewer weeks. The risk of death increases with the length of pregnancy. At 16 to 20 weeks, the mortality rate is 1 per 29,000; at 21 weeks or more, it increases to 1 per 11,000.[53] This higher rate later in the pregnancy is due to the increased risk of uterine perforation, bleeding, infection, and incomplete abortion; these things can happen because the uterine wall becomes thinner as the pregnancy progresses.

Medication Abortions Unlike surgical abortions, **medication abortions** are performed without entry into the uterus. Mifepristone, formerly known as RU-486 and currently sold in the United States under the brand name Mifeprex, is a steroid hormone that induces abortion by blocking the action of progesterone, the hormone produced by the ovaries and placenta that maintains the lining of the uterus. As a result, the uterine lining and the embryo are expelled from the uterus, terminating the pregnancy. Medication abortions must be performed early in the pregnancy, no later than 9 weeks after a woman's last menstrual period.

Mifepristone's nickname, "the abortion pill," implies an easy process. However, this treatment actually involves more steps than a suction curettage abortion, which takes approximately 15 minutes followed by a physical recovery of about 1 day. With mifepristone, a first visit to the clinic involves a physical exam and a dose of three tablets, which may cause minor side effects such as nausea, headaches, weakness, and fatigue. The patient returns 2 days later for a dose of prostaglandins (misoprostol), which causes uterine contractions that expel the fertilized egg. The patient is required to stay under observation at the clinic for 4 hours and to make a follow-up visit 12 days later.[54]

Ninety-seven percent of women who use this method will experience a complete abortion.[55] The side effects are similar to those reported during heavy menstruation and include cramping, minor pain, and nausea. Approximately 1 in 1,000 women requires a blood transfusion because of severe bleeding.[56]

Looking Ahead to Pregnancy and Parenthood

The many methods available to control fertility give you choices that did not exist when your parents—and even you—were born. Today, sexually active people are able to choose if and when they want to have children. Some will remain childless by choice. Others will utilize birth control as a way to delay and space their desired number of children.

As you approach the decision of whether or not to have children, or when to do so, take the time to evaluate your emotions, finances, and physical health.

Emotional Health

First and foremost, consider why you may want to have a child. To fulfill an inner need to carry on the family? To share love? Because it's expected? Then, consider the responsibilities involved with becoming a parent. Are you ready to make all the sacrifices necessary to bear and raise a child? Can you care for this new human being in a loving and nurturing manner? Are you with someone you think would be a good parent? Do you have a strong social support system? Preparing emotionally for parenthood can be as important as preparing physically.

Financial Evaluation

Money isn't the most important thing, but finances are another important consideration. Are you willing to go out to dinner less often, forgo a new pair of shoes, or drive an older car? These are important questions to ask yourself when considering the financial aspects of being a parent. Can you afford to give your child the life you would like him or her to enjoy?

The U.S. Department of Agriculture estimates that it will cost an average of $234,900 to raise a child born in 2011 to age 18, not including college tuition.[57] While housing costs and food are the two largest expenditures, quality child care is also expensive. According to the National Association of Child Care Resource and Referral Agencies (NACCRRA), average full-time child care costs for an infant range from about $4,600 in Mississippi to about $15,000 in Massachusetts.[58]

It is also important to check whether your medical insurance provides pregnancy benefits. If not, you can expect to pay, on average, $18,000 for a normal delivery and up to $28,000 for a cesarean section birth, including prenatal medical care, delivery, and follow-up care.[59] Also, both potential parents should investigate their employers' policies concerning parental leave, including length of leave available and conditions for returning to work.

Physical Health: Paternal Health

It is common wisdom that mothers-to-be, even before they become pregnant, should steer clear of toxic chemicals that can cause birth defects, should eat a healthy diet, and should stop smoking and drinking alcohol. Now, similar precautions are recommended for fathers-to-be. Research suggests that a man's exposure to chemicals, particularly tobacco smoke, but also to many pesticides and solvents, influences not only his ability to father a child, but the health of his future child as well.[60] Chemical exposure can also reduce the number of sperm, reduce the sperms' ability to fertilize an egg, cause miscarriage, or cause health problems in the

baby. The father's age also plays a role; men age 40 and over are more likely to father a child with autism, schizophrenia, or Down syndrome.

Physical Health: Maternal Health

The birth of a healthy baby depends in part on the mother's **preconception care.** Maternal factors that can affect a fetus or infant include drug use (illicit or otherwise), alcohol consumption, and whether the mother smokes or is obese. The key to promoting preconception health is to combine the best medical care, healthy behaviors, strong support, and safe environments at home and at work.[61]

> **preconception care** Medical care received prior to becoming pregnant that helps a woman assess and address potential maternal health issues.

During a preconception care visit, a clinician performs a thorough medical evaluation and talks with the woman about any conditions she might have, such as diabetes or high blood pressure. The clinician will also determine if the woman has had any problems with prior pregnancies, if any genetic disorders run in the family, and if the woman's immunizations are up-to-date. If, for example, she has never had rubella (German measles), a woman needs to be immunized prior to becoming pregnant. A rubella infection can kill the fetus or cause blindness or hearing disorders in the infant. The clinician will encourage the woman to eliminate alcohol consumption and tobacco use, and may adjust some medications, such as antidepressants, to safer levels.

Nutrition counseling is another important part of preconception care. Among the many important nutrition issues is folic acid (folate) intake. When consumed the month before conception and during early pregnancy, folate reduces the risk of spina bifida, a congenital birth defect resulting from failure of the spinal column to close.

Why is preconception care so important? Prenatal care, which usually begins at week 11 or 12 of a pregnancy, comes too late to prevent a number of serious maternal and child health problems in the United States. The fetus is most susceptible to developing certain problems in the first 4 to 10 weeks after conception, before prenatal care normally begins. Because many women are not aware that they are pregnant until after this critical period, they are unable to reduce the risks to their own and to their baby's health unless intervention begins before conception.[62]

> **what do you think?**
> Have you thought about whether or when to have children? Do you think your expectations about parenthood are realistic?
> ● Is there a certain age at which you feel you will be ready to be a parent?
> ● What goals do you hope to achieve before undertaking parenthood?
> ● What are your biggest concerns about parenthood?

Pregnancy

Pregnancy is an important event in a woman's life. The actions taken before, as well as behaviors engaged in during, pregnancy can significantly affect the health of both infant and mother.

The Process of Pregnancy

The process of pregnancy begins the moment a sperm fertilizes an ovum in the fallopian tubes (Figure 6.9). From there, the single fertilized cell, now called a *zygote,* multiplies and becomes a sphere-shaped cluster of cells called a *blastocyst* that travels toward the uterus, a journey that may take 3 to 4 days. Upon arrival, the embryo burrows into the thick, spongy endometrium (implantation) and is nourished from this carefully prepared lining.

human chorionic gonadotropin (HCG) Hormone detectable in blood or urine samples of a woman within the first few weeks of pregnancy.

Pregnancy Testing A pregnancy test scheduled with your doctor or a local family planning clinic will confirm a pregnancy.

Women who wish to know immediately can purchase home pregnancy test kits, sold over the counter in drugstores. A positive test is based on the secretion of **human chorionic gonadotropin (HCG),** which is found in the woman's urine.

Home pregnancy tests vary, but some can be used as early as a week after conception, and many are 99 percent reliable.[63] Instructions must be followed carefully. If the test is done too early in the pregnancy, it may show a false negative. Other causes of false negatives are unclean testing devices, ingestion of certain drugs, and vaginal or urinary tract infections. Accuracy also depends on the quality of the test itself and the user's ability to perform it and interpret the results. Blood tests administered and analyzed in a doctor's office are more accurate than home tests.

Early Signs of Pregnancy A woman's body undergoes substantial changes during the course of a pregnancy (see Figure 6.10 on page 187). The first sign of pregnancy is usually a missed menstrual period (although some women "spot" in early pregnancy, which may be mistaken for a period). Other signs include breast tenderness, emotional upset, extreme fatigue, sleeplessness, and nausea and vomiting (especially in the morning).

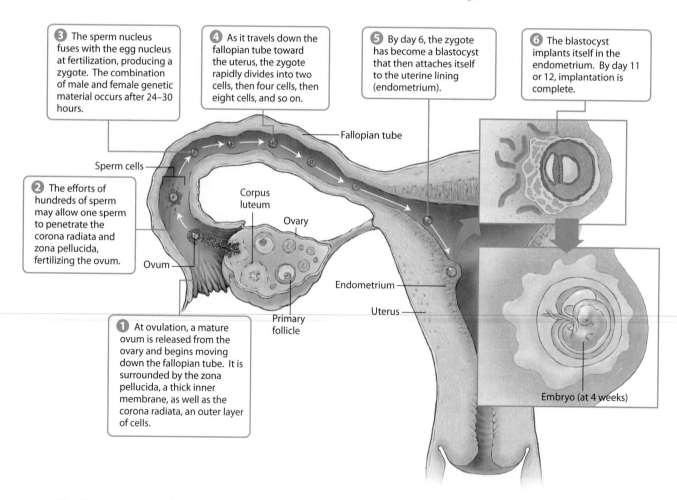

3 The sperm nucleus fuses with the egg nucleus at fertilization, producing a zygote. The combination of male and female genetic material occurs after 24–30 hours.

4 As it travels down the fallopian tube toward the uterus, the zygote rapidly divides into two cells, then four cells, then eight cells, and so on.

5 By day 6, the zygote has become a blastocyst that then attaches itself to the uterine lining (endometrium).

6 The blastocyst implants itself in the endometrium. By day 11 or 12, implantation is complete.

2 The efforts of hundreds of sperm may allow one sperm to penetrate the corona radiata and zona pellucida, fertilizing the ovum.

1 At ovulation, a mature ovum is released from the ovary and begins moving down the fallopian tube. It is surrounded by the zona pellucida, a thick inner membrane, as well as the corona radiata, an outer layer of cells.

Sperm cells

Fallopian tube

Corpus luteum

Ovary

Ovum

Primary follicle

Endometrium

Uterus

Embryo (at 4 weeks)

FIGURE 6.9 **Fertilization**
Fertilization usually occurs in the upper third of the fallopian tube, and implantation in the uterus takes place about 6 days later.

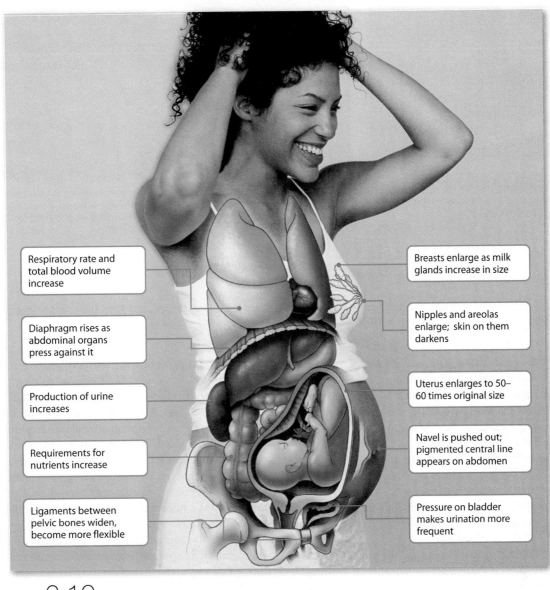

Respiratory rate and total blood volume increase

Diaphragm rises as abdominal organs press against it

Production of urine increases

Requirements for nutrients increase

Ligaments between pelvic bones widen, become more flexible

Breasts enlarge as milk glands increase in size

Nipples and areolas enlarge; skin on them darkens

Uterus enlarges to 50–60 times original size

Navel is pushed out; pigmented central line appears on abdomen

Pressure on bladder makes urination more frequent

FIGURE 6.10 **Changes in a Woman's Body during Pregnancy**

Pregnancy typically lasts 40 weeks and is divided into three phases, or **trimesters,** of approximately 3 months each. The due date is calculated from the expectant mother's last menstrual period.

The First Trimester

During the first trimester, few noticeable changes occur in the mother's body. She may urinate more frequently and experience morning sickness, swollen breasts, or undue fatigue. These symptoms may not be frequent or severe, so women often do not realize they are pregnant right away.

During the first 2 months after conception, the **embryo** differentiates and develops its various organ systems, beginning with the nervous and circulatory systems. At the start of the third month, the embryo is called a **fetus,** indicating that all organ systems are in place. For the rest of the pregnancy, growth and refinement occur in each major body system so that they can function independently, yet in coordination with all the others, at birth. The photos in **Figure 6.11** on page 188 illustrate physical changes during fetal development.

The Second Trimester

At the beginning of the second trimester, the fourth through sixth months of pregnancy, physical changes in the mother become more visible. Her breasts swell, and her waistline thickens. During this time, the fetus makes greater demands on the mother's body. In particular, the **placenta,** the network of blood vessels that carries nutrients and oxygen to the fetus and fetal waste products to the mother, becomes well established.

trimester A 3-month segment of pregnancy; used to describe specific developmental changes that occur in the embryo or fetus.

embryo The fertilized egg from conception until the end of 2 months' development.

fetus The word for a developing baby from the third month of pregnancy until birth.

placenta The network of blood vessels connected to the umbilical cord that carries nutrients, oxygen, and wastes between the developing fetus and the mother.

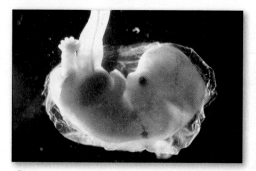

a A human embryo during the first trimester. The embryonic period lasts from the third to the eighth week of development. By the end of the embryonic period, all organs have formed.

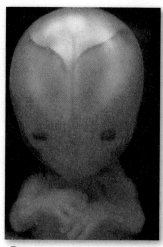

b A human fetus during the second trimester. Growth during the fetal period is very rapid.

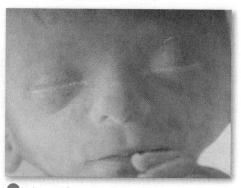

c A human fetus during the third trimester. By the end of the fetal period, the growth rate of the head has slowed relative to the growth rate of the rest of the body.

FIGURE 6.11 Series of Fetoscopic Photographs Showing Development in the First, Second, and Third Trimesters of Pregnancy

The Third Trimester The end of the sixth month through the ninth mark the third trimester. This is the period of greatest fetal growth, when the fetus gains most of its weight. The growing fetus depends entirely on its mother for nutrition and must receive large amounts of calcium, iron, and protein from the mother's diet.

Although the fetus may live if it is born during the seventh month, it needs the layer of fat it acquires during the eighth month and time for the organs (especially the respiratory and digestive organs) to develop fully. Infants born prematurely usually require intensive medical care.

Emotional Changes Of course, the process of pregnancy involves much more than the changes in a woman's body and the developing fetus. Many important emotional changes occur from the time a woman learns she is pregnant through the *postpartum period* (the 6 weeks after the baby is born). Throughout pregnancy, women may experience fear of complications, anxiety about becoming a parent, and wonder and excitement over the developing baby.

history of both parents and their families and note any hereditary conditions that could put a woman or her fetus at risk. Regular checkups to measure weight gain and blood pressure and to monitor the fetus's size and position should continue throughout the pregnancy. The American Congress of Obstetricians and Gynecologists recommends seven or eight prenatal visits for women with low-risk pregnancies.

A woman should carefully choose a practitioner who will attend her pregnancy and delivery. If possible, she should do this before she becomes pregnant. Recommendations from friends and from one's family physician are a good starting point. Also she should consider a practitioner's philosophy about pain management during labor, experience handling complications, and willingness to accommodate her personal beliefs on issues, such as the use of a doula (a trained childbirth assistant) or Lamaze techniques. Several different types of practitioners are qualified to care for a woman through pregnancy, birth, and the postpartum period, including obstetrician-gynecologists, family practitioners, and midwives.

Prenatal Care

A successful pregnancy depends on a mother who takes good care of herself and her fetus. Good nutrition and exercise; avoiding drugs, alcohol, and other harmful substances; and regular medical checkups from the beginning of pregnancy are essential. Early detection of fetal abnormalities, identification of high-risk mothers and infants, and early intervention for possible complications are the major purposes of prenatal care.

Ideally, a woman should begin prenatal appointments within the first 3 months of becoming pregnant. This early care reduces infant mortality and low birth weight. On the first visit, the practitioner should obtain a complete medical

Nutrition and Exercise Pregnant women only need about 300 additional calories a day. Special attention should be paid to getting enough folic acid (found in dark leafy greens, citrus fruits, and beans); iron (dried fruits, meats, legumes, liver, and egg yolks); calcium (nonfat or low-fat dairy products and some canned fish); and fluids. While vitamin supplements can correct some deficiencies, there is no substitute for a well-balanced diet. Babies born to poorly nourished mothers run high risks of substandard mental and physical development.

Weight gain during pregnancy helps nourish a growing baby. For a woman of normal weight before pregnancy, the recommended gain during pregnancy is 25 to 35 pounds.[64] For overweight women, weight gain of 15 to 25 pounds is recommended, and for obese women, 11 to 20. Underweight women should gain 28 to 40 pounds, and women carrying twins should gain about 35 to 45 pounds. Gaining too much or too little weight can lead to complications. With higher weight gain, women may develop gestational diabetes, hypertension, or increased risk of delivery complications. Gaining too little increases the chance of a low birth weight baby.

Exercise is an important factor in overall health during pregnancy, as it is in all other stages of life. Regular exercise is recommended for pregnant women; however, women should consult with their health care provider before starting any exercise program. Exercise can help control weight, make labor easier, and help with a faster recovery as a result of increased strength and endurance. Physical activity includes regular, moderate physical activity such as brisk walking or swimming. Women can usually maintain their customary level of activity during most of a pregnancy, although there are some cautions: a pregnant woman should avoid exercise that puts her at risk of falling or having an abdominal injury; and in the third trimester, exercises that involve lying on the back should be avoided as that can restrict blood flow to the uterus.

Drugs and Alcohol A woman should consult with a health care provider regarding safety of any drugs she might use during pregnancy. Even too much of common over-the-counter medications such as aspirin can damage a developing fetus. During the first 3 months of pregnancy, the fetus is especially subject to the **teratogenic** (birth defect–causing) effects of drugs, environmental chemicals, X rays, or diseases. The fetus can also develop an addiction to or tolerance for drugs that the mother is using.

Maternal consumption of alcohol is detrimental to a growing fetus. Symptoms of **fetal alcohol syndrome (FAS)** include mental retardation, slowed nerve reflexes, and small head size. The exact amount of alcohol that causes FAS is not known; therefore, the American Congress of Obstetricians and Gynecologists recommends total abstinence during pregnancy.[65]

Smoking Tobacco use, and smoking in particular, harms every phase of reproduction. Women who smoke have more difficulty becoming pregnant and have a higher risk of being infertile. Women who smoke during pregnancy have a greater chance of miscarriage, complications, premature births, low

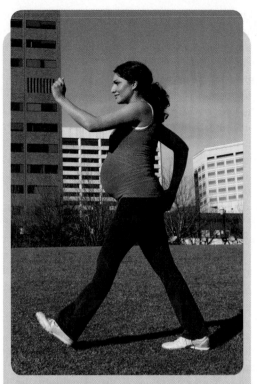

What should I consider before becoming a parent?

Before you decide whether or when to become a parent, you should consider your and your partner's physical health, emotional health, and financial security.

birth weight infants, stillbirth, and infant mortality, specifically due to sudden infant death syndrome (SIDS).[66] Smoking restricts the blood supply to the developing fetus and thus limits oxygen and nutrition delivery and waste removal. Tobacco use appears to be a significant factor in the development of cleft lip and palate.

Other Teratogens A pregnant woman should avoid exposure to X rays, toxic chemicals, heavy metals, pesticides, gases, and other hazardous compounds. She should avoid cleaning cat-litter boxes, if possible, because cat feces can contain organisms that cause **toxoplasmosis.** If a pregnant woman contracts this disease, her baby may be stillborn or suffer mental retardation or other birth defects.

Maternal Age The average age at which a woman has her first child in the United States is 25, up from 21 in 1970. Although births to women in their twenties are declining, the rate of first births to women between the ages of 30 and 39 are the highest reported in four decades, and births to women over 39 have continued to increase slightly over previous years.[67] Statistically, the chances of having a baby with birth defects rise after the age of 35. Researchers believe this is due to a decline in the quality of eggs after this age. Two specific age-related risks are miscarriage and **Down syndrome.** The risk of miscarriage nearly doubles for women 35 to 45 compared to women under 35.[68] The risk of conceiving a baby with Down syndrome also increases, from 1 chance in 1,250 at age 25, to 1 in 400 at age 35, to 1 in 30 at age 45.[69]

While some risks increase with age, many doctors note that older mothers bring some advantages to their pregnancies. They tend to be more conscientious about following medical advice during pregnancy and are more psychologically mature and ready to include an infant in their family than are some younger women.

teratogenic Causing birth defects; may refer to drugs, environmental chemicals, X rays, or diseases.

fetal alcohol syndrome (FAS) A collection of symptoms, including mental retardation, that can appear in infants of women who drink alcohol during pregnancy.

toxoplasmosis A disease caused by an organism found in cat feces that, when contracted by a pregnant woman, may result in stillbirth or an infant with mental retardation or birth defects.

Down syndrome A genetic disorder characterized by mental retardation and a variety of physical abnormalities.

Prenatal Testing and Screening Modern technology enables medical practitioners to detect health defects in a fetus as early as the fourteenth to eighteenth weeks of pregnancy. One common test is ultrasonography or ultrasound, which uses high-frequency sound waves to create a sonogram, or visual image, of the fetus in the uterus. The sonogram is used to determine the fetus's size and position. Knowing the baby's position helps health care providers perform other tests and deliver the infant. Sonograms can also detect birth defects in the central nervous and digestive systems.

Chorionic villus sampling (CVS) involves snipping tissue from the developing fetal sac. Chorionic villus sampling can be used at 10 to 12 weeks of pregnancy. This is an attractive option for couples who are at high risk for having a baby with Down syndrome or a debilitating hereditary disease.

The **triple marker screen (TMS)** is a maternal blood test that is optimally conducted between the sixteenth and eighteenth weeks of pregnancy. The TMS is a screening test, not a diagnostic tool; it can detect susceptibility for a birth defect or genetic abnormality but is not meant to confirm a diagnosis of any condition. The **quad screen** test is also available. Because it screens for an additional protein in maternal blood, it is more accurate than the triple marker screen.[70] Even more precise is the **integrated screen,** which uses the quad screen, plus results from an earlier blood test, plus ultrasound to screen for abnormalities.

Amniocentesis is a common testing procedure that is strongly recommended for women over age 35. This test involves inserting a long needle through the mother's abdominal and uterine walls into the **amniotic sac,** the protective pouch surrounding the fetus. The needle draws out 3 to 4 teaspoons of fluid, which is analyzed for genetic information about the baby. Amniocentesis can be performed between weeks 14 and 18.

If any of these tests reveals a serious birth defect, parents are advised to undergo genetic counseling. In the case of a chromosomal abnormality such as Down syndrome, the parents are usually offered the option of a therapeutic abortion. Some parents choose this option; others research the condition and decide to continue the pregnancy.

Childbirth

Prospective parents need to make several key decisions before the baby is born. These include where to have the baby, whether to use pain medication during labor and delivery,

which childbirth method to choose, and whether to breast-feed or use formula. Answering these questions in advance will help to smooth the passage into parenthood.

Labor and Delivery

During the few weeks preceding delivery, the baby normally shifts to a head-down position, and the cervix begins to dilate (widen). The junction of the pubic bones loosens to permit expansion of the pelvic girdle during birth. The exact mechanisms that initiate labor are unknown. A change in the hormones in the fetus and mother cause strong uterine contractions to occur, signaling the beginning of labor. Another common early signal is the breaking of the amniotic sac, which causes a rush of fluid from the vagina (commonly referred to as "water breaking").

The birth process has three stages, described in **Figure 6.12** on the following page, which can last from several hours to more than a day. In some cases, toward the end of the second stage the attending practitioner may perform an *episiotomy,* a straight incision in the mother's perineum (the area between the vulva and the anus), to prevent the baby's head from tearing vaginal tissues and to speed the baby's exit from the vagina. Upon exit, the baby takes its first breath, which is generally accompanied by a loud wail. After delivery, the attending practitioner assesses the baby's overall condition, cleans the baby's mucus-filled breathing passages, and ties and severs the umbilical cord. The mother's uterus continues to contract in the third stage of labor until the placenta is expelled.

Managing Labor Pain medication given to the mother during labor can cause sluggish responses in the newborn and other complications. For this reason, some women choose drug-free labor and delivery—but it is important to keep a flexible attitude about pain relief, because each labor is different. One person is not a "success" for delivering without medication and another a "failure" for using medical measures. Remember, pain is to be expected. In fact, many experts say that the pain of labor is the most intense in the human experience. There is no one right answer for managing that pain.

The Lamaze method is the most popular technique of childbirth preparation in the United States. It discourages the use of drugs. Prelabor classes teach the mother to control her pain through special breathing patterns, focusing exercises, and relaxation. The partner (or labor coach) assists by giving emotional support, physical comfort, and coaching for proper breath control during contractions.

Cesarean Section (C-section) If labor lasts too long or if a baby is in physiological distress or is about to exit the uterus any way but headfirst, a **cesarean section (C-section)** may be necessary. This surgical procedure involves making an incision across the mother's abdomen and through the uterus to remove the baby. A C-section may also be performed if labor is extremely difficult, maternal blood pressure falls rapidly, the placenta separates from the uterus too

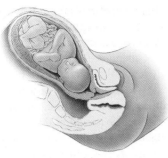

1 **Stage I: Dilation of the cervix** Contractions in the abdomen and lower back push the baby downward, putting pressure on the cervix and dilating it. The first stage of labor may last from a couple of hours to more than a day for a first birth, but it is usually much shorter during subsequent births.

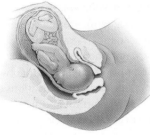

2 **End of Stage I: Transition** The cervix becomes fully dilated, and the baby's head begins to move into the vagina (birth canal). Contractions usually come quickly during transition, which generally lasts 30 minutes or less.

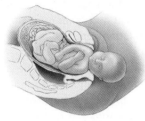

3 **Stage II: Expulsion** Once the cervix has become fully dilated, contractions become rhythmic, strong, and more intense as the uterus pushes the baby headfirst through the birth canal. The expulsion stage lasts 1 to 4 hours and concludes when the infant is finally pushed out of the mother's body.

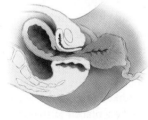

4 **Stage III: Delivery of the placenta** In the third stage, the placenta detaches from the uterus and is expelled through the birth canal. This stage is usually completed within 30 minutes after delivery.

FIGURE 6.12 **The Birth Process**
The entire process of labor and delivery usually takes from 2 to 36 hours. Labor is generally longer for a woman's first delivery and shorter for subsequent births.

soon, the mother has diabetes, or other problems occur. A C-section can be traumatic for the mother if she is not prepared for it. Risks are the same as for any major abdominal surgery, and recovery from birth takes considerably longer after a C-section.

The rate of delivery by C-section in the United States has increased from 5 percent in the mid-1960s to 33 percent in 2011.[71] Although this procedure is necessary in certain cases, some physicians and critics, including the Centers for Disease Control and Prevention (CDC), feel that C-sections are performed too frequently in this country. Natural birth advocates suggest that hospitals driven by profits and worried about malpractice are too quick to intervene in the birth process. Some doctors say that the increase is due to busy mothers who want to schedule their deliveries.

Complications of Pregnancy and Childbirth

Pregnancy carries the risk for potential complications and problems that can interfere with the proper development of the fetus or threaten the health of the mother and child. Some complications may result from a preexisting health condition of the mother, such as diabetes or an STI, whereas others can develop during pregnancy and may result from physiological problems, genetic abnormalities, or exposure to teratogens.

Preeclampsia and Eclampsia **Preeclampsia** is a condition that is characterized by high blood pressure, protein in the urine, and edema (fluid retention), which usually causes swelling of the hands and face. Symptoms may include sudden weight gain, headache, nausea or vomiting, changes in vision, racing pulse, mental confusion, and stomach or right shoulder pain. If preeclampsia is not treated, it can cause strokes and seizures, a condition called *eclampsia*. Potential problems can include liver and kidney damage, internal bleeding, stroke, poor fetal growth, and fetal and maternal death.

This condition tends to occur in the late second or third trimester. The cause is unknown; however, the incidence of preeclampsia is higher in first-time mothers; women over 40 or under 18 years of age; women carrying multiple fetuses; and women with a history of chronic hypertension, diabetes, kidney disorder, or previous history of preeclampsia. Family history of preeclampsia is also a risk factor, whether the history is on the father's or mother's side. Treatment for preeclampsia ranges from bed rest and monitoring for mild cases to hospitalization and close monitoring for more severe cases.

Miscarriage Even when a woman does everything "right," not every pregnancy ends in delivery. In the United States, between 15 to 20 percent of pregnancies end in **miscarriage** (also referred to as *spontaneous abortion*).[72] Most miscarriages occur during the first trimester.

Reasons for miscarriage vary. In some cases, the fertilized egg has failed to divide correctly. In others, genetic abnormalities, maternal illness, or infections are responsible. Maternal hormonal imbalance may also cause a miscarriage, as may a weak cervix, toxic chemicals in the environment, or physical trauma to the mother. In most cases, the cause is not known.

preeclampsia A complication in pregnancy characterized by high blood pressure, protein in the urine, and fluid retention (edema).

miscarriage Loss of the fetus before it is viable; also called *spontaneous abortion*.

ectopic pregnancy Implantation of a fertilized egg outside the uterus, usually in a fallopian tube; a medical emergency that can end in death from hemorrhage or peritonitis.

Ectopic Pregnancy The implantation of a fertilized egg outside the uterus, usually in the fallopian tube or occasionally in the pelvic cavity, is called an **ectopic pregnancy.** Because these structures are not capable of expanding and nourishing a developing fetus, the pregnancy must be

stillbirth Death of a fetus after the twentieth week of pregnancy but before delivery.

postpartum depression Energy depletion, anxiety, mood swings, guilt, and depression that women may feel during the postpartum period.

sudden infant death syndrome (SIDS) The sudden death of an infant under 1 year of age for no apparent reason.

infertility Inability to conceive after a year or more of trying.

terminated surgically, or a miscarriage will occur. If an ectopic pregnancy goes undiagnosed and untreated, the fallopian tube will rupture, putting the woman at great risk of hemorrhage, peritonitis (infection in the abdomen), and even death. Ectopic pregnancy occurs at a rate of 6.4 cases per 1,000 pregnancies in North America and is a leading cause of maternal mortality in the first trimester.[73] Ectopic pregnancy is a potential side effect of pelvic inflammatory disease, which has become increasingly common. The scarring or blockage of the fallopian tubes that occurs with this disease prevents a fertilized egg from passing to the uterus.

Stillbirth One of the most traumatic events a couple can face is a **stillbirth.** Stillbirth is the death of a fetus *after* the twentieth week of pregnancy but before delivery. A stillborn baby is born dead, often for no apparent reason. Each year in the United States, there is about 1 stillbirth in every 160 births.[74] Birth defects, placental problems, poor fetal growth, infections, and umbilical cord accidents are known contributing factors.

The Postpartum Period

The postpartum period lasts 6 weeks after delivery. During this period, many women experience fluctuating emotions. For many new mothers, the physical stress of labor, dehydration and blood loss, and other stresses challenge their stamina. Many new mothers experience what is called the "baby blues," characterized by periods of sadness, anxiety, headache, sleep disturbances, and irritability. For most women, these symptoms disappear after a short while. About 1 in 7 new mothers experience **postpartum depression,** a more disabling syndrome characterized by mood swings, lack of energy, crying, guilt, and depression. It can happen any time within the first year after childbirth. Mothers who experience postpartum depression should seek professional treatment. Counseling is the most common type of treatment, but medication is sometimes recommended.[75]

Breast-Feeding Although the new mother's milk will not begin to flow for 2 or more days after delivery, her breasts secrete a yellow fluid called *colostrum.* Because colostrum contains vital antibodies to help fight infection and boost the baby's immune system, the newborn should be allowed to suckle.

The American Academy of Pediatrics strongly recommends that infants be breast-fed for at least 6 months and as a supplement for 12 months. Scientific findings indicate there are many advantages to breast-feeding. Breast milk is perfectly matched to babies' nutritional needs as they grow. Breast-fed babies have fewer illnesses and a much lower hospitalization rate because breast milk contains maternal antibodies and

immunological cells that stimulate the infant's immune system. When breast-fed babies do get sick, they recover more quickly. They are also less likely to be obese than babies fed on formulas, and they have fewer allergies. They may even be more intelligent. A recent study found that the longer a baby was breast-fed, the higher the IQ was in adulthood. Researchers theorize that breast milk contains substances that enhance brain development.[76] Breast-feeding also has the added benefits of helping mothers lose weight after birth because the production of milk burns hundreds of calories a day and causes the hormone oxytocin to be released, which makes the uterus return to its normal size faster. Long term, breastfeeding may also reduce the risk of breast cancer and ovarian cancer.

Breast milk is not the only way to nourish a baby. Some women are unable or unwilling to breast-feed; women with certain medical conditions or taking certain medications are advised not to breast-feed. Prepared formulas can provide nourishment that allows a baby to grow and thrive. When deciding whether to breast- or bottle-feed, mothers must consider their own desires and preferences, too. Both feeding methods can supply the physical and emotional closeness essential to the parent–child relationship.

Infant Mortality After birth, infant death can be caused by birth defects, low birth weight, injuries, or unknown causes. In the United States, the unexpected death of a child under 1 year of age, for no apparent reason, is called **sudden infant death syndrome (SIDS).** Sudden infant death syndrome is the leading cause of death for children aged 1 month to 1 year and is responsible for about 2,500 deaths a year.[77] It is not a specific disease; rather, it is ruled a cause of death after all other possibilities are ruled out. A SIDS death is sudden and silent; death occurs quickly, often during sleep, with no signs of suffering.

The exact cause of SIDS is unknown, but a few risk factors are known. For example, babies placed to sleep on their stomachs are more likely to die from SIDS than those placed on their backs to sleep, as are babies put to sleep on or covered by soft bedding. Breastfeeding and avoiding exposure to tobacco smoke are known protective factors. Troublingly, African American babies are two times more likely to die from SIDS than white babies, and American Indian babies are three times more likely to die from SIDS than white babies.[78]

Infertility

For the couple desperately wishing to conceive, the road to parenthood may be frustrating. An estimated 1 in 10 American couples experiences **infertility,** usually defined as the inability to conceive after trying for a year or more.[79] Although the focus is often on women, in about 20 percent of cases, infertility is due to a cause involving only the male partner, and in about 30 to 40 percent of cases, infertility is due to causes involving both partners.[80] Because of the likelihood of this, it is important for both partners to be evaluated.

Reasons for the high level of infertility in the United States today include the trend toward delaying childbirth (as a woman gets older, she is less likely to conceive), endometriosis, the rising incidence of pelvic inflammatory disease, and low sperm count. Environmental contaminants known as *endocrine disrupters,* such as some pesticides and emissions from burning plastics, appear to affect fertility in both men and women. Stress and anxiety, both in general and about fertility, can also interfere with getting pregnant. Obesity and diabetes, increasingly common in the United States today, also have reproductive implications.

Causes in Women

Most cases of infertility in women result from problems with ovulation. The most common cause for female infertility is polycystic ovary syndrome (PCOS). A woman's ovaries have follicles, which are tiny, fluid-filled sacs that hold the eggs. When an egg is mature, the follicle breaks open to release the egg so it can travel to the fallopian tubes for fertilization. In women with PCOS, immature follicles bunch together to form large cysts or lumps. The eggs mature within the bunched follicles, but the follicles don't break open to release them. As a result, women with PCOS often don't have menstrual periods, or they have periods infrequently. Because the eggs are not released, women with PCOS have trouble getting pregnant. Researchers estimate that 5 to 10 percent of women of childbearing age—as many as 5 million women in the United States—have PCOS.[81] Although obesity doesn't cause infertility, it is a characteristic of PCOS. It also increases the level of estrogen in the body and can cause ovulatory disorders, both of which interfere with getting pregnant.[82]

In some women the ovaries stop functioning before natural menopause, a condition called *premature ovarian failure.* Another cause of infertility is **endometriosis.** With this very painful disorder, parts of the endometrial lining of the uterus implant themselves outside the uterus and block the fallopian tubes. The disorder can be treated surgically or with hormonal therapy.

Pelvic inflammatory disease (PID) is a serious infection that scars the fallopian tubes and blocks sperm migration. Infection-causing bacteria (chlamydia or gonorrhea) can silently invade the fallopian tubes, causing normal tissue to turn into scar tissue. This scar tissue blocks or interrupts the normal movement of eggs into the uterus. About 1 in 10 women with PID becomes infertile, and if a woman has multiple episodes of PID, her chances of becoming infertile increase.[83]

Causes in Men

Among men, the single largest fertility problem is **low sperm count.**[84] Although only one viable sperm is needed for fertilization, research has shown that all the other sperm in the ejaculate aid in the fertilization process. There are normally 60 to 80 million sperm per milliliter of semen. When the count drops below 20 million, fertility declines. Low sperm count may be attributable to environmental factors (such as exposure of the scrotum to intense heat or cold, radiation, certain chemicals, or altitude), being overweight, or wearing excessively tight underwear or clothing.[85] Other factors, such as the mumps virus, can damage the cells that make sperm, or varicocele (enlarged veins on a man's testicle) can heat the testicles and damage the sperm.[86]

endometriosis A disorder in which uterine lining tissue establishes itself outside the uterus.

pelvic inflammatory disease (PID) An infection that scars the fallopian tubes and consequently blocks sperm migration, causing infertility.

low sperm count A sperm count below 20 million sperm per milliliter of semen; the leading cause of infertility in men.

Infertility Treatments

Medical procedures can identify the cause of infertility in about 90 percent of cases. The chances of becoming pregnant after the cause has been determined range from 30 to 70 percent, depending on the reason for infertility.[87] The numerous tests and the invasion of privacy that are involved in efforts to conceive can put stress on an otherwise strong, healthy relationship. A good physician or fertility team will take the time to ascertain the couple's level of motivation and coping skills.

Workups to determine the cause of infertility can be expensive, and the costs are often not covered by insurance companies. Fertility workups for men include a sperm count, a test for sperm motility, and an analysis of any disease processes present. Women are thoroughly examined by an obstetrician-gynecologist to determine the composition of cervical mucus and evidence of tubal scarring or endometriosis.

Fertility Drugs Fertility drugs stimulate ovulation in women who are not ovulating. Sixty percent to 80 percent of women who use these drugs will begin to ovulate; of those who ovulate, about half will conceive.[88] Fertility drugs can have many side effects, ranging from headaches to abnormal

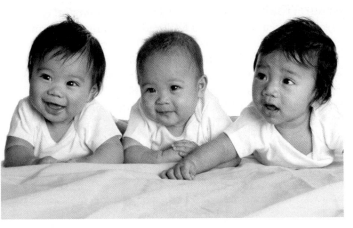

uterine bleeding. Women using fertility drugs are also at increased risk of developing multiple ovarian cysts (fluid-filled growths) and liver damage. The drugs sometimes trigger the release of more than one egg. As many as 1 in 3 women treated with fertility drugs will become pregnant with more than one child.[89]

Alternative Insemination

Another treatment option is **alternative insemination** (also known as *artificial insemination*) of a woman with her partner's sperm. The couple may also choose insemination by an anonymous donor through a sperm bank. Donated sperm are medically screened, classified according to the donor's physical characteristics (such as hair and eye color), and then frozen for future use.

Assisted Reproductive Technology (ART)

Assisted reproductive technology (ART) describes several different medical procedures that help a woman become pregnant. The most common type of ART is **in vitro fertilization (IVF).** During IVF, eggs and sperm are mixed in a laboratory dish to fertilize, and some of the fertilized eggs (zygotes) are then transferred to the woman's uterus.

Other types of assisted reproductive technologies include the following:

- **Intracytoplasmic sperm injection (ICSI),** which involves the injection of a single sperm into an egg. The fertilized egg is then placed in the woman's uterus or fallopian tube. Used with IVF, ICSI is often a successful treatment for men with impaired sperm.
- **Gamete intrafallopian transfer (GIFT),** which involves collecting eggs from the ovaries, then placing them into a thin flexible tube with the sperm. This is then injected into the woman's fallopian tubes, where fertilization takes place.
- **Zygote intrafallopian transfer (ZIFT),** which combines IVF and GIFT. Eggs and sperm are mixed outside of the body. The fertilized eggs (zygotes) are then returned to the fallopian tubes, through which they travel to the uterus.

Other Treatments for Infertility

In *nonsurgical embryo transfer,* a donor egg is fertilized by the man's sperm and implanted in the woman's uterus. In *embryo transfer,* an ovum from a donor is artificially inseminated by the man's sperm, allowed to stay in the donor's body for a time, and then transplanted into the woman's body. Infertile couples have another alternative—embryo adoption programs.

Fertility treatments such as IVF often produce excess fertilized eggs that couples may choose to donate for other infertile couples to adopt.

Gestational Surrogacy

While many infertile couples conceive via infertility treatment, some cannot sustain a pregnancy. Others may not be able to conceive at all. Surrogacy is one road to parenthood for these individuals. With surrogacy, a woman is hired to carry another person's pregnancy to term, at which point the intended parents gain custody. In traditional surrogacy, the gestational carrier is also the biological mother of the child. In gestational surrogacy, the surrogate is not the biological mother. Instead an embryo is created via IVF using the couple's own (or donor) egg and sperm. It is hard to find accurate statistics that track surrogacy, but the practice has become increasingly popular in the past decade. According to one study, over 5,000 babies were born between 2004 and 2008 via gestational surrogacy.[90] Couples considering surrogate motherhood are advised to consult a lawyer before entering into this type of contract.

Adoption

Adoption serves several important purposes in American society. It provides a way for individuals and couples who may not be able or have decided not to have children of their own to form a legal parental relationship with a nonbiological child. It also benefits children whose birth parents are unable or unwilling to raise them. Waiting for a child to adopt can sometimes be a long process. Approximately 2 percent of the adult population has adopted children.[91]

There are two types of adoption: *confidential* and *open.* In confidential adoption, the birth parents and the adoptive parents never know each other. In open adoption, birth parents and adoptive parents know some things about each other. There are different levels of openness. Both parties must agree to this plan, and it is not available in every state.

Increasingly, couples are choosing to adopt children from other countries. In 2011, U.S. families adopted more than 9,000 foreign-born children.[92] The cost of overseas adoption varies widely, but can cost more than $30,000, including agency fees, dossier and immigration processing fees, travel, and court costs.[93] Despite the high cost, it can be a good alternative for many couples, especially those who want to adopt an infant rather than an older child. Some families find it beneficial to serve as foster parents prior to deciding to adopt, and others choose to adopt older children from the foster system in the United States rather than waiting for an infant through international adoption.

Assess yourself

Are You Comfortable with Your Contraception?

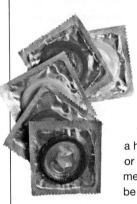

These questions will help you assess whether your current method of contraception or one you may consider using in the future will be effective for you. Answering yes to any of these questions predicts potential problems. If you have more than a few yes responses, consider talking to a health care provider, counselor, partner, or friend to decide whether to use this method or how to use it so that it will really be effective.

Method of contraception you use now or are considering:

_____

		Yes	No
1.	Have I or my partner ever become pregnant while using this method?	Ⓨ	Ⓝ
2.	Am I afraid of using this method?	Ⓨ	Ⓝ
3.	Would I really rather not use this method?	Ⓨ	Ⓝ
4.	Will I have trouble remembering to use this method?	Ⓨ	Ⓝ
5.	Will I have trouble using this method correctly?	Ⓨ	Ⓝ
6.	Does this method make menstrual periods longer or more painful for me or my partner?	Ⓨ	Ⓝ
7.	Does this method cost more than I can afford?	Ⓨ	Ⓝ
8.	Could this method cause serious complications?	Ⓨ	Ⓝ
9.	Am I, or is my partner, opposed to this method because of any religious or moral beliefs?	Ⓨ	Ⓝ
10.	Will using this method embarrass me or my partner?	Ⓨ	Ⓝ
11.	Will I enjoy intercourse less because of this method?	Ⓨ	Ⓝ
12.	Am I at risk of being exposed to HIV or other sexually transmitted infections if I use this method?	Ⓨ	Ⓝ

Total number of yes answers: _____

Source: Adapted from R. A. Hatcher et al., *Contraceptive Technology,* 19th revised ed. Copyright © 2007. Reprinted by permission of Ardent Media, Inc.

YOUR PLAN FOR CHANGE

The **Assess yourself** activity gave you the chance to assess your comfort and confidence with a contraceptive method you are using now or may use in the future. Depending on the results of the assessment, you may consider changing your birth control method.

Today, you can:

○ Visit your local drugstore and study the forms of contraception that are available without a prescription. Think about which of them you would consider using and why.

○ If you are not currently using any contraception or are not in a sexual relationship but might become sexually active, purchase a package of condoms (or pick up a few free samples from your campus health center) to keep on hand just in case.

Within the next 2 weeks, you can:

○ Make an appointment for a checkup with your health care provider. Be sure to ask him or her any questions you have about contraception.

○ Sit down with your partner and discuss contraception. Decide who will be responsible and which form will work best for you.

By the end of the semester, you can:

○ Periodically reevaluate whether your new or continued contraception is still effective for you. Review your experiences, and take note of any consistent problems you may have encountered.

○ Always keep a backup form of contraception on hand. Check this supply periodically and throw out and replace any supplies that have expired.

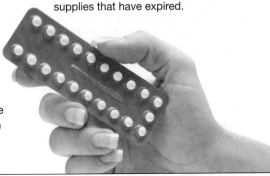

MasteringHealth™

Build your knowledge—and health!—in the Study Area of MasteringHealth with a variety of study tools.

Summary

* Latex or polyurethane male condoms and female condoms, when used correctly for oral sex or intercourse, provide the most effective protection in preventing sexually transmitted infections (STIs). Other contraceptive methods include spermicides, the diaphragm, the cervical cap, the Today Sponge, oral contraceptives, Ortho Evra, Nuva-Ring, Depo-Provera/Depo-subQ Provera, Implanon/Nexplanon, and intrauterine devices. Emergency contraception may be used within 72 hours of unprotected intercourse or the failure of another contraceptive method. Fertility awareness methods rely on altering sexual practices to avoid pregnancy, as do abstinence, outercourse, and withdrawal. Whereas all these methods of contraception are reversible, sterilization is permanent.

* Although controversial, abortion remains legal in the United States. Abortion methods include suction curettage, dilation and evacuation (D&E), intact dilation and extraction (D&X), hysterectomy, induction abortion, and medication abortions.

* Parenting is a demanding job that requires careful planning. Prospective parents must consider emotional health, maternal and paternal health, and financial plans.

* Full-term pregnancy covers three trimesters. Prenatal care includes a complete physical exam within the first trimester, follow-up checkups throughout the pregnancy, healthy nutrition and exercise, and avoidance of all substances that could have teratogenic effects on the fetus, such as alcohol and drugs, smoking, X rays, and harmful chemicals. Prenatal tests, including ultrasonography, chorionic villus sampling and other screening tests, and amniocentesis, can be used to detect birth defects during pregnancy.

* Childbirth occurs in three stages. Partners should jointly choose a labor method early in the pregnancy to be better prepared when labor occurs. Possible complications of pregnancy and childbirth include preeclampsia and eclampsia, miscarriage, ectopic pregnancy, and stillbirth.

* Infertility in women may be caused by pelvic inflammatory disease (PID) or endometriosis. In men, it may be caused by low sperm count. Treatments may include fertility drugs, alternative insemination, in vitro fertilization (IVF), assisted reproductive technology (ART), embryo transfer, and embryo adoption programs. Surrogate motherhood and adoption are also options.

Pop Quiz

1. What type of lubricant could you safely use with a latex condom?
   a. Mineral oil
   b. Water-based lubricant
   c. Body lotion
   d. Petroleum jelly

2. Which of the following is a barrier contraceptive?
   a. Seasonale
   b. FemCap
   c. Ortho Evra
   d. Contraceptive patch

3. What is the most commonly used method of first-trimester abortion?
   a. Suction curettage
   b. Dilation and evacuation (D&E)
   c. Medication abortion
   d. Induction abortion

4. What is meant by the *failure rate* of contraceptive use?
   a. The number of times a woman fails to get pregnant when she wanted to
   b. The number of times a woman gets pregnant when she did not want to
   c. The number of pregnancies that occurs for women using a particular method of birth control
   d. The frequency with which women fail to use a particular method of birth control when having sex

5. Toxic chemicals, pesticides, X rays, and other hazardous compounds that cause birth defects are referred to as
   a. carcinogens.
   b. teratogens.
   c. mutations.
   d. environmental assaults.

6. In an ectopic pregnancy, the fertilized egg usually implants in the woman's
   a. fallopian tube.
   b. uterus.
   c. vagina.
   d. ovaries.

7. What is the recommended pregnancy weight gain for a woman who is at a healthy weight before pregnancy?
   a. 15 to 20 pounds
   b. 20 to 30 pounds
   c. 25 to 35 pounds
   d. 30 to 45 pounds

8. What prenatal test involves snipping tissue from the developing fetal sac?
   a. Fetoscopy
   b. Ultrasound
   c. Amniocentesis
   d. Chorionic villus sampling

9. Why is it recommended not to use condoms made of lambskin?
   a. They are less elastic than latex condoms.

Codependence is often the result of growing up in an environment of addiction. Codependents find it hard to set healthy boundaries and often live in the chaotic, crisis-oriented mode that naturally occurs around addicts. They assume responsibility for meeting others' needs to the point that they subordinate or even cease being aware of their own needs. They may be unable to perceive their needs because they have repeatedly been taught that their needs are inappropriate or less important than someone else's. Although the word *codependent* is used less frequently today, treatment professionals still recognize the importance of helping addicts see how their behavior affects those around them and of working with family and friends to establish healthier relationships and boundaries.

Family and friends can play an important role in getting an addict to seek treatment. They are most helpful when they refuse to be enablers. **Enablers** are people who knowingly or unknowingly protect addicts from the natural consequences of their behavior. If they don't have to deal with the consequences, addicts cannot see the self-destructive nature of their behavior and will therefore continue it. Codependents are the primary enablers of their addicted loved ones, although anyone who has contact with an addict can be an enabler and thus contribute (perhaps powerfully) to continuation of the addictive behavior. Enablers are generally unaware that their behavior has this effect. In fact, enabling is rarely conscious and certainly not intentional.

what do you think?

Why do we tend to protect others from the natural consequences of their destructive behaviors?

● Have you ever confronted someone you were concerned about? If so, was the confrontation successful?

● What tips would you give someone who wants to confront a loved one about an addiction?

Addictive Behaviors

The chemicals in drugs are not the only sources of addiction. People can also become addicted to certain behaviors. **Process addictions** are behaviors known to be addictive because they are mood altering. New knowledge about the brain's reward system suggests that, to the brain, a reward is a reward, whether brought on by a chemical or a behavior, meaning that behaviors can be as addictive as drugs or other substances.[2] The altered or elevated mood is pleasurable to the addict, and he or she learns over time that a certain pattern of behavior leads to that pleasurable feeling. Eventually the addict is compelled to perform the behavior over and over again. Examples of process addictions include disordered gambling, compulsive buying, compulsive exercise, and compulsive Internet or technology use.

Disordered Gambling

Gambling is a form of recreation and entertainment for millions of Americans. Most people who gamble do so casually and moderately to experience the excitement of anticipating a win. However, more than 2 million Americans are *compulsive gamblers,* and 6 million more are considered to be at risk for developing a gambling addiction.[3] The American Psychiatric Association (APA), which previously used the term *pathological gambling,* has proposed the term **disordered gambling** for this addiction and recognizes it as a mental disorder. According to the APA's *Diagnostic and Statistical Manual of Mental Disorders,* 5th edition (*DSM-5*), characteristic behaviors associated with disordered gambling include preoccupation with gambling, unsuccessful efforts to cut back or quit, using gambling to escape problems, and lying to family members to conceal the extent of involvement with gambling.

There is strong evidence for a biological component in disordered gambling. A study of compulsive gamblers found the participants to have decreased blood flow to a key section of the brain's reward system. Similar to people who abuse drugs, it is thought that compulsive gamblers compensate for this deficiency in their brain's reward system by overdoing it and getting hooked.[4] Most compulsive gamblers state that they seek excitement even more than money. They place increasingly larger bets to obtain the desired level of excitement. Like drug addicts, compulsive gamblers live from fix to fix. Their subjective cravings can be as intense as those of drug abusers; they show tolerance in their need to increase the amount of their bets; and they experience highs rivaling that of a drug high. Up to half of pathological gamblers show withdrawal symptoms similar to those of a mild form of drug withdrawal, including sleep disturbance, sweating, irritability, and craving.

Although gambling is illegal for anyone under the age of 21, students have easier access to gambling opportunities than ever before, with a variety of lottery tickets, online poker, and a growing number of casinos in the United States. The percentage of college students who gamble—about 75 percent (both legally and illegally, based on their age)—is consistent with these growing opportunities. About 18 percent of those students reported gambling once a week or more.[5] It is estimated that about 6 percent of U.S. college students have a serious gambling problem that results in psychological difficulties, debt, and failing grades.[6] For more information on student gambling, see the **Student Health Today** box on page 202.

enabler A person who knowingly or unknowingly protects an addict from the consequences of the addict's behavior.

process addiction A condition in which a person is dependent on (addicted to) some mood-altering behavior or process, such as gambling, buying, or exercise.

disordered gambling A set of behaviors including preoccupation with gambling, unsuccessful efforts to cut back or quit, using gambling to escape problems, and lying to family members to conceal the extent of involvement with gambling.

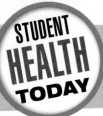
GAMBLING AND COLLEGE STUDENTS

Although many people gamble occasionally without it ever becoming a problem, even model students can find themselves caught up in it. Disordered gambling on college campuses has become a big concern.

A good example is what happens on campuses and across the country each year during March Madness, the National Collegiate Athletic Association men's college basketball tournament. An estimated $12 billion is wagered over the 3 weeks during which the tournament takes place, more than is wagered on the Super Bowl. More and more of these dollars come from the pockets of college students. College athletes in particular are at high risk for sports gambling, and they more frequently bet on sports and play games of chance than do nonathletes.

College students give three main reasons for gambling: risk, excitement, and the chance to make money. But more often than not, they lose enough money to interfere with their financial and academic futures. The most frequent gambling activities are the lottery, followed by card games (such as poker) and sports betting. Gambling seems to go hand-in-hand with other problem behaviors, including binge drinking, smoking, illicit drug use, and unsafe sex after drinking.

Although most college students who gamble are able to do so without developing a problem, warning signs of disordered gambling include the following:

- Frequent talk about gambling; encouraging or challenging others to gamble
- Borrowing money, using financial aid money or other money, or committing crimes to finance gambling
- "Chasing" losses with more gambling
- Secretive about gambling habits, and defensive when confronted.
- Possessing gambling paraphernalia such as lottery tickets or poker items
- Missing or being late for school, work, or family activities due to gambling
- Feeling sad, anxious, fearful, or angry about gambling losses

If any of these warning signs apply to you, consider talking with a counselor to get help.

Sources: Task Force on College Gambling Policies, Division on Addictions at the Cambridge Health Alliance and the National Center for Responsible Gambling, *A Call to Action: Addressing College Gambling: Recommendations for Science-Based Policies and Programs* (Cambridge, MA: Cambridge Health Alliance and the National Center for Responsible Gambling, 2009), Available at

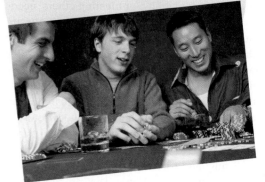

Call, fold, or raise? For increasing numbers of college students, gambling and the debts it can incur are becoming serious problems.

www.ncrg.org; N. Bhullar et al., "The Significance of Gender and Ethnicity in Collegiate Gambling and Drinking," *Addictive Disorders and Their Treatment* 11, no. 3 (2012): 154–164; National Council on Problem Gambling, "College Gambling Facts and Statistics," www.ncpgambling.org; N. Shead et al., "Characteristics of Internet Gamblers among a Sample of Students at a Large, Public University in Southwestern United States," *Journal of College Student Development* 53, no. 1 (2012): 133–148; G. M. Barnes et al., "Comparisons of Gambling and Alcohol Use among College Students and Noncollege Young People in the United States," *Journal of American College Health* 58 no. 5 (2010): 443–452; National Council on Problem Gambling, "March Madness Gambling Brings Out Warnings from NCAA to Tournament Players," 2011, www.ncpgambling.org; Prevention Lane, "Problem Gambling Prevention: College Problem Gambling," 2011, http://preventionlane.org

Compulsive Buying Disorder

In the United States today, many people use shopping as a way to make themselves feel better. But people who regularly engage in "retail therapy" in excess, running credit cards to the limit, may have *compulsive buying disorder.*

Compulsive buying has many of the same characteristics as alcoholism, gambling, and other addictions. Symptoms that a shopper has crossed the line into addiction include buying more than one of the same item, keeping items in the closet with the tags still attached, repeatedly buying much more than they need or can afford, hiding purchases from relatives and loved ones, and experiencing feelings of euphoria and excitement when shopping. The vast majority of compulsive buyers are women, and it is estimated about 5 percent of American adults struggle with this disorder.[7]

Compulsive buying can frequently lead to compulsive borrowing to help support the addiction. Irresponsible investments and purchases lead to debts that the addict tries to repay by borrowing more. Compulsive buyers often borrow money repeatedly from family, friends, or institutions in spite of the problems this causes. (For more information on the perils of credit card debt, see **Focus On: Improving Your Financial Health**.)

Exercise Addiction

Generally speaking, most Americans get too little physical activity, not too much. But exercise, when taken to extremes, can become addictive because of its powerful mood enhancing effects. One indication of exercise addiction's prevalence is that a large portion of Americans with the

MOBILE DEVICES, MEDIA, AND THE INTERNET: COULD YOU UNPLUG?

How hard would it be to give up your mobile devices, media, and the Internet for 24 hours? Judging from the results of a study with participants hailing from 37 different countries on six continents—extremely hard. All students in the study followed the same assignment: give up Internet, TV, radio, phones, iPods/MP3 players, movies, video games, and any other form of electronic or social media for 24 hours. Findings included the following:

❋ Students around the world frequently used the term addiction to speak about their technology habits. "Media is my drug; without it I was lost," said one student from the UK. A student from Argentina observed: "Sometimes I felt 'dead,'" and a student

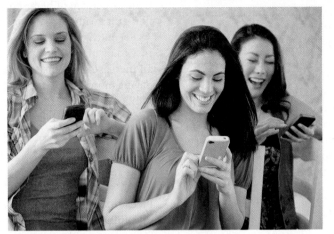

As the world goes wireless, many of us are increasingly attached to our cell phones, laptops, and tablet computers.

from Slovakia noted feeling "sad, lonely and depressed."

❋ Many students view mobile phones as an extension of the self. Going without a phone and easy access to media was disorienting. "It was an unpleasant sur- prise to realize that I am in a state of constant distraction," said a student from Mexico.

Despite the withdrawal symptoms, many students found benefits to unplugging. Some felt they had more time to talk and listen to others. Other students reported feel- ing liberated, and took time to do things they normally did not do, such as visit relatives or do other activities that involve face-to-face contact.

Have you thought about what going "unplugged" might mean for you? What opportu- nities would you have if you did not use electronic media for 24 hours?

Source: The World Unplugged, "Going 24 Hours Without Media," 2011, http://theworldunplugged. wordpress.com

---

eating disorders anorexia nervosa and bulimia nervosa use exercise to purge instead of, or in addition to, self-induced vomiting.[8] Some warning signs of being an **exercise addict** are as follows: always working out alone; always following the same rigid exercise pattern; exercising for more than 2 hours daily, repeatedly; fixation on weight loss or calories burned; exercising when sick or injured; exercising to the point of pain and beyond; and skipping work, class, or social plans for workouts. Addictive exercise results in negative consequences similar to those found in other addictions: alienation of family and friends, injuries from overdoing it, and a craving for more.

Technology Addictions

Have you ever opened your Web browser to quickly check something, and an hour later found yourself still checking your Facebook page? Do you have friends who seem more concerned with texting or surfing the Internet than with eat- ing, going out, studying, or having a face-to-face conversa- tion? These attitudes and behaviors are not unusual; many experts suggest that technology addiction is real and can present serious problems for those addicted. An estimated 1 in 8 Internet users will likely ex- perience **Internet addiction.**[9] Ap- proximately 11 percent of college students report that Internet use and computer games have inter- fered with their academic perfor- mance.[10]

Some online activities, such as gaming and cybersex, seem to be more compelling and potentially addictive than others. Internet addicts typically exhibit symptoms such as general disregard for their health, sleep deprivation, neglecting fam- ily and friends, lack of physical activity, euphoria when on- line, lower grades in school, and poor job performance. In- ternet addicts may feel moody or uncomfortable when they are not online. See the **Tech & Health** box on the struggle one study's participants had unplugging from technology for even a single day.

exercise addict A person who always works out alone, following the same rigid pattern; exercises for more than 2 hours daily, repeatedly, and when sick or injured; focuses on weight loss or calories burned; exer- cises to the point of pain and beyond; and skips work, class, or social activi- ties for workouts.

Internet addiction Compulsive use of the computer, PDA, cell phone, or other form of technology to access the Internet for activities such as e-mail, games, shopping, and blogging.

What Is a Drug?

Drugs are substances other than food that are intended to affect the structure or function of the mind or the body through chemical action. They include prescription medications such as antidepressants and antibiotics; nonprescription or over-the-counter (OTC) medications; legal recreational drugs such as alcohol, caffeine, and tobacco products; and illegal substances such as heroin and methamphetamine. Although many drugs have large benefits, the potential for addiction is great for even the most therapeutic substances due to their potent effects on the brain.

Although illicit psychoactive drugs usually come to mind when we think about drug abuse, prescription medications, OTC medications, and recreational drugs are also abused and misused. **Drug misuse** involves using a drug for a purpose for which it was not intended. For example, taking a friend's high-powered prescription painkiller for your headache is a misuse of that drug. This is not too far removed from **drug abuse,** or the excessive use of any drug, and may cause serious harm.

Drug misuse and abuse are problems of staggering proportions in our society. Approximately 9 percent of Americans report being current (defined as use during the past month) users of illicit drugs.[11] By late adolescence, 42 percent of Americans report having used illicit drugs in their lifetime.[12] Over 21 percent of high school students have taken prescription drugs without a doctor's supervision.[13]

Recently, the overall rate of drug use in the United States rose to its highest level in almost a decade, mostly driven by an increase in the use of marijuana.[14] Drug abuse costs taxpayers more than $193 billion annually in health care costs, public costs related to crime, and lost productivity.[15] It's impossible to put a dollar amount on the pain, suffering, and dysfunction that drugs cause in our everyday lives.

How Drugs Affect the Brain

Pleasure, which scientists call *reward,* is a very powerful biological force for survival. If you do something that feels pleasurable, the brain is wired in such a way that you tend to want to do it again. Life-sustaining activities like eating activate a reward center and "pleasure circuit" of specialized nerve cells devoted to producing and regulating pleasure. One important set of these nerve cells, which uses a chemical **neurotransmitter** called *dopamine,* sits at the very top of the brainstem (see Figure 7.2). These

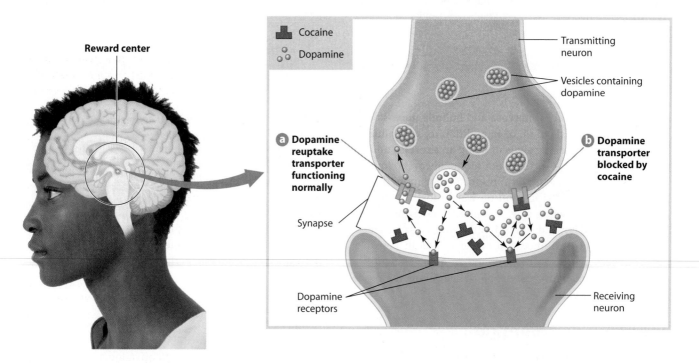

FIGURE 7.2 **The Action of Cocaine at Dopamine Receptors in the Brain, an Example of Psychoactive Drug Action**
(a) In normal neural communication, dopamine is released into the synapse between neurons. It binds temporarily to dopamine receptors on the receiving neuron, and then is recycled back into the transmitting neuron by a transporter.
(b) When cocaine molecules are present, they attach to the dopamine transporter and block the recycling process. Excess dopamine remains active in the synaptic gaps between neurons, creating feelings of excitement and euphoria.
Source: Adapted from *NIDA Research Report—Cocaine Abuse and Addiction* (NIH Publication no. 10-4166, printed May 1999, revised September 2010), www.drugabuse.gov

Video Tutor: Psychoactive Drugs Acting on the Brain

dopamine-containing neurons relay messages about pleasure through their nerve fibers to nerve cells in the limbic system, structures in the brain regulating emotions. Still other fibers connect to a related part of the frontal region of the cerebral cortex, the area of the brain that plays a key role in memory, perception, thought, and consciousness. So, this "pleasure circuit," known as the *mesolimbic dopamine system*, spans the survival-oriented brainstem, the emotional limbic system, and the thinking frontal cerebral cortex.

All drugs that are addicting—in fact, all addictive substances and behaviors—can activate the brain's pleasure circuit. Drug addiction is a biological, pathological process that alters the way in which the pleasure center, as well as other parts of the brain, functions. Almost all **psychoactive drugs** (those that change the way the brain works) do so by affecting chemical neurotransmission, either enhancing it, suppressing it, or interfering with it. Some drugs, such as heroin and LSD, mimic the effects of a natural neurotransmitter. Others, such as PCP, block receptors and thereby prevent neuronal messages from getting through. Still others, such as cocaine, block the *reuptake* of neurotransmitters by neurons, thus producing an increased concentration of the neurotransmitters in the synaptic gap, the space between individual neurons (Figure 7.2). Finally, some drugs, such as methamphetamine, act by causing neurotransmitters to be released in greater amounts than is normal.

Types of Drugs

Scientists divide drugs into six categories: prescription, over-the-counter (OTC), recreational, herbal, illicit, and commercial. These classifications are based primarily on drug action, although some are based on the source of the chemical in question. Each category includes some drugs that stimulate the body, some that depress body functions, and others that produce hallucinations (sounds, images or other sensations that are perceived but are not real). Each category also includes psychoactive drugs.

● **Prescription drugs.** These drugs can be obtained only with a prescription from a licensed physician or dentist. Approximately 47 percent of Americans have reported using at least one prescription medication in the past month.[16]

● **OTC drugs.** These drugs can be purchased without a prescription in many locations such as grocery, drug, and convenience stores. OTC drugs, used to treat everything from headaches to pain, cold, stomach upsets, and athlete's foot, provide an important access to medicine. They create substantial savings for the health care system through decreased visits to health care providers and decreased use of prescription medications.[17] However, there is a risk of OTC drugs being used improperly or misused.[18] (See **Chapter 16** for more information on OTC drugs.)

Using a needle to inject drugs poses health threats beyond the effects of the drug.

● **Recreational drugs.** These belong to a somewhat vague category whose boundaries depend on how the term *recreation* is defined. Generally, recreational drugs contain chemicals used to help people relax or socialize. Most of them are legal even though they are psychoactive. Alcohol, tobacco, and caffeine products are included in this category. (See **Chapter 8** for information on tobacco and alcohol.)

● **Herbal preparations.** Herbals encompass approximately 750 substances, including herbal teas and other products of botanical (plant) origin that are believed to have medicinal properties. (See the Focus On: Understanding Complementary and Alternative Medicine chapter for more on herbal preparations.)

● **Illicit (illegal) drugs.** These are the most notorious type of drug. Although laws governing their use, possession, cultivation, manufacture, and sale differ from state to state, illicit drugs are generally recognized as harmful. All of them are psychoactive.

● **Commercial drugs.** These are drugs found in commercially sold products. More than 1,000 of them exist, including those used in seemingly benign items such as perfumes, cosmetics, household cleansers, paints, glues, inks, dyes, and pesticides.

psychoactive drugs Drugs that affect brain chemistry and have the potential to alter mood or behavior.
oral ingestion Intake of drugs through the mouth.
inhalation The introduction of drugs through the respiratory tract.
injection The introduction of drugs into the body via a hypodermic needle.
transdermal The introduction of drugs through the skin.

Routes of Drug Administration

Route of administration refers to the way in which a given drug is taken into the body. The most common method is by swallowing a tablet, capsule, or liquid (**oral ingestion**). Drugs taken in this manner don't reach the bloodstream as quickly as do drugs introduced to the body by other means. A drug taken orally may not reach the bloodstream for as long as 30 minutes.

Drugs can also enter the body through the respiratory tract via sniffing, snorting, smoking, or inhaling (**inhalation**). Inhaling cigarettes, marijuana, gases, and aerosol sprays are a few examples of ways drugs reach the brain very quickly. Drugs that are inhaled and absorbed by the lungs travel the most rapidly compared to all the routes of drug administration.

Another rapid form of drug administration is by **injection** into the muscles, bloodstream, or just under the skin. Intravenous injection, which involves inserting a hypodermic needle directly into a vein, is the most common method of injection for drug users owing to the rapid speed (within seconds in most cases) with which a drug's effect is felt. It is also the most dangerous method of administration because of the risk of damaging blood vessels and contracting HIV (human immunodeficiency virus) and hepatitis B.

Drugs can also be absorbed through a **transdermal** (i.e., through the skin or tissue

suppositories Mixtures of drugs and a waxy medium designed to melt at body temperature after being inserted into the anus or vagina.

polydrug use Use of multiple medications, vitamins, recreational drugs, or illicit drugs simultaneously.

synergism Interaction of two or more drugs that produces more profound effects than would be expected if the drugs were taken separately; also called *potentiation*.

inhibition A drug interaction in which the effects of one drug are eliminated or reduced by the presence of another drug at the same receptor site.

antagonism A type of interaction in which two or more drugs work at the same receptor site so that one blocks the action of the other.

intolerance A type of interaction in which two or more drugs produce extremely uncomfortable reactions.

cross-tolerance Development of a tolerance to one drug that reduces the effects of another, similar drug.

linings) route. The nicotine patch is a common example of a drug that is administered transdermally. In addition, drugs can enter the body through the vagina or anus in the form of **suppositories.** Suppositories are typically mixed with a waxy medium that melts at body temperature so the drug can be released into the bloodstream. However the drug enters the system, most drugs remain active in the body for several hours.

Drug Interactions

Polydrug use, taking several medications, vitamins, recreational drugs, or illegal drugs simultaneously, can lead to dangerous health problems. Alcohol in particular frequently has dangerous interactions with other drugs. Hazardous interactions include synergism, inhibition, antagonism, intolerance, and cross-tolerance.

Synergism, also called *potentiation*, is an interaction of two or more drugs in which the effects of the individual drugs are multiplied beyond what would normally be expected if they were taken alone. You might think of synergism as $2 + 2 = 10$. A synergistic reaction can be very dangerous and even deadly. Many prescription and OTC medications carry labels that warn the user not to combine the drug with certain other drugs or with alcohol.

Inhibition occurs when the effects of one drug are reduced or eliminated by the presence of another drug at the receptor site. The presence of the second drug partially or completely blocks the first drug.

Antagonism, although usually less serious than synergism, can also produce unwanted and unpleasant effects. In an antagonistic reaction, drugs work at the same receptor site so that one drug blocks the action of the other. The blocking drug occupies the receptor site and prevents the other drug from attaching, thus altering its absorption and action.

Intolerance occurs when drugs combine in the body to produce extremely uncomfortable reactions. The drug Antabuse, used to help alcoholics give up alcohol, works by producing this type of interaction. It binds liver enzymes (the chemicals the liver produces to break down alcohol), making it impossible for the body to metabolize alcohol. As a result, an Antabuse user who drinks alcohol experiences nausea, vomiting, and, occasionally, fever.

Cross-tolerance occurs when a person develops a physiological tolerance to one drug that also

increases the body's tolerance to other substances that act similarly on the body. For example, cross-tolerance can develop between alcohol and barbiturates, two depressant drugs.

Drug Misuse and Abuse

Although drug abuse is usually referred to in connection with illicit psychoactive drugs, many people also abuse and misuse prescription, over-the-counter (OTC), and recreational drugs. In this section, we discuss these drug-related behaviors and focus, in particular, on college students' drug use.

Abuse of Over-the-Counter Drugs

Over-the-counter medications come in many different forms, including pills, liquids, nasal sprays, and topical creams. Although many people assume that no harm can come from drugs that are not illegal or regulated, OTC medications can be abused, with resultant health complications and potential addiction. High doses of certain OTC drugs may cause hallucinations, bizarre sleep patterns, mood changes, and in extreme cases, can lead to death. People who appear to be most vulnerable to abusing OTC drugs are teenagers, young adults, and people over the age of 65.

OTC drugs are abused when taken in more than the recommended dosage or for longer than is recommended. Abuse of and addiction to OTC drugs can be accidental. A person may develop tolerance from continued use, creating an unintended dependence. However, teenagers and young adults sometimes intentionally abuse OTC medications in search of a cheap high, by drinking large amounts of cough medicine, for instance. The following are a few types of OTC drugs that are subject to misuse and abuse:

Over-the-counter cough syrup is frequently abused by young people seeking a high from the ingredient DXM.

- **Sleep aids.** These drugs may be harmful in excess because they can cause problems with the sleep cycle, weaken areas of the body, or induce narcolepsy (a condition of excessive, intrusive sleepiness). Continued use of these products can lead to tolerance and dependence.
- **Cold medicines (cough syrups and tablets).** There are many different ingredients in cough and cold medicines, but one of particular concern is dextromethorphan (DXM), which is present in many types of OTC cold and cough

Medical Marijuana:
TOO LEGAL OR NOT LEGAL ENOUGH?

Currently, 18 states and the District of Columbia have enacted medical marijuana laws. The arguments for and against the legalization of marijuana have been very strong over the past few decades. Below are some of the major points from both sides.

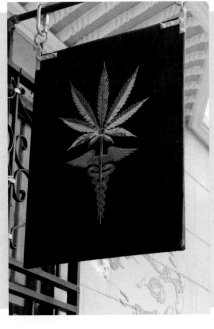

Arguments for Legalization

○ Marijuana is a safe and effective treatment for complications of dozens of conditions, such as cancer, AIDS, multiple sclerosis, pain, migraines, glaucoma, and epilepsy.

○ Legalizing marijuana will save money on law enforcement, and taxing its sale would bring in revenue for the government.

○ Government and U.S. Food and Drug Administration (FDA) oversight would allow for standardization of marijuana growth and production and could promote more responsible cultivation methods.

Arguments against Legalization

○ There are FDA-approved drugs that are just as effective in treating the same conditions that medical marijuana would be used to treat.

○ Marijuana use can cause or worsen respiratory symptoms or conditions such as bronchitis, alters mood and judgment, damages the immune system, and impairs short term memory and motor coordination. These side effects make it inappropriate for FDA approval.

○ Marijuana is known to be addictive and may lead to use of harder drugs.

○ Legalization could make marijuana more available to children and teenagers.

Where Do You Stand?

○ Do you think medical marijuana or marijuana use in general should be legalized by the federal government? What potential problems do you think this would create or solve?

○ What criteria do you think should be used to determine the legality of a particular substance? Who should make those determinations?

○ What are your feelings on drug laws in general—do you think they should be more or less prohibitive? What sort of policies would you propose to protect individuals and their rights?

Sources: Marijuana Policy Project, "Medical Marijuana Overview," 2012 www.mpp.org; Marijuana Policy Project, "Map of State Marijuana Laws," 2012, www.mpp.org; ProCon.org, "Medical Marijuana," 2012, http://medicalmarijuana.procon.org; National Institute on Drug Abuse, "DrugFacts: Is Marijuana Medicine?" July 2012, www.drugabuse.gov

a man's risk of developing testicular cancer. The risk was particularly elevated (about twice that of those who never smoked marijuana) for those who used marijuana at least weekly or who had long-term exposure to the substance beginning in adolescence. The results also suggested that the association with marijuana use might be limited to *nonseminoma*, an aggressive, fast-growing testicular malignancy that tends to strike early, between ages 20 and 35, and accounts for about 40 percent of all testicular cancer cases.[41]

According to the National Survey on Drug Use and Health, teens and young adults who use marijuana are more likely to develop serious mental health problems. A number of studies have shown an association between marijuana use and increased rates of anxiety, depression, suicidal ideation, and schizophrenia.[42] Some of these studies have shown age at first use as an indicator of vulnerability to later problems.

Other risks associated with marijuana use include suppression of the immune system, blood pressure changes, and impaired memory function. Recent studies suggest that pregnant women who smoke marijuana may have children who have subtle brain changes that can cause difficulties with problem-solving skills, memory, and attention, and can more than double the risk of giving birth prematurely.[43]

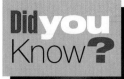
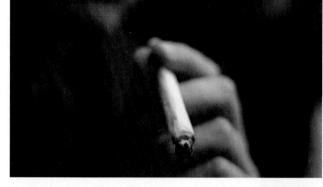

Source: Data from American College Health Association, *American College Health Association-National College Health Assessment (ACHA-NCHA): Reference Group Data Report, Fall 2012* (Hanover, MD: American College Health Association, 2013).

Narcotics and Depressants

Whereas central nervous system stimulants increase muscular and nervous system activity, **depressants** slow down neuromuscular activity and cause sleepiness or calmness. If the dose is high enough, brain function can be slowed to the point of causing death. Forms include opioids, benzodiazepines, and barbiturates, although alcohol is the most widely used central nervous system depressant (see **Chapter 8**).

Opioids cause drowsiness, relieve pain, and produce euphoria. Also called *narcotics,* opioids are derived from the parent drug *opium,* a dark, resinous substance made from the milky juice of the opium poppy seedpod, and they are all highly addictive. Opium and heroin are both illegal in the United States, but some opioids are available by prescription for medical purposes: Morphine is sometimes prescribed for severe pain, and codeine is found in prescription cough syrups and other painkillers. Several prescription drugs, including Vicodin, Percodan, OxyContin, Demerol, and Dilaudid, contain synthetic opioids.

Physical Effects of Opioids
Opioids are powerful depressants of the central nervous system. In addition to relieving pain, these drugs lower heart rate, respiration, and blood pressure. Side effects include weakness, dizziness, nausea, vomiting, euphoria, decreased sex drive, visual disturbances, and lack of coordination.

The human body's physiology could be said to encourage opioid addiction. Opioid-like hormones called **endorphins** are manufactured in the body and have multiple receptor sites, particularly in the central nervous system. When endorphins attach themselves at these points, they create feelings of painless well-being; medical researchers refer to them as "the body's own opioids." When endorphin levels are high, people feel euphoric. The same euphoria occurs when opioids or related chemicals are active at the endorphin receptor sites. Of all the opioids, heroin has the greatest notoriety as an addictive drug. The following section discusses the progression of heroin addiction; addiction to any opioid follows a similar path.

Heroin Addiction *Heroin* is a white powder derived from morphine. *Black tar heroin* is a sticky, dark brown, foul-smelling form of heroin that is relatively pure and inexpensive. Once considered a cure for morphine dependence, heroin was later discovered to be even more addictive and potent than morphine. Today heroin has no medical use.

Heroin is a depressant that produces drowsiness and a dreamy, mentally slow feeling. It can cause drastic mood swings, with euphoric highs followed by depressive lows. Heroin slows respiration and urinary output and constricts the pupils of the eyes. Symptoms of tolerance and withdrawal can appear within 3 weeks of first use.

In 2011, 620,000 Americans reported using heroin in the past year, a considerable increase since 2002.[44] Although heroin is usually injected, the contemporary version of heroin is so potent that users can get high by snorting or smoking the drug. This has attracted a more affluent group of users who may not want to inject, for reasons such as the increased risk of contracting diseases, for example, HIV.

The most common route of administration for heroin addicts is "mainlining"—intravenous injection of powdered heroin mixed in a solution. Many users describe the "rush" they feel when injecting themselves as intensely pleasurable, whereas others report unpredictable and unpleasant side effects. The temporary nature of the rush contributes to the drug's high potential for addiction—many addicts shoot up four or five times a day. Mainlining can cause veins to scar and eventually collapse. Once a vein has collapsed, it can no longer be used to introduce heroin into the bloodstream. Addicts become expert at locating new veins to use: in the feet, the legs, the temples, under the tongue, or in the groin.

Treatment for Heroin Addiction Programs to help people addicted to heroin and other opioids have not been very successful. Some addicts resume drug use even after years of drug-free living because the craving for the injection rush is very strong. It takes a great deal of discipline to seek alternative, nondrug highs.

depressants Drugs that slow down the activity of the central nervous and muscular systems and cause sleepiness or calmness.

opioids Drugs that induce sleep, relieve pain, and produce euphoria; includes derivatives of opium and synthetics with similar chemical properties; also called *narcotics*.

endorphins Opioid-like hormones that are manufactured in the human body and contribute to natural feelings of well-being.

Heroin addicts experience a distinct pattern of withdrawal. Symptoms of withdrawal include intense desire for the drug, sleep disturbance, dilated pupils, loss of appetite, irritability, goose bumps, and muscle tremors. The most difficult time in the withdrawal process occurs 24 to 72 hours following last use. All of the preceding symptoms continue, along with nausea, abdominal cramps, restlessness, insomnia, vomiting, diarrhea, extreme anxiety, hot and cold flashes, elevated blood pressure, and rapid heartbeat and respiration. Once the peak of withdrawal has passed, all these symptoms begin to subside. Still, the recovering addict has many hurdles to jump.

Opium is extracted from opium poppy seed pods like this one.

Methadone maintenance is one treatment available for people addicted to heroin or other opioids. This synthetic narcotic blocks the effects of opioid withdrawal. It is chemically similar enough to opioids to control the tremors, chills, vomiting, diarrhea, and severe abdominal pains of withdrawal. Methadone dosage is decreased over a period of time until the addict is weaned off it.

Methadone maintenance is controversial because of the drug's own potential for addiction. Critics contend that the program merely substitutes one addiction for another. Proponents argue that people on methadone maintenance are less likely to engage in criminal activities to support their habits than heroin addicts are. For this reason, many methadone maintenance programs are financed by state or federal government and are available free of charge or at reduced cost.

A number of new drug therapies for opioid dependence are emerging. Naltrexone (Trexan), an opioid antagonist, has been approved as a treatment. While on naltrexone, recovering addicts do not have the compulsion to use heroin, and if they do use it, they don't get high, so there is no point in using the drug. More recently, researchers have reported promising results with Temgesic (buprenorphine), a mild, nonaddicting synthetic opioid that, like heroin and methadone, bonds to certain receptors in the brain, blocks pain messages, and persuades the brain that its cravings for heroin have been satisfied.

Benzodiazepines and Barbiturates

A *sedative* drug promotes mental calmness and reduces anxiety, whereas a *hypnotic* drug promotes sleep or drowsiness. The most common sedative-hypnotic drugs are **benzodiazepines,** more commonly known as *tranquilizers.* These include prescription drugs such as Valium, Ativan, and Xanax. Benzodiazepines are most commonly prescribed for tension, muscular strain, sleep problems, anxiety, panic attacks, and alcohol withdrawal. **Barbiturates** are sedative-hypnotic drugs that include Amytal and Seconal. Because they are less safe than benzodiazepines, barbiturates are not typically prescribed for medical conditions that call for sedative-hypnotic drug therapy. Today, benzodiazepines have largely replaced barbiturates, which were used medically in the past for relieving tension and inducing relaxation and sleep.

Sedative-hypnotics have a synergistic effect when combined with alcohol, another central nervous system depressant. Taken together, these drugs can lead to respiratory failure and death.

benzodiazepines A class of central nervous system depressant drugs with sedative, hypnotic, and muscle relaxant effects; also called *tranquilizers.*

barbiturates Drugs that depress the central nervous system, have sedative and hypnotic effects, and are less safe than benzodiazepines.

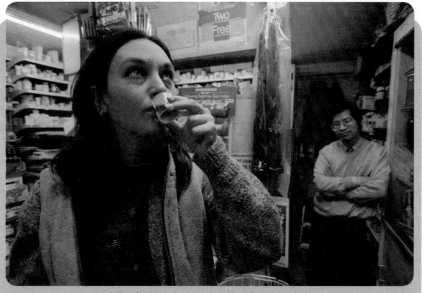

Why is it so hard to quit using heroin?

Heroin's effect on the body is similar to the well-being created by endorphins. Stopping heroin use causes withdrawal symptoms that can be very difficult to manage, which keeps many addicts from attempting to quit. Methadone is a synthetic narcotic that blocks the effects of withdrawal. Although it is still a narcotic and must be administered under the supervision of clinic or pharmacy staff, methadone allows many heroin addicts to lead somewhat normal lives.

All sedative or hypnotic drugs can produce physical and psychological dependence in several weeks. A complication specific to sedatives is cross-tolerance, which occurs when users develop tolerance for one sedative or become dependent on it and develop tolerance for others as well. Withdrawal from sedative or hypnotic drugs may range from mild discomfort to severe symptoms, depending on the degree of dependence.

Rohypnol One benzodiazepine of concern is Rohypnol, a potent tranquilizer similar in nature to Valium but many times stronger. The drug produces a sedative effect, amnesia, muscle relaxation, and slowed psychomotor responses. The most publicized "date rape" drug, Rohypnol has gained notoriety as a growing problem on college campuses. The drug has been added to punch and other drinks at parties, where it is reportedly given to women in hopes of lowering their inhibitions and facilitating potential sexual conquests. (See **Chapter 4** for more on drug-facilitated rape.)

GHB *Gamma-hydroxybutyrate (GHB)* is a central nervous system depressant known to have euphoric, sedative, and anabolic (bodybuilding) effects. It was originally sold over the counter to bodybuilders to help reduce body fat and build muscle. Concerns about GHB led the FDA to ban OTC sales in 1992, and GHB is now a Schedule I drug (Schedule I drugs are classified as having a high potential for abuse, with no currently accepted medical use in the United States).[45] GHB is an odorless, tasteless fluid. Like Rohypnol, GHB has been slipped into drinks without being detected, resulting in loss of memory, unconsciousness, amnesia, and even death. Other dangerous side effects include nausea, vomiting, seizures, hallucinations, coma, and respiratory distress.

Hallucinogens

Hallucinogens, or *psychedelics,* are substances that are capable of creating auditory or visual hallucinations and unusual changes in mood, thoughts, and feelings. The major receptor sites for most of these drugs are in the reticular formation (located in the brain stem at the upper end of the spinal cord), which is responsible for interpreting outside stimuli before allowing these signals to travel to other parts of the brain. When a hallucinogen is present at a reticular formation site, messages become scrambled, and the user may see wavy walls instead of straight ones or may "smell" colors and "hear" tastes. This mixing of sensory messages is known as **synesthesia.** Users may also become less inhibited or recall events long buried in the subconscious mind. The most widely recognized hallucinogens are LSD, Ecstasy, PCP, mescaline, psilocybin, and ketamine. All are illegal and carry severe penalties for manufacture, possession, transportation, or sale.

hallucinogens Substances capable of creating auditory or visual distortions and unusual changes in mood, thoughts, and feelings.

synesthesia An effect, which can be created by a drug, in which sensory messages are incorrectly assigned—for example, the user "hears" a taste or "smells" a sound.

LSD Of all the psychedelics, *lysergic acid diethylamide (LSD)* is the most notorious. First synthesized in the late 1930s by Swiss chemist Albert Hoffman, LSD received media attention in the 1960s when young people used the drug to "turn on, tune in, drop out." Use was banned in the 1970s and had tapered off until recently, when it made a comeback.

Most commonly known as "acid," LSD especially attracts younger users. It's estimated that about 6 percent of Americans between ages 18 and 25 have used LSD at least once in their lifetime.[46] As a comparison, a national survey of college students showed that 5 percent had used the drug at some point in their lives.[47]

The most common and most popular form of LSD is blotter acid—small squares of blotter-like paper that have been impregnated with a liquid LSD mixture. The blotter is swallowed or chewed briefly. LSD also comes in tiny thin squares of gelatin called *windowpane* and in tablets called *microdots,* which are less than an eighth of an inch across (it would take 10 or more to add up to the size of an aspirin tablet). One of the most powerful drugs known to science, LSD can produce strong effects in doses as low as 20 micrograms. (To give you an idea of how small a dose this is, the average postage stamp weighs approximately 60,000 micrograms.) As with any illegal drug, purchasers run the risk of buying an impure product.

In addition to its psychedelic effects, LSD produces several physical effects, including increased heart rate, elevated blood pressure and temperature, goose bumps (roughened skin), increased reflex speeds, muscle tremors and twitches, perspiration, increased salivation, chills, headaches, and mild nausea. The drug also stimulates uterine muscle contractions, so it can lead to premature labor and miscarriage in pregnant women. Research into long-term effects has been inconclusive.

The psychological effects of LSD vary. Euphoria is the common psychological state produced by the drug, but *dysphoria* (a sense of evil and foreboding) may also be experienced. The drug also shortens attention span, causing the mind to wander. Thoughts may be interposed and juxtaposed, so the user experiences several different thoughts simultaneously. Users become introspective, and suppressed memories may surface, often taking on bizarre symbolism. Many more effects are possible, including decreased aggressiveness and enhanced sensory experiences.

LSD causes distortions of ordinary perceptions, such as the movement of stationary objects. "Bad trips," the most publicized risk of LSD, are commonly related to the user's mood. The person, for example, may interpret increased heart rate as a heart attack.

Although there is no evidence that LSD creates physical dependence, it may create psychological dependence. Many LSD users become depressed for 1 or 2 days following a trip and turn to the drug to relieve this depression. The result is a cycle of LSD use to relieve post-LSD depression, which often leads to psychological addiction.

Ecstasy *Ecstasy* is the most common street name for the drug *methylene-dioxymethamphetamine (MDMA),* a synthetic compound with both stimulant and mildly hallucinogenic effects. It is one of the most well-known **club drugs** or "designer drugs," a term applied to synthetic analogs of existing illicit drugs that tend to be popular among teens and young adults at nightclubs, bars, raves, and other all-night parties. Ecstasy creates feelings of extreme euphoria, openness and warmth, an increased willingness to communicate, feelings of love and empathy, increased awareness, and heightened appreciation for music. Young people may use Ecstasy initially to improve their mood or get energized. Like other hallucinogenic drugs, Ecstasy can enhance the sensory experience and distort perceptions, but it does not create visual hallucinations. Effects begin within 20 to 90 minutes and can last for 3 to 5 hours.

Some of the risks associated with Ecstasy use are similar to those of other stimulants. Because of the nature of the drug, Ecstasy users are at greater risk of inappropriate and/or unintended emotional bonding and have a tendency to say things they might feel uncomfortable about later. Physical consequences of Ecstasy use may include mild to extreme jaw clenching, tongue and cheek chewing; short-term memory loss or confusion; increased body temperature as a result of dehydration and heat stroke; and increased heart rate and blood pressure. Individuals with high blood pressure, heart disease, or liver trouble are at greatest danger when using this drug. As the effects of Ecstasy begin to wear off, the user can experience mild depression, fatigue, and a hangover that can last from days to weeks. Chronic use appears to damage the brain's ability to think and to regulate emotion, memory, sleep, and pain. Combined with alcohol, Ecstasy can be extremely dangerous and sometimes fatal. Some studies indicate that the drug may cause long-lasting neurotoxic effects by damaging brain cells that produce serotonin.[48]

> **club drugs** Synthetic analogs that produce similar effects of existing drugs.

PCP *Phencyclidine,* or *PCP,* is a synthetic substance that became a black-market drug in the early 1970s. PCP was originally developed as a dissociative anesthetic, which means that patients receiving this drug could keep their eyes open and apparently remain conscious but feel no pain during a medical procedure. Afterward, patients would experience amnesia for the time the drug was in their system. Such a drug had obvious advantages as an anesthetic, but its unpredictability and drastic effects (postoperative delirium, confusion, and agitation) made doctors abandon it, and it was withdrawn from the legal market.

On the illegal market, PCP is a white, crystalline powder that users often sprinkle onto marijuana cigarettes. It is dangerous and unpredictable regardless of the method of administration. Common street names for PCP are "angel dust" for the crystalline powdered form and "peace pill" and "horse tranquilizer" for the tablet form. The effects of PCP depend on the dose. A dose as small as 5 mg will produce effects similar to those of strong central nervous system depressants—slurred speech, impaired coordination, reduced sensitivity to pain, and reduced heart and respiratory rate. Doses between 5 and 10 mg cause fever, salivation, nausea, vomiting, and total loss of sensitivity to pain. Doses greater than 10 mg result in a drastic drop in blood pressure, coma, muscular rigidity, violent outbursts, and possible convulsions and death.

Psychologically, PCP may produce either euphoria or dysphoria. It also is known to produce hallucinations as well as delusions and overall delirium. Some users experience a prolonged state of "nothingness." The long-term effects of PCP use are unknown.

Mescaline *Mescaline* is one of hundreds of chemicals derived from the peyote cactus, a small, button-like plant that grows in the southwestern United States and in Latin America. Natives of these regions have long used the dried peyote "buttons" for religious purposes.

Users typically swallow 10 to 12 buttons. They taste bitter and generally induce immediate nausea or vomiting. Long-time users claim that the nausea

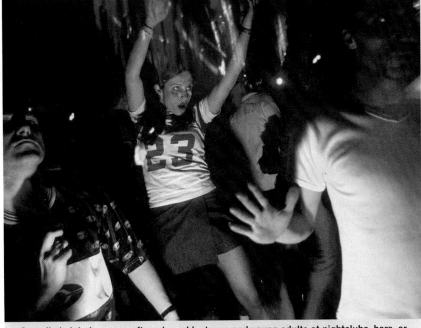

So-called club drugs are often abused by teens and young adults at nightclubs, bars, or all-night dances. Although users may think them relatively harmless, they can produce hallucinations, paranoia, amnesia, dangerous increases in heart rate and blood pressure, coma, and, in some cases, death.

becomes less noticeable with frequent use. Those who are able to keep the drug down begin to feel the effects within 30 to 90 minutes, when mescaline reaches maximum concentration in the brain. (It may persist for up to 9 or 10 hours.) Mescaline is both a powerful hallucinogen and a central nervous system stimulant.

Products sold on the street as mescaline are likely to be synthetic chemical relatives of the true drug. Street names of these products include DOM, STP, TMA, and MMDA. Any of these can be toxic in small quantities.

Mescaline comes from "buttons" of the peyote cactus, like this one.

Psilocybin *Psilocybin* and *psilocin* are the active chemicals in a group of mushrooms sometimes called "magic mushrooms." *Psilocybe* mushrooms, which grow throughout the world, can be cultivated from spores or harvested wild. When consumed, these mushrooms can cause hallucinations. Because many mushrooms resemble the *Psilocybe* variety, people who harvest wild mushrooms for any purpose should be certain of what they are doing. Mushroom varieties can be easily misidentified, and mistakes can be fatal. Psilocybin is similar to LSD in its physical effects, which generally wear off in 4 to 6 hours.

inhalants Chemical vapors that are sniffed or inhaled to produce highs.

anabolic steroids Artificial forms of the hormone testosterone that promote muscle growth and strength.

ergogenic drugs Substances believed to enhance athletic performance.

Ketamine The liquid form of *ketamine,* or Special K, as it is commonly called, is used as an anesthetic in some hospitals and veterinary clinics. After stealing it from hospitals or medical suppliers, dealers typically dry the liquid (usually by cooking it) and grind the residue into powder. Special K causes hallucinations, because it inhibits the relay of sensory input; the brain fills the resulting void with visions, dreams, memories, and sensory distortions. The effects of ketamine are similar to those of PCP—confusion, agitation, aggression, and lack of coordination—and less predictable. Aftereffects of ketamine are less severe than those of ecstasy, so it has grown in popularity as a club drug.

Psilocybe mushrooms produce hallucinogenic effects when ingested.

Inhalants

Inhalants are chemicals that produce vapors that, when inhaled, can cause hallucinations and create intoxicating and euphoric effects. Not commonly recognized as drugs, inhalants are legal to purchase and universally available, but dangerous when used incorrectly. They generally appeal to young people who can't afford or obtain illicit substances. Some products often misused as inhalants include rubber cement, model glue, paint thinner, lighter fluid, varnish, wax, spot removers, and gasoline. Most of these substances are sniffed or "huffed" by users in search of a quick, cheap high. Amyl nitrite and nitrous oxide ("laughing gas") are also sometimes abused.

Because they are inhaled, the volatile chemicals in these products reach the bloodstream within seconds. An inhaled substance is not diluted or buffered by stomach acids or other body fluids and thus is more potent than it would be if swallowed. This characteristic, along with the fact that dosages are extremely difficult to control because everyone has unique lung and breathing capacities, makes inhalants particularly dangerous.

The effects of inhalants usually last fewer than 15 minutes and resemble those of central nervous system depressants. Users may experience dizziness, disorientation, impaired coordination, reduced judgment, and slowed reaction times. Combining inhalants with alcohol produces a synergistic effect and can cause severe liver damage that can be fatal.

An overdose of fumes from inhalants can cause unconsciousness. If the user's oxygen intake is reduced during the inhaling process, death can result within 5 minutes. Whether a user is a first-time or chronic user, *sudden sniffing death syndrome* can be a consequence. This syndrome can occur if a user inhales deeply and then participates in physical activity or is startled.

Anabolic Steroids

Anabolic steroids are artificial forms of the male hormone testosterone that promote muscle growth and strength. Steroids are available in two forms: injectable solutions and pills. These **ergogenic drugs** are used primarily by people who believe the drugs will increase their strength, power, bulk (weight), speed, and athletic performance.

It was once estimated that up to 20 percent of college athletes used steroids. Now that stricter drug-testing policies have been instituted by the National Collegiate Athletic Association (NCAA), reported use of anabolic steroids among intercollegiate athletes has decreased; only about .2 percent of college students report taking them in the past 30 days.[49] Among both adolescents and adults, steroid abuse is higher among men than it is among women. However, steroid abuse is growing most rapidly among young women.[50] The use of steroids among athletes periodically makes the news. Recently, much focus has been placed on Major League Baseball, cycling, and the 2012 Summer Olympic Games where 11 athletes were barred for illegal drug use.

Physical Effects of Steroids Although their primary effects are not psychotropic, anabolic steroids can produce a state of euphoria and diminished fatigue in addition to increased bulk and power in both sexes. These qualities give steroids an addictive quality. When users stop, they can experience psychological withdrawal and sometimes severe depression, in some cases leading to suicide attempts. If untreated, depression associated with steroid withdrawal has been known to last for a year or more after steroid use stops.

Men and women who use steroids experience a variety of adverse effects. These drugs cause mood swings (aggression and violence), sometimes known as "roid rage"; acne; liver tumors; elevated cholesterol levels; hypertension; kidney disease; and immune system disturbances. There is also a danger of transmitting AIDS and hepatitis (a serious liver disease) through shared needles. In women, large doses of anabolic steroids may trigger the development of

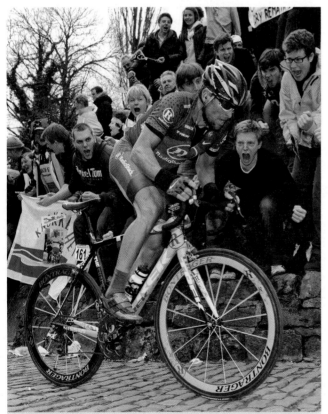

After being stripped of seven Tour de France titles in 2012 and an Olympic medal in 2013, cyclist Lance Armstrong publicly ended his years of denial and admitted to doping. He was banned from cycling for life and has been sued by the U.S. federal government and others for fraud.

masculine attributes such as lowered voice, increased facial and body hair, and male-pattern baldness; they may also result in an enlarged clitoris, smaller breasts, and changes in or absence of menstruation. When taken by healthy men, anabolic steroids shut down the body's production of testosterone, causing men's breasts to grow and testicles to atrophy.

> **detoxification** The process, which involves abstinence, of freeing a drug user from an intoxicating or addictive substance in the body or from dependence on such a substance.

Treatment and Recovery

An estimated 21.6 million Americans aged 12 or older needed treatment for an illicit drug or alcohol use problem in 2011. Of these, only 2.3 million—approximately 11 percent—received treatment.[51] This gap between needing and receiving treatment occurs because the most difficult step in the treatment and recovery process is for the substance abuser to admit that he or she is an addict. Admitting to addiction is difficult because of the power of *denial*—the inability to see the truth. Denial is the hallmark of addiction. It can be so powerful that a planned intervention is sometimes necessary to break down the addict's defenses against recognizing the problem.

Recovery from drug addiction or addiction to a behavior is a long-term process and frequently requires multiple episodes of treatment. The first step generally begins with abstinence—refraining from the behavior. **Detoxification** refers to an early abstinence period during which an addict adjusts physically and cognitively to being free from the addiction's influence. It occurs in virtually every recovering addict, and although it is uncomfortable for most addicts, it can be dangerous for some. This is primarily true for those addicted to chemicals, especially alcohol and heroin, and painkillers such as OxyContin. For these people, early abstinence may involve profound withdrawals that require medical supervision. Because of this, most inpatient treatment programs provide a pretreatment component of supervised detoxification to achieve abstinence safely before treatment begins.

Treatment Approaches

Outpatient behavioral treatment encompasses a wide variety of programs for addicts who visit a clinic at regular intervals. Most of the programs involve individual or group drug counseling. Some programs also offer other forms of behavioral treatment, such as the following:

- Cognitive behavioral therapy, which seeks to help patients recognize, avoid, and cope with the situations in which they are most likely to abuse drugs

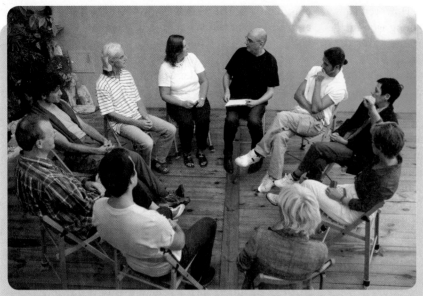

What works in helping people recover from addiction?

Recovery from addiction is a long, difficult process. Treatment and recovery usually begin with a period of detoxification. Recovering addicts usually participate in behavioral or cognitive therapy, which often takes the form of group meetings, to learn how to cope without the addictive behavior or drug and avoid relapse.

- Multidimensional family therapy, which addresses a range of influences on the drug abuse patterns of adolescents and is designed for them and their families
- Motivational interviewing, which is a client-centered, direct method for enhancing intrinsic motivation to change by exploring and resolving ambivalence
- Motivational incentives (contingency management), which uses positive reinforcement to encourage abstinence from drugs

Residential treatment programs can also be very effective, especially for those with more severe problems. For example, therapeutic communities (TCs) are highly structured programs in which addicts remain at a residence, typically for 6 to 12 months. The focus of the TC is on the resocialization of the addict to a drug-free lifestyle.

12-Step Programs The first 12-step program was Alcoholics Anonymous (AA), begun in 1935 in Akron, Ohio. The 12-step program has since become the most widely used approach to dealing with not only alcoholism, but also drug abuse and various other addictive or dysfunctional behaviors. There are more than 200 different recovery programs based on the program, including Narcotics Anonymous, Cocaine Anonymous, Crystal Meth Anonymous, Gamblers Anonymous, and Pills Anonymous.

The 12-step program is nonjudgmental and based on the idea that a program's only purpose is to work on personal recovery. Working the 12 steps includes admitting to having a serious problem, recognizing there is an outside power that could help, consciously relying on that power, admitting and

listing character defects, seeking deliverance from defects, apologizing to those individuals one has harmed in the past, and helping others with the same problem. The 12-step meetings are held at a variety of times and locations in almost every city. There is no membership cost, and the meetings are open to anyone who wishes to attend.

Vaccines against Addictive Drugs Currently, a promising new cocaine vaccine is in development. The vaccine does not eliminate the desire for cocaine; instead, it keeps the user from getting high by stimulating the immune system to attack the drug when it's taken. Clinical human trials are expected to begin soon, and vaccines against nicotine, heroin, and methamphetamine are also in development.

Drug Treatment and Recovery for College Students

For college students who have developed substance or behavioral addictions, early intervention increases the likelihood of successful treatment, successful sobriety, and completion of a college education. Depending on the severity of the abuse or dependence, college students undergoing drug treatment may be required to spend time away from school in a residential drug rehabilitation inpatient facility. The needs of college students seeking drug treatment in rehab do not differ greatly from other adult recovering addicts, but for best results, the community of addicts should include others of a similar age and educational background. Private therapy, group therapy, cognitive training, nutrition counseling, and health therapies can all be used to help with recovery. A growing number of colleges and universities offer special services to students who are recovering from alcohol and other drug addiction and want to stay in school without being exposed to excessive drinking or drug use.

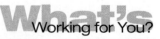
Working for You?

Maybe you already have healthy habits that can help you avoid addictive behaviors. Which of these are you already incorporating into your life?

☐ I have a wide network of friends and family who support me.

☐ I've made the decision not to try drugs in the first place.

☐ I've tried certain drugs but have consciously chosen not to continue using them.

☐ In addition to my studies, I'm pursuing activities that interest me.

Addressing Drug Misuse and Abuse in the United States

Americans are alarmed by the persistent problem of illegal drug use. Respondents in public opinion polls feel that the most important strategy for fighting drug abuse is educating young people. They also endorse strategies such as stricter border surveillance to reduce drug trafficking; longer prison sentences for drug dealers; increased government spending on prevention; antidrug law enforcement; and greater cooperation among government agencies, private groups, and individuals providing treatment assistance.

To address safety concerns, many employers have instituted mandatory drug testing. Despite controversies over accuracy of urinalysis tests, this practice is becoming more common.

All of these approaches will probably help up to a point, but they do not offer a total solution to the problem. Drug abuse has been a part of human behavior for thousands of years, and it is not likely to disappear in the near future. For this reason, it is necessary to educate ourselves and to develop the self-discipline necessary to avoid dangerous drug dependence.

In general, researchers in the field of drug education agree that a multimodal approach is best. Young people should be taught the difference between drug use, misuse, and abuse. Factual information that is free of scare tactics must be presented; lecturing and moralizing have proven not to work.

Harm Reduction Strategies

Harm reduction is a set of practical approaches to reducing negative consequences of drug use, incorporating a spectrum of strategies from safer use to managed use to abstinence. Harm reduction approaches have been widely used in needle exchange programs, where injection drug users receive clean needles and syringes and bleach for cleaning needles; these efforts help reduce the number of HIV and hepatitis B cases. Harm reduction may also involve changing the legal sanctions associated with drug use, increasing the availability of treatment services to drug abusers, and/or attempting to change drug users' behavior through education. Harm reduction strategies meet drug users "where they're at," addressing conditions of use along with the use itself. This strategy recognizes that people always have and always will use drugs and, therefore, attempts to minimize the potential hazards associated with drug use rather than the use itself.

Assess yourself

Do You Have a Problem with Drugs?

Answering the following questions will help you determine whether you have developed a drug problem:

Yes No

○ ○ **1.** In the past year, did you have a hard time paying attention in classes, work, or at home?

○ ○ **2.** Have you ever felt you should cut down on your drug use?

○ ○ **3.** Have you had blackouts or flashbacks as a result of your drug use?

○ ○ **4.** Have people annoyed (irritated, angered, etc.) you by criticizing your drug use?

○ ○ **5.** Have you ever been arrested or in trouble with the law because of your drug use?

○ ○ **6.** Have you lost friends because of your drug use?

○ ○ **7.** Have you ever felt bad or guilty about your drug use?

○ ○ **8.** Have you ever thought you might have a drug problem?

If you answered "yes" to *any* of the questions, you should consider talking to a counselor or health care provider either on campus at your health or counseling center.

Source: Adapted from U.S. Department of Health and Human Services, Substance Abuse and Mental Health Services Administration, Center for Substance Abuse Treatment, "Should You Talk to Someone About a Drug, Alcohol or Mental Health Problem?" 2011, www.samhsa.gov

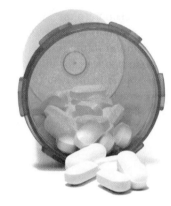

YOUR PLAN FOR CHANGE

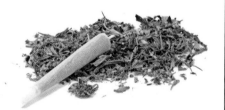

The **Assess yourself** activity describes signs of being controlled by drugs or having a drug problem. Depending on your results, you may need to change certain behaviors that may be detrimental to your health.

Today, you can:

○ Imagine a situation in which someone offers you a drug, and think of several different ways of refusing. Rehearse these scenarios in your head.

○ Stop by your campus health center to find out about drug treatment programs or support groups they may have.

Within the next 2 weeks, you can:

○ Think about the drug use patterns among your social group. Are you ever uncomfortable with these people because of their drug use? Is it difficult to avoid using drugs when you are with them? If the answers are yes, begin exploring ways to expand your social circle.

○ If you are concerned about your own drug use or the drug use of a close friend, make an appointment with a counselor to talk about the issue.

By the end of the semester, you can:

○ Participate in clubs, activities, and social groups that do not rely on substance abuse for their amusement.

○ If you have a drug problem, make a commitment to enter a treatment program. Acknowledge that you have a problem and that you need the assistance of others to help you overcome it.

MasteringHealth™

Build your knowledge—and health!—in the Study Area of MasteringHealth with a variety of study tools.

Summary

* Addiction is the continued involvement with a substance or activity despite ongoing negative consequences of that involvement. Addiction is behavior resulting from compulsion; without the behavior, the addict experiences withdrawal. In contrast, habits can be broken without much discomfort. All addictions share four common symptoms: compulsion, loss of control, negative consequences, and denial.

* Addictive behaviors include disordered gambling, compulsive buying, exercise addiction, and technology addiction. Codependents are typically friends or family members who are controlled by an addict's behavior. Enablers are people who knowingly or unknowingly protect addicts from the consequences of their behavior.

* Drugs are substances other than food that are intended to affect the structure or function of the mind or the body through chemical action. Almost all psychoactive drugs affect neurotransmission in the brain.

* The six categories of drugs are prescription drugs, over-the-counter (OTC) drugs, recreational drugs, herbal preparations, illicit (illegal) drugs, and commercial drugs. Routes of administration include oral ingestion, inhalation, injection (intravenous, intramuscular, and subcutaneous), transdermal, and suppositories.

* OTC medications are drugs that do not require a prescription. Some OTC medications, including sleep aids, cold medicines, and diet pills, can be addictive.

* Prescription drug abuse is at an all-time high, particularly among college students. Only marijuana is more commonly abused. There are a variety of negative consequences associated with prescription drug abuse, including death.

* Illicit drugs, also called *controlled substances,* include cocaine and its derivatives, amphetamines, methamphetamine, marijuana, opioids, depressants, hallucinogens/psychedelics, inhalants, and steroids. Each has its own set of risks and effects.

* People from all walks of life use illicit drugs. Drug use declined from the mid-1980s to the early 1990s but has remained steady since then. However, among young people, use of drugs has been rising in recent years.

* Treatment begins with abstinence from the drug or addictive behavior, usually instituted through intervention by close family, friends, or other loved ones. Treatment programs may be outpatient or residential and may include individual, group, or family therapy, as well as 12-step programs.

* The drug problem reaches everyone through crime and elevated health care costs. Public health and governmental approaches to the problem involve regulation, enforcement, education, and harm reduction.

Pop Quiz

1. Which of the following is not a characteristic of addiction?
   a. Denial
   b. Acknowledgment of self-destructive behavior
   c. Loss of control
   d. Obsession with a substance or behavior

2. An individual who knowingly tries to protect an addict from natural consequences of his or her destructive behaviors is
   a. enabling.
   b. helping the addict to recover.
   c. practicing intervention.
   d. controlling.

3. An example of a process addiction is
   a. a cocaine addiction.
   b. a gambling addiction.
   c. a marijuana addiction.
   d. a caffeine addiction.

4. The excessive use of any drug is called
   a. drug misuse.
   b. drug addiction.
   c. drug tolerance.
   d. drug abuse.

5. Which of the following is not an example of drug misuse?
   a. Developing tolerance to a drug
   b. Taking a friend's prescription medicine
   c. Taking medicine more often than is recommended
   d. Not following the instructions when taking a medicine

6. Rebecca takes a number of medications for various conditions, including Prinivil (an antihypertensive drug), insulin (a diabetic medication), and Claritin (an antihistamine). This is an example of
   a. synergism.
   b. illegal drug use.
   c. polydrug use.
   d. antagonism.

7. Cross-tolerance occurs when
   a. drugs work at the same receptor site so that one blocks the action of the other.
   b. the effects of one drug are eliminated or reduced by the presence of another drug at the receptor site.
   c. a person develops a physiological tolerance to one drug and

shows a similar tolerance to selected other drugs as a result.

d. two or more drugs interact and the effects of the individual drugs are multiplied beyond what normally would be expected if they were taken alone.

8. Which of the following is classified as a stimulant?
   a. Methamphetamine
   b. Alcohol
   c. Marijuana
   d. LSD

9. Freebasing is
   a. mixing cocaine with heroin.
   b. inhaling heroin fumes.
   c. injecting a drug into the veins.
   d. smoking cocaine that has had hydrochloric salt removed from it.

10. The psychoactive drug mescaline is found in what plant?
    a. Mushrooms
    b. Peyote cactus
    c. Marijuana
    d. Belladonna

Answers to these questions can be found on page A-1.

Think about It!

1. What is the current theory that explains how drugs work in the brain?

2. Explain the terms *synergism* and *antagonism*.

3. Why do you think many people today feel that marijuana use is not dangerous? What are the arguments in favor of legalizing marijuana? What are the arguments against legalization?

4. What could you do to help a friend who is fighting a substance abuse problem? What resources on your campus could help you?

5. What types of programs do you think would be effective in preventing drug abuse among high school and college students? How would programs for high school students differ from those for college students?

6. Discuss how addiction affects family and friends. What role do family and friends play in helping the addict get help and maintain recovery?

Accessing Your Health on the Internet

The following websites explore further topics and issues related to personal health. For links to the websites below, visit the Study Area in MasteringHealth.

1. *Join Together.* An excellent site for the most current information related to substance abuse. Also includes information on alcohol and drug policy and provides advice on organizing and taking political action. www.drugfree.org/join-together

2. *National Institute on Drug Abuse (NIDA).* The home page of this U.S. government agency has information on the latest statistics and findings in drug research. www.nida.nih.gov

3. *Substance Abuse and Mental Health Services Administration (SAMHSA).* Outstanding resource for information about national surveys, ongoing research, and national drug interventions. www.samhsa.gov

4. *National Center for Responsible Gambling. College Gambling.org.* A resource for gambling information pertinent to college campuses. www.collegegambling.org

Drinking Alcohol Responsibly and Ending Tobacco Use

8

LEARNING OUTCOMES

✳ Explain the health risks and effects of alcohol consumption.

✳ Discuss the alcohol and tobacco use patterns of college students and overall trends in consumption.

✳ Explain the physiological and behavioral effects of alcohol, including blood alcohol concentration, absorption, and metabolism.

✳ Identify short-term and long-term effects of alcohol consumption.

✳ Describe the symptoms and causes of alcoholism, its cost to society, and effects on the family.

✳ Explore treatment options for alcohol dependence.

✳ Discuss the social and political issues involved in tobacco use.

✳ Explain the scope of tobacco use in the United States.

✳ Describe the health risks and physical impact associated with using tobacco products.

✳ Explain the dangers associated with environmental tobacco smoke.

✳ Assess the effectiveness of tobacco use and prevention policies.

✳ Describe methods and benefits of smoking cessation.

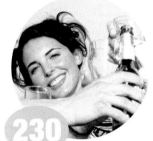

230
How much do college students really drink?

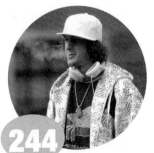

232
Why do people feel the effects of alcohol differently?

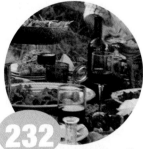

244
Is social smoking really that bad for me?

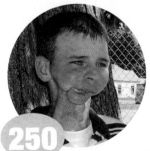

250
Is chewing tobacco as harmful as smoking?

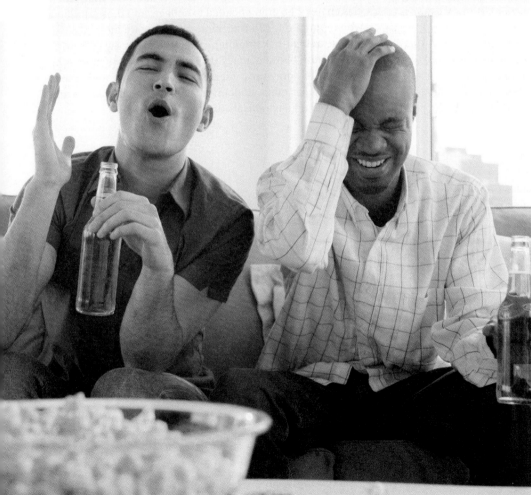

When many of us think of dangerous drugs, illegal substances such as heroin or cocaine often come to mind. But in reality, two socially accepted drugs—alcohol and tobacco—kill far more people. Annually, excessive use of alcohol is responsible for about 80,000 deaths—twice as many as illicit drugs[1]—and tobacco is the single largest preventable cause of death in the United States, claiming a whopping 443,000 lives a year.[2]

90% of the drinking population are infrequent, light, or moderate drinkers.

Alcohol: An Overview

Throughout history, humans have used alcohol during social gatherings, religious ceremonies, and everyday life. The consumption of alcoholic beverages is interwoven with many traditions, and moderate use of alcohol can enhance celebrations or special times. Research shows that very low levels of alcohol consumption, particularly red wine, may actually lower some health risks in older adults.[3] Even though alcohol can play a positive role in some people's lives, it is first and foremost a chemical substance that affects physical and mental behavior. The fact is, alcohol is a drug, and if it is not used responsibly, it can be dangerous.

binge drinking A binge is a pattern of drinking alcohol that brings blood alcohol concentration (BAC) to 0.08 gram-percent or above; for a typical adult, this pattern corresponds to consuming five or more drinks (male) or four or more drinks (female) in about 2 hours.

It is estimated that half of Americans consume alcoholic beverages regularly, and about 21 percent abstain from drinking alcohol altogether.[4] Among those who drink, consumption patterns vary. More men are regular drinkers, and men typically drink more than do women. White drinkers are more likely to drink daily or nearly daily than are nonwhites. As age increases, the number of people who consume alcohol regularly decreases.[5]

Alcohol and College Students

Alcohol is the most popular drug on college campuses: 62 percent of students report having consumed alcoholic beverages in the past 30 days (Figure 8.1).[6] Approximately 39 percent of all college students engage in **binge drinking**[7]—a pattern of drinking that brings blood alcohol concentration (BAC) to 0.08 gram-percent or above. Students who might go out and drink only once a week are considered binge drinkers if they consume five or more drinks (for men) or four or more drinks (for women) within 2 hours.[8] In a new trend on college campuses, women's consumption of alcohol has come close to equaling men's.

College is a critical time to become aware of and responsible for drinking. Many students are away from home, often for the first time, and are excited by their newfound independence. For some students, this independence and the rite of passage into the college culture are symbolized by alcohol use. More than 80 percent of college students drink alcohol to celebrate their twenty-first birthday.[9] In a recent study, nearly half of students celebrating experienced at least one negative consequence of drinking alcohol (e.g., headache, feeling very sick to their stomach, etc.).[10]

The transition into college itself may put first-year students at risk for alcohol misuse. During high school, students who are college bound drink less than their classmates who aren't headed to college, and those students who report a difficult transition to college are more likely to engage in high-risk drinking.[11] Many students say they drink to have fun, but may really be coping with stress, boredom, anxiety, or pressures created by academic and social demands. For other students alcohol lowers inhibitions and is a way to manage social anxiety and shyness.

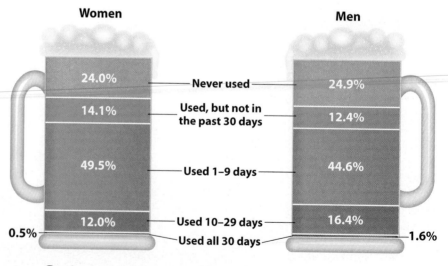

Women   **Men**

	Women	Men
Never used	24.0%	24.9%
Used, but not in the past 30 days	14.1%	12.4%
Used 1–9 days	49.5%	44.6%
Used 10–29 days	12.0%	16.4%
Used all 30 days	0.5%	1.6%

FIGURE 8.1 **College Students' Patterns of Alcohol Use in the Past 30 Days**
Source: Data from American College Health Association, *American College Health Association— National College Health Assessment II: Reference Group Executive Summary, Fall 2012* (Hanover, MD: American College Health Association, 2013).

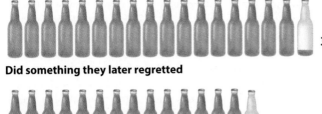

Did something they later regretted 34.1%

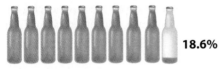

Forgot where they were or what they did 29.6%

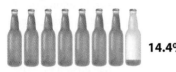

Had unprotected sex 18.6%

Physically injured self 14.4%

3.0%

Got in trouble with the police

1.9%

Physically injured another person

FIGURE 8.2 **Prevalence of Negative Consequences of Drinking among College Students, Past Year**

Source: Data from American College Health Association, *American College Health Association—National College Health Assessment II: Reference Group Executive Summary, Fall 2012* (Hanover, MD: American College Health Association, 2013).

A significant number of students experience negative consequences as a result of their alcohol consumption (Figure 8.2). Nearly 2 percent reported having sex with someone without giving consent, and 0.6 percent reported having sex with someone without getting consent. Women are more likely to have someone use force or the threat of force to have sex with them when alcohol is involved.

Alcohol use among college students also has consequences related to academic performance.[12] Alcohol consumption tends to disrupt sleep, particularly the second half of the night's sleep, and these disruptive effects increase daytime sleepiness and decrease alertness. Research shows that daytime sleepiness as a result of alcohol use and disruptive sleep negatively impacts students'

academic performance and puts them at risk for greater alcohol-related consequences.[13]

Fortunately, many college students report practicing protective behaviors when consuming alcohol to reduce the risk of negative consequences as a result of their alcohol use. The **Skills for Behavior Change** box provides some of these strategies for drinking responsibly.

High-Risk Drinking and College Students

According to a recent study, 1,825 college students die each year because of alcohol-related unintentional injuries, including car accidents.[14] Consumption of alcohol is the number one cause of preventable death among undergraduate college students in the United States today.[15]

Although everyone who drinks is at some risk for alcohol-related problems, college students seem to be particularly vulnerable for the following reasons:

- Alcohol exacerbates their already high risk for suicide, automobile crashes, and falls.
- Many college and university students' customs and celebrations encourage certain dangerous practices and patterns of alcohol use.
- Advertising and promotions from the alcoholic beverage industry heavily target university campuses.
- Beer and other drink specials enable students to consume large amounts of alcohol cheaply.
- College students are particularly vulnerable to peer influence.
- College administrators often deny that alcohol problems exist on their campuses.

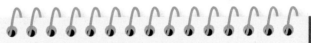

Skills for Behavior Change

Tips for Drinking Responsibly

❯ Eat before and while you drink.
❯ Stay with the same group of friends the entire time you drink.
❯ Don't drink before the party.
❯ Avoid drinking if you are angry, anxious, or depressed.
❯ Pace yourself. Drink one alcoholic drink an hour (or add even more time between drinks).
❯ Alternate alcoholic and nonalcoholic drinks.
❯ Determine ahead of time the number of drinks you will have for the evening.
❯ Avoid drinking games.
❯ Keep track of the number of drinks you drink.
❯ Don't drink and drive. Volunteer to be the sober driver.

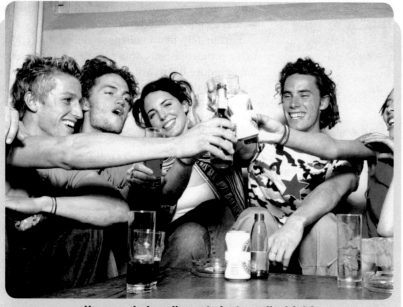

How much do college students really drink?

It may sometimes seem like your campus is crowded with heavy drinkers, but, in fact, most college students—about 60%—drink only occasionally, and 24% don't drink at all. However, college students have high rates of binge drinking; when they do drink, they tend to drink a lot. Irresponsible consumption of alcohol can easily result in disaster, so it is important for you to take control of when you drink, and how much.

Source: American College Health Association, *American College Health Association—National College Health Assessment II (ACHA–NCHA II) Reference Group Data Report, Fall 2012* (Hanover, MD: American College Health Association, 2013).

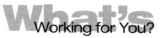

Working for You?

Maybe you already drink responsibly. Which of the following strategies are you already incorporating into your life?

☐ I always have a complete meal before I drink.

☐ I limit myself to two drinks per evening out, and I drink nonalcoholic beverages between drinks.

☐ I'm trying out different clubs and activities that don't involve drinking and encouraging my friends to do the same.

☐ I don't participate in drinking games.

College students are also more likely than their noncollegiate peers to drink recklessly, play drinking games, and engage in other dangerous practices. One such practice is **pre-gaming** (also called pre-loading or front-loading), which involves planned heavy drinking with friends over brief periods of time prior to going out to a bar, party, or sporting event. It is estimated that about 55 percent of both college men and women pre-game before going to a bar or nightclub.[16] Pre-gamers also have higher alcohol consumption during the evening and suffer more negative consequences.

Two-thirds of college students engage in drinking games that involve binge drinking.[17] Those who participate in drinking games are much less likely to monitor

pre-gaming A strategy of drinking heavily, usually with friends, before going out to parties or bars.

drunkorexia A colloquial term to describe the combination of disordered eating, excessive physical activity and heavy alcohol consumption.

or regulate how much they are drinking and are at risk for extreme intoxication. Men more often than women participate in drinking games to consume larger amounts of alcohol,[18] and drinking games have been associated with alcohol-related injuries and deaths from alcohol poisoning. To see whether your alcohol consumption is a problem, complete the **Assess Yourself** quiz at the end of the chapter.

Unfortunately, recent studies confirm what students have been experiencing for a long time—binge drinkers cause problems not only for themselves, but also for those around them. One study indicated that more than 696,000 students between the ages of 18 and 24 were assaulted by another student who had been drinking.[19] Other students report sleep and study disruptions, vandalism of personal property, sexual abuse, and other unwanted sexual advances. Women from colleges with medium to high binge-drinking rates are 1.5 times more at risk of being raped than those from schools with low binge-drinking rates.

Some people use extreme measures to control their eating and/or exercise excessively so that they can save calories, consume more alcohol, and become intoxicated faster.[20] "**Drunkorexia**" is a colloquialism currently being use to describe the combination of two dangerous behaviors: disordered eating and heavy drinking. Early studies have found that college students who restrict the number of calories they consume prior to drinking are more likely to binge drink.[21] One study found that 16 percent of women surveyed "saved" calories for drinking by restricting normal caloric intake.[22] Motivations for drunkorexia include preventing weight gain, getting drunk faster, and saving money that would be spent on food to buy alcohol. Potential risks of drunkorexia include risk of black outs, forced sexual activity, unintended sexual activity, and alcohol poisoning.

Efforts to Reduce Student Drinking

What are colleges currently doing to address the problem of drinking on campus? Programs that have proven particularly effective use cognitive-behavioral skills training with *motivational interviewing,* a nonjudgmental approach to working with students to change behavior. One of these programs is Brief Alcohol Screening and Intervention for College Students (BASICS), which has been effective for heavy-drinking students with already existing or risk for problems related to alcohol. A recent study found that both male and female students significantly changed their behavior with regards to drinking after participating in the program.[23]

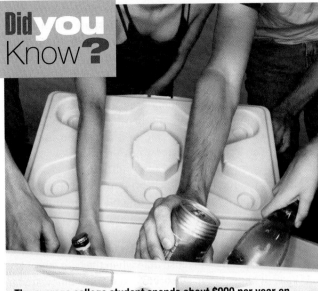

E-interventions—electronically based alcohol education interventions using text messages, e-mails, and podcasts—and Web interventions such as the Alcohol e-Check Up to Go (e-Chug) have shown promise in reducing alcohol-related problems among first-year students.

Web-based education for first-year students, particularly those who are incoming, has become an increasingly important intervention used by universities to reduce both hazardous drinking and alcohol-related problems. Because first-year students are at increased risk for alcohol-related problems, schools ensure that students are made aware of risks and effects of alcohol. Colleges and universities have been using a *social norms* approach to reducing alcohol consumption, sending a consistent message to students about actual drinking behavior on campus. Many students perceive that their peers drink more than they actually do, which may cause them to feel pressured to drink more themselves.

Alcohol in the Body

Learning about the metabolism and absorption of alcohol can help you understand how it affects each person differently and how it is possible to drink safely. It is also key in understanding how to avoid life-threatening circumstances such as alcohol poisoning.

The Chemistry and Potency of Alcohol

The intoxicating substance found in beer, wine, liquor, and liqueurs is **ethyl alcohol,** or **ethanol.** It is produced during a process called **fermentation,** in which yeast organisms break down plant sugars, yielding ethanol and carbon dioxide. Hard liquor is produced through further processing called **distillation,** during which alcohol vapors are condensed and mixed with water to make the final product.

The **proof** of an alcoholic drink is a measure of the percentage of alcohol in the beverage and therefore the strength of the drink. Alcohol percentage is half of the given proof. For example, 80 proof whiskey or scotch is 40 percent alcohol by volume, and 100 proof vodka is 50 percent alcohol by volume. Lower-proof drinks will produce fewer alcohol effects than the same amount of higher-proof drinks. Most wines are between 12 and 15 percent alcohol, and most beers are between 2 and 8 percent, depending on state laws and type of beer.

When discussing alcohol consumption, researchers usually talk in terms of "standard drinks." As defined by the National Institute on Alcohol Abuse and Alcoholism, a **standard drink** is any drink that contains about 14 grams of pure alcohol (about 0.6 fluid ounce or 1.2 tablespoons; see **Figure 8.3** on page 232). The actual size of a standard drink depends on the proof: A 12-oz can of beer and a 1.5-oz shot of vodka are both considered one standard drink because they contain the same amount of alcohol—about 0.6 fluid ounce. If you are estimating your blood alcohol concentration using standard drinks as a measure (see the following sections), you need to keep in mind the size of your drinks as well as their proof. For example, you may have bought only one beer while you were at the ballpark last weekend, but if that beer came in a 22-oz cup, then you actually consumed two standard drinks.

ethyl alcohol (ethanol) An addictive, intoxicating drug produced by fermentation and the main ingredient in alcoholic beverages.

fermentation The process whereby yeast organisms break down plant sugars to yield ethanol.

distillation The process whereby alcohol vapors are condensed and mixed with water to make hard alcohol.

proof A measure of the percentage of alcohol in a beverage. Proof is double the percentage of alcohol in the drink.

standard drink The amount of any beverage that contains about 14 grams of pure alcohol.

Absorption and Metabolism

Unlike the molecules found in most foods and drugs, alcohol molecules are sufficiently small and fat soluble to be absorbed throughout the entire gastrointestinal system. Approximately 20 percent of ingested alcohol diffuses through the stomach lining into the bloodstream, and nearly 80 percent passes through the lining of the upper third of the small intestine. A negligible amount of alcohol is absorbed through the lining of the mouth.

Standard drink equivalent (and % alcohol)		Approximate number of standard drinks in:
Beer = 12 oz (~5% alcohol)		12 oz = 1 16 oz = 1.3 22 oz = 2 40 oz = 3.3
Malt liquor = 8.5 oz (~7% alcohol)		12 oz = 1.5 16 oz = 2 22 oz = 2.5 40 oz = 4.5
Table wine = 5 oz (~12% alcohol)		750-mL (25-oz) bottle = 5
80 proof spirits (gin, vodka, etc.) = 1.5 oz (~40% alcohol)		mixed drink = 1 or more* pint (16 oz) = 11 fifth (25 oz) = 17 1.75 L (59 oz) = 39

FIGURE 8.3 **What Is a Standard Drink?**

*Note: It can be difficult to estimate the number of standard drinks in a single mixed drink made with hard liquor. Depending on factors such as the type of spirits and the recipe, a mixed drink can contain from one to three or more standard drinks. **Source:** Adapted from National Institute on Alcohol Abuse and Alcoholism, *Rethinking Drinking: Alcohol and Your Health,* NIH Publication no. 10-3770 (Bethesda, MD: National Institutes of Health, Revised 2010).

Several factors influence how quickly your body will absorb alcohol: the alcohol concentration in your drink, the amount of alcohol you consume, the amount of food in your stomach, pylorospasm (spasm of the pyloric valve in the digestive system), your metabolism, weight and body mass index, and your mood.

The higher the concentration of alcohol in your drink, the more rapidly it will be absorbed. As a rule, wine and beer are absorbed more slowly than distilled beverages. "Fizzy" alcoholic beverages—such as champagne and carbonated wines—are absorbed more rapidly than those containing no sparkling additives. Carbonated beverages and drinks served with mixers cause the pyloric valve—the opening from the stomach into the small intestine—to relax, thereby emptying the contents of the stomach more rapidly into the small intestine. Because the small intestine is the site of the greatest absorption of alcohol, carbonated beverages increase the rate of absorption.

The more alcohol you consume, the longer absorption takes. Alcohol can irritate the digestive system, which causes pylorospasm. When the pyloric valve is closed, nothing can move from the stomach to the upper third of the small intestine, which slows absorption. If the irritation continues, it can cause vomiting. Alcohol also takes longer to absorb if there is food in your stomach, because the surface area exposed to alcohol is smaller, and because a full stomach retards the emptying of alcoholic beverages into the small intestine. The **Student Health Today** box on the following page discusses the effects of mixing energy drinks with alcohol.

Mood is another factor in absorption, because emotions affect how long it takes for the contents of the stomach to empty into the intestine. Powerful moods like stress and tension are likely to cause the stomach to dump its contents into the small intestine, meaning alcohol is absorbed much more rapidly when people are tense than when they are relaxed.

Once it has been absorbed into the bloodstream, alcohol circulates throughout the body and is metabolized in the liver, where it is converted to *acetaldehyde*—a toxic chemical that can cause nausea and vomiting as well as long-term effects such as liver damage—by the enzyme *alcohol dehydrogenase*. It is then rapidly oxidized to *acetate,* converted to carbon dioxide and water, and eventually excreted from the body. A very small portion of alcohol is excreted unchanged by the kidneys, lungs, and skin.

Alcohol contains 7 calories (kcal) per gram (you will learn more about calories in **Chapter 9**). This means that the average regular beer contains about 150 calories. Mixed drinks may contain more if they are combined with sugary soda or fruit juice. The body uses the calories in alcohol in the same manner it uses those found in carbohydrates: for immediate energy or for storage as fat if not immediately needed.

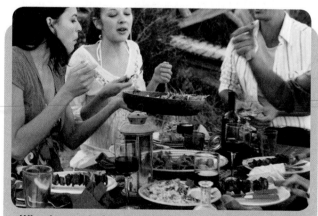

Why do people feel the effects of alcohol differently?

Many factors influence how rapidly a person's body absorbs alcohol, and thus how quickly that person feels the effects of the alcohol. For example, eating while drinking slows down the absorption of alcohol into your bloodstream. Other relevant factors include gender, body weight, body composition, and mood.

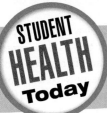
ALCOHOL AND ENERGY DRINKS: A DANGEROUS MIX

Thirty-four percent of 18- to 24-year-olds are regular energy drink consumers, and the alcohol industry has used the popularity of energy drinks to promote its own caffeinated alcoholic beverages (CABs)—premixed alcohol and energy drink products like Sparks, Rockstar 21, and Tilt. In addition, energy drink companies promote mixing energy drinks with alcohol products. Red Bull, for example, promotes a top drinks list suggesting "Jaegerbombs" and "Tucker Death mix."

Because students often mix energy drinks with alcohol for the sake of masking the taste or effects, these drinks can be particularly dangerous. One study found that students drinking alcohol with energy drinks consumed more than those who drank other types of alcoholic beverages (8.3 drinks vs. 6.1 drinks, respectively).

Students also report not noticing the signs of intoxication (dizziness, fatigue, headache, or lack of coordination) when they had consumed alcohol-mixed energy drinks. Caffeine may delay the onset of normal sleepiness, increasing the amount of time a person would normally stay awake and drink. The caffeine in energy drinks also reduces the subjective feeling of drunkenness without actually reducing alcohol-related impairment. Students who reported drinking alcohol-mixed energy drinks were more likely to be taken advantage of sexu-ally; they were also twice as likely to take advantage of someone sexually, ride with a drunk driver, be hurt or injured, or require medical treatment. They were more than twice as likely than non–energy drink drinkers to meet the criteria for alcohol dependency. Weekly or daily energy drink consumption is also strongly associated with alcohol dependency.

More than 20,000 emergency room visits related to highly caffeinated beverages were reported in the past year, according to researchers from the U.S. Substance Abuse and Mental Health Services Administration (SAMHSA). Approximately 42 percent of the cases involving energy drinks were in combination with alcohol or drugs, such as Ritalin or Adderall, and 18- to 25-year-olds were the most common age group seeking emergency treatment for energy drink emergencies.

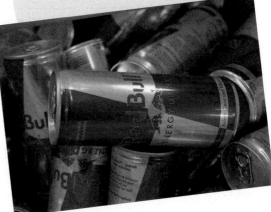

Mixing alcohol with energy drinks, such as Red Bull, can have serious consequences.

Sources: D. L. Thombs et al., "Event-level Analyses of Energy Drink Consumption and Alcohol Intoxication in Bar Patrons," *Addictive Behaviors* 35, no. 4 (2010): 325–330; S. Snipes et al., "High-Risk Cocktails and High Risk Sex: Examining the Relation between Alcohol Mixed with Energy Drink Consumption, Sexual Behavior, and Drug Use in College Students," *Addictive Behaviors* 38 (2013): 1418–1423 (in press); Join Together, "Combining Energy Drinks with Alcohol More Dangerous Than Drinking Alcohol Alone," The Partnership at Drug Free.org, www.drugfree.org; A.M. Arria et al., "Energy Drink Consumption and Increased Risk for Alcohol Dependence," *Alcoholism: Clinical and Experimental Research* 35, no. 2 (2011): 365–375; W. I. William et al., "Energy Drinks: Psychological Effects and Impact on Well-Being and Quality of Life: A Literature Review," *Innovations in Clinical Neuroscience* 9, no. 1 (2012): 25–34; Substance Abuse and Mental Health Services Administration, Center for Behavioral Health Statistics and Quality, *The DAWN Report: Update on Emergency Department Visits Involving Energy Drinks: A Continuing Public Health Concern.* (Rockville, MD: Substance Abuse and Mental Health Services Administration, January 10, 2013).

The breakdown of alcohol occurs at a fairly constant rate of 0.5 ounce per hour (approximately equivalent to one standard drink). This amount of alcohol is equivalent to 12 ounces of 5 percent beer, 5 ounces of 12 percent wine, or 1.5 ounces of 40 percent (80 proof) liquor. Unmetabolized alcohol circulates in the bloodstream until enough time passes for the body to break it down.

Blood Alcohol Concentration

Blood alcohol concentration (BAC) is the ratio of alcohol to total blood volume. It is the factor used to measure the physiological and behavioral effects of alcohol. Despite individual differences, alcohol produces some general behavioral effects, depending on BAC (see **Figure 8.4** on page 234). At a BAC of 0.02 percent, a person feels slightly relaxed and in a good mood. At 0.05, relaxation increases, there is some motor impairment, and a willingness to talk becomes apparent. At 0.08, the person feels euphoric, and there is further motor impairment. The legal limit for BAC is 0.08 percent in all states and the District of Columbia. At 0.10, the depressant effects of alcohol become apparent, drowsiness sets in, and motor skills are further impaired, followed by a loss of judgment. Thus, a driver may not be able to estimate distance or speed, and some drinkers may do things they would not do when sober. As BAC increases, the drinker suffers increasingly negative physiological and psychological effects.

A drinker's BAC depends on weight and body fat, the water

blood alcohol concentration (BAC) The ratio of alcohol to total blood volume; the factor used to measure the physiological and behavioral effects of alcohol.

Blood Alcohol Concentration (BAC)	Psychological and Physical Effects
Not Impaired	
<0.01%	Negligible
Sometimes Impaired	
0.01–0.04%	Slight muscle relaxation, mild euphoria, slight body warmth, increased sociability and talkativeness
Usually Impaired	
0.05–0.07%	Lowered alertness, impaired judgment, lowered inhibitions, exaggerated behavior, loss of small muscle control
Always Impaired	
0.08–0.14%	Slowed reaction time, poor muscle coordination, short-term memory loss, judgment impaired, inability to focus
0.15–0.24%	Blurred vision, lack of motor skills, sedation, slowed reactions, difficulty standing and walking, passing out
0.25–0.34%	Impaired consciousness, disorientation, loss of motor function, severely impaired or no reflexes, impaired circulation and respiration, uncontrolled urination, slurred speech, possible death
0.35% and up	Unconsciousness, coma, extremely slow heartbeat and respiration, unresponsiveness, probable death

FIGURE 8.4 **The Psychological and Physical Effects of Alcohol**

content in body tissues, the concentration of alcohol in the beverage consumed, the rate of consumption, and the volume of alcohol consumed. Heavier people have larger body surfaces through which to diffuse alcohol; therefore, they have lower concentrations of alcohol in their blood than do thin people after drinking the same amount. Because alcohol does not diffuse as rapidly into body fat as into water, alcohol concentration is higher in a person with more body fat. Because a woman is likely to have proportionately more body fat and less water in her body tissues than does a man of the same weight, she will be more intoxicated than a man after drinking the same amount of alcohol.

learned behavioral tolerance The ability of heavy drinkers to modify behavior so that they appear to be sober even when they have high BAC levels.

Body fat is not the only contributor to the differences in alcohol's effects on men and women. Compared with men, women have half as much *alcohol dehydrogenase,* the enzyme that breaks down alcohol in the stomach before it reaches the bloodstream and the brain. Therefore, if a man and a woman drink the same amount of alcohol, the woman's BAC will be approximately 30 percent higher than the man's, leaving her more vulnerable to slurred speech, careless driving, and other drinking-related impairments. Hormonal differences can also play a role: Certain points in the menstrual cycle and the use of oral contraceptives are likely to contribute to longer periods of intoxication. Figure 8.5 compares blood alcohol levels in men and women by weight and consumption.

Both breath analysis (breathalyzer tests) and urinalysis are used to determine whether an individual is legally intoxicated, but blood tests are more accurate measures of BAC. An increasing number of states are requiring blood tests for people suspected of driving under the influence of alcohol. In some states, refusal to take the breath or urine test results in immediate revocation of a person's driver's license.

People can develop physical and psychological tolerance to the effects of alcohol through regular use. The nervous system adapts over time, so greater amounts of alcohol are required to produce the same physiological and psychological effects. Though BAC may be quite high, the individual has learned to modify his or her behavior to appear sober. This ability is called **learned behavioral tolerance**.

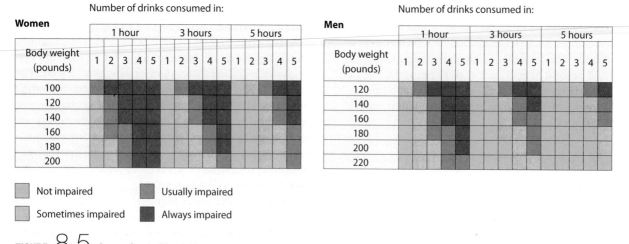

FIGURE 8.5 **Approximate Blood Alcohol Concentration (BAC) and the Physiological and Behavioral Effects**
Remember that there are many variables that can affect BAC, so this is only an estimate of what your BAC would be.

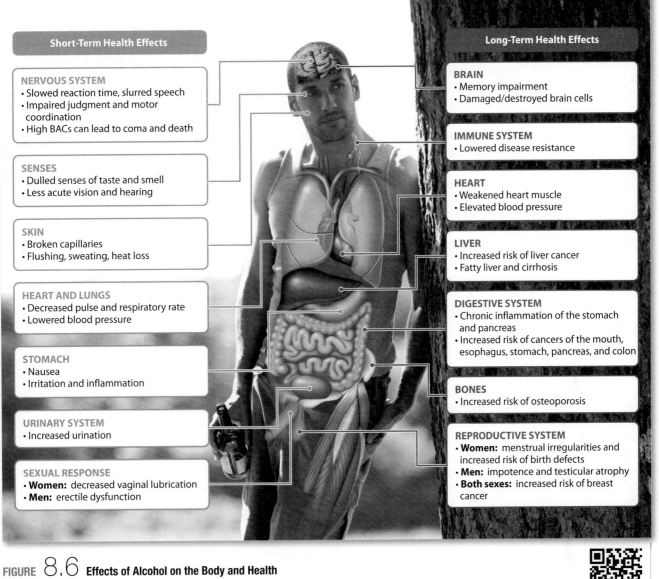

Short-Term Health Effects

NERVOUS SYSTEM
• Slowed reaction time, slurred speech
• Impaired judgment and motor coordination
• High BACs can lead to coma and death

SENSES
• Dulled senses of taste and smell
• Less acute vision and hearing

SKIN
• Broken capillaries
• Flushing, sweating, heat loss

HEART AND LUNGS
• Decreased pulse and respiratory rate
• Lowered blood pressure

STOMACH
• Nausea
• Irritation and inflammation

URINARY SYSTEM
• Increased urination

SEXUAL RESPONSE
• **Women:** decreased vaginal lubrication
• **Men:** erectile dysfunction

Long-Term Health Effects

BRAIN
• Memory impairment
• Damaged/destroyed brain cells

IMMUNE SYSTEM
• Lowered disease resistance

HEART
• Weakened heart muscle
• Elevated blood pressure

LIVER
• Increased risk of liver cancer
• Fatty liver and cirrhosis

DIGESTIVE SYSTEM
• Chronic inflammation of the stomach and pancreas
• Increased risk of cancers of the mouth, esophagus, stomach, pancreas, and colon

BONES
• Increased risk of osteoporosis

REPRODUCTIVE SYSTEM
• **Women:** menstrual irregularities and increased risk of birth defects
• **Men:** impotence and testicular atrophy
• **Both sexes:** increased risk of breast cancer

FIGURE 8.6 **Effects of Alcohol on the Body and Health**

Video Tutor: Long- and Short-Term Effects of Alcohol

Alcohol and Your Health

The immediate and long-term effects of alcohol consumption can vary greatly (Figure 8.6). Whether or not you experience any immediate or long-term consequences as a result of your alcohol use depends on you as an individual, the amount of alcohol you consume, and your circumstances.

Immediate and Short-Term Effects of Alcohol

The most dramatic effects produced by ethanol occur within the central nervous system (CNS). Alcohol depresses CNS functions, which decreases respiratory rate, pulse rate, and blood pressure.

As CNS depression deepens, vital functions become noticeably affected. In extreme cases, coma and death can result.

Alcohol is a diuretic that causes increased urinary output. Although this effect might be expected to lead to automatic **dehydration,** the body actually retains water, most of it in the muscles or in the cerebral tissues.

dehydration Loss of water from body tissues.

Because water is usually pulled out of the *cerebrospinal fluid* (fluid within the brain and spinal cord), drinkers may suffer symptoms that include "morning-after" headaches.

Alcohol irritates the gastrointestinal system and may cause indigestion and heartburn if consumed on an empty stomach. In addition, people who engage in brief drinking sprees during which they consume unusually high amounts of alcohol put themselves at risk for irregular heartbeat or

hangover The physiological reaction to excessive drinking, including headache, upset stomach, anxiety, depression, diarrhea, and thirst.

congeners Forms of alcohol that are metabolized more slowly than ethanol and produce toxic by-products.

alcohol poisoning (acute alcohol intoxication) A potentially lethal blood alcohol concentration that inhibits the brain's ability to control consciousness, respiration, and heart rate; usually occurs as a result of drinking a large amount of alcohol in a short period of time.

even total loss of heart rhythm, which can disrupt blood flow and damage the heart muscle.

Hangover

A **hangover** is often experienced the morning after a drinking spree. Its symptoms are familiar to most people who drink: headache, muscle aches, upset stomach, anxiety, depression, diarrhea, and thirst. Hangovers kick in for more than half of people after their blood alcohol content reaches 0.11. Approximately 20 to 25 percent of those who drink enough to get a hangover do not experience them.[24] Smoking while drinking may also worsen hangovers. The more people smoke on the day they drink alcohol heavily, the more likely they are to have a hangover, and heavy drinking paired with heavy smoking leads to more intense hangovers.[25] **Congeners,** forms of alcohol that are metabolized more slowly than ethanol and are more toxic, are thought to play a role in the development of a hangover. The body metabolizes the congeners after the ethanol is gone from the system, and their toxic by-products may contribute to the hangover. Alcohol also upsets the water balance in the body, which results in excess urination, dehydration, and thirst the next day. Increased production of hydrochloric acid can irritate the stomach lining and cause nausea. Recovery from a hangover usually takes 12 hours. Bed rest, solid food, and aspirin or ibuprofen may help relieve a hangover's discomforts, but the only sure way to avoid one is to abstain from excessive alcohol use in the first place.

Alcohol and Injuries

Alcohol use plays a significant role in the types of injuries people experience. Hospitalizations for alcohol overdoses among 18- to 24-year-olds rose by 25 percent over the last 10 years, and about 30 percent of young adults hospitalized for overdoses involve excessive alcohol consumption.[26] Alcohol use is involved in approximately 70 percent of fatal injuries during activities such as swimming and boating. A person with a BAC over 0.1 who operates a boat is 16 times more likely to be killed in an accident than a person who had not been drinking.[27] Alcohol is involved in 40 percent of fatal injuries due to house fires.[28]

Alcohol use is also a key risk factor for suicide—playing a role in approximately one third of suicides in the United States. Alcohol may increase suicide risk by increasing the intensity of depressive thoughts, lowering inhibitions to harm oneself, and interfering with the ability to assess future consequences of one's actions.[29]

Alcohol and Sexual Decision Making

Alcohol has a clear influence on one's ability to make good decisions about sex because it lowers inhibitions, and you may do things you might not do when sober. Students who are intoxicated are less likely to use safer sex practices and are more likely to engage in high-risk sexual activity. About 1 in 5 college students reports engaging in sexual activity, including having sex with someone they just met and having unprotected sex, after drinking.[30] The chance of acquiring a sexually transmitted infection or experiencing an unplanned pregnancy also increases as students drink more heavily.

Alcohol and Sexual Assault and Violence

In a recent survey, almost 20 percent of undergraduate women reported experiencing some type of sexual assault since entering college—with most incidents involving alcohol or unknowingly consuming a drug placed in their drinks.[31] Another study of college students showed heavy drinking to be associated with dating violence by men in their first year of college. Among women, heavy drinking in their sophomore year predicted dating violence in their junior year.[32] (For more on sexual assault, see **Chapter 4**.)

Alcohol and Weight Gain

The "freshman 15" and other college-year weight gain may have more to do with alcohol consumption than the food served in the dining halls. Alcohol has 7 calories per gram—nearly as much as fat (9 calories per gram) and more than carbohydrates or protein (4 calories per gram)—and the calories from alcohol provide few nutrients. A standard drink contains 12 to 15 grams of alcohol, meaning a single drink can add about 100 calories to your daily intake. By drinking an extra 150 calories a day more than you need, you can gain 1 pound a month and up to 12 pounds a year.[33]

Alcohol Poisoning

Alcohol poisoning (also known as **acute alcohol intoxication**) occurs much more frequently than people realize and can all too often be fatal. Alcohol, used either alone or in combination with other drugs, is responsible for more toxic overdose deaths than any other substance.

The amount of alcohol that causes a person to lose consciousness is dangerously close to the lethal dose. Death from alcohol poisoning can be caused by either central nervous system and respiratory depression or by the inhalation of vomit or fluid into the lungs. Alcohol depresses the nerves that control involuntary actions such as breathing and the gag reflex (which prevents choking). As BAC levels reach higher concentrations, eventually these functions can be completely suppressed. If a drinker becomes unconscious and vomits, there is a danger of asphyxiation through choking to death on one's own vomit.

Blood alcohol concentration can continue rising even after a drinker becomes unconscious, because alcohol in the stomach and intestine continues to empty into the bloodstream. Signs of alcohol poisoning include inability to be roused; a weak, rapid pulse; an unusual or irregular breathing pattern; and cool (possibly damp), pale, or bluish skin. If you are with someone who has been drinking heavily and who exhibits these symptoms, or if you are unsure about the person's condition, call your local emergency number (9-1-1 in most areas) for immediate assistance.

236 | PART THREE | AVOIDING RISKS FROM HARMFUL HABITS

Long-Term Effects of Alcohol

Alcohol is distributed throughout most of the body and may affect many organs and tissues. Problems associated with long-term, habitual use of alcohol include diseases of the nervous system, cardiovascular system, and liver, as well as some cancers.

Effects on the Nervous System
The nervous system is especially sensitive to alcohol. Even people who drink moderately experience shrinkage in brain size and weight and a loss of some degree of intellectual ability.

Research suggests that developing brains in adolescents are much more prone to brain damage than was previously thought. Alcohol appears to damage the frontal areas of the adolescent brain, which are crucial for controlling impulses and thinking through consequences of intended actions.[34] In addition, researchers suggest that people who begin drinking at an early age are at much higher risk of experiencing alcohol abuse or dependence, drinking five or more drinks per drinking occasion, and at least weekly driving under the influence of alcohol.[35]

Cardiovascular Effects
Alcohol affects the cardiovascular system in a number of ways. Numerous studies have associated light to moderate alcohol consumption (no more than two drinks a day) with a reduced risk of coronary artery disease.[36] Several mechanisms have been proposed to explain how this might happen. The strongest evidence points to an increase in high-density lipoprotein (HDL) cholesterol, which is known as "good" cholesterol. Studies have shown that moderate drinkers have higher levels of HDL.[37] Alcohol's effects on blood clotting, insulin sensitivity, and inflammation are also thought to play a role in protecting against heart disease.

However, alcohol consumption is not a preventive measure against heart disease—it causes many more cardiovascular health hazards than benefits. Drinking too much alcohol contributes to high blood pressure and higher calorie intake, both of which are risk factors for cardiovascular disease.[38]

Liver Disease
One result of heavy drinking is that the liver begins to store fat—a condition known as *fatty liver*. If there is insufficient time between drinking episodes, this fat cannot be transported to storage sites, and the fat-filled liver cells stop functioning. Continued drinking can cause a further stage of liver deterioration called *fibrosis*, in which the damaged area of the liver develops fibrous scar tissue. Cell function can be partially restored at this stage with proper nutrition and abstinence from alcohol. If the person continues to drink, however, **cirrhosis** results **(Figure 8.7)**. Among the top 10 causes of death in the United States, cirrhosis occurs as liver cells die and damage becomes permanent. **Alcoholic hepatitis** is another serious condition resulting from prolonged use of alcohol. A chronic inflammation of the liver develops, which may be fatal in itself or progress to cirrhosis.

cirrhosis The last stage of liver disease associated with chronic heavy use of alcohol, during which liver cells die and damage becomes permanent.

alcoholic hepatitis Condition resulting from prolonged use of alcohol, in which the liver is inflamed; can be fatal.

Cancer
Alcohol is considered a carcinogen. The repeated irritation caused by long-term use of alcohol has been linked to cancers of the esophagus, stomach, mouth, tongue, and liver. In one study, National Institute on Alcohol Abuse and Alcoholism scientists discovered a possible link between acetaldehyde and DNA damage that could help explain the connection between drinking and certain types of cancer.[39]

There is substantial evidence that women who consume even low levels of alcohol (three to six drinks per week) have a higher risk of breast cancer compared with those who abstain, and the risk is even higher for women who consume more than 2 drinks per day.[40] Girls and young women who drink alcohol also increase their risk of benign (noncancerous)

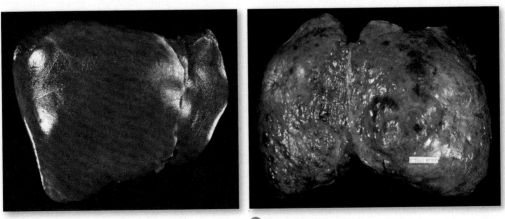

ⓐ A normal liver　　　　ⓑ A liver with cirrhosis

FIGURE 8.7 **Comparison of a Healthy Liver with a Cirrhotic Liver**
In cirrhosis, healthy liver cells are replaced with scar tissue that interferes with the liver's ability to perform its many vital functions.

breast disease, which in turn increases the risk for developing breast cancer. In a recent study, girls and young women who drank 6 or 7 days a week were 5.5 times more likely to have benign breast disease than those who didn't drink or who had less than one drink per week.[41]

Other Effects Alcohol abuse is a major cause of chronic inflammation of the pancreas, the organ that produces digestive enzymes and insulin. Chronic abuse of alcohol inhibits enzyme production, which further inhibits the absorption of nutrients. Drinking alcohol can block the absorption of calcium, a nutrient that strengthens bones. This should be of particular concern to women because of their risk for osteoporosis (see **Chapter 14**), as heavy consumption of alcohol worsens this condition. Evidence also suggests that alcohol impairs the body's ability to recognize and fight foreign bodies, such as bacteria and viruses.

Alcohol and Pregnancy

Teratogenic substances cause birth defects. Of the 30 known teratogens in the environment, alcohol is one of the most dangerous and common. If a woman ingests alcohol while pregnant, it will pass through the placenta and enter the growing fetus's bloodstream. A study found that more than 7.6 percent of children have been exposed to alcohol *in utero,* and 1.4 percent of pregnant women reported binge drinking.[42] It is well-known that consuming four or more drinks a day during pregnancy may significantly increase the risk of childhood mental health and learning problems. There is more research now that points to even moderate use (small glass of wine, half a pint of beer or shot of liquor) of alcohol once or twice a week during pregnancy can cut a baby's intelligence by several points.[43] The best advice to women who are pregnant is that any use may result in varying degrees of effects, ranging from mild learning disabilities to major physical, mental, and intellectual impairment. Alcohol consumed during the first trimester poses the greatest threat to organ development; exposure during the last trimester, when the brain is developing rapidly, is most likely to affect CNS development.

A disorder called **fetal alcohol syndrome (FAS)** is associated with alcohol consumption during pregnancy and is the most common, preventable cause of mental impairment in the Western world. FAS is the third most common birth defect and the second leading cause of mental

fetal alcohol syndrome (FAS) A disorder involving physical and mental impairment that may affect the fetus when the mother consumes alcohol during pregnancy.

Characteristic facial features of FAS include a small, upturned nose with a low bridge and a thin upper lip.

retardation in the United States, with an estimated incidence of 1 to 2 in every 1,000 live births.[44]

Among the symptoms of FAS are mental retardation, small head, tremors, and abnormalities of the face, limbs, heart, and brain. Children with FAS may experience problems such as poor memory and impaired learning, reduced attention span, impulsive behavior, and poor problem-solving abilities, among others.

Children who do not have all of the physical or behavioral symptoms of FAS may be diagnosed with disorders such as partial fetal alcohol syndrome or alcohol-related neurodevelopmental disorder; all of these disorders (including FAS) fall under the umbrella term *fetal alcohol spectrum disorders* (FASD). An estimated 40,000 infants in the United States are affected by FASD each year—more than those affected by spina bifida, Down syndrome, and muscular dystrophy combined.[45] Infants whose mothers habitually consumed more than 3 oz of alcohol (approximately six drinks) in a short time period when pregnant are at high risk for FASD. Risk levels for babies whose mothers consume smaller amounts are uncertain. To avoid any chance of harming her fetus, any woman of childbearing age who is or may become pregnant is advised to refrain from consuming any amount of alcohol.

Drinking and Driving

Traffic accidents are the leading cause of accidental death for all age groups from 1 to 44 years old.[46] Approximately 31 percent of all traffic fatalities in 2010 involved at least one alcohol-impaired driver (having a BAC of 0.08 percent or higher).[47] Unfortunately, college students are overrepresented in alcohol-related crashes. A recent survey reported that 15.1 percent of college students have driven after drinking alcohol and 1.7 percent of students said that, in the past 30 days, they had driven after drinking five or more drinks.[48]

In 2010, there were 10,228 alcohol-impaired driving fatalities in the United States—an average of one alcohol-related fatality approximately every 51 minutes.[49] Over the past 20 years, the percentage of intoxicated drivers involved in fatal

3 in 10

Americans will be involved in an alcohol-related accident at some time in their lives.

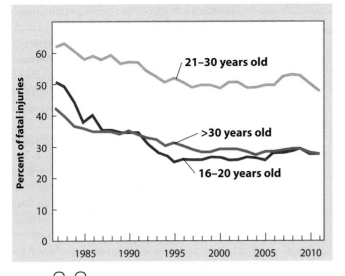

FIGURE 8.8 Percentage of Fatally Injured Drivers with BACs Greater Than 0.08%, by Driver Age, 1982–2011
Source: Insurance Institute for Highway Safety, "Fatality Facts 2011: Alcohol," Copyright © 2013. Reprinted by permission of Insurance Institute of Highway Safety.

crashes decreased for all age groups (Figure 8.8). Laws that raised the drinking age to 21, stricter law enforcement, laws prohibiting anyone under 21 from driving with any detectable BAC, increased automobile safety, and educational programs designed to discourage drinking and driving all likely contributed to the reduction in fatalities. Furthermore, all states have zero-tolerance laws for driving while intoxicated, and the penalty is usually suspension of the driver's license.[50]

Despite all these measures, the risk of being involved in an alcohol-related automobile crash remains substantial. Laboratory and test track research shows that the vast majority of drivers are impaired even at 0.08 BAC with regard to critical driving tasks. The likelihood of a driver being involved in a fatal crash rises significantly with a BAC of 0.05 percent and even more rapidly after 0.08 percent.[51]

Alcohol-related fatal crashes occur more often at night than during the day, and the hours between 9:00 P.M. and 6:00 A.M. are the most dangerous. Seventy-five percent of fatally injured drivers involved in nighttime single-vehicle crashes had detectable levels of alcohol in their blood.[52] The risk of being involved in an alcohol-related crash also varies with the day of the week. In 2010, 26 percent of all fatal crashes during the week were alcohol related, compared with 45 percent on weekends.[53]

Abuse and Dependence

Alcohol use becomes **alcohol abuse** when it interferes with work, school, or social and family relationships, or when it entails any violation of the law, including driving under the influence (DUI). **Alcoholism**, or **alcohol dependence**, results when personal and health problems related to alcohol use are severe, and stopping alcohol use results in withdrawal symptoms.

Identifying an Alcoholic

As with other drug addictions, craving, loss of control, tolerance, psychological dependence, and withdrawal symptoms must be present to qualify a drinker as an addict (see **Chapter 7**). Irresponsible and problem drinkers, such as people who get into fights or embarrass themselves or others when they drink, are not necessarily alcoholics. Alcoholics can be found at all socioeconomic levels and in all professions, ethnic groups, geographical locations, religions, and races. Data indicate that about 15 percent of people in the United States are problem drinkers, and about 5 to 10 percent of male drinkers and 3 to 5 percent of females would be diagnosed as alcohol dependent.[54]

Recognizing and admitting the existence of an alcohol problem is often extremely difficult. Alcoholics deny their problem, often making statements such as, "I can stop any time I want to. I just don't want to right now." The fear of being labeled a "problem drinker" often prevents people from seeking help. People who recognize alcoholic behaviors in themselves may wish to seek professional help to determine whether alcohol has become a controlling factor in their lives. (The **Skills for Behavior Change** box on the following page gives tips for cutting down on drinking.)

Among full-time college students, 1 in 4 experienced alcohol abuse or dependence in the past year.[55] In a recent study, the progression to alcohol dependency based on college students' drinking patterns when they entered showed that 1.9 percent of nondrinkers, 4.3 percent of light drinkers, 12.8 percent of moderate drinkers, and 19 percent of heavy drinkers developed alcohol dependency.[56]

> **alcohol abuse** Use of alcohol that interferes with work, school, or personal relationships or that entails violations of the law.
>
> **alcoholism (alcohol dependence)** Condition in which personal and health problems related to alcohol use are severe and stopping alcohol use results in withdrawal symptoms.

The Causes of Alcohol Abuse and Alcoholism

We know that alcoholism is a disease with biological and social/environmental components, but we do not know what role each component plays in the disease.

Biological and Family Factors Research into the hereditary and environmental causes of alcoholism has found higher rates of alcoholism among children of alcoholics than in the general population. The development of alcoholism among individuals with a family history of alcoholism is about four to eight times more common than it is among individuals with no such family history.[57]

Despite evidence of heredity's role in alcoholism, scientists do not yet understand the precise role of genes in increased risk for alcoholism, nor have they identified a specific "alcoholism" gene. Alcohol use disorders are between 50 percent and 60 percent heritable. Anxiety and depression, by comparison, are around 20 to 40 percent heritable, respectively.[58] Adoption studies have helped demonstrate a strong link between

Cut Down on Your Drinking

If you have a severe drinking problem, alcoholism in your family, or other medical problems, you should stop drinking completely. If you need to cut down on your drinking, these steps can help you:

❱ **If you suspect that you drink too much, talk with a counselor or a clinician at your student health center.** That person can advise you about what is right for you.

❱ **Write your reasons for cutting down or stopping.** You may want to improve your health, sleep better, or get along better with your family or friends.

❱ **Set a drinking limit.** Determine a limit for how much you will drink. If you aren't sure what goal is right for you, talk with your counselor. Once you determine your goal, write it down and put it where you can see it, such as on your refrigerator or bathroom mirror.

❱ **Keep a diary of your drinking.** Write down every time you have a drink. Try to keep your diary for 3 or 4 weeks. This will show you how much you drink and when.

❱ **Keep little or no alcohol at home.** You don't need the temptation.

❱ **Drink slowly.** When you drink, sip slowly. Take a break of 1 hour between drinks. Drink a nonalcoholic beverage after every alcoholic drink you consume.

❱ **Learn how to say no.** You do not have to drink when other people are or take a drink when offered one. Practice ways to say no politely. Stay away from people who give you a hard time about not drinking.

❱ **Stay active.** Use the time and money once spent on drinking to do something fun with your family or friends.

❱ **Get support.** Ask your family and friends for support to help you reach your goal. Talk to your counselor if you are having trouble cutting down.

❱ **Avoid temptations.** Watch out for people, places, or times that make you drink, even if you do not want to. Plan ahead of time what you will do to avoid drinking when you are tempted.

❱ **Remember, don't give up!** Most people don't give up drinking all at once. If you don't reach your goal the first time, try again. Get support from people who care about you and want to help.

Source: National Institutes of Health from National Institute on Alcohol Abuse and Alcoholism, "How to Cut Down on Your Drinking," NIH Pub no. 96-3770, 1996, www.niaaa.nih.gov

biological parents' substance use and their children's risk for addiction. Recently, scientists have found a gene that, by controlling the way that alcohol stimulates the brain to release dopamine, can trigger feelings of reward. Alcohol gives individuals with the gene a stronger sense of reward from alcohol, making it more likely for them to be heavy drinkers.[59] However, there is nothing deterministic about the genetic basis for addiction. Although no single gene causes addiction, multiple genes can affect the ability to develop addiction.

Social and Cultural Factors Some people begin drinking as a way to dull the pain of an acute loss or an emotional or social problem even if they are not genetically predisposed to alcoholism. Unfortunately, they become even sadder as the depressant effect of the drug begins to take its toll, sometimes causing them to antagonize friends and other social supports. Eventually, the drinker becomes physically dependent on the drug.

Family attitudes toward alcohol also seem to influence whether a person will develop a drinking problem. It has been clearly demonstrated that people who are raised in cultures where drinking is a part of religious or ceremonial activities or part of the family meal are less prone to alcohol dependence. In contrast, societies where alcohol purchase is carefully controlled and drinking is regarded as a rite of passage to adulthood appear to have greater tendency for abuse. The **Health in a Diverse World** box on the following page discusses some of the patterns of alcohol use and abuse around the world.

The amount of alcohol a person consumes seems to be directly related to the drinking habits of that individual's social group. A recent study found that those whose friends and relatives drank heavily were 50 percent more likely to drink heavily themselves.[60] Moreover, even having friends of friends who drank heavily appeared to influence individual alcohol consumption. The opposite is also true, that people who were friends with abstinent individuals or had family members who were abstinent were less likely to drink themselves. This finding has increased importance for individuals who are in treatment or have been in treatment and their need to sever ties with heavy drinkers to successfully maintain their abstinence.

Women and Alcoholism

Women tend to become alcoholics at later ages and after fewer years of heavy drinking than do men. With greater risks for cirrhosis, excessive memory loss and shrinkage of the brain, heart disease, and cancers of the mouth, throat, esophagus, liver, and colon than male alcoholics, women suffer the consequences of alcoholism more profoundly and become addicted faster with less alcohol use.[61]

Highest risks for alcoholism occur among women who are unmarried but living with a partner, are in their twenties or early thirties, or have a husband or partner who drinks heavily. Other risk factors for women

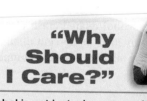

"Why Should I Care?"

Alcohol is not just a beverage—it's a drug that can interact with other drugs you may be using. When alcohol and prescription drugs are taken together, severe medical problems can result, including alcohol poisoning, unconsciousness, respiratory depression, and death.

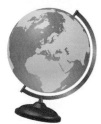
GLOBAL HEALTH AND ALCOHOL USE

Alcohol consumption comes with many serious social and developmental issues, including violence, child neglect and abuse, and absenteeism in the workplace. Throughout the world, alcohol is a factor in 60 types of diseases and injuries and a component cause in 200 others. Almost 4 percent of all deaths worldwide are attributed to alcohol, greater than deaths caused by HIV/AIDS, violence, or tuberculosis. Worldwide, the impact of alcohol use is as follows:

✳ The use of alcohol results in 2.5 million deaths each year.

✳ 320,000 people ages 15 to 29 die from alcohol-related causes annually—9 percent of all deaths for that age group.

✳ Alcohol is the world's third largest risk factor for disease burden.

✳ It is the leading risk factor for disease burden in the Western Pacific and the Americas and the second leading risk factor in Europe.

A large variation exists in adult per capita consumption. The highest consumption levels can be found in the developed world, mostly the Northern Hemisphere, but also in Argentina, Australia, and New Zealand. Medium

consumption levels can be found in southern Africa, with Namibia and South Africa having the highest levels, and in North and South America. Low consumption levels can be found in the countries of North Africa and sub-Saharan Africa, the Eastern Mediterranean region, and southern Asia and the Indian Ocean. These regions represent large populations of Muslims, who have high rates of abstention.

Source: World Health Organization, *Global Status Report on Alcohol and Health*, (Geneva: WHO Press, 2011) Available at www.who.int

---

include a family history of drinking problems, pressure to drink from a peer or spouse, depression, and stress.

Alcohol and Prescription Drug Abuse

When alcohol and prescription drugs are taken together, severe medical problems can result, including alcohol poisoning, unconsciousness, respiratory depression, and death. The greatest risks from drug mixing occur when alcohol is mixed with prescription painkillers. Both drugs slow breathing rates in unique ways and inhibit the coughing reflex; when combined, they can stop breathing altogether. Alcohol also interacts with antianxiety medications (e.g., Xanax), antipsychotics, antidepressants, sleep medications, and muscle relaxants, causing dizziness and drowsiness and making falls and unintentional injuries more likely. The prescription drugs that are most commonly combined with alcohol include opioids (e.g., Vicodin, OxyContin, Percocet), stimulants (e.g., Ritalin, Adderall, Concerta), sedative/anxiety medications (e.g., Ativan, Xanax), and sleeping medications (e.g., Ambien, Halcion).

Costs to Society

Alcohol-related costs to society are estimated to be well over $223.5 billion when health insurance, criminal justice costs, treatment costs, and lost productivity are considered.[62] Reportedly, alcoholism is directly or indirectly responsible for over 25 percent of the nation's medical expenses and lost earnings.[63] A recent study estimated that underage drinking alone costs society $61.9 billion annually.[64] The largest costs

were related to violence ($35 billion) and drunken driving accidents ($9.5 billion), followed by high-risk sex (nearly $5 billion), property crime ($3 billion), and addiction treatment programs (nearly $2.5 billion). By dividing the cost of underage drinking by the estimated number of underage drinkers, the study estimated that every underage drinker costs society an average of over $2,000 a year.[65]

Treating Alcoholism

Despite growing recognition of our national alcohol problem, only a very small percentage of alcoholics ever receive care in special treatment facilities. Numerous factors contribute to this low treatment utilization, including high costs or inability to pay for treatment, lack of insurance, inability or unwillingness to admit to an alcohol problem, the social stigma attached to alcoholism, potential loss of income, breakdowns in referral and delivery systems, and failure of the professional medical establishment to recognize and diagnose alcoholic symptoms among patients.[66] Student efforts to fit in by drinking can escalate into alcohol abuse behavior and put their health, well-being, and chances of academic success at risk. Of the nearly 12,000 college students admitted into treatment for substance abuse, approximately 47 percent report alcohol as their primary substance of abuse.[67]

Alcoholics who decide to quit drinking will experience *detoxification*, the process by which addicts end their dependence on a drug. Withdrawal symptoms include hyperexcitability, confusion and agitation, sleep disorders, convulsions and tremors of the hands, depression, headache, and seizures. For a small percentage of people, alcohol withdrawal results in a severe syndrome known as **delirium tremens (DTs)**, characterized by confusion, delusions, agitated behavior, and hallucinations.

Treatment Programs

The alcoholic who is ready for help has several avenues of treatment: psychologists and psychiatrists specializing in the treatment of alcoholism, private treatment centers, hospitals specifically designed to treat alcoholics, community mental health facilities, and support groups such as **Alcoholics Anonymous (AA)**.

Private Treatment Facilities Upon admission to a private treatment facility, the patient receives a complete physical exam to determine whether underlying medical problems will interfere with treatment. Shortly after detoxification, alcoholics begin their treatment for psychological addiction. Most treatment facilities keep their patients from 3 to 6 weeks. Treatment at private centers can cost several thousand dollars, but some insurance programs or employers will assume most of this expense.

Therapy Several types of therapy, including family therapy, individual therapy, and group therapy, are commonly used in alcoholism recovery programs. In family therapy, the person and family members examine the psychological reasons underlying the addiction and environmental factors enabling it. In individual and group therapy with fellow addicts, alcoholics learn positive coping skills for situations that have regularly caused them to turn to alcohol.

On some college campuses, the problems associated with alcohol abuse are so great that student health centers are opening their own treatment programs. For example, the University of Texas offers a support service called Complete Recovery 101, and at other schools students in recovery live together in special housing. Because it can be difficult to recover from an alcohol abuse problem in college, support programs such as these hope to offer the support and comfortable environment recovering students need.

Relapse

Success in recovery varies with the individual. Over half of all alcoholics relapse (resume drinking) within the first 3 months of treatment. Why is the relapse rate so high? Treating an addiction requires more than getting the addict to stop using a substance; it also requires getting the person to break a pattern of behavior that has dominated his or her life. Many alcoholics refer to themselves as "recovering" throughout their lifetime; they never use the word *cured.*

People who are seeking to regain a healthy lifestyle must not only confront their addiction, but must also guard against the tendency to relapse. Identifying situations in their lives that could trigger relapse—such as becoming angry or frustrated, or being around others drinking—are important for alcoholics. It can help to join a support group; maintain stability (resisting the urge to move, travel, assume a new job, or make other drastic life changes); set aside time each day for reflection; and assume responsibility for their own actions. To be effective, recovery programs must offer alcoholics ways to increase self-esteem and resume personal growth.

Tobacco Use in the United States

Tobacco use is the single most preventable cause of death in the United States: Nearly 443,000 Americans die each year of tobacco-related diseases.[68] Moreover, another 10 million people will suffer from health disorders caused by tobacco. To date, tobacco is known to cause about 20 diseases, and about half of all regular smokers die of smoking-related diseases.

While tobacco usage has steadily declined in the past decades, millions of people continue to light up. In 2011, about 43 million U.S. adults smoked cigarettes.[69] A particular bright spot in the fight against smoking is the declining prevalence of the habit among 18- to 24-year-olds. In 2005, young adults had the highest percentage of current smokers in the United States, but by 2011 they had the lowest percentage of any age group (from 24.4 percent to 18.9 percent, respectively).[70] Nonetheless, tobacco is a stubborn problem throughout the world due to its highly addictive nature and the environmental and social factors that make quitting difficult. Table 8.1 on the following page shows the percentages of Americans who smoke by demographic group.

Tobacco and Social Issues

U.S. and state governments have waged a long war on tobacco. But production and distribution of tobacco products involve many political and economic issues. Tobacco-growing states derive substantial income from tobacco production, and federal, state, and local governments benefit enormously from cigarette taxes.

Advertising The tobacco industry spends an estimated $36 million per day on advertising and promotional material.[71] With the number of smokers declining by about 1 million each year, the industry must actively recruit new smokers. Tobacco advertising also plays an important role in encouraging young people to begin a lifelong addiction to smoking before they are old enough to fully understand its long-term health risk.[72] Ninety percent of adults who smoke started by the age of 21, and half of them became regular smokers by their eighteenth birthday. Tobacco companies also target children and teens with tobacco products that

TABLE 8.1	Percentage of Population That Smokes (Age 18 and Older) among Select Groups in the United States	
		Percentage
United States overall		9.9
Race		
Asian		12.0
Black, non-Hispanic		19.4
Hispanic		12.9
Native American/AI		31.5
White, non-Hispanic		20.6
Age		
18–24		18.9
25–44		22.1
45–64		21.4
65+		7.9
Gender		
Male		21.6
Female		16.5
Education		
Undergraduate		9.3
Some college		22.3
High school		23.8
Income Level		
Below poverty level		29.0
At or above poverty level		17.9

Source: Adapted from Centers for Disease Control and Prevention, "Current Cigarette Smoking among Adults–United States 2011," *Morbidity and Mortality Weekly Report* 61, no. 44 (2012): 889–894.

are candy, fruit, or alcohol flavored, thus making them more palatable to young people.[73]

Advertisements in women's magazines imply that smoking is the key to financial success, thinness, independence, and social acceptance—and they have apparently been working. From the mid-1970s through the early 2000s, cigarette sales to women increased dramatically. Not coincidentally, by 1987 cigarette-induced lung cancer had surpassed breast cancer as the leading cancer killer among women and has remained the leading cancer killer in every year since.[74]

Women are not the only targets of gender-based cigarette advertisements. Men are depicted in locker rooms, charging over rugged terrain in off-road vehicles, or riding stallions into the sunset in blatant appeals to a need to feel and appear masculine. Minorities are also often targeted. Recent studies have shown a higher concentration of tobacco advertising in magazines aimed at African Americans, such as *Jet* and *Ebony*, than in similar magazines aimed at broader audiences, such as *Time* and *People*. Billboards and posters aiming the cigarette message at Latinos have dotted the landscape and store windows in Latino communities for many years, especially in low-income areas. Recent innovations by tobacco companies have included sponsorship of community-based events such as festivals and annual fairs.

Financial Costs to Society Estimates show that tobacco use causes more than $193 billion in annual health-related economic losses. The economic burden of tobacco use totals more than $96 billion in medical expenditures and $97 billion in indirect costs (absenteeism, added cost of fire insurance, training costs to replace employees who die prematurely, disability payments, etc.).[75] The economic costs of smoking are estimated to be about $3,100 per smoker per year.[76] These costs far exceed the tax revenues on the sale of tobacco products, even though the average cigarette tax in 2012 was $1.48 per pack and is rising in some states.[77]

College Students and Tobacco Use

Being placed in a new and often stressful social and academic environment makes college students especially vulnerable to outside influences. On top of targeted advertising, peer influence can prompt students to start smoking, and many colleges and universities still sell tobacco products in campus stores. College men and women have nearly identical rates of cigarette smoking, but men use more cigars and smokeless tobacco.[78] On the plus side, cigarette smoking among U.S. college students has decreased in recent years (see **Figure 8.9**).[79]

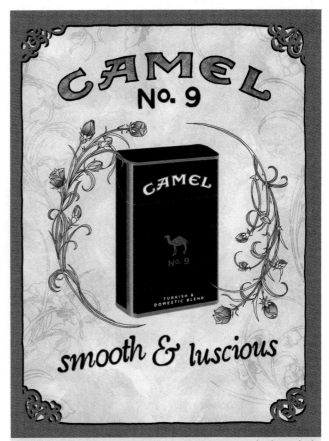

Cigarette companies market to women with glamorous packaging and ad campaigns borrowed from cosmetics, perfume (such as the famous Chanel scents evoked by this Camel No. 9 brand), and the fashion industry.

nicotine The primary stimulant chemical in tobacco products; nicotine is highly addictive.

See the **Points of View** box on the following page for a discussion of banning smoking on campuses.

Why Do College Students Smoke?
Some of the reasons students smoke are to relax or to reduce stress. Smokers are more likely to have higher levels of perceived stress than nonsmokers. Other key reasons students smoke are to fit in or because they are addicted.

For some students weight control is an important motivator, and fear of weight gain is a common reason for smoking relapse among those who quit. Students diagnosed or treated for depression are much more likely to use tobacco compared to students who are not.

Social Smoking
Many college smokers identify themselves as "social smokers"—those who smoke only when they are with people, rather than alone. Half of college smokers deny being smokers, even though they reported smoking in the past 30 days. Many of these students smoke in social situations where they also drink alcohol. Like regular smokers, social smokers engage in more alcohol use, illicit drug use, and higher sexual risk-taking behaviors than do nonsmokers.[80] Even occasional smoking is not without risks of damaging health effects. Social smoking in college can lead to a complete dependence on nicotine and all the associated health risks.

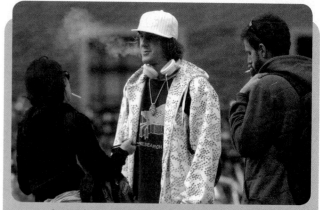

Is social smoking really that bad for me?

An occasional puff once in a while when you are out with friends can't hurt, right? Wrong! There is no "safe" amount of tobacco use—any smoking or exposure to smoke increases your risks for negative health effects such as heart disease and lung cancer. And even if you only smoke once or twice a week and consider yourself a social smoker, chances are you're on the road to dependence and a more frequent smoking habit.

nicotine, as well as 7,000 other chemical substances, including arsenic, formaldehyde, and ammonia, directly to the lungs. Among these chemicals are more than 69 known or suspected carcinogens.[81] The heat from tobacco smoke is also harmful. Inhaling hot toxic gases exposes sensitive mucous membranes to irritating chemicals that weaken the tissues and contribute to cancers of the mouth, larynx, and throat.

Tobacco and Its Effects

Smoking, the most common form of tobacco use, delivers a strong dose of

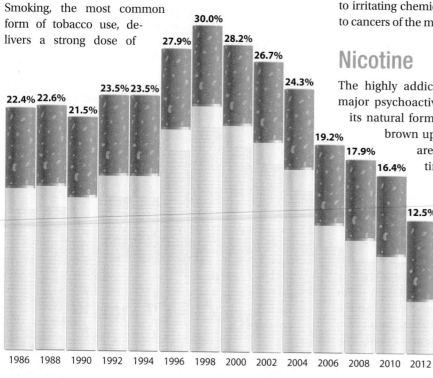

Nicotine

The highly addictive chemical stimulant **nicotine** is the major psychoactive substance in all tobacco products. In its natural form, nicotine is a colorless liquid that turns brown upon exposure to air. When tobacco leaves are burned in a cigarette, pipe, or cigar, nicotine is released and inhaled into the lungs. Sucking or chewing tobacco releases nicotine into the saliva, and the nicotine is then absorbed through the mucous membranes in the mouth.

Nicotine is a powerful central nervous system stimulant that produces a variety of physiological effects. In the cerebral cortex, it produces an aroused, alert mental state. Nicotine stimulates the adrenal glands, which increases the production of adrenaline. It also increases heart and respiratory rates, constricts blood vessels, and, in turn, increases blood pressure because the heart must work harder to pump blood through the narrowed vessels.

FIGURE 8.9 Trends in Prevalence of Cigarette Smoking in the Past Month among College Students

Source: Data from L. D. Johnston et al., "Monitoring the Future National Survey Results on Drug Use, 1975–2011, Volume II: College Students and Adults Ages 19–50" (Ann Arbor: Institute for Social Research, The University of Michigan, 2013).

Smoking on College & University Campuses:
SHOULD IT BE BANNED?

In recent years hundreds of campuses implemented all-out prohibitions or significant restrictions on tobacco use, with many more campuses pursuing becoming smoke-free. It is estimated that currently 17 percent of all U.S. campuses are tobacco or smoke-free, and the number is rapidly growing. The debate regarding tobacco-free campuses is contentious at many schools. Below are some of the major points for both sides of the question.

Arguments for Banning Tobacco on Campuses

○ The majority of college students—4 out of 5—do not smoke.

○ Two thirds of students and most employees prefer to attend classes held on a smoke-free campus.

○ One in five students say they have experienced some immediate health impact from exposure to environmental tobacco smoke.

○ Nonsmokers are 40 percent less likely to become smokers if they live in smoke-free dorms.

Arguments against Banning Tobacco on Campuses

○ There are so many other causes of potentially harmful fumes on campus—from diesel trucks, for example—that banning smoking wouldn't really affect the overall health and air quality on campus.

○ The policy would be difficult if not impossible to enforce.

○ Smokers forced outside to light up are possibly being put in danger at night or in other situations when they would have to leave residence halls.

○ Smoking bans in public and private places violate the rights of smokers and encourage discriminatory treatment of people addicted to nicotine.

Where Do You Stand?

○ Is smoking on a college campus a threat to public health?

○ Do you think that smokers have the right to smoke in dorms, in campus buildings, in adjacent parks, or in other public places on campus? Why or why not?

○ How do you feel when you are walking across campus and someone is smoking close to you? Do you feel as though you could or should ask smokers to put out their cigarettes?

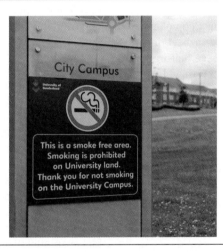

○ Would banning smoking be discriminatory? A violation of individual rights? Should student smokers be singled out for exclusion on college campuses?

Sources: University of Michigan, National Tobacco Free Campus Initiative, http://sph.umich.edu; American Smokers' Rights Foundation, U.S. Colleges and Universities with Smoke-free and Tobacco-Free Policies, January 2, 2013, U.S. Surgeon General's June 2012 webinar on tobacco-free college campuses.

what do you think?

Because nicotine is highly addictive, should it be regulated as a controlled substance?

● How could tobacco be regulated effectively?

● Should more resources be used for research into nicotine addiction? Why or why not?

Tar and Carbon Monoxide

Cigarette smoke is a complex mixture of chemicals and gases produced by the burning of tobacco and its additives. Particulate matter condenses in the lungs to form a thick, brownish sludge called **tar**, which contains various carcinogenic agents, such as benzopyrene, and chemical irritants, such as phenol. Phenol has the potential to combine with other chemicals that contribute to developing lung cancer.

In healthy lungs, millions of tiny hairlike projections (*cilia*) on the surfaces lining the upper respiratory passages sweep away foreign matter, which is expelled from the lungs by coughing. However, the cilia's cleansing function is impaired in smokers' lungs by nicotine, which paralyzes the cilia for up to 1 hour following a single cigarette. This allows tars and other solids in tobacco smoke to accumulate and irritate sensitive lung tissue.

Cigarette smoke also contains poisonous gases, the most dangerous of which is **carbon monoxide,** the deadly gas that comes out of

tar A thick, brownish sludge condensed from particulate matter in smoked tobacco.

carbon monoxide A gas found in tobacco smoke that reduces the ability of blood to carry oxygen.

exhaust pipes in cars. In the human body, carbon monoxide reduces the oxygen-carrying capacity of the red blood cells by binding with the receptor sites for oxygen; this causes oxygen deprivation in many body tissues. It is at least partly responsible for increased risk of heart attacks and strokes in smokers.

Tobacco Addiction

Smoking is a complicated behavior. Somewhere between 60 and 80 percent of people have tried a cigarette. Of those who try smoking, there is a 68 percent chance that sooner or later they will become nicotine dependent.[82] Why do some walk away from cigarettes while others get hooked?

Beginning smokers usually feel the effects of nicotine with their first puff. Smoking is a very efficient drug-delivery system, getting the drug to the brain in just a few seconds. These symptoms, called **nicotine poisoning,** include dizziness, light-headedness, rapid and erratic pulse, clammy skin, nausea, vomiting, and diarrhea. These unpleasant effects cease as tolerance to the chemical develops, which happens almost immediately in new users, perhaps after the second or third cigarette. In contrast, tolerance to most other drugs, such as alcohol, develops over a period of months or years. Regular smokers often no longer experience the "buzz" of smoking, but continue to smoke simply because stopping is too difficult

A pack-a-day smoker experiences 300 "hits," or **pairings,** a day. In pairing, an environmental cue triggers a craving for nicotine.[83] Simple pairings, such as drinking a cup of coffee, sitting in a car, finishing a meal, or sipping a beer, induce nicotine craving. The brain gets used to these pairings and cries out in displeasure when the association is missing.

Tobacco Products

Tobacco comes in several forms.

Cigarettes *Filtered cigarettes,* which are designed to reduce levels of gases such as hydrogen cyanide and carbon monoxide, may actually deliver more hazardous gases to the user than do nonfiltered brands. Some smokers use low-tar and low-nicotine products as an excuse to smoke more cigarettes. This practice is self-defeating because they wind up exposing themselves to more harmful substances than they would with regular-strength cigarettes.

Clove cigarettes contain about 40 percent ground cloves (a spice) and about 60 percent tobacco. Many users mistakenly believe that these products are made entirely of ground cloves and that smoking them eliminates the risks associated with tobacco. In fact, clove cigarettes contain higher levels of tar, nicotine, and carbon monoxide than do regular cigarettes—and the numbing effect of eugenol, the active ingredient in cloves, allows smokers to inhale the smoke more deeply. The same effect is true of *menthol cigarettes:* The throat-numbing effect of the menthol allows for deeper inhalation.

nicotine poisoning Symptoms often experienced by beginning smokers, including dizziness, diarrhea, light-headedness, rapid and erratic pulse, clammy skin, nausea, and vomiting.

pairing An environmental cue that triggers nicotine cravings.

bidis Hand-rolled flavored cigarettes.

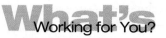

Maybe you've tried smoking and quit, or never started. Which of these nonsmoking strategies are you already incorporating into your life?

☐ When I'm stressed out, I go for a run, do yoga, or talk with a good friend about what's bothering me.

☐ I avoid people who smoke and places where people are smoking.

☐ My friends and I don't need to smoke to be cool or fit in; we're well aware of how toxic that habit is.

Cigars Many people believe that cigars are safer than cigarettes, when in fact nothing could be further from the truth. Cigar smoke contains 23 poisons and 43 carcinogens. Most cigars contain as much nicotine as several cigarettes, and when cigar smokers inhale, nicotine is absorbed as rapidly as it is with cigarettes. For those who don't inhale, nicotine is still absorbed through the mucous membranes in the mouth.

While cigar use has declined in recent years, the sale of little cigars has increased approximately 240 percent.[84] About the same size and shape as cigarettes, little cigars come in packs of 20, can be candy or fruit flavored, and cost much less than cigarettes. In a recent study, users of little cigars were more likely to be younger, male, black, and current cigarette, cigar, hookah, or marijuana smokers. Users also tended to have a lower perception of harm, greater sensation-seeking behaviors, and higher perceived levels of stress.[85]

Bidis Generally made in India or Southeast Asia, **bidis** are small, hand-rolled cigarettes that come in a variety of flavors, such as vanilla, chocolate, and cherry. They have become increasingly popular with college students, because they are viewed to be safer and cheaper than cigarettes. However, they are far more toxic than cigarettes. A study found that bidis produced three times more carbon monoxide and nicotine and five times more tar than cigarettes.[86] The leaf wrappers are nonporous, which means that smokers have to pull harder to inhale and inhale more to keep the bidi lit. During testing, it took an average of 28 puffs to smoke a bidi, compared to only 9 puffs for a regular cigarette. This results in much more exposure to higher amounts of tar, nicotine, and carbon monoxide.[87]

Pipes and Hookahs Pipes have had a long history of use throughout the world, including ritualistic and ceremonial use in many cultures. Hookahs—a type of water pipe with a long hose for inhaling—originated in the Middle East, but has become particularly popular among college-aged adults in the United States recently. While water pipes may cut down on the throat irritation users feel by cooling smoke before it is inhaled, it's important to realize two things: first, the main ingredient in hookahs remains tobacco; and second, a hookah does not filter out any harmful chemicals found in tobacco smoke. According to the National Cancer Institute and the American Cancer Society, pipe smoking carries risks similar to cigar smoking.[88]

Smokeless Tobacco There are two types of smokeless tobacco: chewing tobacco and snuff.

Chewing tobacco comes in three forms—loose leaf, plug, or in a pouch—and contains tobacco leaves treated with molasses and other flavorings. The user dips the tobacco by placing a small amount between the lower lip and teeth to stimulate the flow of saliva and release the nicotine. **Dipping** rapidly releases nicotine into the bloodstream. Use of chewing tobacco by teenagers, especially white males, has increased in recent years.[89]

Snuff is a finely ground form of tobacco that can be inhaled, chewed, or placed against the gums. It comes in dry or moist powdered form or sachets (tea bag–like pouches). In 2009, "snus" became the latest form of smokeless tobacco to hit the market in the United States. Popular for more than 100 years in Sweden, these small sachets of tobacco are placed inside the cheek and sucked. Some people prefer snus to chewing tobacco because it doesn't require the user to spit frequently.

Smokeless tobacco is just as addictive as cigarettes and actually contains more nicotine—holding an average-sized dip or chew in the mouth for 30 minutes delivers as much nicotine as smoking four cigarettes. A two-can-a-week snuff user gets as much nicotine as a ten-pack-a-week smoker.

Dental problems are common among users of smokeless tobacco. Contact with tobacco juice causes receding gums, tooth decay, bad breath, and discolored teeth. Damage to both the teeth and jawbone can contribute to early loss of teeth.

Health Hazards of Tobacco Products

Each day, cigarettes contribute to approximately 1,170 deaths from cancer, cardiovascular disease, and respiratory disorders.[90] In addition, tobacco use can negatively impact the health of almost every system in your body. **Figure 8.10** summarizes some of the physiological and health effects of smoking.

chewing tobacco A stringy type of tobacco that is placed in the mouth and then sucked or chewed.

dipping Placing a small amount of chewing tobacco between the lower lip and teeth for rapid nicotine absorption.

snuff A powdered form of tobacco that is sniffed and absorbed through the mucous membranes in the nose or placed inside the cheek and sucked.

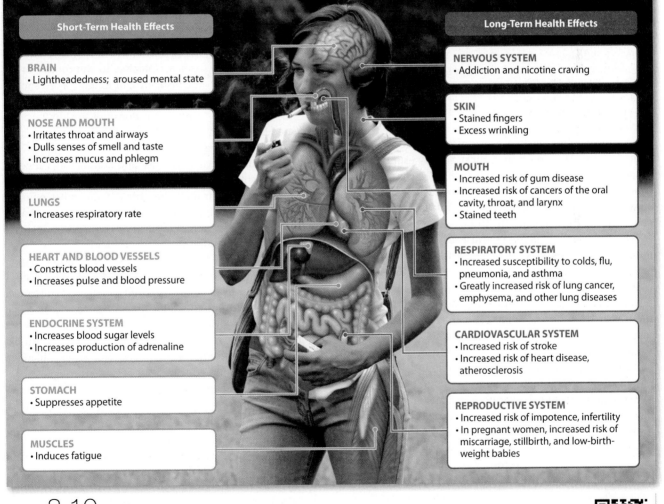

Short-Term Health Effects

BRAIN
• Lightheadedness; aroused mental state

NOSE AND MOUTH
• Irritates throat and airways
• Dulls senses of smell and taste
• Increases mucus and phlegm

LUNGS
• Increases respiratory rate

HEART AND BLOOD VESSELS
• Constricts blood vessels
• Increases pulse and blood pressure

ENDOCRINE SYSTEM
• Increases blood sugar levels
• Increases production of adrenaline

STOMACH
• Suppresses appetite

MUSCLES
• Induces fatigue

Long-Term Health Effects

NERVOUS SYSTEM
• Addiction and nicotine craving

SKIN
• Stained fingers
• Excess wrinkling

MOUTH
• Increased risk of gum disease
• Increased risk of cancers of the oral cavity, throat, and larynx
• Stained teeth

RESPIRATORY SYSTEM
• Increased susceptibility to colds, flu, pneumonia, and asthma
• Greatly increased risk of lung cancer, emphysema, and other lung diseases

CARDIOVASCULAR SYSTEM
• Increased risk of stroke
• Increased risk of heart disease, atherosclerosis

REPRODUCTIVE SYSTEM
• Increased risk of impotence, infertility
• In pregnant women, increased risk of miscarriage, stillbirth, and low-birth-weight babies

FIGURE 8.10 **Effects of Smoking on the Body and Health**

Video Tutor: Long- and Short-Term Effects of Tobacco

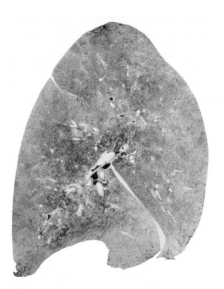

a A healthy lung

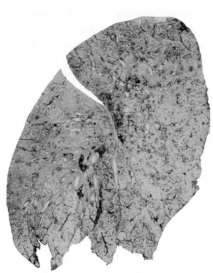

b A smoker's lung permeated with deposits of tar

FIGURE 8.11 **Lung Damage from Chemical in Tobacco Smoke**
Smoke particles irritate lung pathways, causing extra mucus production, and nicotine paralyzes the cilia that normally function to keep the lungs clear of excess mucus. The result is difficulty breathing, "smoker's cough," and chronic bronchitis. At the same time, tar collects within the alveoli (air sacs), ultimately causing their walls to break, leading to emphysema. Tar and other carcinogens in tobacco smoke also cause cellular mutations that lead to cancer.

Cancer

Lung cancer is the leading cause of cancer deaths in the United States. The American Cancer Society estimates that tobacco smoking causes 85 to 90 percent of all cases of lung cancer; fewer than 10 percent of cases occur among nonsmokers. There were an estimated 228,190 *new* cases of lung cancer in the United States in 2013 alone, and an estimated 159,480 Americans died from the disease in 2013.[91] Figure 8.11 illustrates how tobacco smoke damages the lungs.

Lung cancer can take 10 to 30 years to develop, and the outlook for its victims is poor. Most lung cancer is not diagnosed until it is fairly widespread in the body; at that point, the 5-year survival rate is only 16 percent. When a malignancy is diagnosed and recognized while still localized, the 5-year survival rate rises to 52 percent.[92]

If you are a smoker, your risk of developing lung cancer depends on several factors. First, the amount you smoke per day is important. Someone who smokes two packs a day is 15 to 25 times more likely to develop lung cancer than a nonsmoker. Also, smoking as little as one cigar per day can double the risk of several cancers, including that of the oral cavity (lip, tongue, mouth, and throat), esophagus, larynx, and lungs. A second factor is when you started smoking; if you started in your teens, you

leukoplakia A condition characterized by leathery white patches inside the mouth; produced by contact with irritants in tobacco juice.

have a greater chance of developing lung cancer than do people who start later. And a third risk factor is if you inhale deeply when you smoke. Smokers are also more susceptible to the cancer-causing effects of exposure to other irritants, such as asbestos and radon, than are nonsmokers.

A major health risk of chewing tobacco is **leukoplakia,** a condition characterized by leathery white patches inside the mouth that are produced by contact with irritants in tobacco juice. Three to 17 percent of diagnosed leukoplakia cases develop into oral cancer. There were over 41,000 cases of oral cancer diagnosed in 2013—the vast majority of which were caused by smokeless tobacco or cigarettes.[93] Users of smokeless tobacco are 50 times more likely to develop oral cancers than are nonusers.[94] Warning signs include lumps in the jaw or neck; color changes or lumps inside the lips; white, smooth, or scaly patches in the mouth or on the neck, lips, or tongue; a red spot or sore on the lips or gums or inside the mouth that does not heal in 2 weeks; repeated bleeding in the mouth; and difficulty or abnormality in speaking or swallowing.

The lag time between first use and contracting cancer is shorter for smokeless tobacco users than for smokers, because absorption through the gums is the most efficient route of nicotine administration. Many smokeless tobacco users eventually "graduate" to cigarettes and further increase their risk for developing additional problems.

Tobacco is linked to other cancers as well. The rate of pancreatic cancer is more than twice as high for smokers as nonsmokers. Typically, people diagnosed with pancreatic cancer live only about 3 months after their diagnosis. Cancers of the lip, tongue, salivary glands, and esophagus are five times more likely to occur among smokers than among nonsmokers. Smokers are also more likely to develop kidney, bladder, and larynx cancers. A growing body of evidence suggests that long-term use of smokeless tobacco also increases the risk of cancer of the larynx, esophagus, nasal cavity, pancreas, colon, kidney, and bladder.[95]

Cardiovascular Disease

Over a third of all tobacco-related deaths occur from heart disease.[96] Smokers have a 70 percent higher death rate from heart disease than nonsmokers do, and heavy smokers have a 200 percent higher death rate than moderate smokers do. In fact, smoking cigarettes poses as great a risk for developing heart disease as high blood pressure and high cholesterol levels do (see **Chapter 12**). Daily cigar smoking, especially for people who inhale, also increases the risk of heart disease (cigar smokers double their risk of heart attack and stroke).[97]

Smoking contributes to heart disease by adding the equivalent of 10 years of aging to the arteries.[98] One explanation for the mechanism behind this is that smoking and exposure to environmental tobacco smoke (ETS) encourage and accelerate the buildup of fatty deposits (plaque) in the heart and major blood vessels (*atherosclerosis*). Smokers can experience a 50 percent increase in plaque accumulation in the arteries, compared with ex-smokers, and a 20 percent increase in plaque buildup for nonsmokers regularly exposed to ETS. For unknown reasons, smoking decreases blood levels of HDLs, the "good cholesterol" that helps protect against heart attacks.

Smoking also contributes to **platelet adhesiveness**, the sticking together of red blood cells that is associated with blood clots. The oxygen deprivation associated with smoking decreases the oxygen supplied to the heart and can weaken tissues. Smoking also contributes to irregular heart rhythms, which can trigger a heart attack. Both carbon monoxide and nicotine in cigarette smoke can precipitate angina attacks (pain spasms in the chest when the heart muscle does not get the blood supply it needs).

A stroke occurs when a small blood vessel in the brain bursts or is blocked by a blood clot, denying oxygen and nourishment to vital portions of the brain, and smokers are twice as likely to suffer strokes as nonsmokers.[99] Depending on the area of the brain affected, stroke can result in paralysis, loss of mental functioning, or death. Smoking contributes to strokes by raising blood pressure, which increases the stress on vessel walls, and platelet adhesiveness contributes to blood clot formation.

Respiratory Disorders

Smoking quickly impairs the respiratory system. Smokers can feel its impact in a relatively short period of time—they are more prone to breathlessness, chronic cough, and excess phlegm production than are nonsmokers their age. Over time, cumulative lung damage can lead to chronic obstructive pulmonary disease (COPD), including chronic bronchitis and emphysema (see **Focus On: Reducing Risks and Coping with Chronic Diseases and Conditions**). Ultimately, smokers are up to 18 times more likely to die of lung disease than are nonsmokers.[100]

Chronic bronchitis may develop in smokers because their inflamed lungs produce more mucus, which they constantly try to expel along with foreign particles. This results in the persistent cough known as "smoker's hack." Smokers are also more prone than nonsmokers to respiratory ailments such as influenza, pneumonia, and colds.

Emphysema is a chronic disease in which the alveoli (the tiny air sacs in the lungs) are destroyed, impairing the lungs' ability to obtain oxygen and remove carbon dioxide. Where healthy people expend only about 5 percent of their energy in breathing, people with advanced emphysema expend nearly 80 percent. Because the heart has to work harder to do even the simplest tasks, it may become enlarged, and death from heart damage may result. There is no known cure for emphysema, and the damage is irreversible. Approximately 80 percent of all cases are related to cigarette smoking.[101]

Sexual Dysfunction and Fertility Problems

Despite attempts by tobacco advertisers to make smoking appear sexy, research shows it can actually cause impotence in men. Studies have found that male smokers are much more likely to experience erectile dysfunction than are nonsmokers.[102] Toxins in cigarette smoke damage blood vessels, reducing blood flow to the penis and leading to an inadequate erection. It is thought that impotence may indicate oncoming cardiovascular disease.

In women, smoking can lead to infertility and problems with pregnancy. Women who smoke increase their risk for infertility, ectopic pregnancy, miscarriage, and stillbirth. Smoking during pregnancy also increases risk of sudden infant death syndrome and the chances of the baby being born with a cleft lip or cleft palate.[103] Smoking while pregnant accounts for approximately 30 percent of premature births and increases the risk of low birth weight (less than 5.5 pounds), which in turn increases babies' likelihood of illness or death.[104]

Unique Risks for Women

Today, 16.5 percent of women—slightly more than 1 in 6—smoke, compared with 21.6 percent of men. Women who smoke now are just as likely to die of cancer and other smoking related diseases as men, and both active and passive smoking increase chances of breast cancer.[105] Accordingly, women have assumed a much larger burden of smoking-related diseases than they did in the past. Women are 26 times more likely to die from lung cancer than non-smoking women compared to 30 years ago.[106]

Higher rates of osteoporosis, depression, and thyroid-related diseases are just some of the risks that women who smoke take. Women who smoke (particularly those who also use oral contraceptives) are also at increased risk for blood clots, on top of heavier menstrual bleeding, longer duration of cramps, and less predictable length of menstrual cycle.

platelet adhesiveness Stickiness of red blood cells associated with blood clots.

emphysema A chronic lung disease in which the tiny air sacs in the lungs are destroyed, making breathing difficult.

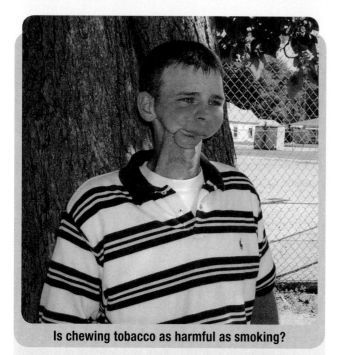

Is chewing tobacco as harmful as smoking?

No matter in what form you use it—cigar, pipe, bidi, dip, snuff, or cigarette—tobacco is hazardous to your health. Chewing tobacco and snuff actually contain more nicotine than cigarettes and just as many toxic and carcinogenic chemicals. This young cancer survivor began using smokeless tobacco at age 13; by age 17, he was diagnosed with squamous cell carcinoma. He has undergone surgery to remove neck muscles, lymph nodes, and his tongue, and he now educates others about the dangers of chewing tobacco.

Other Health Effects

Studies have shown tobacco use to be a serious risk factor in the development of gum disease.[107] In addition, smoking increases risk of macular degeneration, one of the most common causes of blindness in older adults. It also causes premature skin wrinkling, staining of the teeth, yellowing of the fingernails, and bad breath. Nicotine speeds up the process by which the body uses and eliminates drugs, making medications less effective. In addition, recent research suggests that smoking significantly increases the risk for Alzheimer's disease.[108]

environmental tobacco smoke (ETS) Smoke from tobacco products, including secondhand and mainstream smoke.

mainstream smoke Smoke that is drawn through tobacco while inhaling.

sidestream smoke The cigarette, pipe, or cigar smoke breathed by nonsmokers; commonly called *secondhand smoke.*

Environmental Tobacco Smoke

Even though fewer than 30 percent of Americans smoke, air pollution from smoking in public places continues to be a problem. **Environmental tobacco smoke (ETS)** is divided into two categories: mainstream and sidestream smoke. **Mainstream smoke** refers to smoke drawn through tobacco while inhaling; **sidestream smoke** (commonly called *secondhand smoke*) refers to smoke from the burning end of a cigarette or smoke exhaled by a smoker. People who breathe smoke from someone else's smoking product are said to be *involuntary* or *passive* smokers. Between 1988 and 2008, detectable levels of nicotine exposure in nonsmoking Americans has decreased from 87.9 percent to 40.1 percent.[109] The decrease in exposure to secondhand smoke is due to the growing number of laws that ban smoking in work and public places.

Children are more heavily exposed to ETS than adults. Over 53 percent of U.S. children aged 3 to 11 years—or 22 million children—are exposed.[110] Disparities in ETS also occur among ethnic and racial lines and among income levels. African Americans have been found to have higher levels of exposure to ETS than whites and Latinos. ETS exposure is also higher among low-income persons.[111]

Risks from Environmental Tobacco Smoke

Although involuntary smokers breathe less tobacco than active smokers do, they still face risks from exposure. According to the American Lung Association, secondhand smoke has about 2 times more tar and nicotine, 5 times more carbon monoxide, and 50 times more ammonia than mainstream smoke. Every year, ETS is estimated to be responsible for approximately 3,400 lung cancer deaths in nonsmoking adults, 46,000 coronary and heart disease deaths in nonsmoking adults who live with smokers, and higher risk of death in newborns from sudden infant death syndrome.[112]

The Environmental Protection Agency has designated secondhand smoke as a known carcinogen. There are more than 50 cancer-causing agents found in secondhand smoke.[113] There is also strong evidence that secondhand smoke interferes with normal functioning of the heart, blood, and vascular systems, significantly increasing the risk for heart disease and having immediate effects on the cardiovascular system. Studies indicate that nonsmokers exposed to secondhand smoke were 20 to 30 percent more likely to have coronary heart disease than those who were not.[114]

Tobacco Use and Prevention Policies

It has been more than 40 years since the government began warning that tobacco use is hazardous to the health of the nation. Despite all the education on the health hazards of tobacco use, health care spending and lost productivity associated with smoking still exceeds $193 billion each year.[115]

In the late 1990s, the tobacco industry reached a Master's Settlement Agreement with 40 states: This legal agreement requires tobacco companies to pay out approximately $206 billion over 25 years. The agreement also included a variety of measures to support antismoking education and advertising and to fund research to determine effective smoking cessation strategies.

Unfortunately, most of the money designated for tobacco control and prevention at the state level has not been used for this purpose. Facing budget woes, many states have drastically cut spending on antismoking programs. In the few states that have spent the settlement money on smoking cessation programs, there has been some reported success in decreasing cigarette use.[116] The Family Smoking Prevention and Tobacco Control Act signed into law in 2009 allows the U.S. Food and Drug Administration (FDA) to forbid advertising geared toward children, to lower the amount of nicotine in tobacco products, to ban sweetened cigarettes that appeal to young people, and to prohibit labels such as "light" and "low tar."[117] One of the most significant impacts of the law is that it requires more prominent health warnings on advertising of tobacco products. Smokeless tobacco ads now must contain a warning that fills 20 percent of the advertising space. Cigarette packages and advertising were required to have bigger, stronger warnings that must cover the top half of the front and back of each package and include "color graphics depicting the negative health consequences of smoking" (Figure 8.12). The FDA created graphics modeled after ads already used in Canada, Australia, and New Zealand, but lawsuits brought on by tobacco companies prevented their implementation in 2012.

Quitting

Smokers must break both the physical addiction to nicotine and the habit of lighting up at certain times of day. Approximately 70 percent of adult smokers in the United States want to quit smoking, and up to 44 percent make a serious attempt to quit each year. However, only somewhere between 4 and 7 percent succeed.[118] Quitting is often a lengthy process involving several unsuccessful attempts before success is finally achieved; even successful quitters suffer occasional slips. For those smokers unable to quit, they can expect to lose at least one decade of life compared to those who do not smoke. Cessation before the age of 40 years reduces the risk of death associated with continued smoking by about 90 percent.[119]

The person who wishes to quit smoking has several options. Most people who are successful quit "cold turkey"—that is, they decide simply not to smoke again. Others focus on gradual reduction in smoking levels, which can reduce risks over time. Still others resort to short-term programs, such as those offered by the American Cancer Society, which are based on behavior modification and a system

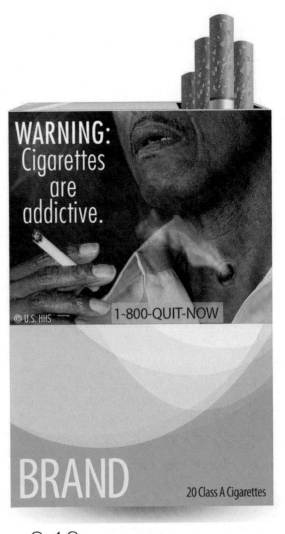

FIGURE 8.12 **Proposed New Cigarette Product Warning Labels**
The U.S. Food and Drug Administration proposed that graphic warning images, such as this one, be placed on all cigarette packages and advertisements. However, lawsuits prevented their implementation, and the FDA is now in the process of creating new warning labels.
Source: U.S. Food and Drug Administration, "Proposed Cigarette Product Warning Labels," Accessed May 23, 2011, www.fda.gov

of self-rewards. Treatment centers, community outreach plans sponsored by a local medical clinic, and telephone quit lines are helpful for some, whereas some people work privately with their physicians to reach their goal. Programs that combine several approaches have shown the most promise.

Breaking the Nicotine Addiction

Nicotine addiction may be one of the toughest addictions to overcome. Symptoms of **nicotine withdrawal** include irritability, restlessness, nausea, vomiting,

nicotine withdrawal Symptoms, including nausea, headaches, irritability, and intense tobacco cravings, suffered by nicotine-addicted individuals who cease using tobacco.

TABLE 8.2 Coping Strategies for Common Smoking Withdrawal Problems

Withdrawal Challenge	Estimated Length of Symptoms	Coping Strategies*
Anger, frustration, and irritability	Peaks in first week after quitting, but can last 2–4 weeks.	Avoid caffeine, which can amp up an already agitated mood. Get a massage; try deep breathing or exercise.
Anxiety	Builds over the first 3 days and may last up to 2 weeks.	Same strategies as above. Also remind yourself that the symptoms usually pass by themselves over time.
Mild depression	One month or less.	Be with supportive friends, increase physical activity, make a list of things that are upsetting you and write down possible solutions. If depression lasts longer than a month, seek medical advice.
Weight gain	Usually begins in the early weeks and continues through the first year after quitting.	Studies show nicotine replacement products such as gum and lozenges can help counter weight gain. You may also ask your doctor about the drug bupropion (brand names Wellbutrin or Zyban), which has also been shown to counter weight gain.

*Asking your doctor for nicotine replacement products or other medications is a valid coping strategy for any of the withdrawal challenges listed here.
Source: Adapted from National Cancer Institute, "Handling Withdrawal Symptoms When You Decide to Quit," National Cancer Institute Fact Sheet, 2010, www.cancer.gov

and intense cravings for tobacco (see Table 8.2). The evidence is strong that consistent pharmacological treatments can help a smoker quit: An estimated 25 to 33 percent of people who have used nicotine replacement therapy or smoking-cessation medications continue to abstain from cigarettes for over 6 months.[120] The **Skills for Behavior Change** box presents one of the American Cancer Society's approaches for quitting smoking.

Nicotine Replacement Products Nontobacco products that replace depleted levels of nicotine in the bloodstream have helped some people stop using tobacco. The two most common are nicotine chewing gum and the nicotine patch, both of which are available over the counter. The FDA has also approved a nicotine nasal spray, a nicotine inhaler, and nicotine lozenges. Another product called an e-cigarette is also available, although it comes with its own health concerns. See the **Tech & Health** box on the following page.

Nicotine gum delivers about as much nicotine as a cigarette does, but because it is absorbed through the mucous membrane of the mouth, it doesn't produce the same rush. Users experience no withdrawal symptoms and fewer cravings for nicotine as the dosage is reduced until they are completely weaned—users chew up to 20 pieces of gum a day for 1 to 3 months. Nicotine-containing lozenges are available in two strengths, and a 12-week program of use is recommended to allow users to taper off the drug.

The nicotine patch is generally used in conjunction with a comprehensive smoking-behavior cessation program. A small, thin patch placed on the smoker's upper body delivers a continuous flow of nicotine through the skin, helping to relieve cravings. Patches can be bought with or without a prescription and are available in different dosages. The FDA recommends using the patch for a total of 3 to 5 months.

During this time, the dose of nicotine is gradually reduced until the smoker is fully weaned from the drug. The patch costs less than a pack of cigarettes—about $4—and some insurance plans will pay for it.[121]

Tips for Quitting Smoking

If you're a smoker and you're ready to quit, try these tips to help kick the habit:

❭ Use the four Ds to fight the urge to smoke:
> ❭ Delay—put off smoking for 10 minutes; when the 10 minutes are up, put it off for another 10 minutes.
> ❭ Deep breathing.
> ❭ Drink water.
> ❭ Do something else.

❭ Keep "mouth toys" handy: hard candy, gum, toothpicks, and carrot sticks can help.

❭ If you've had trouble stopping before, ask your doctor about nicotine chewing gum, patches, nasal sprays, inhalers, or lozenges.

❭ Make an appointment with your dental hygienist to have your teeth cleaned.

❭ Examine those associations that trigger your urge to smoke.

❭ Tell your family and friends that you've stopped smoking so they won't offer you a cigarette.

❭ Aim to spend your time in places that don't allow smoking.

❭ Take up a new sport, exercise program, hobby, or organizational commitment. This will help shake up your routine and distract you from smoking.

E-CIGARETTES: HEALTH RISKS AND CONCERNS

Electronic cigarettes, also called e-cigarettes, are increasingly popular worldwide. They consist of a battery, atomizer, and a cartridge containing nicotine and other chemicals. The cartridge vaporizes the nicotine and allows users to inhale it. Because there is no smoke, some feel e-cigarettes must be safe compared to regular cigarettes. They are often marketed as antismoking devices. Unfortunately, e-cigarettes still have a host of worries associated with them.

While the lack of smoke may reduce some risks, nicotine—the main component of cigarettes that causes cardiovascular damage—makes e-cigarettes far from healthy. The U.S. Food and Drug Administration (FDA) analyzed samples of two popular

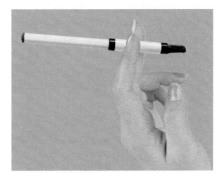

Electronic cigarette, or e-cigarette.

brands and found variable amounts of nicotine and traces of known carcinogens. Almost always manufactured in China, the devices are built without real safety or quality controls. Defective parts and leaky cartridges are par for

the course. There is also no safe way to dispose of e-cigarette products and accessories, potentially resulting in nicotine exposure to children, other adults, or pets, as well as contamination of water or soil. Currently, e-cigarettes do not contain any health warnings, and health professionals continue to urge for more action to regulate these products.

Sources: University of California, Riverside, "Electronic Cigarettes Are Unsafe and Pose Health Risks, UC Riverside Study Finds," 2010, http://newsroom.ucr.edu; U.S. Food and Drug Administration, "FDA and Public Health Experts Warn about Electronic Cigarettes," 2010, www .fda.gov; L. Dale, Mayo Clinic, "Electronic Cigarettes: A Safe Way to Light Up?" 2011, www.mayoclinic.com; E. Sohn, Discovery News, "How Safe Are E-Cigarettes?" 2011, http://news .discovery.com; A. Norton, "Are E-Cigarettes Bad for Health?" 2012, www.huffingtonpost.com

---

The nasal spray, which requires a prescription, is much more powerful and delivers nicotine to the bloodstream faster than gum or the patch. Patients are warned to be careful not to overdose; as little as 40 mg nicotine taken at once could be lethal. The FDA has advised that it should be used for no more than 3 months and never for more than 6 months, so that smokers don't find themselves as dependent on nicotine in spray form as they were on cigarettes. The FDA also advises that no one who experiences nasal or sinus problems, allergies, or asthma should use it.

The nicotine inhaler, which also requires a prescription, consists of a mouthpiece and cartridge. By puffing on the mouthpiece, the smoker inhales air saturated with nicotine, which is absorbed through the lining of the mouth, not the lungs. This nicotine enters the body much more slowly than the nicotine in cigarettes does. Using the inhaler mimics the hand-to-mouth actions used in smoking and causes the back of the throat to feel as it would when inhaling tobacco smoke.

"Why Should I Care?"

If the life-threatening health consequences aren't enough to make you give up smoking, consider the negative impact smoking can have on your social (and romantic!) life. Popular media may make smoking seem glamorous and sexy, but in reality, smoking makes your breath, hair, and clothing smell bad; it causes your skin to age prematurely; it yellows your teeth; and it can interfere with a man's ability to achieve and maintain an erection.

Smoking Cessation Medications Bupropion (brand names Zyban and Wellbutrin), an antidepressant, is FDA approved as a smoking-cessation aid. Varinicline (brand name Chantix) reduces nicotine cravings and the urge to smoke, and blocks the effects of nicotine at nicotine receptor sites in the brain. Both these drugs may sometimes cause changes in behavior such as agitation, depression, hostility, and suicidal thoughts. If someone experiences these things while on a smoking cessation drug, they should stop taking it and contact their health care professional.[122]

Benefits of Quitting

Many tissues damaged by smoking can repair themselves. As soon as a smoker stops, the body begins the repair process (Figure 8.13). Within 8 hours, carbon monoxide and oxygen levels return to normal, and "smoker's breath" disappears. Circulation and the senses of taste and smell improve within weeks. Often, within a month of quitting, the mucus that clogs airways is broken up and eliminated. The risk of dying from a heart attack falls by half after only 1 year without smoking and declines steadily thereafter. At the end of 10 smoke-free years, the ex-smoker can expect to live out his or her normal life span, and after about 15 years without smoking, the ex-smoker's risk of coronary heart disease is similar to that of people who have never smoked.[123]

A recent study suggested women who quit smoking before age 40 may avoid more than 90 percent of the added risk of dying early. Women who quit before 30 could avoid 97 percent of that risk.[124] Women who quit are also less likely to bear babies with low birth weight.

Another significant benefit of quitting smoking is the money saved. A pack of cigarettes averages $6.00, including taxes.[125] Using this number, a pack-a-day smoker burns through about $42.00 per week, or $2,184.00 per year. That is money that could otherwise have gone toward a car payment or a much-earned vacation over spring break.

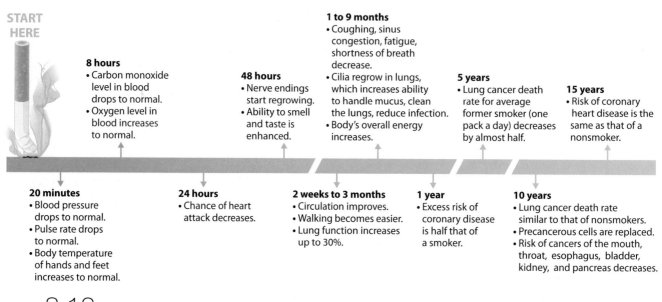

START HERE

8 hours
- Carbon monoxide level in blood drops to normal.
- Oxygen level in blood increases to normal.

48 hours
- Nerve endings start regrowing.
- Ability to smell and taste is enhanced.

1 to 9 months
- Coughing, sinus congestion, fatigue, shortness of breath decrease.
- Cilia regrow in lungs, which increases ability to handle mucus, clean the lungs, reduce infection.
- Body's overall energy increases.

5 years
- Lung cancer death rate for average former smoker (one pack a day) decreases by almost half.

15 years
- Risk of coronary heart disease is the same as that of a nonsmoker.

20 minutes
- Blood pressure drops to normal.
- Pulse rate drops to normal.
- Body temperature of hands and feet increases to normal.

24 hours
- Chance of heart attack decreases.

2 weeks to 3 months
- Circulation improves.
- Walking becomes easier.
- Lung function increases up to 30%.

1 year
- Excess risk of coronary disease is half that of a smoker.

10 years
- Lung cancer death rate similar to that of nonsmokers.
- Precancerous cells are replaced.
- Risk of cancers of the mouth, throat, esophagus, bladder, kidney, and pancreas decreases.

FIGURE 8.13 When Smokers Quit

Within 20 minutes of smoking that last cigarette, the body begins a series of changes that continues for years. However, by smoking just one cigarette a day, the smoker loses all these benefits, according to the American Cancer Society.

Alcohol and Tobacco: Are Your Habits Placing You at Risk?

1 Why Do You Smoke?

Identifying why you smoke can help you develop a plan to quit. Answer the following questions and evaluate your reasons for smoking.

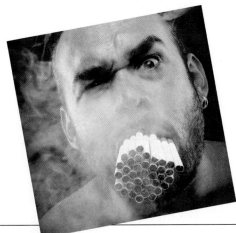

1. I smoke to keep from slowing down.
   ☐ Often   ☐ Sometimes   ☐ Never

2. I feel more comfortable with a cigarette in my hand.
   ☐ Often   ☐ Sometimes   ☐ Never

3. Smoking is pleasant and enjoyable.
   ☐ Often   ☐ Sometimes   ☐ Never

4. I light up a cigarette when something makes me angry.
   ☐ Often   ☐ Sometimes   ☐ Never

5. When I run out of cigarettes, it's almost unbearable until I get more.
   ☐ Often   ☐ Sometimes   ☐ Never

6. I smoke cigarettes automatically without even being aware of it.
   ☐ Often   ☐ Sometimes   ☐ Never

7. I reach for a cigarette when I need a lift.
   ☐ Often   ☐ Sometimes   ☐ Never

8. Smoking relaxes me in a stressful situation.
   ☐ Often   ☐ Sometimes   ☐ Never

Interpreting Part 1

Use your answers to identify some of the key reasons why you smoke, then use the tips presented in this chapter to develop a plan for quitting.

Source: Abridged and adapted from National Institutes of Health, *Why Do You Smoke?* NIH Pub. No. 93-1822. (Washington, DC: U.S. Department of Health and Human Services, 1990).

YOUR PLAN FOR CHANGE

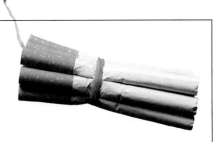

This **Assess** yourself activity gave you the chance to evaluate your current smoking habits. Regardless of your current level of nicotine addiction, if you smoke at all, now is the time to take steps toward kicking the habit.

Today, you can:

◯ Develop a plan to kick the tobacco habit. The first step in quitting smoking is to identify why you want to quit. Write your reasons down and carry a copy of it with you. Every time you are tempted to smoke, go over your reasons for stopping.

◯ Think about the times and places you usually smoke. What could you do instead of smoking at those times? Make a list of positive tobacco alternatives.

Within the next 2 weeks, you can:

◯ Pick a day to stop smoking, fill out the Behavior Change Contract (available in the front of this text and online), and have a family member or friend sign it.

◯ Throw away all your cigarettes, lighters, and ashtrays.

By the end of the semester, you can:

◯ Focus on the positives. Now that you have stopped smoking, your mind and your body will begin to feel better. Make a list of the good things about not smoking. Carry a copy with you, and look at it whenever you have the urge to smoke.

◯ Reward yourself for stopping. Go to a movie, go out to dinner, or buy yourself a gift.

2 What's Your Risk of Alcohol Abuse?

Many college students engage in potentially dangerous drinking behaviors. Do you have a problem with alcohol use? Take the following quiz to see.

1. **How often do you have a drink containing alcohol?**
   - ⓪ Never
   - ① Monthly or less
   - ② 2 to 4 times a month
   - ③ 2 to 3 times a week
   - ④ 4 or more times a week

2. **How many alcoholic drinks do you have on a typical day when you are drinking?**
   - ⓪ 1 or 2
   - ① 3 or 4
   - ② 5 or 6
   - ③ 7 to 9
   - ④ 10 or more

3. **How often do you have six drinks or more on one occasion?**
   - ⓪ Never
   - ① Less than monthly
   - ② Monthly
   - ③ Weekly
   - ④ Daily or almost daily

4. **How often during the past year have you been unable to stop drinking once you had started?**
   - ⓪ Never
   - ① Less than monthly
   - ② Monthly
   - ③ Weekly
   - ④ Daily or almost daily

5. **How often during the past year have you failed to do what was normally expected from you because of drinking?**
   - ⓪ Never
   - ① Less than monthly
   - ② Monthly
   - ③ Weekly
   - ④ Daily or almost daily

6. **How often during the past year have you needed a first drink in the morning to get yourself going after a heavy drinking session?**
   - ⓪ Never
   - ① Less than monthly
   - ② Monthly
   - ③ Weekly
   - ④ Daily or almost daily

7. **How often during the past year have you had a feeling of guilt or remorse after drinking?**
   - ⓪ Never
   - ① Less than monthly
   - ② Monthly
   - ③ Weekly
   - ④ Daily or almost daily

8. **How often during the past year have you been unable to remember what happened the night before because you had been drinking?**
   - ⓪ Never
   - ① Less than monthly
   - ② Monthly
   - ③ Weekly
   - ④ Daily or almost daily

9. **Have you or someone else been injured as a result of your drinking?**
   - ⓪ No
   - ① Yes, but not in the past year
   - ② Yes, during the past year

10. **Has a relative, friend, or a doctor or other health care professional been concerned about your drinking or suggested you cut down?**
    - ⓪ No
    - ① Yes, but not in the past year
    - ② Yes, during the past year

Interpreting Part 2

Scores below 6: Congratulations! You are in control of your drinking behaviors and do a good job of consuming alcohol responsibly and in moderation.

Scores between 6 and 8: Your alcohol consumption is possibly risky. Try taking steps to change your drinking behavior and make some positive changes for your health and safety.

Scores above 8: Your drinking patterns are putting you at high risk for illness, unsafe sexual situations, or alcohol-related injuries, and may even affect your academic performance.

Source: T. Babor et al., "The Alcohol Use Disorders Identification Test: Interview Version," *Audit: The Alcohol Use Disorders Identification Test,* 2nd Edition. Copyright © 2001 World Health Organization. Reprinted with permission.

YOUR PLAN FOR CHANGE

This **Assessyourself** activity gave you the chance to evaluate your alcohol consumption. If some of your answers surprised you or if you were unsure how to answer some of the questions, consider taking steps to change your behavior.

Today, you can:

◯ Start a diary of your drinking habits. Keeping track of how much you drink—as well as how much money you spend on drinks and how you feel when you are drinking—will make you more aware of your true drinking habits.

◯ Spend some time thinking about the ways your family members use alcohol. Is there a family history of alcohol abuse or addiction? Did your family's alcohol consumption have any effect on you while you were growing up? Consider whether your current alcohol use is healthy, or whether it is likely to create problems for you in the future.

Within the next 2 weeks, you can:

◯ Make your first drink a glass of water or another nonalcoholic beverage the next time you go to a party. Intersperse alcoholic drinks with nonalcoholic beverages to help you pace your consumption.

◯ Challenge yourself and a few close friends to get together at least once a week for a nonalcoholic social occasion, such as a sports event or movie night.

By the end of the semester, you can:

◯ Commit yourself to limiting your alcohol intake at every social function you attend. Decide ahead of time whether you want to drink and, if so, what your limit will be; then stick to it.

◯ Cultivate friendships and explore activities that do not center on alcohol. If your current group of friends drinks heavily, and it is becoming a problem for you, you may need to step back from the group for a while.

MasteringHealth™

Build your knowledge—and health!—in the Study Area of MasteringHealth with a variety of study tools.

Summary

* Alcohol is a chemical substance that affects your physical and mental behavior. It is regularly used by about 50 percent of all Americans, while 25 percent completely abstain. Over 44 percent of all college students are binge drinkers.

* Negative consequences associated with alcohol use among college students are academic problems, sleep disruptions, doing something they regretted later, forgetting where they were or what they did, unprotected or nonconsensual sex, physical injury to self or others, trouble with the police, automobile accidents, and increased risk of suicide.

* Alcohol's effect is measured by the blood alcohol concentration (BAC), the ratio of alcohol to total blood volume. The higher the BAC, the greater drowsiness and impaired judgment and coordination will be.

* Alcohol is a central nervous system (CNS) depressant. Long-term alcohol overuse can cause damage to the nervous system, cardiovascular damage, liver disease, increased risk for cancer, damage to the pancreas, and increased risk of osteoporosis. Drinking during pregnancy can cause fetal alcohol syndrome (FAS) and fetal alcohol spectrum disorders (FASDs).

* Alcohol use becomes alcoholism when it interferes with school, work, or social and family relationships, or entails violations of the law. Causes of alcoholism include biological, family, social, and cultural factors.

* Most alcoholics do not admit to a problem until reaching a major life crisis or having their families intervene. Treatment options include treatment facilities, therapy, and self-help programs. Most alcoholics relapse because alcoholism is a behavioral addiction as well as a chemical addiction.

* Tobacco use involves many social and political issues, including advertising targeted at youth and women, the fastest growing populations of smokers. Health care and lost productivity resulting from smoking costs the nation as much as $193 billion per year.

* Smoking delivers over 7,000 chemicals to the lungs of smokers. Tobacco is available in smoking and smokeless forms. Both contain nicotine, an addictive psychoactive substance.

* Health hazards of smoking include markedly higher rates of cancer, heart and circulatory disorders, respiratory diseases, sexual dysfunction, fertility problems, and gum diseases. Smoking during pregnancy increases risk of miscarriage and low birth weight. Smokeless tobacco increases risks for oral cancer and other oral problems. Environmental tobacco smoke puts nonsmokers at risk for cancer and heart disease.

* To quit, smokers must kick a chemical addiction and a behavioral habit. Nicotine-replacement products or drugs such as Zyban and Chantix can help wean smokers off nicotine. Therapy methods can also help.

Pop Quiz

1. Which of the following is false?
   a. College students drink in an effort to deal with stress and boredom.
   b. College students tend to underestimate the amount that their peers drink.
   c. Rape is linked to binge drinking.
   d. Consumption of alcohol is the number one cause of preventable death among undergraduates.

2. When Amanda goes out on the weekends, she usually has four to five beers in a row. This type of high-risk drinking is called
   a. tolerance.
   b. alcoholic addiction.
   c. alcohol overconsumption.
   d. binge drinking.

3. Blood alcohol concentration (BAC) is the
   a. concentration of plant sugars in the bloodstream.
   b. percentage of alcohol in a beverage.
   c. amount you can drink and still legally drive.
   d. ratio of alcohol to the total blood volume.

4. If a man and a woman drink the same amount of alcohol, the woman's blood alcohol concentration (BAC) will be approximately
   a. the same as the man's BAC.
   b. 60% higher than the man's BAC.
   c. 30% higher than the man's BAC.
   d. 30% lower than the man's BAC.

5. Which of the following is *not* a potential long-term effect of alcohol abuse?
   a. Increased risk of some cancers
   b. Increased risk of liver damage
   c. Increased risk of eye disorders
   d. Increased risk of nervous system damage

6. Which of the following does *not* contribute to college students' vulnerability to tobacco?
   a. Targeting by tobacco marketers
   b. The new, stressful environment of college
   c. Presence of tobacco products on campus
   d. Lack of information about the dangers of smoking

7. What is the major psychoactive ingredient in tobacco products?
   a. Carbon monoxide
   b. Tar
   c. Formaldehyde
   d. Nicotine

8. What does nicotine do to the cilia hairs found in the lungs?
   a. Instantly destroys them
   b. Thickens them
   c. Paralyzes them
   d. Accumulates on them

9. What effect does carbon monoxide have on a smoker's body?
   a. It accumulates on the alveoli in the lungs, making breathing difficult.
   b. It increases heart rate.
   c. It interferes with the ability of red blood cells in the blood to carry oxygen.
   d. It dulls taste and smell.

10. How quickly will an individual begin to see health benefits after quitting smoking?
    a. Within 8 hours
    b. Within a month
    c. Within a year
    d. Never

Answers to these questions can be found on page A-1.

Think about It!

1. When it comes to drinking alcohol, how much is too much? How can you avoid drinking amounts that will affect your judgment? If you see a friend having too many drinks at a party, what actions could you take?

2. What are some of the most common negative consequences college students experience as a result of drinking? What negative impacts do students experience as a result of other students' excessive drinking?

3. Describe the difference between a problem drinker and an alcoholic. What factors can cause someone to become an alcoholic? What effect does alcoholism have on an alcoholic's family?

4. Discuss health hazards associated with tobacco. Who should be responsible for the medical expenses of smokers? Insurance companies? Smokers themselves?

5. Describe the various methods of tobacco cessation. Which would be most effective for you? Why?

Accessing Your Health on the Internet

The following websites explore further topics and issues related to personal health. For links to the websites, visit the Study Area in MasteringHealth.

1. *Alcoholics Anonymous.* Provides general information about AA and the 12-step program. www.aa.org

2. *American Lung Association.* This site offers a wealth of information regarding smoking trends, environmental smoke, and advice on smoking cessation. www.lungusa.org

3. *ASH (Action on Smoking and Health).* The nation's oldest and largest antismoking organization, ASH takes legal actions and does other work to fight smoking and protect nonsmokers' rights. www.ash.org

4. *College Drinking: Changing the Culture.* This online resource center targets three audiences: the student population as a whole, the college and its surrounding environment, and the individual at risk or alcohol-dependent drinker. www.collegedrinkingprevention.gov

5. *The Tobacco Atlas.* This book and website, a joint production of the World Lung Foundation and the American Cancer Society, cover a range of topics including the history of tobacco use, prevalence of use, youth smoking, secondhand smoke, quitting, and more. www.tobaccoatlas.com

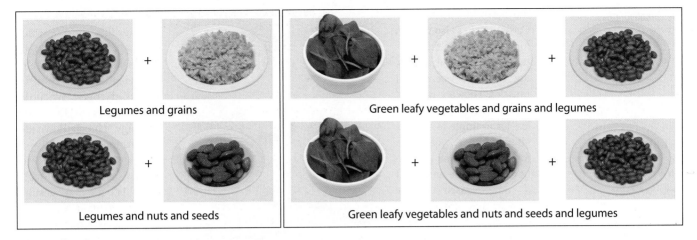

| Legumes and grains | Green leafy vegetables and grains and legumes |
| Legumes and nuts and seeds | Green leafy vegetables and nuts and seeds and legumes |

FIGURE 9.2 **Foods Providing Complementary Amino Acids**
Eaten in the right combinations, plant-based foods can provide all the essential amino acids. In some cases you might need to combine three sources of protein to put together a complete meal. Two of the limiting amino acids in leafy green vegetables are supplied by either grains or nuts and seeds, and the third is found in legumes.

sources of plant protein (Figure 9.2). Plant sources of protein fall into three general categories: *legumes* (beans, peas, peanuts, and soy products), *grains* (e.g., wheat, corn, rice, and oats), and *nuts and seeds.* Certain vegetables, such as leafy green vegetables and broccoli, also contribute valuable plant proteins. Mixing two or more foods from each of these categories during the same meal will provide all the essential amino acids necessary to ensure adequate protein absorption.

The average American consumes more than 79 grams of protein daily, and much of this comes from high-fat animal flesh and dairy products.[6] (In contrast, protein deficiency poses a threat to the global population.) The recommended daily protein intake for adults is only 0.8 grams (g) per kilogram (kg) of body weight (0.36 grams per pound of body weight). To calculate your protein needs: Divide your body weight in pounds by 2.2 to get your weight in kilograms, then multiply by 0.8. The result is your recommended protein intake per day. For example, the protein recommendation for a normal weight college aged female who weighs 125 lb or 57 kg, would be 56 grams of protein per day. Another way to present protein recommendations is as a percentage of your calories. The typical recommendation is that in a 2,000-calorie diet, 10 to 35 percent of calories should come from lean protein, for an average of 50 to 175 grams per day. A 6-ounce steak contains 53 grams of protein—almost the same as the daily needs of an average-sized woman! Table 9.2 compares what percentages of your diet should come from protein, carbohydrates, and fats.

Individuals might need to eat extra protein if they are fighting off a serious infection, recovering from surgery or blood loss, or recovering from burns, and a woman might need to eat extra protein if she is pregnant. In these instances, proteins that are lost to cellular repair and development need to be replaced. There is considerable controversy over whether someone in high-level physical training needs additional protein to build and repair muscle fibers or whether normal

daily requirements should suffice. In addition, a sedentary person or one who gets little exercise may find it easier to stay in energy balance if more of his calories come from protein and fewer come from carbohydrates. Why? Because proteins make a person feel full and satisfied for a longer period of time.

carbohydrates Basic nutrients that supply the body with glucose, the energy form most commonly used to sustain normal activity.

Carbohydrates

Carbohydrates supply us with the energy needed to sustain normal daily activity. For a quick source of energy, the human body metabolizes carbohydrates faster and more efficiently than protein. Carbohydrates are easily converted to glucose,

T A B L E 9.2 | **Recommended Intake for Carbohydrates, Proteins, and Fats for Adults Ages 19–70 (as a percentage of total calories)**

Nutrient	Percentage of Total Calories
Carbohydrate	45–65%
Total Fat	20–35%
Saturated fat	7–10%
Omega-6 fatty acids	5–10%
Omega-3 fatty acids	0.6–1.2%
Protein	10–35%

Note: These values represent the Acceptable Macronutrient Distribution Range (AMDR) for the three energy nutrients. This range of intake is associated with a lowered risk of chronic disease. Consuming in excess of the AMDR may lead to an increased risk and unbalanced intake of sufficient essential nutrients.

Source: Adapted from The National Academies, *Dietary Reference Intakes for Energy, Carbohydrate, Fiber, Fat, Fatty Acids, Cholesterol, Protein, and Amino Acids*, Food and Nutrition Board of the Institute of Medicine, 2005, www.nap.edu

simple carbohydrates A major type of carbohydrate, which provides short-term energy; also called simple sugars.

complex carbohydrates A major type of carbohydrate, which provides sustained energy.

monosaccharides Simple sugars that contain only one molecule of sugar.

disaccharides Sugars that contain a combination of two monosaccharides.

starch A complex carbohydrate form that is the storage form of glucose in plants.

glycogen The complex carbohydrate form of glucose stored in the liver and, to a lesser extent, in muscles.

fiber The indigestible portion of plant foods that helps move food through the digestive system and softens stools by absorbing water.

whole grains Grains that are milled in their complete form, and so include the bran, germ, and endosperm, with only the husk removed.

the fuel for the body's cells. Carbohydrates also play an important role in the functioning of internal organs, the nervous system, and muscles. They are the best fuel for endurance athletics, for example at the beginning and the end of a race because they provide both an immediate and a time-released energy source; they are digested easily and then consistently metabolized in the bloodstream. Carbohydrates are also the fuel for your brain.

Like proteins, carbohydrates provide 4 calories per gram. The RDA for adults is 130 grams per day. There are two major types of carbohydrates: **simple carbohydrates** and **complex carbohydrates.**

Simple Carbohydrates
A typical American diet contains large amounts of simple carbohydrates, or *simple sugars*, found naturally in fruits, vegetables, and dairy. The most common form of simple carbohydrates is *glucose*. Fruits and berries contain *fructose* (commonly called *fruit sugar*). Both glucose and fructose are examples of single sugars called **monosaccharides.** Two single sugars combined, such as *sucrose* (granulated table sugar) that you put on cereal or in a cup of coffee, are referred to as a **dissacharide** (di = two). *Lactose* (milk sugar) found in milk and dairy products and *maltose* found in germinating grains such as barley, are two more examples of common disaccharides. Eventually, the human body converts all types of simple sugars to *glucose* to provide energy to cells.

Complex Carbohydrates
Starches, glycogen, and fiber are the main types of complex carbohydrates, which are found in grains, cereals, and vegetables.

Starches make up the majority of the complex carbohydrate group and come from flours, breads, pasta, rice, corn, oats, barley, potatoes, and related foods. The body breaks

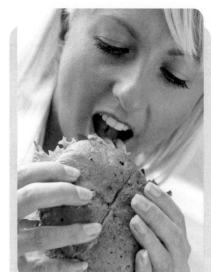

Why are whole grains better than refined grains?

Whole-grain foods contain fiber, a crucial form of carbohydrate that protects against some gastrointestinal disorders and reduces risk for certain cancers. Fiber is also associated with lowered blood cholesterol levels; studies have shown that eating 2.5 servings of whole grains per day can reduce cardiovascular disease risk by as much as 21%. But are people getting the message? One nutrition survey showed that only 4.8% of U.S. adults consume three or more servings of whole grains each day, and 72% ate less than one serving of whole grains per day.

Sources: C. E. O'Neil et al., "Whole Grain Consumption Is Associated with Diet Quality and Nutrient Intake in Adults: The National Health and Nutrition Examination Survey 1999–2004," *Journal of the American Dietetic Association* 110, no. 10 (2010): 1461–1468, doi: 10.1016/j.jada.2010.07.012; P. Mellen, T. Walsh, and D. Herrington, "Whole Grain Intake and Cardiovascular Disease: A Meta-Analysis," *Nutrition, Metabolism, and Cardiovascular Diseases: NMCD* 18, no. 4, (2008): 283–290.

down these complex carbohydrates into glucose, which can be easily absorbed by cells and used as energy or stored in the muscles and the liver as **glycogen.** When the body requires a sudden burst of energy, it breaks down glycogen into glucose.

Fiber, sometimes referred to as "bulk" or "roughage," is the indigestible portion of plant foods that helps move foods through the digestive system, delays absorption of cholesterol and other nutrients, and softens stools by absorbing water. Dietary fiber is found only in plant foods, such as fruits, vegetables, nuts, and grains. The Food and Nutrition Board of the Institute of Medicine makes three fiber distinctions: dietary fiber, functional fiber, and total fiber.[7] *Dietary fiber* comprises the nondigestible parts of plants—the leaves, stems, and seeds. *Functional fiber* consists of nondigestible forms of carbohydrates that may come from plants or may be manufactured in the laboratory and have known health benefits. *Total fiber* is the sum of dietary fiber and functional fiber in a person's diet. Another classification of fiber types is either *soluble* or *insoluble*. Soluble fibers, such as pectins, gums, and mucilages, dissolve in water, form gel-like substances, and can be digested easily by bacteria in the colon. Major food sources of soluble fiber include citrus fruits, berries, oat bran, dried beans (e.g., kidney, garbanzo, pinto, and navy beans), and some vegetables. Insoluble fibers, such as lignins and cellulose, are those that typically do not dissolve in water and cannot be fermented by bacteria in the colon.

Which Carbohydrates Should I Eat?
Despite growing evidence that supports the benefits of **whole grains** and high-fiber diets, intake among the general public remains low. Whole

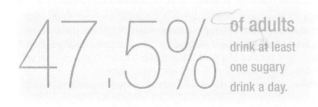

47.5% of adults drink at least one sugary drink a day.

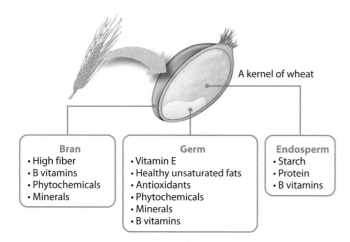

A kernel of wheat

Bran	Germ	Endosperm
• High fiber	• Vitamin E	• Starch
• B vitamins	• Healthy unsaturated fats	• Protein
• Phytochemicals	• Antioxidants	• B vitamins
• Minerals	• Phytochemicals	
	• Minerals	
	• B vitamins	

FIGURE 9.3 **Anatomy of a Whole Grain**
Whole grains are more nutritious than refined grains because they contain the bran, germ, and endosperm of the seed—sources of fiber, vitamins, minerals, and beneficial phytochemicals (chemical compounds that occur naturally in plants).

Source: Adapted from Joan Salge Blake, Kathy D. Munoz, and Stella Volpe, *Nutrition: From Science to You*, 1st ed. © 2010. Printed and electronically reproduced by permission of Pearson Education, Inc., Upper Saddle River, New Jersey.

Bulk Up Your Fiber Intake!

❭ Whenever possible, select whole-grain breads, especially those low in fat and sugars. Choose breads with three or more grams of fiber per serving. Read labels—just because bread is brown doesn't mean it is better for you.

❭ Eat whole, unpeeled fruits and vegetables rather than drinking their juices. The fiber in the whole fruit tends to slow blood sugar increases and helps you feel full longer.

❭ Substitute whole-grain pastas, bagels, and pizza crust for the refined, white flour versions.

❭ Add wheat crumbs or grains to meat loaf and burgers to increase fiber intake.

❭ Enhance your fiber intake with quinoa, an edible seed that is also high in protein.

❭ Toast grains to bring out their nutty flavor and make foods more appealing.

❭ Sprinkle ground flaxseed on cereals, yogurt, and salads, or add to casseroles, burgers, and baked goods. Flaxseeds have a mild flavor and are also high in beneficial fatty acids.

grains are found in foods such as brown rice, wheat, bran, and whole-grain breads and cereals (see Figure 9.3). Fiber protects against obesity, colon and rectal cancers, heart disease, constipation, and possibly even type 2 diabetes, so most experts believe that Americans should double their current consumption of dietary fiber—to 25 grams per day for women and 38 grams per day for men.[8] What's the best way to increase your intake of dietary fiber? Eat fewer refined or processed carbohydrates in favor of more whole grains, fruits, vegetables, legumes, nuts, and seeds. As with most nutritional advice, however, too much of a good thing can pose problems. Sudden increases in dietary fiber may cause flatulence (intestinal gas), cramping, or bloating. Consume plenty of water or other (sugar-free!) liquids to reduce such side effects. Find out more about the benefits of fiber in the **Skills for Behavior Change** box.

Americans typically consume far too many refined carbohydrates (i.e., carbohydrates containing only sugars and starches), which have few health benefits and are a major factor in our growing epidemic of overweight and obesity. Many of the simple sugars in these foods come from *added sugars,* sweeteners that are put in during processing to flavor foods, make sodas taste good, and ease our craving for sweets. A classic example is the amount of added sugar in one can of soda: more than 10 teaspoons per 12 ounce can. All that refined sugar can cause tooth decay and may put on pounds.

Sugar is found in high amounts in a wide range of food products. High-sugar beverages such as soda, juice drinks, and even some energy drinks contain more than 30 grams of sugar in a 12-ounce serving. Even such diverse items as ketchup, barbecue sauce, and flavored coffee creamers derive 30 to 65 percent of their calories from sugar. Knowing what foods contain these sugars, considering the amounts you consume each day that are hidden in foods, and then trying to reduce these levels can be a great way to reduce excess weight. Read food labels carefully before purchasing. If *sugar* or one of its aliases (including *high fructose corn syrup* and *cornstarch*) appears near the top of the ingredients list, then that product contains a lot of sugar and is probably not your best nutritional bet. Also, most labels list the amount of sugar as a percentage of total calories.

Fats

Fats are perhaps the most misunderstood of the body's required nutrients. In our diet, fats are the most energy-dense source of calories, providing 9 calories per gram. Fats play a vital role in maintaining healthy skin and hair, insulating body organs against shock, maintaining body temperature, and promoting healthy cell function. Fats make foods taste better and carry the fat-soluble vitamins A, D, E, and K to the cells. They also provide a concentrated form of energy in the absence of sufficient amounts of carbohydrates and make you feel full after eating. But despite the fact that fat performs all these

fats Basic nutrients composed of carbon and hydrogen atoms; needed for the proper functioning of cells, insulation of body organs against shock, maintenance of body temperature, and healthy skin and hair.

functions, we are constantly urged to cut back on them because excessive consumption can lead to weight gain and cardiovascular disease.

Triglycerides, which make up about 95 percent of total body fat, are the most common form of fat in foods. When we consume too many calories from any source, the liver converts the excess into triglycerides, which are stored throughout our bodies.

The remaining 5 percent of body fat is composed of substances such as **cholesterol.** The ratio of total cholesterol to a group of compounds called **high-density lipoproteins (HDLs)** is important in determining risk for heart disease. Lipoproteins facilitate the transport of cholesterol in the blood. High-density lipoproteins are capable of transporting more cholesterol than are **low-density lipoproteins (LDLs).** Whereas LDLs transport cholesterol to the body's cells, HDLs transport circulating cholesterol to the liver for metabolism and elimination from the body. People with a high percentage of HDLs appear to be at lower risk for developing cholesterol-clogged arteries. (See **Chapter 12** for more on the role cholesterol plays in cardiovascular health.)

Types of Dietary Fats

Fat molecules include *fatty acid* chains of carbon and hydrogen atoms. Fatty acid chains that cannot hold any more hydrogen in their chemical structure are called **saturated fats.** They generally come from animal sources, such as meat, dairy, and poultry products and are solid at room temperature. **Unsaturated fats** have room for additional hydrogen atoms in their chemical structure and are liquid at room temperature. They come from plants and include most vegetable oils. Unsaturated fats are considered better for your health than saturated fats.

The terms *monounsaturated fatty acids* (*MUFAs*) and *polyunsaturated fatty acids* (*PUFAs*) refer to the relative number of hydrogen atoms that are missing in a fatty acid chain. Peanut and olive oils are high in monounsaturated fats. Corn, sunflower, and safflower oils are high in polyunsaturated fats. There is currently a great deal of controversy about which type of unsaturated fat is most beneficial. Monounsaturated fatty acids, such as olive oil, seem to lower LDL levels and increase HDL levels and thus are currently the preferred, or least harmful, fats. They are also resistant to oxidation, a process that leads to cell and tissue damage. For a breakdown of the types of fats in common vegetable oils, see **Figure 9.4.**

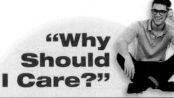

"Why Should I Care?"

Cholesterol can accumulate on the inner walls of arteries and narrow the channels through which blood flows. This buildup, called plaque, is a major cause of *atherosclerosis*, a component of cardiovascular disease.

Polyunsaturated fatty acids come in two forms: *omega-3 fatty acids* (found in many types of fatty fish) and *omega-6 fatty acids* (found in corn, soybean, and cottonseed oils). Some nutritional researchers believe that PUFAs may decrease levels of both harmful LDL cholesterol and beneficial HDL cholesterol. However, two PUFAs are classified as *essential fatty acids*—that is, we must receive them from our diets. These two fats, *linoleic acid*, an omega-6 fatty acid, and *alpha-linolenic acid,* an omega-3 fatty acid, are needed to make hormone-like compounds that control immune function, pain perception, and inflammation, to name a few key benefits.[9] You may have also heard of EPA and DHA. These are derivatives of alpha-linolenic acid that are found abundantly in oily fish such as

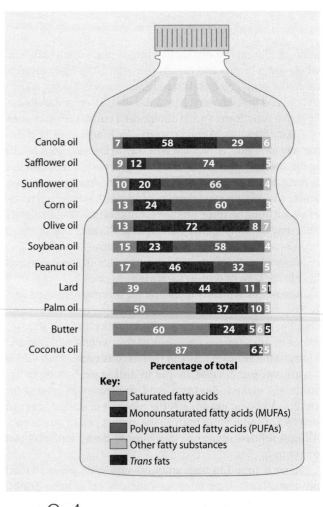

FIGURE 9.4 **Percentages of Saturated, Polyunsaturated, Monounsaturated, and Trans Fats in Common Vegetable Oils**

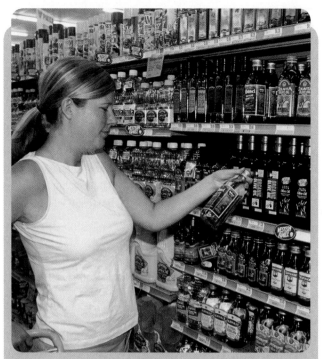

Are all fats bad for me?

All fats are not the same, and your body needs some fat to function healthily. Try to reduce saturated fats from meat, dairy, and poultry products; avoid *trans* fats, those that can come in stick margarine, commercially baked goods, and deep-fried foods. Replace these with monounsaturated fats, such as those in peanut and olive oils, and polyunsaturated fats, commonly found in fatty fish like salmon.

salmon and tuna and are associated with reduced risk for heart disease.[10] While consuming fish oil tablets may increase your omega-3 fatty acid levels in the same way eating fresh salmon does, the salmon has other major benefits that can't be found in a supplement.[11] Generally, about 20 to 35 percent of calories should come from fat, with 5 to 10 percent coming from omega-6 fatty acids.

Avoiding *Trans* Fatty Acids

For decades, Americans shunned butter, certain cuts of red meat, and other foods because of the saturated fats found in them. What they didn't know is that foods low in saturated fat, such as margarine, could be just as harmful. These processed foods contain a form of fat known as *trans* fats. In one study, researchers concluded that just a 2 percent caloric intake of *trans* fats was associated with a 23 percent increased risk for heart disease and a 47 percent increased chance of sudden cardiac death.[12]

What are **trans** fats (**trans** fatty acids)? *Trans* fats are fatty acids that are produced by adding hydrogen molecules to liquid oil to make the oil into a solid. Unlike regular fats and oils, these "partially hydrogenated" fats stay solid or semisolid at room temperature. *Trans* fats have been used in margarines, many commercial baked goods, and restaurant deep-fried foods.

Today, *trans* fats are being removed from most foods, and if they are present, they must be clearly indicated on food packaging. Some cities and states have banned their use in restaurants. If you see the words *partially hydrogenated oils, fractionated oils, shortening, lard,* or *hydrogenation* on a food label, then *trans* fats are present.

New Fat Advice: Is More Fat Ever Better?

Some researchers worry that we have gone too far in our anti-fat frenzy. In fact, some studies have shown that when comparing low-fat diets to other diets, there are few improvements in weight loss and blood fat measures.[13] The bottom line for fat intake is that moderation is the key. No more than 7 to 10 percent of your total calories should come from saturated fat and that no more than 35 percent should come from all forms of fat. In general, switching to beneficial fats without increasing total fat intake is a good idea.

Enjoying a healthy intake of dietary fat doesn't have to be difficult or confusing. Follow these guidelines to add more healthy fats to your diet:

- Eat fatty fish (herring, mackerel, salmon, sardines, or tuna) at least twice weekly. The **Be Healthy, Be Green** box on page 268 provides tips for making sustainable seafood choices to fulfill your need for omega-3 fatty acids.
- Use soy, olive, peanut, and canola oils instead of lard or butter.
- Add healthy amounts of green leafy vegetables, walnuts, walnut oil, and ground flaxseed to your diet.

Follow these guidelines to help reduce your overall intake of less healthy fats:

- Read the nutrition facts panel on foods to find out how much fat is in your food. Remember that no more than 10 percent of your total calories should come from saturated fat, and no more than 35 percent should come from all forms of fat.
- Chill meat-based soups and stews, scrape off any fat that hardens on top, and then reheat to serve.
- Fill up on fruits and vegetables.
- Hold the creams and sauces.
- Avoid margarine products with *trans* fatty acids. Whenever possible, opt for other healthy toppings on your bread, such as fresh vegetable spreads, sugar-free jams, fat-free cheese, etc.
- Choose lean meats, fish, or skinless poultry. Broil or bake whenever possible. Drain off fat after cooking.
- Choose fewer cold cuts, bacon, sausages, hot dogs, and organ meats.
- Select nonfat and low-fat dairy products.
- When cooking, use substitutes for butter, margarine, oils, sour cream, mayonnaise, and full-fat salad dressings. Chicken or beef broth, fresh herbs, wine, vinegar, and low-calorie dressings provide flavor with less fat.

trans fats (trans fatty acids) Fatty acids that are produced when polyunsaturated oils are hydrogenated to make them more solid.

BE HEALTHY, BE GREEN

TOWARD SUSTAINABLE SEAFOOD

The U.S. Department of Agriculture recommends consuming fish two or three times per week to reduce saturated fat and cholesterol levels and to increase omega-3 fatty acid levels. However, there are many environmental concerns surrounding the seafood industry today that call into question the sustainability and safety of such consumption. More than 70 percent of the world's natural fishing grounds have been overfished, and whole stretches of the oceans are, in fact, dead zones, where fish and shellfish can no longer live.

The FDA continues to keep a close eye on the safety of fish and shellfish in areas affected by the 2010 Gulf of Mexico oil spill. Commercial fishing was allowed to resume in federal waters in April 2011, although several coastal areas still remain closed. The long-term effects on seafood and fishing grounds remain unknown. Fish and shellfish from areas not affected by the oil disaster are considered safe for consumers to eat.

In an effort to counteract the loss of wild fish populations, increasing numbers of fish are being farmed, which poses additional health risks and environmental concerns. Some farmed fish are laden with antibiotics, while highly concentrated levels of parasites and bacteria from fish farm runoff may enter the ocean and river fish populations through adjacent waterways. There are other reasons to think carefully about your farmed fish alternatives. Farmed salmon, for example, are often fed wild fish, resulting in a net loss of fish from the sea.

At the same time that fish populations are threatened, high levels of chemicals, parasites, bacteria, and toxins are also being found in many of the fish available on the market. Mercury, a waste product of many industries, binds to proteins and stays in an animal's body, accumulating as it moves up the food chain. In humans, mercury can damage the nervous system and kidneys and cause birth defects and developmental problems in fetuses and children. Polychlorinated biphenyls (PCBs), chemicals that can build up in the fatty tissue of fish, are another cause of major concern.

So what is a savvy fish consumer to do? Knowing where your fish are caught and the methods by which they are caught is important. Several major environmental groups have developed guides to inform consumers of safe and sustainable seafood choices. The Monterey Bay Aquarium in California provides a national guide for seafood available for purchase in the United States. You can find the guide online at www.montereybayaquarium.org. This guide is also available as a free iPhone or Android app, or can be accessed on other mobile devices at http://mobile.seafoodwatch.org. Another great resource is the FishPhone service offered by the Blue Ocean Institute. Simply send a text message to 30644 with the word *FISH* and the type of fish you want to know about, and it will send you information about whether it is safe to eat. Remember: Your consumer choices make a difference. Purchasing seafood from environmentally responsible sources will support fisheries and fish farms that are healthier for you and the environment.

Sources: U.S. Food and Drug Administration, "Deep Water Horizon Oil Spill: Questions and Answers," updated April 2013, www.fda.gov; M. Schleifstein, "Research Scientists Hear That Some Remain Skeptical of Seafood Safety in Aftermath of BP Deep Horizon Oil Spill," NOLA.com: *The Times-Picayune*, January 23, 2013, www.nola.com

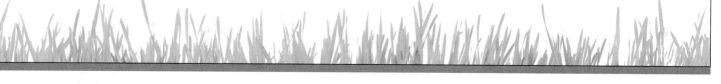

Vitamins

Vitamins are potent and essential organic compounds that promote growth and help maintain life and health. Every minute of every day, vitamins help maintain nerves and skin, produce blood cells, build bones and teeth, heal wounds, and convert food energy to body energy—and they do all this without adding any calories to your diet.

Vitamins can be classified as either *fat soluble,* which means they are absorbed through the intestinal tract with the help of fats, or *water soluble,* which means they are dissolved easily in water. Vitamins A, D, E, and K are fat-soluble; B-complex vitamins and vitamin C are water soluble. Fat-soluble vitamins tend to be stored in the body, and toxic accumulations in the liver may cause cirrhosis-like symptoms. Water-soluble vitamins generally are excreted and cause few toxicity problems. See Table 9.3 and 9.4 on pages 269 and 270 for more information on the functions and potential dangers of specific vitamins.

Antioxidants The old adage "you are what you eat" is indeed a motto to live by. Beneficial foods termed **functional foods** are based on the ancient belief that eating the right foods may not only prevent disease, but also cure some diseases (see the **Health Headlines** box on page 271). Some of the most popular functional foods today are items containing **antioxidants** or other *phytochemicals* (from the Greek word meaning *plant*). Among the nutrients commonly cited as providing a protective antioxidant effect are vitamin C, vitamin E, and beta-carotene, a precursor to

vitamins Essential organic compounds that promote growth and reproduction and help maintain life and health.

functional foods Foods believed to have specific health benefits and/or to prevent disease.

antioxidants Substances believed to protect against tissue damage at the cellular level.

Do It! Nutritools

Complete the **Know Your Fat Sources** activity in the Study Area of MasteringHealth™

TABLE

9.3   A Guide to Water-Soluble Vitamins

Vitamin Name and Recommended Intake	Reliable Food Sources	Primary Functions	Toxicity/Deficiency Symptoms
Thiamin (vitamin B_1) RDA: Men = 1.2 mg/day Women = 1.1 mg/day	Pork, fortified cereals, enriched rice and pasta, peas, tuna, legumes	Required as enzyme cofactor for carbohydrate and amino acid metabolism	**Toxicity:** none known **Deficiency:** beriberi, fatigue, apathy, decreased memory, confusion, irritability, muscle weakness
Riboflavin (vitamin B_2) RDA: Men = 1.3 mg/day Women = 1.1 mg/day	Beef liver, shrimp, milk and dairy foods, fortified cereals, enriched breads and grains	Required as enzyme cofactor for carbohydrate and fat metabolism	**Toxicity:** none known **Deficiency:** ariboflavinosis, swollen mouth and throat, seborrheic dermatitis, anemia
Niacin, nicotinamide, nicotinic acid RDA: Men = 16 mg/day Women = 14 mg/day UL = 35 mg/day	Beef liver, most cuts of meat/fish/poultry, fortified cereals, enriched breads and grains, canned tomato products	Required for carbohydrate and fat metabolism; plays role in DNA replication and repair and cell differentiation	**Toxicity:** flushing, liver damage, glucose intolerance, blurred vision differentiation **Deficiency:** pellagra; vomiting, constipation, or diarrhea; apathy
Vitamin B_6 (pyridoxine, pyridoxal, pyridoxamine) RDA: Men and women 19–50 = 1.3 mg/day Men > 50 = 1.7 mg/day Women > 50 = 1.5 mg/day UL = 100 mg/day	Chickpeas (garbanzo beans), most cuts of meat/fish/poultry, fortified cereals, white potatoes	Required as enzyme cofactor for carbohydrate and amino acid metabolism; assists synthesis of blood cells	**Toxicity:** nerve damage, skin lesions **Deficiency:** anemia; seborrheic dermatitis; depression, confusion, and convulsions
Folate (folic acid) RDA: Men = 400 µg/day Women = 400 µg/day UL = 1,000 µg/day	Fortified cereals, enriched breads and grains, spinach, legumes (lentils, chickpeas, pinto beans), greens (spinach, romaine lettuce), liver	Required as enzyme cofactor for amino acid metabolism; required for DNA synthesis; involved in metabolism of homocysteine	**Toxicity:** masks symptoms of vitamin B_{12} deficiency, specifically signs of nerve damage **Deficiency:** macrocytic anemia; neural tube defects in a developing fetus; elevated homocysteine levels
Vitamin B_{12} (cobalamin) RDA: Men = 2.4 µg/day Women = 2.4 µg/day	Shellfish, all cuts of meat/fish/poultry, milk and dairy foods, fortified cereals	Assists with formation of blood; required for healthy nervous system function; involved as enzyme cofactor in metabolism of homocysteine	**Toxicity:** none known **Deficiency:** pernicious anemia; tingling and numbness of extremities; nerve damage; memory loss, disorientation, and dementia
Pantothenic acid AI: Men = 5 mg/day Women = 5 mg/day	Meat/fish/poultry, shiitake mushrooms, fortified cereals, egg yolks	Assists with fat metabolism	**Toxicity:** none known **Deficiency:** rare
Biotin RDA: Men = 30 µg/day Women = 30 µg/day	Nuts, egg yolks	Involved as enzyme cofactor in carbohydrate, fat, and protein metabolism	**Toxicity:** none known **Deficiency:** rare
Vitamin C (ascorbic acid) RDA: Men = 90 mg/day Women = 75 mg/day Smokers = 35 mg more per day than RDA UL = 2,000 mg	Sweet peppers, citrus fruits and juices, broccoli, strawberries, kiwi	Antioxidant in extracellular fluid and lungs; regenerates oxidized vitamin E; assists with collagen synthesis; enhances immune function; assists in synthesis of hormones, neurotransmitters, and DNA; enhances iron absorption	**Toxicity:** nausea and diarrhea, nosebleeds, increased oxidative damage, increased formation of kidney stones in people with kidney disease **Deficiency:** scurvy, bone pain and fractures, depression, and anemia

Note: RDA = Recommended Dietary Allowance; AI = Adequate Intakes; UL = Tolerable Upper Level Intakes. Values are for all adults aged 19 and older, except as noted. Values increase among women who are pregnant or lactating.
Source: J. Thompson and M. Manore, *Nutrition: An Applied Approach,* 2nd ed., © 2009. Printed and electronically reproduced by permission of Pearson Education, Inc., Upper Saddle River, New Jersey.

TABLE
9.4 | A Guide to Fat-Soluble Vitamins

Vitamin Name and Recommended Intake	Reliable Food Sources	Primary Functions	Toxicity/Deficiency Symptoms
Vitamin A (retinol, retinal, retinoic acid) RDA: Men = 900 µg Women = 700 µg UL = 3,000 µg/day	Preformed retinol: beef and chicken liver, egg yolks, milk Carotenoid precursors: spinach, carrots, mango, apricots, cantaloupe, pumpkin, yams	Required for ability of eyes to adjust to changes in light; protects color vision; assists cell differentiation; required for sperm production in men and fertilization in women; contributes to healthy bone and healthy immune system	**Toxicity:** fatigue; bone and joint pain; spontaneous abortion and birth defects of fetuses in pregnant women; nausea and diarrhea; liver damage; nervous system damage; blurred vision; hair loss; skin disorders **Deficiency:** night blindness, xerophthalmia; impaired growth, immunity, and reproductive function
Vitamin D (cholecalciferol) AI (assumes that person does not get adequate sun exposure): Adult 19–70 = 15 µg/day 600 IU/day Adult > 70 = 20 µg/day 800 IU/day UL = 50 µg/day 4,000 IU/day	Canned salmon and mackerel, milk, fortified cereals	Regulates blood calcium levels; maintains bone health; assists cell differentiation	**Toxicity:** hypercalcemia **Deficiency:** rickets in children; osteomalacia and/or osteoporosis in adults
Vitamin E (tocopherol) RDA: Men = 15 mg/day Women = 15 mg/day UL = 1,000 mg/day	Sunflower seeds, almonds, vegetable oils, fortified cereals	As a powerful antioxidant, protects cell membranes, polyunsaturated fatty acids, and vitamin A from oxidation; protects white blood cells; enhances immune function; improves absorption of vitamin A	**Toxicity:** rare **Deficiency:** hemolytic anemia; impairment of nerve, muscle, and immune function
Vitamin K (phylloquinone, menaquinone, menadione) AI: Men = 120 µg/day Women = 90 µg/day	Kale, spinach, turnip greens, Brussels sprouts	Serves as a coenzyme during production of specific proteins that assist in blood coagulation and bone metabolism	**Toxicity:** none known **Deficiency:** impaired blood clotting; possible effect on bone health

Note: RDA = Recommended Dietary Allowance; AI = Adequate Intakes; UL = Tolerable Upper Level Intakes. Values are for all adults aged 19 and older, except as noted. Values increase among women who are pregnant or lactating.
Source: Adapted from J. Thompson and M. Manore, *Nutrition: An Applied Approach*, 2nd ed., © 2009. Printed and electronically reproduced by permission of Pearson Education, Inc., Upper Saddle River, New Jersey; The National Academies, "Dietary Reference Intakes for Calcium and Vitamin D," 2011, available at www.iom.edu

vitamin A. These substances may protect people from damage caused by *free radicals*, which are unstable molecules formed during metabolism that can damage or kill healthy cells, cell proteins, and DNA. Free radical formation is a natural process that cannot be avoided, but antioxidants can neutralize free radicals, slow their formation, and may even repair the damage.

To date, many claims about the benefits of antioxidants in reducing the risk of heart disease, improving vision, and slowing the aging process have not been fully investigated, and conclusive statements about their true benefits are difficult to find. Large, longitudinal epidemiological studies suggest that antioxidants in whole foods, mostly fruits and vegetables, help protect against certain diseases, but so far no protection through use of antioxidant supplements has been documented.[14] People who consume diets rich in vitamin C seem to develop fewer cancers, but meta-analysis studies detect no effect from dietary vitamin C.[15] Recent studies report that high-dose vitamin C given intravenously, rather than orally, may be effective in treating cancer and protecting from diseases affecting the central nervous system.[16]

Possible effects of vitamin E intake are even more controversial. Researchers have long theorized that because many cancers result from DNA damage, and because vitamin E

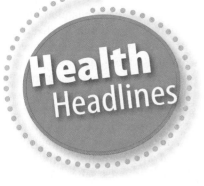

Health Headlines

HEALTH CLAIMS OF FUNCTIONAL FOODS

Functional foods contain an active compound that may provide a health benefit beyond basic nutrition. Functional foods are similar to traditional foods, such as soy, chocolate, or flax seeds, with a beneficial ingredient that may improve overall health, reduce disease, or minimize health concerns.

✱ Yogurt and kefir, and other fermented milk products, contain living, beneficial bacteria called probiotics. You will see them labeled as *Lactobacillus* or *Bifidobacterium* in a product's list of ingredients. Probiotics colonize the large intestine, where they are thought to reduce the risk of diarrhea, irritable bowel syndrome, and inflammatory bowel disease.

✱ Cocoa is particularly rich in a class of chemicals called flavanols that have been shown in many studies to reduce the risk for cardiovascular disease, diabetes, and even arthritis. Dark chocolate has a higher level of flavonols than does milk chocolate.
✱ Whole-grain cereals, breads, and pastas may reduce the risk of cardiovascular disease and some types of cancer and may help maintain healthy blood glucose levels.
✱ Soy proteins, whether from soy milk, tofu, or other soy products, have been associated with a reduced risk for cardiovascular disease.

Want to incorporate more functional foods in your diet? They don't have to come in fancy packages. For example, fruits, vegetables, and fish are all considered functional foods.

There are a few things you should know about labeling. In the United States, the Food and Drug Administration (FDA) does not currently provide a specific definition or regulation for functional foods. However, the FDA does regulate health claims on the labels of food products sold in the United States. See the Read Food Labels section on page 277 in this chapter for the types of health claims that the FDA allows food manufacturers to make.

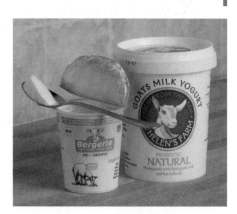

Yogurt and kefir (a fermented milk drink) are dairy products containing beneficial bacteria called probiotics.

Sources: L. Vitetta et al., "A Review of Pharmacobiotic Regulation of Gastrointestinal Inflammation by Probiotics, Commensal Bacteria, and Prebiotics," *Inflammopharmacology* 20, no. 5 (2012): 251–266, doi: 10.1007/s10787-012-0126-8; L. Hooper et al., "Effects of Chocolate, Cocoa, and Flavan-3-ols on Cardiovascular Health: A Systematic Review and Meta-Analysis of Randomized Trials," *American Journal of Clinical Nutrition* 95, no. 3 (2012): 740–753, doi: 10.3945/ajcn.111.023457; D. Grassi et al., "Protective Effects of Flavanol-Rich Dark Chocolate on Endothelial Function and Wave Reflection During Acute Hyperglycemia," *Hypertension* 60, no. 3 (2012): 827–832, doi: 10.1161/HYPERTENSIONAHA.112.193995; S. Ramos-Romero et al., "Effect of a Cocoa Flavonoid-Enriched Diet on Experimental Autoimmune Arthritis," *British Journal of Nutrition* 107, no. 4 (2012): 523–532, doi: 10.1017/S000711451100328X.

---

appears to protect against DNA damage, vitamin E would also reduce cancer risk. Surprisingly, the great majority of studies have demonstrated no effect or, in some cases, a negative effect.[17] However, it can be difficult to compare studies on vitamin E because several different forms of vitamin E exist.

Carotenoids are part of the red, orange, and yellow pigments found in fruits and vegetables. Beta-carotene, the most researched carotenoid, is a precursor of vitamin A, meaning that vitamin A can be produced in the body from beta-carotene. Like vitamin A, beta-carotene has antioxidant properties.

Although there are over 600 carotenoids in nature, two that have received a great deal of attention are *lycopene* (found in tomatoes, papaya, pink grapefruit, and guava) and *lutein* (found in green leafy vegetables such as spinach, broccoli, kale, and Brussels sprouts). The National Cancer Institute and the American Cancer Society have

endorsed lycopene as a possible factor in reducing the risk of cancer. A landmark study assessing the effects of tomato-based foods reported that men who ate 10 or more servings of lycopene-rich foods per week had a 45 percent lower risk of prostate cancer.[18] Research on the benefits of lycopene-rich foods continues for both cancer and other conditions, including heart disease.[19] Lutein is most often cited as a means of protecting the eyes, particularly from age-related macular degeneration (ARMD), a leading cause of blindness for people aged 65 and older.

carotenoids Fat-soluble plant pigments with antioxidant properties.

Blueberries are a great source of antioxidants.

Vitamin D Vitamin D, the sunshine vitamin, is formed in the skin when exposed to ultraviolet rays from the sun. An adequate amount of vitamin D can be obtained with 5 to 30 minutes of sun on your face, neck, hands, back, and legs twice a week, without sunscreen.[20] However, not everyone can or should rely on the sun to meet their daily vitamin D needs. Consuming vitamin D fortified milk and yogurt, eating fatty fish such as salmon, and eating vitamin D fortified cereals can meet your daily recommendations for this vitamin. Vitamin D improves bone strength, helps fight infections, lowers blood pressure, reduces the risk of developing diabetes mellitus, and may reduce the growth of cancer cells. Too little vitamin D may have serious consequences. *Rickets* in children, and its adult version, *osteomalacia,* are on the rise worldwide, causing muscle and bone weakness and pain.[21] Inadequate vitamin D reduces the absorption of calcium, promoting *osteoporosis,* a condition in which the bones lose density and become brittle. Breast and prostate cancer, heart disease, and stroke have also been connected to inadequate vitamin D.

More is not always better, however.[22] Too much vitamin D, generally from excess use of vitamin D supplements, can reduce appetite and cause nausea, vomiting, and constipation. Excess vitamin D can also affect the nervous system, cause depression, and deposit calcium in the soft tissues of the kidneys, lungs, blood vessels, and heart.

Folate

One of the B vitamins, folate is needed for the production of compounds necessary for DNA synthesis in body cells. It is particularly important for proper cell division during embryonic development; folate deficiencies during the first few weeks of pregnancy, typically before a woman even realizes she is pregnant, can prompt a neural tube defect such as spina bifida, in which the primitive tube that eventually forms the brain and spinal cord fails to close properly. The FDA requires that all bread, cereal, rice, and pasta products sold in the United States be fortified with folic acid, the synthetic form of folate, to reduce the incidence of neural tube defects.

Folate is also important for the synthesis of several amino acids and for the production of healthy red blood cells. The DRI for folate is 400 micrograms daily for both males and females throughout adulthood. During pregnancy, this increases to 600 micrograms per day.

Minerals

Minerals are inorganic, indestructible elements that aid physiological processes within the body. Without minerals, vitamins could not be absorbed. Minerals are readily excreted and, with a few exceptions, usually not toxic.

minerals Inorganic, indestructible elements that aid physiological processes.

Major minerals are the minerals that the body needs in fairly large amounts: sodium, calcium, phosphorus, magnesium, potassium, sulfur, and chloride. *Trace minerals* include iron, zinc, manganese, copper, and iodine. Only very small amounts of trace minerals are needed, and serious problems may result if excesses or deficiencies occur (see Table 9.5 and Table 9.6 on pages 273 and 274).

Sodium

Sodium is necessary for the regulation of blood and body fluids, transmission of nerve impulses, heart activity, and certain metabolic functions. It enhances flavors, balances the bitterness of certain foods, acts as a preservative, and tenderizes meats, so it's often present in high quantities in many of the foods we eat. A common misconception is that salt and sodium are the same thing. However, table salt accounts for only 15 percent of sodium intake. The majority of sodium in our diet comes from highly processed foods that are infused with sodium to enhance flavor and preservation. Pickles, fast foods, salty snack foods, processed cheeses, canned soups and frozen dinners, many breads and bakery products, and smoked meats and sausages often contain several hundred milligrams of sodium per serving.

Many health professionals believe there is evidence that Americans need to reduce sodium.[23] The Institute of Medicine, the American Heart Association, the FDA, and the U.S. Department of Agriculture (USDA) are among the professional and governmental organizations that recommend that healthy people consume fewer than 2,300 milligrams of sodium each day. What does that really mean? For most of us, less than 1 teaspoon of table salt per day is all we need! The latest National Health and Nutrition Examination Survey (NHANES) estimated that the average American over 2 years of age consumes 3,463 milligrams per day.[24]

Why is high sodium intake a concern? Many experts believe that there is a link between excessive sodium intake and hypertension (high blood pressure). Although this theory is controversial, researchers recommend that hypertensive Americans cut back on sodium to reduce their risk for cardiovascular disorders, including stroke, debilitating bone fractures, and other health problems.[25]

Calcium

Calcium plays a vital role in building strong bones and teeth, muscle contraction, blood clotting, nerve impulse transmission, regulating heartbeat, and fluid balance within cells. The issue of calcium consumption has gained national attention with the rising incidence of osteoporosis among older adults. Most Americans do not consume the recommended 1,000 to 1,200 milligrams of calcium per day.[26]

Milk is one of the richest sources of dietary calcium. Calcium-fortified orange juice and soy milk are good alternatives if you do not drink dairy milk. Many green leafy vegetables are good sources of calcium, but some contain oxalic acid, which makes their calcium harder to absorb. Spinach, chard, and beet greens are not particularly good sources of calcium, whereas broccoli, cauliflower, and many peas and beans offer good supplies.

It is generally best to take calcium throughout the day, consuming it with foods containing protein, vitamin D, and vitamin C for optimal absorption.

Even if you never use table salt, you still may be getting excess sodium in your diet.

TABLE

9.5

A Guide to Major Minerals

Mineral Name and Recommended Intake	Reliable Food Sources	Primary Functions	Toxicity/Deficiency Symptoms
Sodium AI: Adults = 1.5 g/day (1,500 mg/day)	Table salt, pickles, most canned soups, snack foods, cured luncheon meats, canned tomato products	Fluid balance; acid–base balance; transmission of nerve impulses; muscle contraction	**Toxicity:** water retention, high blood pressure, loss of calcium **Deficiency:** muscle cramps, dizziness, fatigue, nausea, vomiting, mental confusion
Potassium AI: Adults = 4.7 g/day (4,700 mg/day)	Most fresh fruits and vegetables: potato, banana, tomato juice, orange juice, melon	Fluid balance; transmission of nerve impulses; muscle contraction	**Toxicity:** muscle weakness, vomiting, irregular heartbeat **Deficiency:** muscle weakness, paralysis, mental confusion, irregular heartbeat
Phosphorus RDA: Adults = 700 mg/day	Milk/cheese/yogurt, soy-milk and tofu, legumes (lentils, black beans), nuts (almonds, peanuts), poultry	Fluid balance; bone formation; component of ATP, which provides energy for our bodies	**Toxicity:** muscle spasms, convulsions, low blood calcium **Deficiency:** muscle weakness, muscle damage, bone pain, dizziness
Chloride AI: Adults = 2.3 g/day (2,300 mg/day)	Table salt	Fluid balance; transmission of nerve impulses; component of stomach acid (HCL); antibacterial	**Toxicity:** none known **Deficiency:** dangerous blood acid–base imbalances, irregular heartbeat
Calcium RDA: Adult males 19–70 = 1,000 mg/day Adult females 19–50 = 1,000 mg/day Adult females 51–70 = 1,200 mg/day Adults > 70 = 1,200 mg/day UL = 2,500 mg/day for adults 19–50; adults > 50 = 2,000 mg/day	Milk/yogurt/cheese (best absorbed form of calcium), sardines, collard greens and spinach, calcium-fortified juices	Primary component of bone; acid–base balance; transmission of nerve impulses; muscle contraction	**Toxicity:** mineral imbalances, shock, kidney failure, fatigue, mental confusion **Deficiency:** osteoporosis, convulsions, heart failure
Magnesium RDA: Men 19–30 = 400 mg/day Men > 30 = 420 mg/day Women 19–30 = 310 mg/day Women > 30 = 320 mg/day UL = 350 mg/day	Greens (spinach, kale, collards), whole grains, seeds, nuts, legumes (navy and black beans)	Component of bone; muscle contraction; assists more than 300 enzyme systems	**Toxicity:** none known **Deficiency:** low blood calcium; muscle spasms or seizures; nausea; weakness; increased risk of chronic diseases such as heart disease, hypertension, osteoporosis, and type 2 diabetes
Sulfur No DRI	Protein-rich foods	Component of certain B vitamins and amino acids; acid–base balance; detoxification in liver	**Toxicity:** none known **Deficiency:** none known

Note: RDA = Recommended Dietary Allowance; AI = Adequate Intakes; UL = Tolerable Upper Level Intake. Values are for all adults aged 19 and older, except as noted.

Source: Adapted from J. Thompson and M. Manore, *Nutrition: An Applied Approach,* 2nd ed., © 2009. Printed and electronically reproduced by permission of Pearson Education, Inc., Upper Saddle River, New Jersey; The National Academies, "Dietary Reference Intakes for Calcium and Vitamin D," www.iom.edu, 2011.

Mineral Name and Recommended Intake	Reliable Food Sources	Primary Functions	Toxicity/Deficiency Symptoms
Selenium RDA: Adults = 55 µg/day UL = 400 µg/day	Nuts, shellfish, meat/fish/poultry, whole grains	Required for carbohydrate and fat metabolism	**Toxicity:** brittle hair and nails, skin rashes, nausea and vomiting, weakness, liver disease **Deficiency:** specific forms of heart disease and arthritis, impaired immune function, muscle pain and wasting, depression, hostility
Fluoride AI: Men = 4 mg/day Women = 3 mg/day UL = 2.2 mg/day for children 4–8 years; children > 8 years = 10 mg/day	Fluoridated water and other beverages made with this water	Development and maintenance of healthy teeth and bones	**Toxicity:** fluorosis of teeth and bones **Deficiency:** dental caries, low bone density
Iodine RDA: Adults = 150 µg/day UL = 1,100 µg/day	Iodized salt and foods processed with iodized salt	Synthesis of thyroid hormones; temperature regulation; reproduction and growth	**Toxicity:** goiter **Deficiency:** goiter, hypothyroidism, cretinism in infant of mother who is iodine deficient
Chromium AI: Men 19–50 = 35 µg/day Men > 50 = 30 µg/day Women 19–50 = 25 µg/day Women > 50 = 20 µg/day	Grains, meat/fish/poultry, some fruits and vegetables	Glucose transport; metabolism of DNA and RNA; immune function and growth	**Toxicity:** none known **Deficiency:** elevated blood glucose and blood lipids, damage to brain and nervous system
Manganese AI: Men = 2.3 mg/day Women = 1.8 mg/day UL = 11 mg/day for adults	Whole grains, nuts, legumes, some fruits and vegetables	Assists many enzyme systems; synthesis of protein found in bone and cartilage	**Toxicity:** impairment of neuromuscular system **Deficiency:** impaired growth and reproductive function, reduced bone density, impaired glucose and lipid metabolism, skin rash
Iron RDA: Men = 8 mg/day Women 19–50 = 18 mg/day Women > 50 = 8 mg/day	Meat/fish/poultry (best absorbed form of iron), fortified cereals, legumes, spinach	Component of hemoglobin in blood cells; component of myoglobin in muscle cells; assists many enzyme systems	**Toxicity:** nausea, vomiting, and diarrhea; dizziness, confusion; rapid heartbeat; organ damage; death **Deficiency:** iron-deficiency microcytic anemia, hypochromic anemia
Zinc RDA: Men = 11 mg/day Women = 8 mg/day UL = 40 mg/day	Meat/fish/poultry (best absorbed form of zinc), fortified cereals, legumes	Assists more than 100 enzyme systems; immune system function; growth and sexual maturation; gene regulation	**Toxicity:** nausea, vomiting, and diarrhea; headaches; depressed immune function; reduced absorption of copper **Deficiency:** growth retardation, delayed sexual maturation, eye and skin lesions, hair loss, increased incidence of illness and infection
Copper RDA: Adults = 900 µg/day UL = 10 mg/day	Shellfish, organ meats, nuts, legumes	Assists many enzyme systems; iron transport	**Toxicity:** nausea, vomiting, and diarrhea; liver damage **Deficiency:** anemia, reduceable levels of white blood cells, osteoporosis in infants and growing children

Note: RDA = Recommended Dietary Allowance; AI = Adequate Intakes; UL = Tolerable Upper Intake Level. Values are for all adults aged 19 and older, except as noted.
Source: Adapted from J. Thompson and M. Manore, *Nutrition: An Applied Approach*, 2nd ed., © 2009. Printed and electronically reproduced by permission of Pearson Education, Inc., Upper Saddle River, New Jersey.

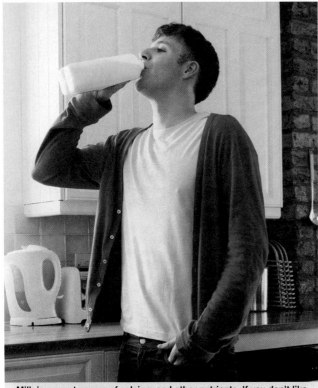

Milk is a great source of calcium and other nutrients. If you don't like milk or can't drink it, make sure to get enough calcium—at least 1,000 milligrams a day—through other sources.

Many dairy products are both excellent sources of calcium and fortified with vitamin D, which is known to improve calcium absorption.

Do you consume carbonated soft drinks? Be aware that the added phosphoric acid (phosphate) in these drinks can cause you to excrete extra calcium, which may result in calcium loss from your bones. One study of 2,500 men and women found that in women who consumed at least three cans of cola per week, even diet cola, bone density of the hip was 4 to 5 percent lower than in women who drank fewer than one cola per month. Colas did not seem to have the same effect on men.[27] There may also be a "milk displacement" effect, meaning that people who drank soda were not drinking milk, thereby decreasing their calcium intake.

Iron Worldwide, iron deficiency is the most common nutrient deficiency, affecting more than 2 billion people, nearly 30 percent of the world's population.[28] In the United States, iron deficiency is less prevalent, but it is still the most common micronutrient deficiency.[29] How much iron do we need? Women aged 19 to 50 need about 18 milligrams per day, and men aged 19 to 50 need about 8 milligrams.

Iron deficiency frequently leads to *iron-deficiency anemia*. **Anemia** results from the body's inability to produce hemoglobin (the oxygen-carrying component of the blood). When iron-deficiency anemia occurs, body cells receive less oxygen, and carbon dioxide wastes are removed less

efficiently. As a result, the iron-deficient person feels tired. Iron deficiency in the diet is not the only cause of anemia; anemia can also result from blood loss, cancer, ulcers, and other conditions.

Iron overload or iron toxicity due to ingesting too many iron-containing supplements is the leading cause of accidental poisoning in small children in the United States. Symptoms of toxicity include nausea, vomiting, diarrhea, rapid heartbeat, weak pulse, dizziness, shock, and confusion. Excess iron intake from high meat consumption, iron fortification, and supplementation has also been associated with other problems such as cardiovascular disease and cancer.[30]

How Can I Eat More Healthfully?

Americans today overall eat more food than ever before. From 1970 to 2010, average calorie consumption increased from 2,169 to 2,614 calories per day (see **Figure 9.5** on page 276).[31] In general, it isn't the actual amounts of food, but the number of calories in the foods we choose to eat that has increased. When these trends are combined with our increasingly sedentary lifestyle, it is not surprising that we have seen a dramatic rise in obesity.[32]

Two dietary tools have been created for consumers to make eating healthfully simple and easy: the Dietary Guidelines for Americans and the MyPlate Guidance System.

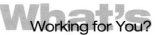

Working for You?

Maybe you already eat a healthful, balanced diet. Below are a few aspects of a healthful approach to eating. Which of these are you already incorporating into your life?

☐ I choose whole-grain breads and cereals.

☐ I try to avoid eating saturated fats.

☐ I limit my salt intake.

☐ I carry whole fruit with me for a snack during the day.

Dietary Guidelines for Americans, 2010

The Dietary Guidelines for Americans are a set of recommendations for healthy eating created by the U.S. Department of Health and Human Services and the USDA. These guidelines are revised every 5 years. The 2010 Dietary Guidelines for Americans are designed to help bridge the gap between the standard American diet and the key recommendations that

anemia Condition that results from the body's inability to produce hemoglobin.

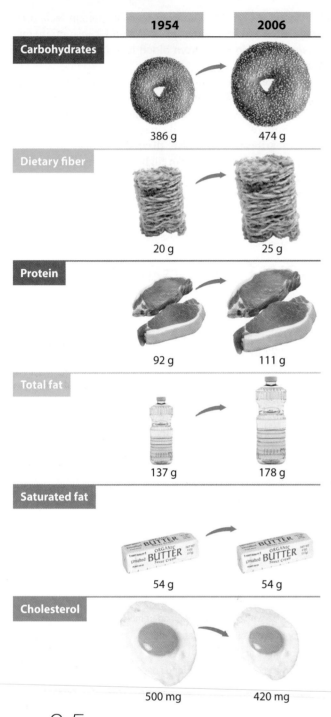

	1954	2006

Carbohydrates

386 g → 474 g

Dietary fiber

20 g → 25 g

Protein

92 g → 111 g

Total fat

137 g → 178 g

Saturated fat

54 g → 54 g

Cholesterol

500 mg → 420 mg

FIGURE 9.5 **Trends in Per Capita Nutrient Consumption**
Since 1954, Americans' daily caloric intake has increased by about 25%, as has daily consumption of carbohydrates, fiber, and protein. Daily total fat intake has increased by 30%.

Source: Data from USDA Economic Research Service, "Nutrient Availability," Updated August 2012, www.ers.usda.gov

aim to combat the growing obesity epidemic by balancing calories with adequate physical activity.[33] The dietary recommendations are transformed into an easy-to-follow graphic and guidance system called MyPlate, which can be found at www.choosemyplate.gov and is illustrated in **Figure 9.6.**

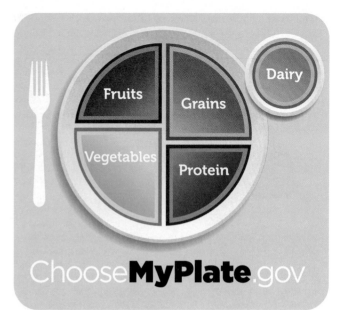

FIGURE 9.6 **MyPlate Plan**
The USDA MyPlate plan takes a new approach to dietary and exercise recommendations. Each colored section of the plate represents a food group. An interactive tool helps you analyze and track your foods and physical activity and provides helpful tips to personalize your plan.
Source: U.S. Department of Agriculture, 2011, www.choosemyplate.gov

MyPlate Food Guidance System

The MyPlate food guidance system takes into consideration the dietary and caloric needs of a wide variety of individuals, such as pregnant or breast-feeding women, those trying to lose weight, and adults with different activity levels. The interactive website www.choosemyplate.gov can create personalized dietary and exercise recommendations based on the individual information you enter.

MyPlate also encourages consumers to eat for health through three general areas of recommendation:

1. Balance calories:
- Enjoy your food, but eat less.
- Avoid oversized portions.

2. Increase foods:
- Make half your plate fruits and vegetables.
- Make at least half your grains whole.
- Switch to fat-free or 1% milk.

3. Reduce foods:
- Compare sodium in foods like soup, bread, and frozen meals—and choose the foods with lower numbers.
- Drink water instead of sugary drinks.

Understand Serving Sizes MyPlate presents personalized dietary recommendations in terms of numbers of servings of particular nutrients. But how much is one serving? Is it different from a portion? Although these two terms are often used interchangeably, they actually mean very different things. A *serving* is the recommended amount you should consume, whereas a *portion* is the amount you choose to eat at any one time. The saying "your eyes are bigger than your stomach" is rooted in truth—most of us select portions that are much bigger than recommended servings. See Figure 9.7 for a handy pocket guide with tips on recognizing serving sizes.

Unfortunately, we don't always get a clear picture from food producers and advertisers about what a serving really is. Consider a bottle of soda: The food label may list one serving size as 8 fluid ounces and 100 calories. However, note the size of the entire bottle: If the bottle holds 20 ounces, drinking the whole thing serves up 250 calories.

Eat Nutrient-Dense Foods Although eating the proper number of servings from MyPlate is important, it is also important to recognize that there are large caloric, fat, and energy differences among foods within a given food group. For example, fish and hot dogs provide vastly different nutrient levels per calorie. If you had a portion of fish and a portion of hot dogs, both containing the same amount of calories, the fish will provide less fat and more nutritional value than would the hot dogs, making it more nutrient dense. It is important to eat foods that have a high nutritional value for their caloric content.

Reduce Empty Calorie Foods Avoid *empty calories*, that is, high-calorie foods and drinks with little nutritional value. MyPlate recommends we limit sugar- and fat-laden items as part of a healthy diet, including the following:[34]

- **Cakes, cookies, pastries, and donuts:** Just one slice of chocolate cake contains 77 percent empty calories.
- **Sodas, energy drinks, sports drinks, and fruit drinks:** 12 fluid ounces of soda contains 192 calories or 100 percent empty calories.
- **Cheese:** Switching from whole milk mozzarella cheese to nonfat mozzarella cheese saves you 76 empty calories per ounce.
- **Pizza:** 1 slice of pepperoni pizza adds 139 empty calories to your meal.
- **Ice cream:** 76 percent of the 275 calories are empty calories.
- **Sausages, hot dogs, bacon, and ribs:** Adding a sausage link to your breakfast adds 96 empty calories.
- **Wine, beer, and all alcoholic beverages:** A whopping 155 empty calories are consumed with each 12 fluid ounces of beer.
- **Refined grains, including crackers, cookies, and white rice:** Switching from snack crackers to whole wheat can save you 25 fat laden empty calories per serving.

Physical Activity Strive to be physically active for at least 30 minutes daily, preferably with moderate to vigorous activity levels on most days. Physical activity does not mean you have to go to the gym, jog 3 miles a day, or hire a personal trainer. Any activity that gets your heart pumping (e.g., gardening, playing basketball, heavy yard work, and dancing) is a good way to get moving. MyPlate personalized plans

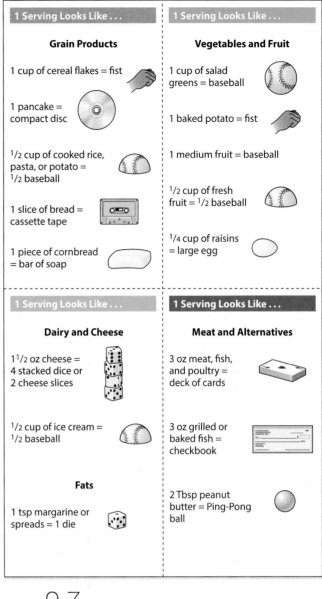

FIGURE 9.7 Serving Size Card
One of the challenges of following a healthy diet is judging how big a portion size should be and how many servings you are really eating. The comparisons on this card can help you recall what a standard food serving looks like. For easy reference, photocopy or cut out this card, fold on the dotted lines, and keep it in your wallet. You can even laminate it for long-term use.
Source: National Heart, Lung and Blood Institute, a department of National Institutes of Health, "Serving Size Card," Available at http://www.nhlbi.nih.gov

will offer recommendations for weekly physical activity. (For more on physical fitness, see **Chapter 11.**)

Choose Foods Wisely— Read the Labels

How do you know if the packaged foods you eat contain sufficient levels of any of the nutrients recommended as part of a healthy diet? To help consumers evaluate the nutritional

% Daily Value (%DV) The value on a food label that lets you know how much of a nutrient is provided by eating one serving of the food.

values of packaged foods, the FDA and the USDA developed the **% Daily Value (%DV)** that you can see on food and supplement labels. The %DV lets you know how a serving of food will contribute to the nutrient levels in your diet. The %DV values are calculated using a 2,000 calorie/day diet, so if your calorie needs differ, some of the %DV values may actually be different for you (lower if you need a higher calorie diet and higher if you need a lower calorie diet). In addition to the percentage of nutrients found in a serving of food, labels also include information on the serving size, calories, calories from fat per serving, and percentage of *trans* fats in a food. **Figure 9.8** walks you through a typical food label.

Food labels can contain other information as well, such as health claims. Health claims may assist you in selecting functional foods that meet your nutritional needs. The FDA allows for five types of health-related claims on food and dietary supplements:[35]

- **Nutrient content claims** that indicate a specific nutrient is present at a certain level. For example, a product might say "High in fiber" or "Low in fat" or "This product contains 100 calories per serving." Nutrient content claims can use the following words: *More, Less, Fewer, Good Source of, Free, Light, Lean, Extra Lean, High, Low, Reduced.*
- **Structure and function claims** that describe the effect that a dietary component has on the body. An example of a structure/function claim is "Calcium builds strong bones."
- **Dietary guidance claims** describe health benefits or health effects of a broad category of foods rather than a specific nutrient. An example is "Diets rich in fruits and vegetables may reduce the risks of some types of cancer."

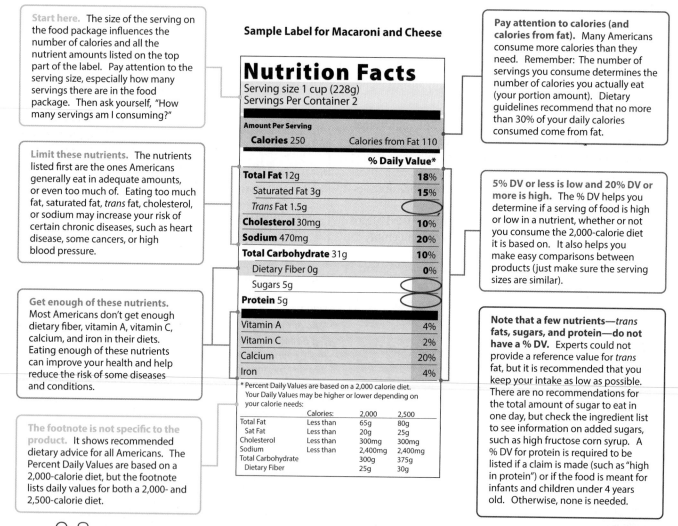

FIGURE 9.8 Reading a Food Label

Source: The U.S. Food and Drug Administration Center for Food Safety and Applied Nutrition, "A Key to Choosing Healthful Foods: Using the Nutrition Facts on the Food Label," Updated March 2013, www.fda.gov

Video Tutor: Understanding Food Labels

● **Qualified health claims** convey a relationship between diet and the risk for disease. These must be approved by the FDA and supported by scientific research. You will find qualified health claims about cancer risk, cardiovascular disease, cognitive function, diabetes, and hypertension, for example, "Diets low in *sodium* may reduce the risk of high blood pressure, a disease associated with many factors."

● **Health claims** confirm a relationship between components in the diet and the risk of disease or health. These must be approved by the FDA and supported by evidence. There are a number of health claims that are approved. For example, a whole-grain bread package may state, "In a low-fat diet, whole-grain foods like this bread may reduce the risk of heart disease."

Vegetarianism: A Healthy Diet?

According to a poll conducted by the Vegetarian Resource Group, more than 4 percent of U.S. adults, approximately 9 million people, are vegetarians.[36] Other surveys have shown that nearly 23 million Americans are "vegetarian inclined," or "flexitarians," meaning that they are omnivores who are trying to eat more vegetarian meals and are reducing meat consumption in favor of other "faceless" forms of protein.[37] The word **vegetarian** means different things to different people. Strict vegetarians, or *vegans*, avoid all foods of animal origin, including dairy products and eggs. Their diet is based on vegetables, grains, fruits, nuts, seeds, and legumes. Far more common are *lacto-vegetarians*, who eat dairy products but avoid flesh foods and eggs. *Ovo-vegetarians* add eggs to a vegan diet, and *lacto-ovo-vegetarians* eat both dairy products and eggs. *Pesco-vegetarians* eat fish, dairy products, and eggs, and *semivegetarians* eat chicken, fish, dairy products, and eggs. Some people in the semivegetarian category prefer to call themselves "non–red meat eaters."

Common reasons for pursuing a vegetarian lifestyle include concern for animal welfare, improving health, environmental concerns, natural approaches to wellness, food safety, weight loss, and weight maintenance. Generally, people who follow a balanced vegetarian diet weigh less and have better cholesterol levels, fewer problems with irregular bowel movements (constipation and diarrhea), and a lower risk of heart disease than do nonvegetarians. The benefits of vegetarianism also include a reduced risk of some cancers, particularly colon cancer, and a reduced risk of kidney disease.[38]

Although in the past vegetarians often suffered from vitamin deficiencies, most vegetarians today are adept at combining the right types of foods and eating a variety of different foods to ensure proper nutrient intake. Vegan diets may be deficient in vitamins B_2 (riboflavin), B_{12}, and D. Vegans are also at risk for deficiencies of calcium, iron, zinc, and other

minerals but can obtain these nutrients from supplements. Strict vegans have to pay much more attention to what they eat than the average person does, but by eating complementary combinations of plant products, they can receive adequate amounts of essential amino acids. In fact, whereas vegans typically get 50 to 60 grams of protein per day, lacto-ovo-vegetarians normally consume between 70 and 90 grams per day, well beyond the recommended amounts. Pregnant women, older adults, sick people, and children who are vegans need to take special care to ensure that their diets are adequate. In all cases, seek advice from a health care professional if you have questions.

vegetarian A person who follows a diet that excludes some or all animal products.

dietary supplements Vitamins and minerals taken by mouth that are intended to supplement existing diets.

what do you think?

Why are so many people becoming vegetarians?
● How easy is it to be a vegetarian on your campus?
● What concerns about vegetarianism would you be likely to have, if any?

Supplements: Research on the Daily Dose

Dietary supplements are products—usually vitamins and minerals—taken by mouth and intended to supplement existing diets. Ingredients range from vitamins, minerals, and herbs to enzymes, amino acids, fatty acids, and organ tissues.

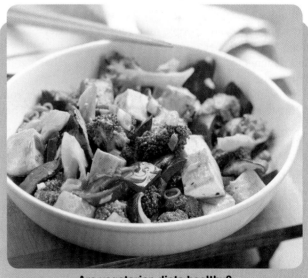

Are vegetarian diets healthy?

Adopting a vegetarian diet can be a very healthy way to eat. Take care to prepare your food healthfully by avoiding added sugars and excessive sodium. Make sure you get all the essential amino acids by eating meals like this tofu and vegetable stir-fry. To further enhance it, add a whole grain, such as brown rice.

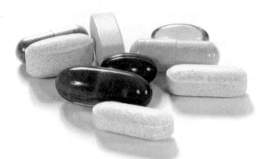

See It! Videos

How accurate are restaurant calorie counts? Watch **Menu Calorie Counts** in the Study Area of MasteringHealth™

They can come in tablet, capsule, liquid, powder, and other forms. Because of dietary supplements' potential for influencing health, their sales have skyrocketed.

It is important to note that all dietary supplements are not regulated like other food and drug products. The FDA does not evaluate the safety and efficacy of supplements prior to their marketing; it can take action to remove a supplement from the market only after it has been proved harmful. Currently, the United States has no formal guidelines for supplement sale and safety, and supplement manufacturers are responsible for self-monitoring their activities.

Do you really need to buy any of the myriad dietary supplements that are available? The Office of Dietary Supplements, part of the National Institutes of Health, states that some supplements may help ensure that you get adequate amounts of essential nutrients if you don't consume a variety of foods, as recommended in the Dietary Guidelines for Americans. However, dietary supplements are not intended to prevent or treat disease, and they should be used under the guidance of your health care provider.[39] Populations that may benefit from using supplements include pregnant and breast-feeding women, older adults, vegans, people on a very low-calorie weight–loss diet, alcohol-dependent individuals, and patients with malabsorption problems or other significant health problems.

Recently, researchers raised a concern about toxicity from taking high-dose supplements of fat-soluble vitamins. They recommended that the fat-soluble vitamins A, D, and E, as well as the B vitamins folic acid and niacin, be categorized as over-the-counter medications and that vitamin A should be removed from multivitamins.[40] The Academy of Nutrition and Dietetics recommends that, whereas there are benefits for some people in taking supplements, a healthy diet is the best way to give your body what it needs.[41]

Choosing Organic or Locally Grown Foods

organic Grown without use of pesticides, chemicals, or hormones.

locavore A person who primarily eats food grown or produced locally.

Concerns about food safety, genetically modified foods, and the health impacts of chemicals used in the growth and production of food have led many people to turn to foods that are **organic**—foods and beverages developed, grown, or raised without the use of synthetic pesticides, chemicals, or hormones. Any food sold in the United States as organic has to meet criteria set by the USDA under the National Organic Rule and can carry a USDA seal verifying products as "certified organic." Under this rule, a product that is certified may carry one of the following terms: "100 percent Organic" (100% compliance with organic criteria), "Organic" (must contain at least 95% organic materials), "Made with Organic Ingredients" (must contain at least 70% organic ingredients), or "Some Organic Ingredients" (contains less than 70% organic ingredients—usually listed individually). To be labeled with any of the above terms, the foods must be produced without hormones, antibiotics, herbicides, insecticides, chemical fertilizers, genetic modification, or germ-killing radiation. However, reliable monitoring systems to ensure credibility are still under development.

The market for organics has been increasing by more than 20 percent per year—five times faster than food sales in general. Whereas only a small subset of the population once bought organic, nearly all U.S. consumers now occasionally reach for something labeled organic. In 2011, annual organic food sales were estimated to be $31 billion.[42]

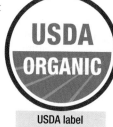

USDA label for organic foods.

Is eating organic food better for you, though? A review of the research published over the past 50 years found no evidence of a difference in nutrient quality of organic versus traditionally grown foods.[43] While pesticide residues do remain on conventionally grown produce, the USDA reports that the foods they tested contain much lower levels of pesticides than the tolerance levels set by the Environmental Protection Agency. The USDA report released in 2013 suggested these pesticide residues do not pose a safety concern. The USDA still advises, however, that consumers always rinse fruits and vegetables before cooking or consuming them.[44]

The word **locavore** has been coined to describe people who eat only food grown or produced locally, usually within close proximity to their homes. Farmers' markets or home-grown foods or those grown by independent farmers are thought to be fresher and to require far fewer resources to get them to market and keep them fresh for longer periods of time. Locavores believe that locally grown organic food is preferable to foods produced by large corporations or supermarket-based organic foods because they make a smaller impact on the environment. Although there are many reasons why organic farming is better for the environment, the fact that pesticides, herbicides, and other products are not used is perhaps the greatest benefit.

See It! Videos

Is organic produce better for you? Watch **Organic Produce** in the Study Area of MasteringHealth™

Eating Well in College

Many college students may find it hard to fit a well-balanced meal into the day, but eating breakfast and lunch are important if you are to keep energy levels up and get the most out of your classes. Eating a complete breakfast that includes complex carbohydrates, protein, and healthy, unsaturated fat (such as a banana, peanut butter, and whole-grain bread sandwich or a dry fruit and nut mix without added sugar or salt) is key. If you are short on time, you can bring these items to class to ensure that your meals fit into your day. Generally speaking, you can eat more healthfully and for less money if you bring food from home or your campus dining hall. However, if your campus is like many others, you've probably noticed a move toward fast-food restaurants in your student unions. If you must eat fast food, follow the tips below to get more nutritional bang for your buck:

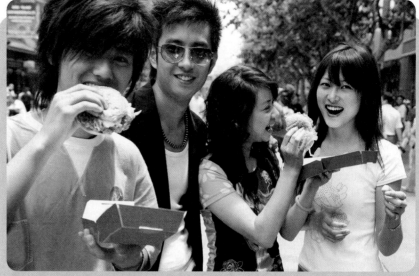

How can I eat well when I don't have enough time?

Fast food may be convenient, but it is high in fat, calories, sodium, and refined carbohydrates. Even when you are short on time and money, it is possible—and worthwhile—to make healthier choices. If you are ordering fast food, opt for foods prepared by baking, roasting, or steaming; ask for the leanest meat option; and request that sauces, dressings, and gravies be served on the side.

- Ask for nutritional analyses of items. Most fast-food chains now have them.
- Order salads, but be careful about what you add to them. Taco salads and Cobb salads are often high in fat, calories, and sodium. Ask for dressing on the side, and use it sparingly. Try the vinaigrette or low-fat dressings. Stay away from eggs and other high-fat add-ons, such as bacon bits, croutons, and crispy noodles.
- If you crave fries, try baked "fries," which may be lower in fat.
- Avoid giant sizes, and refrain from ordering extra sauce, bacon, cheese, dressings, and other extras that add additional calories, sodium, carbohydrates, and fat.
- Limit beverages and foods that are high in added sugars.
- At least once per week, swap a vegetable-based meat substitute into your fast-food choices.

In the dining hall, try these ideas:

- Choose lean meats, grilled chicken, fish, or vegetable dishes. Avoid fried chicken, fatty cuts of red meat, or meat dishes smothered in creamy or oily sauce.
- Hit the salad bar and load up on leafy greens, beans, tuna, or tofu. Choose items such as avocado or nuts for a little "good" fat. Go easy on the dressing, or substitute vinaigrette or low-fat dressings.
- Get creative. Choose items such as a baked potato with salsa, or add grilled chicken to your salad. Top toast with veggies, hummus, or grilled chicken or tuna.
- When choosing items from a made-to-order food station, ask the preparer to hold the butter or oil, mayonnaise, sour cream, or cheese- or cream-based sauces.
- Avoid going back for seconds and consuming large portions.
- Pass on high-calorie, low-nutrient foods such as sugary cereals, ice cream, and other sweet treats. Choose fruit or low-fat yogurt to satisfy your sweet tooth.

Maintaining a nutritious diet within the confines of student life can be challenging. However, if you take the time to

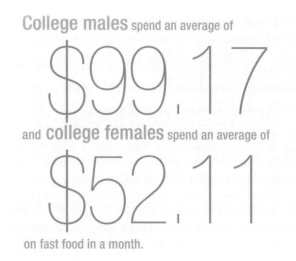

College males spend an average of

$99.17

and college females spend an average of

$52.11

on fast food in a month.

Do It! Nutritools

Ever wondered how your favorite meal stacks up, nutrition-wise? Complete the **Build a Meal, Build a Salad, Build a Pizza,** and **Build a Sandwich** activities in the Study Area of MasteringHealth™

Healthy Eating Simplified

When messages from nutrition experts, marketing campaigns, and media blitzes leave you scratching your head about what to eat, try following these simple tips for health-conscious eating:

❭ You don't need foods from fancy packages to improve your health. Fruits, vegetables, and whole grains should make up the bulk of your diet. Shop the perimeter of the store and shop the bulk foods aisle.

❭ Let the plate method guide you. Your plate should be half vegetables, a quarter lean protein, and a quarter whole grains/bread. A serving of fruit should be dessert.

❭ Avoid or limit processed foods/packaged foods. This will assist you in limiting added sodium, sugar, and fat. If you can't make sense of the ingredients, don't eat it.

❭ Eat natural snacks such as dried fruit, nuts, fresh fruits, string cheese, yogurt without added sugar, hard-boiled eggs, and vegetables.

❭ Be mindful of your eating. Eat until you are satisfied but not overfull.

❭ Bring healthful foods with you when you head out the door. Whether you go to class, on a road trip, or to work, you *can* control the foods that are available. Don't put yourself in a position to buy from a vending machine or convenience store.

Source: M. Pollan, *Food Rules: An Eater's Manual* (New York: Penguin Books, 2010).

plan healthy meals, you will find that you are eating better, enjoying it more, and actually saving money. The **Skills for Behavior Change** box boils down healthy eating into some simple tips to follow, and the **Money & Health** box on the following page examines ways to include fruits and vegetables in your diet without breaking the bank.

Food Safety: A Growing Concern

Eating unhealthy food is one thing. Eating food that has been contaminated with a pathogen, toxin, or other harmful substance is quite another. As outbreaks of foodborne illness (commonly known as food poisoning) make the news, the food industry has come under fire. The new Food Safety Modernization Act, passed into law in 2011, strengthens these safeguards and gives the FDA more authority to inspect food manufacturing facilities and to recall contaminated foods.[45]

Foodborne Illnesses

Are you concerned that the chicken you are buying doesn't look pleasingly pink or that your "fresh" fish smells a little *too* fishy? You may have good reason to be worried. In increasing numbers, Americans are becoming sick from what they eat, and many of these illnesses are life threatening. Scientists estimate that foodborne pathogens sicken 1 in 6 Americans, or 48 million people, and cause some 128,000 hospitalizations and 3,000 deaths in the United States annually.[46] These numbers have remained fairly constant since 2004, despite increased attention to prevention in the United States.[47] Because most of us don't go to the doctor every time we feel ill, we may not make a connection between what we eat and later symptoms.

Most foodborne infections and illnesses are caused by several common types of bacteria and viruses. Foodborne illnesses can also be caused by a toxin in food that was originally produced by a bacterium or other microbe in the food. These toxins can produce illness even if the microbes that produced them are no longer there. For example, botulism is caused by a deadly toxin produced by the bacterium *Clostridium botulinum*. This bacterium is widespread in soil, water, plants, and intestinal tracts, but it can grow only in environments with limited or no oxygen. Potential food sources include improperly canned food and vacuum-packed or tightly wrapped foods. Though rare, this illness is fatal if untreated, as the powerful neurotoxin causes paralysis and can lead to the cessation of breathing.

Signs of foodborne illnesses vary tremendously and usually include one or several symptoms: diarrhea, nausea,

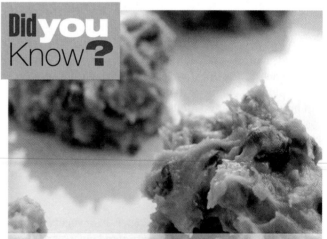

Did you Know?

In a survey conducted by the American Dietetic Association, college students indicated a high degree of confidence in their ability to handle food safely, yet, in the same survey 53% of students admitted to eating raw homemade cookie dough (which contains uncooked eggs, a potential source of salmonella), 33% said they ate fried eggs with soft or runny yolks, and 7% said they ate pink hamburger.

Source: Data from C. Byrd-Bredbenner et al., "Risky Eating Behaviors of Young Adults—Implications for Food Safety Education," *Journal of the American Dietetic Association* 108, no. 3 (2008): 549–552.

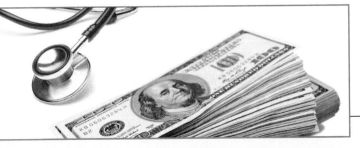

Money&Health

ARE FRUITS AND VEGGIES BEYOND YOUR BUDGET?

Many people on a tight budget, including college students, think that fruits and vegetables are beyond their budget. Maybe a carton of orange juice and a package of carrots are affordable, but five to nine servings a day? No way.

If that sounds like you, it's time for some facts. In 2011, the U.S. Department of Agriculture published data showing that the average American family spends more money on food than is necessary to consume a nutritious diet—one that includes the recommended servings of fruits and vegetables. The report concluded that, contrary to popular opinion, people on a tight budget can eat healthfully, including plenty of fruits and vegetables, and spend less on food.

So how do you do it? Here are some tips:

✳ Focus on five fresh favorites. Throughout the United States, five of the least expensive, perennially available fresh vegetables are carrots, eggplant, lettuce, potatoes, and summer squash. Five fresh fruit options are apples, bananas, pears, pineapple, and watermelon.

✳ Buy small amounts frequently. Most items of fresh produce keep only a few days, so buy amounts that you know you'll be able to eat or freeze.

✳ Celebrate the season. From apples to zucchini, when fruits and veggies are in season, they cost less. If you can freeze them, stock up. If not, enjoy them fresh while you can.

✳ Do it yourself. Avoid prewashed, precut fruits and vegetables, including salad greens. They cost more and often spoil faster. Also choose frozen 100% juice concentrate and add the water yourself.

✳ Buy canned or frozen on sale, in bulk. Canned and frozen produce, especially when it's on sale, may be much less expensive than fresh. Most frozen items are just as nutritious as fresh, and can be even more so, depending on how long ago the fresh food was harvested. For canned items, choose fruits without added sugars and vegetables without added salt or sauces. Bear in mind that beans are legumes and count as a vegetable choice. Low-sodium canned beans are one of the most affordable, convenient, and nutritious foods you can buy.

✳ Fix and freeze. Make large batches of homemade soup, vegetable stews, and pasta sauce and store them in single-serving containers in your freezer.

✳ Grow your own. All it takes is one sunny window, a pot, soil, and a packet of seeds. Lettuce, spinach, and fresh herbs are particularly easy to grow indoors in small spaces.

Sources: U.S. Department of Agriculture, "Eating Healthy on a Budget: The Consumer Economics Perspective," September 2011, www.choosemyplate .gov; U.S. Department of Agriculture, "Smart Shopping for Veggies and Fruits," Center for Nutrition Policy and Promotion, June 2011, www.choosemyplate.gov; U.S. Centers for Disease Control and Prevention, "30 Ways in 30 Days to Stretch Your Fruit & Vegetable Budget," Fruits & Veggies: More Matters, September 2011, www.fruitsandveggiesmatter.gov

---

cramping, and vomiting. Depending on the amount and virulence of the pathogen, symptoms may appear as early as 30 minutes after eating contaminated food or as long as several days or weeks later. Most of the time, symptoms occur 5 to 8 hours after eating and last only a day or two. For certain populations, such as the very young; older adults; or people with severe illnesses such as cancer, diabetes, kidney disease, or AIDS, foodborne diseases can be fatal.

Several factors may contribute to the increase in foodborne illnesses. The movement away from a traditional meat-and-potato American diet to heart-healthy eating—increasing consumption of fruits, vegetables, and grains—has spurred demand for fresh foods that are not in season most of the year. This means that we must import fresh fruits and vegetables, thus putting ourselves at risk for ingesting exotic pathogens or even pesticides that have been banned in the United States for safety reasons. Depending on the season, 34 percent of the imported fruits and vegetables consumed in the United States come from Mexico.[48] Although we are told when we travel to developing countries to "boil it, peel it, or don't eat it," we bring imported foods into our kitchens at home and eat them, often without even washing them.

Food can become contaminated by being watered with tainted water, fertilized with animal manure, picked by people who have not washed their hands properly after using the toilet, or by not being subjected to the same rigorous pesticide regulations as American-raised produce. To give you an idea of the implications, studies have shown that *Escherichia coli* can survive in cow manure for up to 70 days and can multiply in foods grown with manure unless heat or additives such as salt or preservatives are used to kill the microbes.[49] There are no regulations that prohibit farmers from using animal manure to fertilize crops. In addition, *E. coli* actually increases in summer months as cows await slaughter in crowded, overheated pens. This increases the chances of meat coming to market already contaminated.

Other key factors associated with the increasing spread of foodborne diseases include the inadvertent introduction

food allergy Overreaction by the body to normally harmless proteins, which are perceived as allergens. In response, the body produces antibodies, triggering allergic symptoms.

celiac disease An inherited autoimmune disorder affecting the digestive process of the small intestine and triggered by the consumption of gluten, a protein found in certain grains.

food intolerance Adverse effects resulting when people who lack the digestive chemicals needed to break down certain substances eat those substances.

of pathogens into new geographic regions and insufficient education about food safety. Globalization of the food supply, climate change, and global warming are also contributing factors.

Avoiding Risks in the Home

Part of the responsibility for preventing foodborne illness lies with consumers—more than 30 percent of all foodborne illnesses result from unsafe handling of food at home. Fortunately, consumers can take several steps to reduce the likelihood of contaminating their food. Among the most basic precautions are to wash your hands and to wash all produce before eating it. Also, avoid cross-contamination in the kitchen by using separate cutting boards and utensils for meats and produce. Temperature control is also important—refrigerators must be set at 40 degrees or less. Be sure to cook meats to the recommended temperature to kill contaminants before eating. Hot foods must be kept hot and cold foods kept cold in order to avoid unchecked bacterial growth. Eat leftovers within 3 days, and if you're unsure how long something has been sitting in the fridge, don't take chances. When in doubt, throw it out. See the **Skills for Behavior Change** box for more tips about reducing risk of foodborne illness when shopping for and preparing food.

Food Sensitivities

About 33 percent of people today *think* they have an allergy or avoid a certain food because they think they are allergic to it; however, it is estimated that only 4 to 8 percent of children and 2 percent of adults have a true food allergy. Still, there may be reason to be concerned. The prevalence of reported food allergies is on the rise. Data suggests the prevalence of peanut allergies among children tripled between 1997 and 2008.[50]

A **food allergy,** or hypersensitivity, is an abnormal response to a food that is triggered by the immune system. Symptoms of an allergic reaction vary in severity and may include a tingling sensation in the mouth; swelling of the lips, tongue, and throat; difficulty breathing; hives; vomiting; abdominal cramps; diarrhea; drop in blood pressure; loss of consciousness; and death. Approximately 150 deaths per year occur from anaphylaxis (the acute systemic immune and inflammatory response) that occurs with allergic reactions. These symptoms may appear within seconds to hours after eating the foods to which one is allergic.[51]

The Food Allergen Labeling and Consumer Protection Act (FALCPA) requires food manufacturers to label foods clearly to indicate the presence of (or possible contamination by) any of the eight major food allergens: milk, eggs, peanuts, wheat, soy, tree nuts (walnuts, pecans, etc.), fish, and shellfish. Although over 160 foods have been identified as allergy triggers, these 8 foods account for 90 percent of all food allergies in the United States.[52]

Celiac disease is an inherited autoimmune disorder that affects digestive activity in the small intestine. Affecting over 3 million Americans, most of whom are undiagnosed, it is a growing problem, particularly for those under the age of 20.[53] When a person with celiac disease consumes gluten, a protein found in wheat, rye, and barley, the person's immune system attacks the small intestine and stops nutrient absorption. Pain, cramping, and other symptoms often follow in the short term. Untreated, celiac disease can lead to other health problems, such as osteoporosis, nutritional deficiencies, and cancer. Once a person is diagnosed with celiac disease, the best treatment is to avoid breads, pastas, and other foods containing gluten.

Food intolerance can cause you to have symptoms of digestive upset, but the upset is not the result of an immune system response. Probably the best example of a food intolerance is *lactose intolerance,* a problem that affects about 1

Skills for Behavior Change

Reduce Your Risk for Foodborne Illness

❭ When shopping for fish, buy from markets that get their supplies from state-approved sources; check for cleanliness at the salad bar and at the meat and fish counters.

❭ Keep most cuts of meat, fish, and poultry in the refrigerator no more than 1 or 2 days. Check the shelf life of all products before buying. Use the sniff test—if fish smells really fishy, don't eat it.

❭ Use a meat thermometer to ensure that meats are completely cooked. Beef and lamb steaks and roasts should be cooked to at least 145°F; ground meat, pork chops, ribs, and egg dishes to 160°F; ground poultry and hot dogs to 165°F; chicken and turkey breasts to 170°F; and chicken and turkey legs, thighs, and whole birds to 180°F. Fish is done when the thickest part becomes opaque and the fish flakes easily when poked with a fork.

❭ Never leave cooked food standing on the stove or table for more than 2 hours.

❭ Never thaw frozen foods at room temperature. Put them in the refrigerator for a day to thaw or thaw in cold water, changing the water every 30 minutes.

❭ Wash your hands and countertop with soap and water when preparing food, particularly after handling meat, fish, or poultry.

❭ When freezing chicken or other raw foods, make sure juices can't spill over into ice cubes or into other areas of the refrigerator.

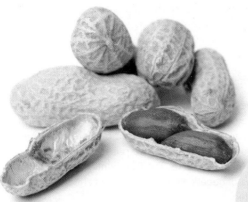

Genetically Modified Food Crops

Genetic modification involves the insertion or deletion of genes into the DNA of an organism. In the case of **genetically modified (GM) foods**, this genetic cutting and pasting is done to enhance production; for example, by making disease- or insect-resistant plants, improving yield, or controlling weeds. In addition, GM foods are sometimes created to improve the color and appearance of foods or to enhance specific nutrients. For example, in regions where rice is a staple and vitamin A deficiency and iron-deficiency anemia are leading causes of morbidity and mortality, GM technology has been used to create varieties of rice high in vitamin A and iron. Another use under development is the production and delivery of vaccines through GM foods.

> **genetically modified (GM) foods**
> Foods derived from organisms whose DNA has been altered using genetic engineering techniques.

U.S. farmers have widely accepted GM crops.[55] Soybeans and cotton are the most common GM crops, followed by corn. On our supermarket shelves, an estimated 75 percent of processed foods are genetically modified.[56]

The long-term safety of GM foods is still a big question. In one report, three strains of maize (corn) showed signs of causing liver and kidney toxicity, but these claims have been refuted by producers.[57] However, unintentional transfer of potentially allergy-provoking proteins has occurred, and rigorous, validated tests of crops are necessary to protect allergic consumers.[58] But according to the World Health Organization, no effects on human health have been shown from consumption of GM foods in countries that have approved their use.[59] The debate surrounding GM foods is not likely to end soon; see the **Points of View** box on page 286 for more on this debate.

> **Peanuts** are among the eight most common food allergens: 1.4% of the general population are allergic to them, with higher rates in children.

in every 10 adults. Lactase is an enzyme in the lining of the gut that degrades the sugar lactose, which is in dairy products. If you don't have enough lactase, you cannot digest lactose, and it remains in the gut to be used by bacteria. Gas is formed, and you experience bloating, abdominal pain, and sometimes diarrhea. Populations in which fresh milk consumption continues into adulthood typically have rates of lactose intolerance as low as 2 to 3 percent, whereas 80 percent or more of non–milk-drinking populations are lactose intolerant.[54] Food intolerance also occurs in response to some food additives, such as the flavor enhancer MSG, certain dyes, sulfites, gluten, and other substances. In some cases, the food intolerance may have psychological triggers.

If you suspect that you have an actual allergic reaction to food, see an allergist to be tested to determine the source of the problem. Because several diseases share symptoms with food allergies (ulcers and cancers of the gastrointestinal tract can cause vomiting, bloating, diarrhea, nausea, and pain), clinical diagnosis is essential.

Genetically Modified Foods:
BOON OR BANE?

Genetically modified crop farming is expanding rapidly around the world. State governments, industry, and scientists tout the benefits of genetically modified foods for health, agriculture, and the ecosystem, including feeding the world's population. In contrast, consumer activists, environmental organizations, religious groups, and health advocates, warn of unexpected health risks and environmental and socioeconomic consequences. Consumers question whether genetically modified plants are safe to eat and if they pose dangers to conventional crops. They have urged the Food and Drug Administration to update labeling regulations similar to legislation proposed by more than 12 states. None of these state initiatives have passed, including the 2012 Proposition 37 in California. The FDA continues to evaluate the safety issues of genetically modified foods and future regulations to protect the world's food supply.

Below are some of the main points for and against the development of GM food.

Arguments for the Development of GM Foods

○ People have been manipulating food crops—primarily through selective breeding—since the beginning of agriculture. Genetic modification is fundamentally the same thing, just more precise.

○ Genetically modified seeds and products are tested for safety, and there has never been a substantiated claim for a human illness resulting from consumption of a GM food.

○ Genetically modified crops can have a positive impact on the environment. Current agricultural practices are very environmentally damaging, whereas insect- and weed-resistant GM crops will allow farmers to use far fewer chemical insecticides and herbicides.

○ Genetically modified crops have the potential to reduce world hunger: They can be created to grow more quickly than conventional crops, increasing productivity and allowing for faster cycling of crops, which means more food yield. In addition, nutrient-enhanced crops can address malnutrition, and crops engineered to resist spoiling or damage can allow for transportation to areas affected by drought or natural disaster.

Arguments against the Development of GM Foods

○ Genetic modification is fundamentally different from and more problematic than selective breeding because it transfers genes between species in ways that could never happen naturally.

○ There haven't been enough independent studies of GM products to confirm that they are safe for consumption. Also, there are potential health risks if GM products approved for animal feed or other uses are mistakenly or inadvertently used in the production of food for human consumption.

○ The use of GM crops cannot be completely controlled, so they have the potential to damage the environment. Inadvertent cross-pollination could lead to the creation of "super weeds"; insect-resistant crops could harm insect species that are not pests; and insect- and disease-resistant crops could prompt the evolution of even more virulent species, which would then require more aggressive control measures, such as the increased use of chemical sprays.

○ Because corporations create and patent GM seeds, they will control the market, meaning that poor farmers in the developing world would become reliant on these corporations. This circumstance would be more likely to increase world hunger than to alleviate it.

Where Do You Stand?

○ Do you think GM foods are more helpful or harmful?

○ What are your greatest concerns over GM foods? What do you think are their greatest benefits?

○ In what ways could the creators of GM foods address the concerns of those opposed to them?

○ What sort of regulation do you think the government should have with regard to the creation, cultivation, and sale of GM foods?

○ Currently, there are no GM livestock; however, many livestock are fed GM feed or feed that includes additives and vaccines produced by GM microorganisms. Do you feel any differently about directly consuming GM crops versus eating the flesh, milk, or eggs of an animal that has been fed on GM crops?

○ If scientists were to develop GM livestock, would that alter your stance on any of these questions?

How Healthy Are Your Eating Habits?

1 Keep Track of Your Food Intake

Keep a food diary for 5 days, writing down everything you eat or drink. Be sure to include the approximate amount or portion size. Add up the number of servings from each of the major food groups on each day and enter them into the chart below.

Number of Servings:						
	Day 1	Day 2	Day 3	Day 4	Day 5	Average
Fruits						
Vegetables						
Grains						
Protein Foods						
Dairy						
Fats and Oils						
Sweets						

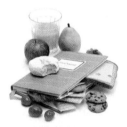

1A Does Your Diet Have Proportionality?

	Yes	No
1. Are grains the main food choice at all your meals?	○	○
2. Do you often forget to eat vegetables?	○	○
3. Do you typically eat fewer than three pieces of fruit daily?	○	○
4. Do you often have fewer than 3 cups of milk daily?	○	○
5. Is the portion of meat, chicken, or fish the largest item on your dinner plate?	○	○

Scoring 1A

If you answered yes to three or more of these questions, then your diet probably lacks proportionality. Review the recommendations in this chapter, particularly the MyPlate guidelines, to learn how to balance your diet.

2 Evaluate Your Food Intake

Now compare your consumption patterns to the MyPlate recommendations. Look at **Table 9.1** (page 262) and **Figure 9.6** (page 276) and visit www.choosemyplate.gov to evaluate your daily caloric needs and the recommended consumption rates for the different food groups. How does your diet match up?

	Less than the recommended amount	About equal to the recommended amount	More than the recommended amount
1. How does your daily fruit consumption compare to the recommendation for you?	○	○	○
2. How does your daily vegetable consumption compare to the recommendation for you?	○	○	○
3. How does your daily grain consumption compare to the recommendation for you?	○	○	○
4. How does your daily protein food consumption compare to the recommendation for you?	○	○	○
5. How does your daily dairy food consumption compare to the recommendation for you?	○	○	○
6. How does your daily calorie consumption compare to the recommendation for your age and activity level?	○	○	○

Scoring 2

If you found that your food intake is consistent with the MyPlate recommendations, congratulations! If you are falling short in a major food group or are overdoing it in certain categories, consider taking steps to adopt healthier eating habits. Following are some additional assessments to help you figure out where your diet is lacking.

2A Are You Getting Enough Fat-Soluble Vitamins in Your Diet?

	Yes	No
1. Do you eat at least 1 cup of deep yellow or orange vegetables, such as carrots and sweet potatoes, or dark green vegetables, such as spinach, every day?	◯	◯
2. Do you consume at least two glasses (8 ounces each) of milk daily?	◯	◯
3. Do you eat a tablespoon of vegetable oil, such as corn or olive oil, daily? (Tip: Salad dressings, unless they are fat free, count!)	◯	◯
4. Do you eat at least 1 cup of leafy green vegetables in your salad and/or put lettuce in your sandwich every day?	◯	◯

Scoring 2A

If you answered yes to all four questions, you are on your way to acing your fat-soluble vitamin needs! If you answered no to any of the questions, your diet needs some fine-tuning. Deep orange and dark green vegetables are excellent sources of vitamin A, and milk is an excellent choice for vitamin D. Vegetable oils provide vitamin E, and if you put them on top of your vitamin K–rich leafy green salad, you'll hit the vitamin jackpot.

2B Are You Getting Enough Water-Soluble Vitamins in Your Diet?

	Yes	No
1. Do you consume at least 1/2 cup of rice or pasta daily?	◯	◯
2. Do you eat at least 1 cup of a ready-to-eat cereal or hot cereal every day?	◯	◯
3. Do you have at least one slice of bread, a bagel, or a muffin daily?	◯	◯
4. Do you enjoy a citrus fruit or fruit juice, such as an orange, a grapefruit, or orange juice every day?	◯	◯
5. Do you have at least 1 cup of vegetables throughout your day?	◯	◯

Scoring 2B

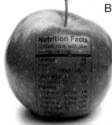

If you answered yes to all of these questions, you are a vitamin B and C superstar! If you answered no to any of the questions, your diet could use some refinement. Rice, pasta, cereals, bread, and bread products are all excellent sources of B vitamins. Citrus fruits are a ringer for vitamin C. In fact, all vegetables can contribute to meeting your vitamin C needs daily.

Source: J. S. Blake, K. D. Munoz, and S. Volpe, *Nutrition and You*, 1st ed., © 2010. Reprinted and electronically reproduced by permission of Pearson Education, Inc., Upper Saddle River, New Jersey.

YOUR PLAN FOR CHANGE

The **Assess yourself** activity gave you the chance to evaluate your current nutritional habits. Now that you have considered these results, you can decide whether you need to make changes in your daily eating for long-term health.

Today, you can:

◯ Start keeping a more detailed food log. The easy-to-use SuperTracker at www.supertracker.usda.gov can help you keep track of your food intake and analyse what you eat. Take note of the nutritional content of the foods you eat, and write down the details about the number of calories, grams of fat, grams of sugar, milligrams of sodium, and so on of each food. Try to find specific weak spots: Are you consuming too many calories or too much salt or sugar? Does what you eat contain too little calcium or iron? Use the SuperTracker to plan a healthier food intake to overcome these weak spots.

◯ Take a field trip to the grocery store. Forgo your fast-food dinner and instead spend time in the produce section of the supermarket. Purchase your favorite fruits and vegetables, and try something new to expand your tastes.

Within the next 2 weeks, you can:

◯ Plan at least three meals that you can make at home or in your dorm room, and purchase the ingredients you'll need ahead of time. Something as simple as a chicken sandwich on whole-grain bread will be more nutritious, and probably cheaper, than heading out for a fast-food meal.

◯ Start reading labels. Be aware of the amount of calories, sodium, sugars, and fats in prepared foods; aim to buy and consume prepared foods that are lower in all of these and higher in calcium and fiber.

By the end of the semester, you can:

◯ Get in the habit of eating a healthy breakfast every morning. Combine whole grains, proteins, and fruit in your breakfast—for example, eat a bowl of cereal with milk and bananas or a cup of yogurt combined with granola and berries. Eating a healthy breakfast will jump-start your metabolism, prevent drops in blood glucose levels, and keep your brain and body performing at their best through your morning classes.

◯ Commit to one or two healthful changes to your eating patterns for the rest of the semester. You might resolve to eat five servings of fruits and vegetables every day, switch to low-fat or nonfat dairy products, stop drinking soft drinks, or use only olive oil in your cooking. Use your food diary to help you spot places where you can make healthier choices on a daily basis.

MasteringHealth™

Build your knowledge—and health!—in the Study Area of MasteringHealth with a variety of study tools.

Summary

* Nutrition is the science of the relationship between physiological function and the essential elements of the foods we eat.

* The essential nutrients include water, proteins, carbohydrates, fats, vitamins, and minerals. Water makes up 50 to 70 percent of our body weight and is necessary for nearly all life processes. Proteins are major components of our cells and are key elements of antibodies, enzymes, and hormones. Carbohydrates are our primary sources of energy. Fats play important roles in maintaining body temperature, cushioning and protecting organs, and promoting healthy cell function. Vitamins are organic compounds, and minerals are inorganic compounds. We need both in relatively small amounts to promote growth and maintain healthy body function.

* A healthful diet is adequate, moderate, balanced, varied, and nutrient dense. The Dietary Guidelines for Americans and the MyPlate plan provide guidelines for healthy eating. These recommendations, developed by the USDA, place emphasis on balancing calories and understanding which foods to increase and which to decrease. Vegetarianism can provide a healthy alternative for people wishing to eat less or no meat. Although some people may benefit from taking vitamin and mineral supplements, a healthy diet is the best way to give your body the nutrients it needs.

* Food labels provide information on the serving size, as well as the number of calories in a serving, amounts of various nutrients in a serving, and the percentage of recommended daily values those amounts represent.

* Organic foods are grown and produced without the use of synthetic pesticides, chemicals, or hormones. The USDA offers certification of organics.

* College students face unique challenges in eating healthfully. Learning to make better choices at fast-food restaurants and to eat nutritionally in the campus cafeteria is possible when you use the information in this chapter.

* Food safety and health concerns are becoming increasingly important to health-wise consumers. Recognizing potential risks and taking steps to prevent problems are part of a sound nutritional plan.

Pop Quiz

1. What is the most crucial nutrient for life?
   a. Water
   b. Fiber
   c. Minerals
   d. Starch

2. Which of the following nutrients are most important for the repair and growth of body tissue?
   a. Carbohydrates
   b. Proteins
   c. Vitamins
   d. Fats

3. Which of the following nutrients moves food through the digestive tract?
   a. Water
   b. Fiber
   c. Minerals
   d. Starch

4. What substance plays a vital role in maintaining healthy skin and hair, insulating body organs against shock, maintaining body temperature, and promoting healthy cell function?
   a. Fats
   b. Fibers
   c. Proteins
   d. Carbohydrates

5. Triglycerides make up about ___ percent of total body fat.
   a. 5
   b. 35
   c. 55
   d. 95

6. Which of the following fats is a healthier fat to include in the diet?
   a. *Trans* fat
   b. Saturated fat
   c. Unsaturated fat
   d. Hydrogenated fat

7. Which vitamin maintains bone health?
   a. B_{12}
   b. D
   c. B_6
   d. Niacin

8. What is the most common nutrient deficiency worldwide?
   a. Fat deficiency
   b. Iron deficiency
   c. Fiber deficiency
   d. Calcium deficiency

9. Which of the following foods would be considered a healthy, *nutrient-dense* food?
   a. Nonfat milk
   b. Cheddar cheese
   c. Soft drink
   d. Potato chips

10. Carrie eats dairy products and eggs, but she does not eat fish or red meat. Carrie is considered a(n)
    a. vegan.
    b. lacto-ovo-vegetarian.
    c. ovo-vegetarian.
    d. pesco-vegetarian.

Answers to these questions can be found on page A-1.

Think about It!

1. What factors have been the greatest influences on your eating behaviors?
2. What does the MyPlate graphic look like? Approximately what percent of the plate is taken up by each food group? What can you do to increase or decrease your intake of selected food groups?
3. What are the major types of nutrients? What happens if you fail to get enough of some of them? Are there significant differences between men and women in particular areas of nutrition?
4. Distinguish between the different types of vegetarianism. Which types are most likely to lead to nutrient deficiencies? What can be done to ensure that vegetarians receive enough of the major nutrients?
5. What are the major problems that many college students face when trying to eat the right foods? List five actions that you and your classmates could take immediately to improve your eating.
6. What are the major risks for food-borne illnesses, and what can you do to protect yourself?
7. How do food intolerances differ from true food allergies?

Accessing Your Health on the Internet

The following websites explore further topics and issues related to personal health. For links to these websites, visit the Study Area in MasteringHealth.

1. *Academy of Nutrition and Dietetics (ANA).* The ANA provides information on a full range of dietary topics, including sports nutrition, healthful cooking, and nutritional eating; the site also links to scientific publications and information on scholarships and public meetings. www.eatright.org
2. *U.S. Food and Drug Administration (FDA).* The FDA provides information for consumers and professionals in the areas of food safety, supplements, and medical devices. www.fda.gov
3. *Food and Nutrition Information Center.* This site offers a wide variety of information related to food and nutrition. http://fnic.nal.usda.gov
4. *National Institutes of Health: Office of Dietary Supplements.* This is the site of the International Bibliographic Database of Information on Dietary Supplements (IBDIDS), updated quarterly. http://ods.od.nih.gov
5. *U.S. Department of Agriculture (USDA).* The USDA offers a full discussion of the USDA's *Dietary Guidelines for Americans.* www.usda.gov
6. *U.S. Department of Agriculture, USDA: Choose MyPlate.* This is the home of *Choose MyPlate,* a visual representation and interactive site that promotes the five food groups to encourage healthy eating. www.choosemyplate.gov

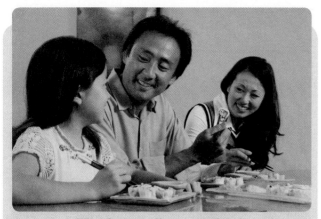

What factors affect my weight?

Many factors help determine weight and body type, including heredity and genetic makeup, environment, and learned eating patterns, which are often connected to family habits.

Metabolic Rates Several aspects of your metabolism also help determine whether you gain, maintain, or lose weight. Each of us has an innate energy-burning capacity called **basal metabolic rate (BMR)**, the minimum rate at which the body uses energy to maintain basic vital functions. A BMR for the average, healthy adult is usually between 1,200 and 1,800 calories per day. Technically, to measure BMR, a person would be awake, but all major stimuli (including stressors to the sympathetic nervous system and digestion) would be at rest. Usually, the best time to measure BMR is after 8 hours of sleep and after a 12-hour fast.

A more practical way of assessing your energy expenditure levels is the **resting metabolic rate (RMR).** Slightly higher than the BMR, the RMR includes the BMR plus any additional energy expended through daily sedentary activities such as food digestion, sitting, studying, or standing. The **exercise metabolic rate (EMR)** accounts for the remaining percentage of all daily calorie expenditures and refers to the energy expenditure that occurs during physical activity. For most of us, these calories come from light daily activities, such as walking, climbing stairs, and mowing the lawn.

Your BMR (and RMR) fluctuates throughout your life, and it is highest during infancy, puberty, and pregnancy. Generally the younger you are, the higher your BMR, partly because cells undergo rapid subdivision during periods of growth, and that consumes lots of energy. After age 30, a person's BMR slows down 1 to 2 percent a year, and older people commonly find they must work harder to burn off an extra helping of ice cream. Slower BMR, coupled with less activity, age-related muscle loss, and priorities shifting from fitness to family obligations or career, contribute to the weight gain of many middle-aged people.

Some sources indicate the brain's hypothalamus—the structure that regulates appetite—signals hunger when levels of certain nutrients in the blood fall. According to one theory, the monitoring system in obese people does not work properly, so the desire to eat is more frequent and intense than in normal-weight individuals. Another theory is that thin people send more effective messages to the hypothalamus. This concept, called **adaptive thermogenesis,** states that thin people can consume large amounts of food without gaining weight because the appetite center of their brains speeds up metabolic activity to compensate for consumption.

> **basal metabolic rate (BMR)** The rate of energy expenditure by a body at complete rest in a neutral environment.
>
> **resting metabolic rate (RMR)** The energy expenditure of the body under BMR conditions plus other daily sedentary activities.
>
> **exercise metabolic rate (EMR)** The energy expenditure that occurs during exercise.
>
> **adaptive thermogenesis** Theoretical mechanism by which the brain regulates metabolic activity according to caloric intake.

may increase risks of obesity in individuals.[17] New research indicates that people with certain genetic variations may tend to graze for food more often, eat more meals, and consume more calories every day, as well as display patterns of seeking out high-fat food groups.[18] This doesn't mean those who struggle with weight are doomed to be overweight or obese. If genes make you crave certain foods, you may be able to reduce your genetic risk by consciously changing certain eating behaviors. Another study found that the effects of an obesity-linked gene are diminished among physically active adults. Individuals who exercised 90 minutes per day seemed to be beating their genetically enhanced obesity tendency, compared to those who exercised a half hour daily.[19]

One potential genetic basis for obesity comes from observational studies of certain Native American and African tribes. Labeled by researchers as the *thrifty gene theory*, they note higher body fat and obesity levels in some of these tribes today than in the general population.[20] Researchers theorize that because the current tribe's ancestors struggled through centuries of famine, they appear to have survived by adapting metabolically to periods of famine with slowed metabolism. Over time, ancestors may have passed on a genetic, hormonal, or metabolic predisposition toward fat storage that makes losing fat more difficult. If this thrifty gene hypothesis is true, certain people may be genetically programmed to burn fewer calories. Nevertheless, there is growing consensus that only 2 to 5 percent of childhood obesity cases are caused by a defect that impairs function in a gene; common forms of childhood obesity seem to result from obesogenic behaviors in an obesogenic environment.[21]

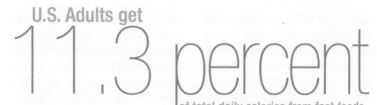

U.S. Adults get **11.3 percent** of total daily calories from fast foods.

On the other side of the BMR equation is the **set point theory,** which proposes that our bodies fight to maintain weight around a narrow range or set fat point. If we go on a drastic starvation diet or fast, BMR slows to conserve energy. Set point theory suggests our bodies may sabotage weight loss efforts by holding on to calories. This would have been very helpful for human survival during days of famine, but in food-rich modern society, it exacerbates the problem of obesity. The good news is that set points can be changed; however, these changes may take time to become permanent. Healthy diet, steady weight loss, and exercise appear to be the best methods of sustaining weight loss.

Yo-yo diets are when people cycle between periods when they lose pounds and then gain them back. When dieters resume eating after weight loss, BMR is reset lower due to earlier calorie restrictions, making it almost certain that they will regain the pounds they just lost. Repeated cycles of dieting and regaining weight may actually promote the trend of people getting heavier and heavier over time.

Hormonal Influences: Ghrelin and Leptin

Obese people may be more likely than thin people to satisfy their appetite and eat for reasons other than nutrition.[22] In some instances, the problem with overconsumption may be related more to **satiety** than it is to appetite or hunger. People generally feel satiated, or full, when they have satisfied their nutritional needs and their stomach signals "no more."

Over the years, many people have attributed obesity to thyroid gland problems and resultant hormone imbalances that cause fatigue, impede the way calories burn and energy is used, and a number of other functions. Many experts now believe that less than 2 percent of the obese population actually have thyroid issues.[23] Today, researchers realize that several other hormones, dietary proteins, and other chemicals can also affect caloric expenditure and a person's ability to lose weight, control appetite, and sense fullness. More research on the thyroid-obesity connection as well as how hormones may interact to affect energy balance is necessary.

One hormone produced in the stomach that researchers suspect may influence satiety and play a role in keeping weight off is *ghrelin,* sometimes referred to as "the hunger hormone." Researchers at the University of Washington studied a small group of obese people who had lost weight over a 6-month period.[24] They noted ghrelin levels rose before every meal and fell drastically shortly afterward, suggesting that the hormone plays a role in appetite stimulation. Since that early research, ghrelin has been shown to be an important growth hormone that plays a key role in the regulation of appetite and food intake control, gastrointestinal motility,

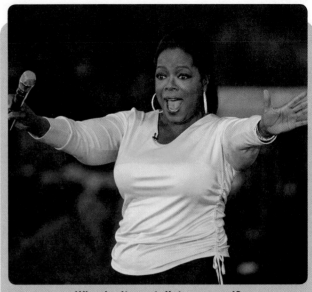

Why don't most diets succeed?

Just about any calorie-cutting diet can produce weight loss in the short term, often through water-weight loss. However, without improved nutrition and sustained exercise and activity, lost weight will return and the overall dieting process will have failed.

gastric acid secretion, endocrine and exocrine pancreatic secretions, glucose and lipid metabolism, and cardiovascular and immunological processes.[25]

Another hormone gaining increased attention and research is *leptin*—an appetite regulator produced by fat cells in mammals. As fat tissue increases, levels of leptin in the blood increase, and when leptin blood levels rise, appetite drops. Scientists believe leptin serves as a satiety signal, telling the brain when you are full.[26] For unknown reasons, obese people seem to have faulty leptin receptors, although it may be that environmental cues are stronger than biological signals in some individuals.

Fat Cells and Predisposition to Fatness

Some obese people may have excessive numbers of fat cells. Whereas an average-weight adult has approximately 25 to 35 billion fat cells and a moderately obese adult 60 to 100 billion, an extremely obese adult has as many as 200 billion.[27] This type of obesity, **hyperplasia,** usually appears in early childhood and perhaps, due to the mother's dietary habits, even prior to birth. The most critical periods for the development of hyperplasia are the last 2 to 3 months of fetal development, the first year of life, and the period between ages 9 and 13. Central to this theory is the belief that the number of fat cells in a body does not increase appreciably during adulthood. However, the ability of each of these cells to swell **(hypertrophy)** and shrink does carry over into adulthood. People with large numbers of fat cells may be able to lose weight by decreasing the size of each cell in adulthood, but with the next calorie binge, the cells swell

set point theory Theory that a form of internal thermostat controls our weight and fights to maintain this weight around a narrowly set range.

yo-yo diets Cycles in which people diet and regain weight.

satiety The feeling of fullness or satisfaction at the end of a meal.

hyperplasia A condition characterized by an excessive number of fat cells.

hypertrophy The act of swelling or increasing in size, as with cells.

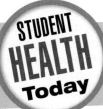
BEWARE OF PORTION INFLATION AT RESTAURANTS

Would you be surprised to learn that today's serving portions are significantly larger than those of past decades? From burgers and fries to meat-and-potato or pasta meals, today's popular restaurant foods dwarf their earlier counterparts. For example, a 25-ounce prime rib dinner served at one steak chain contains nearly 3,000 calories and 150 grams of fat! That's almost twice as many calories and more than three times the fat that most adults need in a whole day, and it's just the meat part of the meal.

Many researchers believe that the main reason Americans are gaining weight is that people no longer recognize a normal serving size. "Biggie" size has become the new normal for many, with larger sizes equated with better value. The National Heart, Lung, and Blood Institute has developed a pair of "portion distortion" quizzes that show how today's portions compare with those of 20 years ago. Test yourself online at http://hp2010.nhlbihin .net/portion to see whether you can guess the differences between today's meals and those previously considered normal.

To make sure you're not over-eating when you dine out, follow these strategies:

* Order the smallest size available. Focus on taste, not quantity. Get used to eating less, eating slowly, and enjoying what you eat.
* Take your time, and let your fullness indicator have a chance to kick in while there is still time to quit.
* Dip your food in dressings, gravies, and sauces on the side rather than pouring these extra calories over the top.
* Order an appetizer as your main meal and order a small size salad or veggie to add nutritional value.
* Split your main entrée with a friend, and order a side salad for each of you. Alternatively, order a take out box immediately, put one half of your meal in it to eat another day and finish the rest at the restaurant.
* Avoid buffets and all-you-can-eat establishments. If you go to them, use

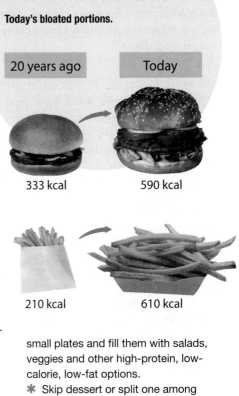

Today's bloated portions.

20 years ago	Today
333 kcal	590 kcal
210 kcal	610 kcal

small plates and fill them with salads, veggies and other high-protein, low-calorie, low-fat options.
* Skip dessert or split one among several people.

---

and sabotage weight-loss efforts. Weight gain may be tied to both the number of fat cells in the body and the capacity of individual cells to enlarge.

Environmental Factors

Environmental factors have come to play a large role in weight maintenance. Automobiles, remote controls, desk jobs, and long sessions on computers and other devices all cause us to sit more and move less, and this lack of physical activity causes a decrease in energy expenditure. Time our grandparents may have spent going for a walk after dinner is now more frequently devoted to watching television, playing video games, texting, or reading online. Coupled with our culture of eating more, it's a recipe for weight gain.

Greater Access to High-Calorie Foods More foods that are high in calories and low in nutrients exist today compared to the past. There are many environmental factors that can prompt us to consume them:

● Advertising constantly bombards us with messages that promote eating—emphasizing good taste over the poor nutritional value of most of what is being sold.
● Super-sized portions are now the norm (see the **Student Health Today** box above), as larger dishes, cups, and serving utensils mask serving sizes and lead to increased calorie and fat intake.
● Drinks like lattes and extra large sodas add many extra calories.
● Families have increased reliance on restaurant and store-bought convenience foods, which tend to be higher in calories than food made from scratch.
● Bottle-feeding infants may increase energy intake relative to breast-feeding.
● Misleading food labels confuse consumers about serving sizes.
● Fast-food restaurants, cafes, vending machines, and quick-stop markets are everywhere, offering easy access to food at all hours.

The good news is that between the years 2003 and 2010 Americans consumed nearly 75 fewer calories per day than during the previous decade. Some believe that a greater awareness of the perils of consuming too many high-sugar soft drinks and beverages has caused people to eat fewer calories. Others worry that we should be seeing weight loss if we are consuming fewer calories. One possibility is that we are exercising less than ever, thereby offsetting any potential weight loss.[28]

Early Sabotage: A Youthful Start on Obesity

Children have always loved junk food. However, today's youth have easy access to a vast array of high-fat, high-calorie foods, exercise less, have fewer physical education requirements in schools, and are more obese than ever before. Over 17 percent of all children and adolescents are now obese, and rates are three times higher than for their parent's generation.[29] Sedentary activities such as social media sites, video games, and television have replaced vigorous physical play for many, and school policies have also been a factor in the growth of childhood obesity. For decades the trend was to eliminate recess and physical education classes while cafeterias were much more likely to serve students pizza and fries than healthy food. The classic American suburb, with its high-speed roads and lack of sidewalks, has also impacted childhood obesity. Even when parks or schools are near home, it may be too dangerous for children to walk to them.

In addition, youth are at risk because of factors that are only beginning to be understood. Several studies have suggested that maternal nutrition, diabetes, and obesity—particularly where there is high fat consumption during pregnancy—may play a role in predisposing the fetus to becoming overweight or obese prior to puberty and early onset puberty.[30] Research also shows that race and ethnicity seem to be intricately interwoven with environmental factors in increasing risks to young people.[31]

On top of potential physical problems of obesity, obese kids often face weight-related stigma and vicious comments about their size from their peers. Obesity stigma is a major threat to overweight and obese children's self-esteem; it increases risk of suicidal thoughts, anxiety, and depression, contributes to low grades in school, and decreases likelihood of physical activity. Obese youth may feel a lack of social acceptance, be bullied by classmates, and develop feelings of mistrust and fear of others.[32]

Psychosocial and Socioeconomic Factors

The relationship of weight problems to emotional insecurities, needs, and wants remains difficult to assess. What we do know is that eating tends to be a focal point of people's lives and is in part a social ritual associated with companionship, celebration, and enjoyment. It can also be used to soothe fears, sadness, and worry—hence the term *comfort food*. What's more, your weight can even be linked to your friends and partners (see the **Student Health Today** box on the following page). The psychosocial aspect of the eating experience can be a major obstacle to successful weight control.

Socioeconomic status can have a significant effect on risk for obesity. When tough economic times hit, people tend to eat more inexpensive, high-calorie foods. People living in poverty may live in communities with less access to fresh, nutrient-dense foods and have less time to cook nutritious meals owing to shiftwork, longer commutes, or multiple jobs.[33] Additionally, unsafe neighborhoods and poor infrastructure, such as lack of sidewalks or parks, can make it difficult for less-affluent people to exercise.[34]

Lack of Physical Activity

Although heredity, metabolism, and environment all have an impact on weight management, the increasingly high rate of overweight and obesity in the past decades is largely due to the way we live our lives. In general, Americans are eating more and moving less than ever before, and becoming overfat as a result. Weight management can be much harder when it feels like a chore (the **Skills for Behavior Change** box on the following page offers some ideas for making exercising and healthy eating more fun).

Although the many advertisements for sports equipment and the popularity of athletes may give the impression that Americans love a good workout, for many, moderate or high-levels of physical activity are rare events. One big problem in determining real activity levels of Americans is that data are largely based on self-reporting, and people tend to overestimate their daily exercise level

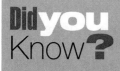

Did you Know?

Obesity has increased dramatically among U.S. youth in the last three decades, nearly tripling previous rates. Over one in six children is obese and one out of every three children are overweight or obese. Young boys are more likely to be obese than girls (19 percent versus 15 percent) and Hispanic and black youth have the highest rates of obesity overall (at 21 % and 24 % respectively).

Source: C. L. Ogden et al., "Prevalence of Obesity and Trends in Body Mass Index among U.S. Children and Adolescents, 1999–2010," *Journal of the American Medical Association* 307 (2012): 483–490.

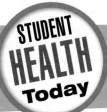

STUDENT HEALTH Today

Do Overfat Family and Friends Influence Your Weight?

According to some research, young adults who are overweight or obese tend to befriend and date people who are similarly sized and also tend to have more overweight relatives. It remains unknown whether this occurs because overweight people attract more overweight friends or because someone of healthy weight gains pounds as he or she socializes with overweight friends or partners.

It makes sense that we are more likely to become overweight if the behaviors of those around us reinforce it through high calorie intake

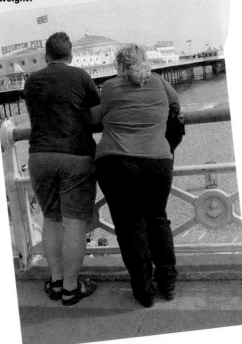

Does who you "hang out" with affect your weight?

and little physical activity. The upside, according to the study's author, is that younger people seem to be influenced by the weight-loss intentions of their social networks as well. By focusing on common goals and engaging friends as potential supporters, you may be able to increase your chances of weight-loss success.

Source: T. Leahey et al., "Social Influences Are Associated with BMI and Weight Loss Intentions in Young Adults," *Obesity* 19, no. 6 (2011): 1157–1162, doi:10.1038/oby.2010.301

Skills for Behavior Change

Finding the Fun in Healthy Eating and Exercise

With a little creativity, you can make healthy weight control a fun, positive part of your life that you look forward to:

❱ Cook and eat with friends. You can share the responsibility for making the meal while you spend time with people you like.

❱ Experiment with new foods: Try one new food or dish each week—variety is the spice of life!

❱ Invite an international student over for dinner and cook together.

❱ Vary your exercise routine: Either change the exercise itself or change your location. Even small changes can breathe life into an old routine.

❱ Try something new: Join a team for the social aspects in addition to exercise, or decide to run a long foot race for the challenge, or learn how to skateboard for fun.

and intensity. There is also a hodgepodge of terminology for determining activity levels, and more than one fitness measure, so defining yourself as "active" can mean very different things for different people. Data from the National Health Interview Survey show that over one third of U.S. adults never engage in any leisure time physical activity (sessions of light or moderate physical activity that last at least 10 minutes). Women are less active than men (33.2 percent vs. 29.9 percent). Inactivity is highest among non-Hispanic blacks (41.2 percent) and Hispanic adults (42.2 percent).[35]

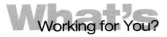

What's Working for You?

Perhaps you've already adopted some habits that help with weight management. Which of the following do you do?

☐ I try to listen to my body's cues, and stop eating when I'm full.

☐ I eat five to seven servings of vegetables a day.

☐ I get out for a walk or a jog three or four times a week.

☐ I eat desserts only when I have extra calories to "spend."

Assessing Body Weight and Body Composition

Everyone has his or her own ideal weight, based on individual variables such as body structure, height, and fat distribution. Traditionally, experts used measurement techniques such as height–weight tables to determine whether an individual was at ideal weight, overweight, obese, or morbidly obese. However, these charts can mislead because they fail to take body composition—that is, a person's ratio of fat to lean muscle—or fat distribution into account. For example, many extremely muscular athletes would be considered overweight based on traditional height–weight charts, whereas women might think their weight is normal based on charts, only to be shocked to discover that 35 to 40 percent of their weight is body fat! More accurate measures of evaluating healthy weight and disease risk focus on a person's percentage of body fat, and how that fat is distributed in his or her body.

Many people worry about becoming fat, but some fat is essential for healthy body functioning. Fat regulates body temperature, cushions and insulates organs and tissues, and is the body's main source of stored energy. Body fat is composed of two types: essential fat and storage fat. *Essential fat* is that fat necessary for maintenance of life and reproductive functions. *Storage fat,* the nonessential fat that many of us try to shed, makes up the remainder of our fat reserves. Being *underweight,* or having extremely low body fat, can cause a host of problems, including hair loss, visual disturbances, skin problems, a tendency to fracture bones easily, digestive system disturbances, heart irregularities, gastrointes-

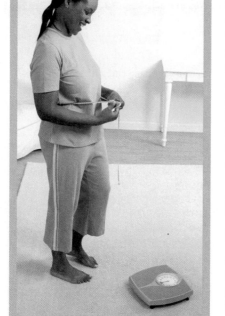

How can I tell if I am overweight or overfat?

Observing the way you look and how your clothes fit can give you a general idea of whether you weigh more or less than in the past. But in order to really evaluate how your weight and body fat might affect your personal health risks, it's best to use more scientific measures, such as BMI, waist circumference, waist-to-hip ratio, or a technician-administered body composition test.

tinal problems, difficulties in maintaining body temperature, and loss of menstrual period in women. Since the early 1960s, the percentages of underweight adults aged 20 to 74 has declined in men (2.2 to 1.0 percent) and women (5.7 to 2.5 percent) as percentages of overweight and obesity have increased. Nearly 3.5 percent of children and adolescents are underweight.[36] (See **Focus On: Enhancing Your Body Image** on page 318 for an in-depth discussion of eating disorders and body image issues.)

Body Mass Index (BMI)

Although people have a general sense that BMI is an indicator of how "fat" a person is, most do not really know that it is not a direct assessment of "fatness." Instead, **body mass index (BMI)** is a description of body weight relative to height—numbers that are highly correlated with your total body fat.

Find your BMI in inches and pounds using **Figure 10.4** on the following page, or calculate your BMI now by dividing your weight in kilograms by height in meters squared. The mathematical formula is

$$\text{BMI} = \text{weight (kg)}/\text{height squared (m}^2)$$

A BMI calculator is also available at the National Heart, Lung, and Blood Institute's website at http://nhlbisupport.com/bmi/bmicalc.htm.

Desirable BMI levels may vary with age and by sex; however, most BMI tables for adults do not account for such variables. *Healthy weights* are defined as those with BMIs of 18.5 to 24.9, the range of lowest statistical health risk.[37] BMIs below 18.5 indicate **underweight.** A BMI of 25 to 29.9 indicates **overweight** and potentially significant health risks. A BMI of 30 or above is classified as **obese,** whereas a BMI of 40 or higher is **morbidly obese.**[38] Nearly 3 percent of obese men and almost 7 percent of obese women are morbidly obese.[39] A new category for BMI of 50 or higher, known as **super obese,** has been added to obesity designations.[40]

Limitations of BMI Like other assessments of fatness, BMI has its limitations. Water, muscle, and bone mass are not included in BMI calculations, and BMI levels don't account for the fact that muscle weighs more than fat, meaning a well-muscled person could weigh enough to be classified as obese according to his or her BMI. For people who are under 5 feet tall or are older and have little muscle mass, BMI levels can also be inaccurate. Although a combination

body mass index (BMI) A number calculated from a person's weight and height that is used to assess risk for possible present or future health problems.

underweight Having a body weight more than 10 percent below healthy recommended levels; in an adult, having a BMI below 18.5.

overweight Having a body weight more than 10 percent above healthy recommended levels; in an adult, having a BMI of 25 to 29.9.

obesity A body weight more than 20 percent above healthy recommended levels; in an adult, a BMI of 30 or more.

morbidly obese Having a body weight 100 percent or more above healthy recommended levels; in an adult, having a BMI of 40 or more.

super obese Having a body weight that is 150 pounds or more above healthy recommended levels; in an adult, having a BMI of 50 or more.

BMI	17	18	18.5	19	20	21	22	23	24	25	26	27	28	29	30	31	32	33	34	35	36	37	38	39	40	41	42
Height														**Weight in pounds**													
4'10"	81	86	89	91	96	100	105	110	115	119	124	129	134	138	143	148	153	158	162	167	172	177	181	186	191	196	201
4'11"	84	89	92	94	99	104	109	114	119	124	128	133	138	143	148	153	158	163	168	173	178	183	188	193	198	203	208
5'	87	92	95	97	102	107	112	118	123	128	133	138	143	148	153	158	163	168	174	179	184	189	194	199	204	209	215
5'1"	90	95	98	100	106	111	116	122	127	132	137	143	148	153	158	164	169	174	180	185	190	195	201	206	211	217	222
5'2"	93	98	101	104	109	115	120	126	131	136	142	147	153	158	164	169	175	180	186	191	196	202	207	213	218	224	229
5'3"	96	102	104	107	113	118	124	130	135	141	146	152	158	163	169	175	180	186	191	197	203	208	214	220	225	231	237
5'4"	99	105	108	110	116	122	128	134	140	145	151	157	163	169	175	180	186	192	197	204	209	215	221	227	232	238	244
5'5"	102	108	111	114	120	126	132	138	144	150	156	162	168	174	180	186	192	198	204	210	216	222	228	234	240	246	252
5'6"	105	112	115	118	124	130	136	142	148	155	161	167	173	179	186	192	198	204	210	216	223	229	235	241	247	253	260
5'7"	109	115	118	121	127	134	140	146	153	159	166	172	178	185	191	198	204	211	217	223	230	236	242	249	255	261	268
5'8"	112	118	122	125	131	138	144	151	158	164	171	177	184	190	197	204	210	216	223	230	236	243	249	256	262	269	276
5'9"	115	122	125	128	135	142	149	155	162	169	176	182	189	196	203	210	216	223	230	236	243	250	257	263	270	277	284
5'10"	119	126	129	132	139	146	153	160	167	174	181	188	195	202	209	216	222	229	236	243	250	257	264	271	278	285	292
5'11"	122	129	133	136	143	150	157	165	172	179	186	193	200	208	215	222	229	236	243	250	257	265	272	279	286	293	301
6'	125	133	136	140	147	154	162	169	177	184	191	199	206	213	221	228	235	242	250	258	265	272	279	287	294	302	309
6'1"	129	137	140	144	151	159	166	174	182	189	197	204	212	219	227	235	242	250	257	265	275	280	288	295	302	310	318
6'2"	132	140	144	148	155	163	171	179	186	194	202	210	218	225	233	241	249	256	264	272	280	287	295	303	311	319	326
6'3"	136	144	148	152	160	168	176	184	193	200	208	216	224	232	240	248	256	264	272	279	287	295	303	311	319	327	335
6'4"	140	148	152	156	164	172	180	189	197	205	213	221	230	238	246	254	263	271	279	287	295	304	312	320	328	336	344

| Under-weight BMI <18.5 | Healthy weight BMI 18.5–24.9 | | | | | | | Overweight BMI 25–29.9 | | | | | Obese BMI 30–39.9 | | | | | | | | | | | Extreme obesity BMI ≥40 | | |

FIGURE 10.4 **Body Mass Index (BMI)**

Locate your height, read across to find your weight, then scan up to determine your BMI. Chart colors indicate if your BMI is considered healthy, overweight, obese, or morbidly obese.

Source: National Institutes of Health/National Heart, Lung, and Blood Institute (NHLBI), *Evidence Report of Clinical Guidelines on the Identification, Evaluation, and Treatment of Overweight and Obesity in Adults,* 1998, www.nhlbi.nih.gov

of measures might be most reliable in assessing fat levels, researchers conclude that as a quick, fairly inexpensive measure, BMI continues to be an a useful and valid tool for developing basic health recommendations.[41]

Youth and BMI Today over 17 percent of youth in America are obese—three times higher than rates in the 1980s.[42]

Although the labels *obese* and *morbidly obese* have been used for years for adults, there is growing concern about the long-term consequences of pinning these potentially stigmatizing labels on children.[43] BMI ranges above a normal weight for children and teens are often labeled differently, as "at risk of overweight" and "overweight," to avoid the sense of shame such words may cause. In addition, BMI ranges for children and teens are defined so that they take into account normal differences in body fat between boys and girls and the differences in body fat that occur at various ages. Specific guidelines for calculating youth BMI are available at the Centers for Disease Control and Prevention website, www.cdc.gov.

Waist Circumference and Ratio Measurements

Knowing where your fat is carried may be more important than knowing how much you carry. Men and postmenopausal women tend to store fat in the upper regions of the body, particularly in the abdominal area. Premenopausal women usually store fat in the lower regions of their bodies, like the hips, buttocks, and thighs. Waist circumference measurement is a useful tool in assessing abdominal fat, which is considered more threatening to health than fat in other regions of the body. In particular, as waist circumference increases, there is a greater risk for diabetes, cardiovascular disease, and stroke.[44] A waistline greater than 40 inches (102 centimeters) in men and 35 inches (88 centimeters) in women may be particularly indicative of greater health risk.[45] If a person is less than 5 feet tall or has a BMI of 35 or above, waist circumference standards used for the general population might not apply.

waist-to-hip ratio Waist circumference divided by hip circumference; a high ratio indicates increased health risks due to unhealthy fat distribution.

The **waist-to-hip ratio** measures regional fat distribution. A waist-to-hip ratio greater than 1 in men and 0.8 in women indicates increased health risks.[46] Waist-to-hip ratios have been used extensively in the past, and the popularity of this technique is increasing. It is relatively inexpensive and accurate and provides some of the same advantages as BMI and waist circumference measurements.

Measures of Body Fat

There are numerous ways besides BMI calculations and waist measurements to assess whether your body fat levels are too high. One low-tech way is simply to look in the mirror or consider how your clothes fit now compared with how they fit last year. More accurate techniques are also available, several of which are described in Figure 10.5 on the following page. These methods usually involve the help of a skilled professional and typically must be done in a lab or clinical setting.

Although opinion varies somewhat, most experts agree that men's bodies should contain between 8 and 20 percent total body fat, and women should be within the range of 20 to 30 percent (see Table 10.1). Generally, men who exceed 22 percent body fat and women who exceed 35 percent are considered overweight, but these ranges vary with age and stages of life. In addition, there are percentages of body fat below which a person is considered underweight, and health is compromised. In men, this lower limit is approximately

TABLE 10.1 | Body Fat Percentage Norms for Men and Women*

Men Age	Very Lean	Excellent	Good	Fair	Poor	Very Poor
20–29	<7%	7%–10%	11%–15%	16%–19%	20%–23%	>23%
30–39	<11%	11%–14%	15%–18%	19%–21%	22%–25%	>25%
40–49	<14%	14%–17%	18%–20%	21%–23%	24%–27%	>27%
50–59	<15%	15%–19%	20%–22%	23%–24%	25%–28%	>28%
60–69	<16%	16%–20%	21%–22%	23%–25%	26%–28%	>28%
70–79	<16%	16%–20%	21%–23%	24%–25%	26%–28%	>28%

Women Age	Very Lean	Excellent	Good	Fair	Poor	Very Poor
20–29	<14%	14%–16%	17%–19%	20%–23%	24%–27%	>27%
30–39	<15%	15%–17%	18%–21%	22%–25%	26%–29%	>29%
40–49	<17%	17%–20%	21%–24%	25%–28%	29%–32%	>32%
50–59	<18%	18%–22%	23%–27%	28%–30%	31%–34%	>34%
60–69	<18%	18%–23%	24%–28%	29%–31%	32%–35%	>35%
70–79	<18%	18%–24%	25%–29%	30%–32%	33%–36%	>36%

*Assumes nonathletes. For athletes, recommended body fat is 5 to 15 percent for men and 12 to 22 percent for women. Please note that there are no agreed-upon national standards for recommended body fat percentage.
Source: Based on data from the Cooper Institute, Dallas TX, www.cooperinstitute.org

Underwater (hydrostatic) weighing:
Measures the amount of water a person displaces when completely submerged. Fat tissue is less dense than muscle or bone, so body fat can be computed within a 2%–3% margin of error by comparing weight underwater and out of water.

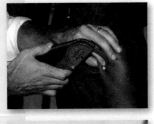

Skinfolds:
Involves "pinching" a person's fold of skin (with its underlying layer of fat) at various locations of the body. The fold is measured using a specially designed caliper. When performed by a skilled technician, it can estimate body fat with an error of 3%–4%.

Bioelectrical impedance analysis (BIA):
Involves sending a very low level of electrical current through a person's body. As lean body mass is made up of mostly water, the rate at which the electricity is conducted gives an indication of a person's lean body mass and body fat. Under the best circumstances, BIA can estimate body fat with an error of 3%–4%.

Dual-energy X-ray absorptiometry (DXA):
The technology is based on using very-low-level X ray to differentiate between bone tissue, soft (or lean) tissue, and fat (or adipose) tissue. The margin of error for predicting body fat is 2%–4%.

Bod Pod:
Uses air displacement to measure body composition. This machine is a large, egg-shaped chamber made from fiberglass. The person being measured sits in the machine wearing a swimsuit. The door is closed and the machine measures how much air is displaced. That value is used to calculate body fat, with a 2%–3% margin of error.

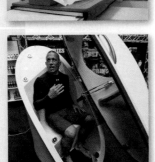

FIGURE 10.5 **Overview of Various Body Composition Assessment Methods**
Source: Adapted from J. Thompson and M. Manore, *Nutrition: An Applied Approach,* 2nd edition, © 2009. Printed and electronically reproduced by permission of Pearson Education, Inc., Upper Saddle River, New Jersey.

3 to 7 percent of total body weight and in women it is approximately 8 to 15 percent.

Before undergoing any body composition or body fat assessment, make sure you understand the expense, potential for accuracy, risks, and training of the tester. Also, consider why you are seeking this assessment and what you plan to do with the results.

See It! Videos
A new strategy to keep off the weight? Watch **Keeping It Off** in the Study Area of
MasteringHealth™

Managing Your Weight

At some point in our lives, almost all of us will decide to lose weight or modify our diet. Many will have mixed success. Failure is often related to thinking about losing weight in terms of short-term "dieting" rather than adjusting long-term eating behaviors (such as developing the habit of healthy snacking; see the **Skills for Behavior Change** box below). There is no magic cure for years of overconsumption. Careful attention to portions, healthy choices from all of the food groups, and regular exercise are the best options for sustained weight loss. If you see diets that allow unlimited quantities of certain foods, like the egg or grapefruit diet—beware! Although fad and low-calorie diets often produce significant immediate weight loss, they are often difficult to maintain and almost always result in regained weight. Repeated bouts of restrictive dieting may be physiologically harmful; moreover, the sense of failure we ex-

Tips for Sensible Snacking

❭ **Keep healthy munchies around.** Buy 100 percent whole-wheat breads, and if you need something to spice that up, use low-fat or soy cheese, low-fat cream cheese, peanut butter, hummus, or other healthy favorites. Some baked crackers or chips are low in fat and calories and high in fiber. Look for these on your grocery shelves. Look for 100-calorie individual packages to help you with portion control

❭ **Keep "crunchies" on hand.** Apples, pears, green pepper sticks, popcorn, carrots, and celery all are good choices. Wash the fruits and vegetables and cut them up to carry with you; eat them when a snack attack comes on.

❭ **Quench your thirst with hot drinks.** Hot tea, heated milk, plain or decaffeinated coffee, hot chocolate made with nonfat milk or water, or soup broths will help keep you satisfied.

❭ **Choose natural beverages.** Drink plain water, 100 percent juice in small quantities, or other low-sugar choices to satisfy your thirst. Avoid juices, energy drinks, and soft drinks that have added sugars, low fiber, and no protein. Avoid supersizing anything you put in your mouth.

❭ **Eat nuts instead of candy or high-calorie energy bars.** Although nuts are relatively high in calories, they are also loaded with healthy fats and make a healthy snack when consumed in moderation.

❭ **If you must have a piece of chocolate, keep it small.** Dark chocolate is better than milk chocolate or white chocolate because of its antioxidant content.

TRACK YOUR DIET AND ACTIVITY: THERE'S AN APP FOR THAT!

A recent study found people who kept detailed food journals lost more weight than people who did not. In the past, keeping a physical journal could be a pain, but today there are many diet-tracking applications for smart phones available for free or low cost. The best programs combine food and physical activity logs, so if you splurge on dessert, you can figure out how many miles you'll need to jog to burn it off. These apps often feature calculators for determining daily calorie intake goals as well as barcode scanners that allow you to quickly add packaged foods to your log. In some cases, the apps include discussion boards where you can talk about weight loss or fitness with other users.

Here are a few options worth trying:

* **Lose It!** (Free) www.loseit.com
* **MyFitnessPal Calorie Counter & Diet Tracker.** (Free) www.myfitnesspal.com
* **Restaurant Weight Loss.** (Free for restricted version and modest cost for full version) http://ellisapps.com
* **MyNetDiary.** (Free trial of basic version, and modest cost for full features) www.mynetdiary.com

Source: A. Kong et al., "Self-monitoring and Eating-Related Behaviors Are Associated with 12-Month Weight Loss in Postmenopausal Overweight-to-Obese Women," *Journal of the Academy of Nutrition and Dietetics* 112, no. 9 (2012): 1428–1435. Link to www.MyNetDiary.com courtesy of My Net Diary.com.

---

perience each time we don't meet our goal can exact far-reaching psychological costs. Drugs and intensive counseling can contribute to weight loss, but even then, many people regain weight after treatment. Maintaining a healthful body takes constant attention and nurturing over the course of your lifetime.

Improving Your Eating Habits

Before you can change a behavior, you must first determine what causes (or "triggers") it. When it comes to unhealthy eating habits, many people find it helpful to keep a chart of their eating patterns: when they feel like eating, where they are when they decide to eat, the amount of time they spend eating, other activities they engage in during the meal (watching television or reading), whether they eat alone or with others, what and how much they consume, and how they felt before they took their first bite. If you keep a detailed daily log of eating triggers for at least a week, you will discover useful clues about what in your environment or your emotional makeup causes you

"Why Should I Care?"

It may be easy to grab a fast-food meal and go, but unless you are very physically active, your body will likely store that super-sized meal as fat, which is anything but easy to lose. Remember—it takes only 3,500 unused calories to create a pound of body fat, so eating 500 extra calories a day—less than the average hamburger—can lead to a pound of weight gain in just a week's time.

85% **of customers** consuming weight-loss products and services are female.

to want food. Many people eat compulsively when stressed; however, for other people, the same circumstances diminish their appetite. See **Figure 10.6** on the following page for ways you can adjust your eating triggers and snack more healthfully in order to manage your weight.

Once you have evaluated your behaviors and determined your triggers, you can begin to devise a plan for improved eating that is nutritious and easy to follow. If you are unsure of where to start, seek assistance from reputable sources, such as the MyPlate plan at www.choosemyplate.gov. Registered dietitians, some physicians (not all doctors have a strong background in nutrition), health educators and exercise physiologists with nutritional training, and other health professionals can provide reliable information. Beware of people who call themselves nutritionists or nutritional life "coaches." There is no such official credential for these titles. Check the formal nutritional credentials of people who want to give advice. Avoid weight-loss programs that promise quick, "miracle" results or that are run by "trainees," often people with short courses on nutrition and exercise who are designed to sell products or services. (See the **Tech & Health** box above for tips on more tools you can use to stay in control of your consumption).

Assess the nutrient value of any prescribed diet; verify that dietary guidelines are consistent with reliable nutrition research; and analyze the suitability of the diet

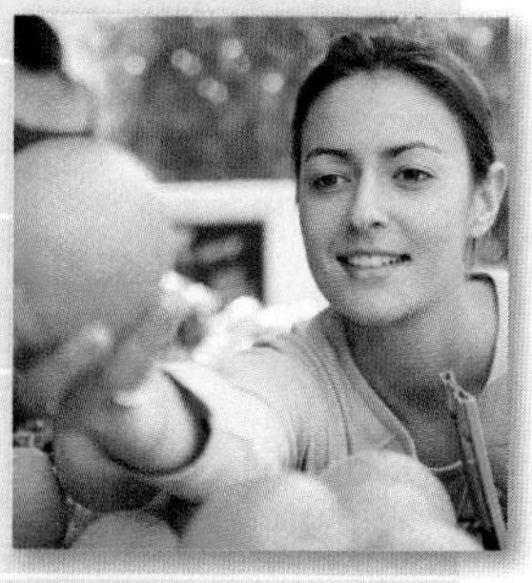

If your trigger is . . .	then try this strategy . . .
A stressful situation	Acknowledge and address feelings of anxiety or stress, and develop stress management techniques to practice daily.
Feeling angry or upset	Analyze your emotions and look for a noneating activity to deal with them, such as taking a quick walk or calling a friend.
A certain time of day	Change your eating schedule to avoid skipping or delaying meals and overeating later; make a plan of what you'll eat ahead of time to avoid impulse or emotional eating.
Pressure from friends and family	Have a response ready to help you refuse food you do not want, or look for healthy alternatives you can eat instead when in social settings.
Being in an environment where food is available	Avoid the environment that causes you to want to eat: Sit far away from the food at meetings, take a different route to class to avoid passing the vending machines, shop from a list and only when you aren't hungry, arrange nonfood outings with your friends.
Feeling bored and tired	Identify the times when you feel low energy and fill them with activities other than eating, such as exercise breaks; cultivate a new interest or hobby that keeps your mind and hands busy.
The sight and smell of food	Stop buying high-calorie foods that tempt you to snack, or store them in an inconvenient place, out of sight; avoid walking past or sitting or standing near the table of tempting treats at a meeting, party, or other gathering.
Eating mindlessly or inattentively	Turn off all distractions, including phones, computers, television, and radio, and eat more slowly, savoring your food and putting your fork down between bites so you can become aware of when your hunger is satisfied.
Spending time alone in the car	Get a book on tape to listen to, or tape your class notes and use the time for studying. Keep your mind off food. Don't bring money into the gas station where snacks are tempting.
Alcohol use	Drink plenty of water and stay hydrated. Seek out healthy snack choices. After a night out, brush your teeth immediately upon getting home and stay out of the kitchen.
Feeling deprived	Allow yourself to eat "indulgences" in moderation, so you won't crave them; focus on balancing your calorie input to calorie output.
Eating out of habit	Establish a new routine to circumvent the old, such as taking a new route to class so you don't feel compelled to stop at your favorite fast-food restaurant on the way.
Watching television	Look for something else to occupy your hands and body while your mind is engaged with the screen: Ride an exercise bike, do stretching exercises, doodle on a pad of paper, or learn to knit.

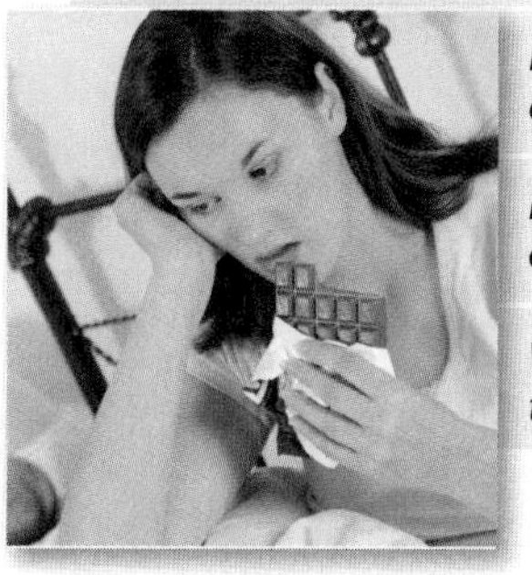

FIGURE 10.6 **Avoid Trigger-Happy Eating**
Learn what triggers your "eat" response—and what stops it—by keeping a daily log.

to your tastes, budget, and lifestyle. Any diet that requires radical behavior changes or prepackaged meals that don't teach you how to eat healthfully is likely to fail. The most successful plans allow you to make food choices in real-world settings and do not ask you to sacrifice everything you enjoy. See Table 10.2 on the following page for an analysis of some of the popular diets being marketed today. For information on other plans, check out the regularly updated list of the diet book reviews on the Academy of Nutrition and Dietetics website at www.eatright.org.

Understanding Calories and Energy Balance

A *calorie* is a unit of measure that indicates the amount of energy gained from food or expended through activity. Each time you consume 3,500 calories more than your body needs to maintain weight, you gain a pound of storage fat. Conversely, each time your body expends an extra 3,500 calories, you lose a pound of fat. If you consume 140 calories

Diet Name	Basic Principles	Good for Diabetes and Heart Health?	Weight Loss Effectiveness	Pros, Cons, and Other Things to Consider
DASH (Dietary Approaches to Stop Hypertension)	A balanced plan developed to fight high blood pressure. Eat fruits, veggies, whole grains, lean protein, and low-fat dairy. Avoid sweets, fats, red meat, and sodium.	Yes	Not specifically designed for weight loss.	A safe and healthy diet that can be complicated to learn. Although not designed for weight reduction, it is regarded as very effective in improving cholesterol levels and other biomarkers long term.
Mediterranean	A plan that emphasizes fruits, vegetables, fish, whole grains, beans, nuts, legumes, olive oil, and herbs and spices. Poultry, eggs, cheese, yogurt, and red wine can be enjoyed in moderation, whereas sweets and red meat are saved for special occasions.	Yes	Effective	Widely considered to be one of the more healthy, safe, and balanced diets. Weight loss may not be as dramatic but long-term health benefits have been demonstrated.
Weight Watchers	The program assigns every food a point value based on its nutritional values and how hard your body has to work to burn it off. Total points allowed depend on someone's activity level and their personal weight goals. In-person group meetings or online membership are options.	Yes (depending on individual choices)	Effective	Experts consider Weight Watchers effective and easy to follow for both short- and long-term weight loss. Other pluses include an emphasis on group support and room for occasional indulgences. But while not as expensive as some plans, there are membership fees.
Jenny Craig	Prepackaged meals do the work of restricting calorie intake. Members get personalized meal and exercise plans, plus weekly counseling sessions.	Yes	Effective short term, long-term results dependent on adopting healthful eating later	Support and premade meals make weight loss easier, however, it may be difficult to maintain for long run. Cons include cost, which will run hundreds of dollars per month for food alone, plus membership fees. Lactose- and gluten-intolerant individuals cannot join due to available foods.
Biggest Loser	Four servings a day of fruits and vegetables, three of protein foods, two of whole grains, and no more than 200 calories of "extras" like desserts. Exercise, food journals, portion control, and calculating personal calorie allowances are all stressed.	Yes	Effective	This diet is effective at weight loss. Also helps reduce blood glucose levels and reduces other biomarkers such as cholesterol, triglycerides, etc.
Slim-Fast	Users eat 1,200 calories per day using two Slim-Fast meal replacements (a bar or a shake) plus one regular meal and a few snacks.	No for heart health, but probably helps diabetics	Effective short term, long-term results dependent on adopting healthful eating later	Experts say Slim-Fast is good for short-term weight loss (up to 20 pounds over a few months). But it scores lower than many other diets on heart health.
Nutrisystem	Low-calorie, prepackaged meals are ordered online and delivered to your home.	No for heart health, but probably helps diabetics	Effective short-term, long-term results dependent on adopting healthful eating later	Nutrisystem is quite safe, easier to follow than many other diets, and has few nutritional deficiencies, according to experts. As a heart diet, it's off the mark. It is also expensive (similar to Jenny Craig) due to the cost of ordering food and may not help you learn to eat healthfully after diet is done.

Diet Name	Basic Principles	Good for Diabetes and Heart Health?	Weight Loss Effectiveness	Pros, Cons, and Other Things to Consider
Medifast	Dieters eat six meals a day, five of them 100-calorie Medifast products. After goal weight loss, people wean from Medifast food and gradually add back in starchy veggies, whole grains, fruit, and low-fat dairy products.	Likely yes	Effective in short term; long-term results unproven	Medifast scored above average in short-term weight loss but gets lower marks for keeping weight off. Because of the extremely low calorie intakes on the program, it is hard to stay on the program for long; doesn't teach healthy eating as part of plan.
Atkins	Carbs—sugars and "simple starches" like potatoes, white bread, and rice—are avoided in this plan and protein and fat from chicken, meat, and eggs are embraced.	Not likely with so much fat eaten	Effective in short term, mixed long-term results	Atkins is extremely effective at short-term weight loss, but many experts worry that fat intake is up to three times higher than standard daily recommendations.
Paleo	Based on the theory that digestive systems have not evolved to deal with many modern foods such as diary, legumes, grains and sugar, this plan emphasizes meats, fish, poultry, fruits, and vegetables.	Unknown (too few studies)	Unknown (too few studies)	Gets low marks by health and nutrition experts due to avoidance of grains, legumes, and dairy and higher fat than the government recommends. Missing essential nutrients, costly to maintain. It can be hard to follow long term and has had only a few very small studies done to document effectiveness.

Source: Opinions on diet pros and cons are based on *U.S. News & World Report* "Best Diets Overall Rankings," 2012, http://health.usnews.com; Dietary reviews available online from registered dieticians at the Academy of Nutrition and Dietetics, 2013. www.eatright.org

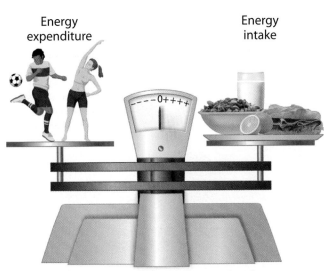

Energy expenditure   Energy intake

Energy expenditure = Energy intake

FIGURE 10.7 **The Concept of Energy Balance**
If you consume more calories than you burn, you will gain weight. If you burn more than you consume, you will lose weight. If both are equal, your weight will not change, according to this concept.

(the amount in one can of regular soda) more than you need every single day and make no other changes in diet or activity, you would gain 1 pound in 25 days (3,500 calories ÷ 140 calories ÷ day = 25 days). Conversely, if you walk for 30 minutes each day at a pace of 15 minutes per mile (172 calories burned) in addition to your regular activities, you would lose 1 pound in 20 days (3,500 calories ÷ 172 calories ÷ day = 20.3 days). This is an example of the concept of energy balance described in Figure 10.7. Of course, these are generic formulas. If you weigh more, you will burn more calories moving your body through the same exercise routine than will someone who is thinner.

Including Exercise

Increasing BMR, RMR, or EMR levels will help burn calories. What can you do to increase your basal or resting metabolic rates? A key is to increase your muscle-to-fat ratio because lean tissue (muscle) is more metabolically active than fat tissue. This means that theoretically, even at rest, a pound of muscle would burn more calories than a pound of fat. How much more? Exact estimates vary, with experts reporting between 2 and 50 calories more per day per pound of muscle. Lifting weights and engaging in other physical activity can build your muscle mass and increase your BMR and RMR. In addition, any increase in the intensity, frequency, and duration of daily exercise levels can have a significant impact on total calorie expenditure.

The energy spent on physical activity is the energy used to move the body's muscles and the extra energy used to speed up heartbeat and respiration rate. The number of calories spent depends on three factors:

1. The number and proportion of muscles used
2. The amount of weight moved
3. The length of time the activity takes

An activity involving both the arms and legs burns more calories than one involving only the legs. An activity performed by a heavy person burns more calories than the same activity performed by a lighter person. And an activity performed for 40 minutes requires twice as much energy as the same activity performed for only 20 minutes. Thus, an obese person walking for 1 mile burns more calories than does a slim person walking the same distance. It also may take overweight people longer to walk the mile, which means that they are burning energy for a longer time and therefore expending more overall calories than thinner walkers.

Some Perspective on Weight Control Efforts

Being overweight does not mean people are weak willed or lazy. Weight loss is difficult for many people and may require lots of effort, as well as supportive friends, relatives, and community resources. People of the same age, sex, height, and weight can have differences of as much as 1,000 calories a day in RMR; this may explain why one person's gluttony is another's starvation. In addition, many social factors can influence your ability to lose weight.

To reach and maintain the weight at which you will be healthy and feel your best, you must develop a program of exercise and healthy eating behaviors that will work for you now and over the long term. Remember that you didn't gain your weight in 1 week, so you're not likely to lose it all in the week or two before spring break. It is unrealistic and potentially dangerous to punish your body by trying to lose weight in a short

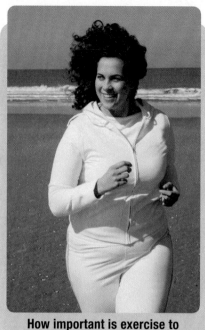

How important is exercise to weight management?

Participating in daily physical activity is key to managing your weight, as well as overall fitness and health.

period of time. Instead, try to lose a healthy 1 to 2 pounds during the first week, and stay with this slow and easy regimen. Making permanent changes to your lifestyle by adding exercise and cutting back on calories to expend about 500 calories more than you consume each day will help you lose weight at a rate of 1 pound per week. See the **Skills for Behavior Change** box on the following page for strategies to make your weight management program succeed.

Considering Drastic Weight-Loss Measures

When nothing seems to work, people often become frustrated and may take significant risks to lose weight. Dramatic weight loss may be recommended in cases of extreme health risk. Even in such situations, drastic dietary, pharmacological, or surgical measures should be considered carefully and discussed with several knowledgeable health professionals.

Very-Low-Calorie Diets In severe cases of obesity that are not responsive to traditional dietary strategies, medically supervised, powdered formulas with daily values of 400 to 700 calories plus vitamin and mineral supplements may be given to patients. Such **very-low-calorie diets (VLCDs)** should

Extreme dieting can pose many serious health risks for the unsuspecting dieter.

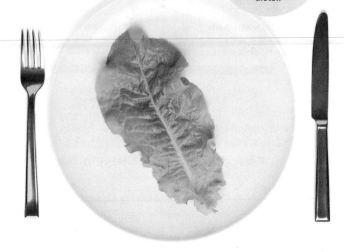

very-low-calorie diets (VLCDs)
Diets with a daily caloric value of 400 to 700 calories.

Keys to Successful Weight Management

MAKE A PLAN

❭ Establish short- and long-term plans. What are the diet and exercise changes you can make this week? Once you do 1 week, plot a course for 2 weeks, and so on.

❭ Look for balance. Remember that it is calories taken in and burned over time that make the difference. If you're going to eat that 200-calorie snack, think about how long you will have to exercise to burn those calories.

CHANGE YOUR HABITS

❭ Be adventurous. Expand your usual foods to enjoy a wider variety.

❭ Rather than deprive yourself of foods you love, eat small portions less often and savor the flavor.

❭ Notice whether you are hungry before starting a meal. Eat slowly, noting when you start to feel full, and *stop* before you are full. Drink water before or during the meal to help you feel full faster.

❭ Eat breakfast. This will prevent you from being too hungry and overeating at lunch. Remember that smaller meals, eaten more often during the day, are a better way to keep the "hungries" at bay.

❭ Keep healthful snacks on hand for when you get hungry.

INCORPORATE EXERCISE

❭ Be active and slowly increase your time, speed, distance, or resistance levels. Remember that even small exercise bouts add up throughout the week.

❭ Vary your physical activity. Find activities that you really love and try things you haven't tried before.

❭ Find an exercise partner to help you stay motivated.

❭ Make it a fun break. Go for a walk in a place that interests you. Tune in to your surroundings to take your mind off of your sweating and heavy breathing!

never be undertaken without strict medical supervision. These severe diets do not teach healthy eating, and persons who manage to lose weight on them may experience significant weight regain. Problems associated with any form of severe caloric restriction include blood sugar imbalance, cold intolerance, constipation, decreased BMR, dehydration, diarrhea, emotional problems, fatigue, headaches, heart irregularities, kidney infections and failure, loss of lean body tissue, weakness, and the potential for coma and death.

One particularly dangerous potential complication of VLCDs is *ketoacidosis.* After a prolonged period of inadequate carbohydrate or food intake, the body will have depleted its immediate energy stores and will begin metabolizing fat stores through *ketogenesis* in order to supply the brain and nervous system with an alternative fuel known as *ketones.* Ketogenesis is one of the body's normal processes for metabolizing fat and may help provide energy to the brain during times of fasting, low carbohydrate intake, or vigorous exercise. However, ketones may also suppress appetite and cause dehydration at a time when a person should feel hungry and seek out food. The condition of having increased levels of ketones in the body is *ketosis*; if enough ketones accumulate in the blood, it may lead to *ketoacidosis,* in which the blood becomes more acidic. People with untreated type 1 diabetes and individuals with anorexia nervosa or bulimia nervosa are at risk of developing ketoacidotic symptoms as damage to body tissues begins.

If fasting continues, the body will turn to its last resort—protein—for energy, breaking down muscle and organ tissue to stay alive. As this occurs, the body loses weight rapidly. At the same time, it also loses significant water stores. Eventually, the body begins to run out of liver tissue, heart muscle, and so on. Within about 10 days after the typical adult begins a complete fast, the body will have depleted its energy stores, and death may occur.

Drug Treatment Individuals looking for help in losing weight often turn to thousands of commercially marketed, over-the-counter weight-loss supplements. Remember, U.S. Food and Drug Administration (FDA) approval is not required for over-the-counter "diet aids" or supplements, and many manufacturers simply feed off people's desperation. Most of these supplements contain stimulants such as caffeine or diuretics, and their effectiveness in promoting weight loss has been largely untested and unproven by any scientific studies. In many cases, the only thing that users lose is money. Virtually all persons who used diet pills in review studies regained their weight once they stopped taking them.[47]

By contrast, FDA-approved diet pills have historically been available only by prescription. These lines blurred when in 2007 the FDA approved the first over-the-counter weight loss pill—a half-strength version of the prescription drug orlistat (brand name Xenical), marketed as Alli. This drug inhibits the action of lipase, an enzyme that helps the body to digest fats, causing about 30 percent of fats consumed to pass through the digestive system undigested, leading to reduced overall caloric intake. Known side effects of orlistat include gas with watery fecal discharge; oily stools

See It! Videos

What makes one diet plan work better than another? Watch **Best Diet Plan Apparently Works** in the Study Area of MasteringHealth™

and spotting; frequent, often unexpected, bowel movements; and possible deficiencies of fat-soluble vitamins. There have also been several FDA warnings issued about fake Alli products being sold at reduced prices online.

When used as part of a long-term, comprehensive weight-loss program, weight-loss drugs can potentially help those who are severely obese lose up to 10 percent of their weight and maintain the loss. The challenge is to develop an effective drug that can be used over time without adverse effects or abuse, and no such drug currently exists. A classic example of supposedly safe drugs that were later found to have dangerous side effects are Pondimin and Redux, known as *fen-phen* (from their chemical names fenfluramine and phentermine), two of the most widely prescribed diet drugs in U.S. history.[48] When they were found to damage heart valves and contribute to pulmonary hypertension, a massive recall and lawsuit ensued.

Surgery In spite of criticisms of weight-loss surgery by health professionals, the rate of bariatric surgeries has grown. Generally, these surgeries fall into one of two major categories: *restrictive surgeries,* such as gastric banding, that limit food intake, and *malabsorption surgeries* that decrease the absorption of food into the body, such as *gastric bypass.* Each type of surgery has its own benefits and risks. To select the best option, a physician will consider that operation's benefits and risks along with many other factors, including the patient's BMI, eating behaviors, obesity-related health conditions, and previous operations. Some health advocates have proposed that obesity be classified as a disability (see the **Points of View** box on the following page), which could potentially affect a physician's decision on recommending surgery.

In gastric banding and other restrictive surgeries, the surgeon uses an inflatable band to partition off part of the stomach. The band is wrapped around that part of the stomach and is pulled tight, like a belt, leaving only a small opening between the two parts of the stomach. The upper part of the stomach is smaller, so the person feels full more quickly, and food digestion slows so that the person also feels full longer. Although the bands are designed to stay in place, they can be removed surgically. They can also be inflated to different levels to adjust the amount of restriction.

In contrast to the restrictive surgeries, gastric bypass is designed to drastically decrease the amount of food a person can eat and absorb. Results are fast and dramatic, but there are many risks, including blood clots in the legs, a leak in a staple line in the stomach, pneumonia, infection, bowel obstruction, diarrhea, and death. According to the Agency for Healthcare Research and Quality, 19 percent of patients experience *dumping syndrome,* which is involuntary vomiting or defecation.[49] Infections, poor wound health, and other issues can occur. Because the stomach pouch that remains after surgery is so small (about the size of a lime), the person can initially drink only a few tablespoons of liquid and consume only a very small amount of food at a time. For

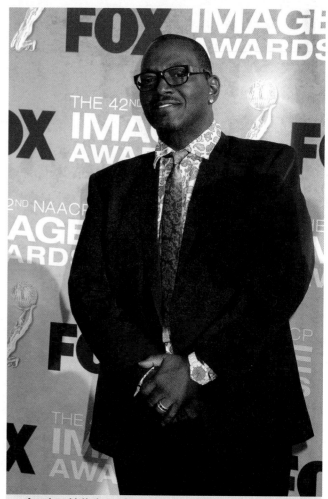

American Idol judge and record producer Randy Jackson and NBC weatherman Al Roker each have undergone gastric bypass surgery to shed well over 100 pounds and reduce the risks of serious chronic diseases such as type 2 diabetes.

this reason, possible side effects include nausea and vomiting (if the person consumes too much), vitamin and mineral deficiencies, and dehydration. As gastric bypass techniques continue to improve and become less invasive, their popularity will continue to grow. Patients have seen remarkable cures for type 2 diabetes, with 95 to 99 percent cure rates even before weight loss begins and dramatic reductions in blood sugar in others.[50] These impressive and unexpected results have caused great excitement among doctors, diabetes researchers, and the public. For those who are morbidly obese, the choice for a higher risk surgery may be similar to the risk of maintaining their weight.

what do you think?

If you wanted to lose weight, what strategies would you most likely choose?
● Which strategies, if any, have worked for you before?
● What factors might serve to help or hinder your weight-loss efforts?

Obesity:
IS IT A DISABILITY?

A person who is 150 to 200 pounds overweight can have difficulty walking, running, getting out of a chair, and doing simple daily tasks. Some people feel obesity should be considered a legal disability that entitles sufferers to certain accommodations. Others believe such a label would add to obesity's stigma and create more problems than it solves.

The federal Americans with Disabilities Act (ADA) defines *disability* as "a physical or mental impairment that substantially limits one or more of the major life activities of [an] individual." To be covered by the ADA, an obese person must have a body mass index (BMI) of over 40 or be at least 100 pounds overweight, as well as have an underlying disorder that caused the obesity. These strict criteria mean that the ADA currently receives few complaints relating to obesity.

Arguments Favoring Disability Status for Obese People

◯ Labeling obesity as a disability would provide obese individuals with better insurance coverage.

◯ A disability label would protect the rights of obese individuals against discrimination based on their weight.

◯ An obese person can have many related medical conditions including arthritis, increased blood pressure, diabetes, diabetic-related vascular diseases, and a weakened cardiovascular system. These conditions can lead to the need for walkers, wheelchairs, and other mobility devices, as well as special health accommodations at home or in the workplace.

Arguments Opposing Disability Status for Obese People

◯ Some doctors worry that defining obesity as a disability would make them vulnerable to lawsuits from obese patients who don't want their doctors to discuss their weight.

◯ Issues of unfair insurance or job practices could be handled with antidiscrimination laws, not by changing obesity's health classification to an official disability.

◯ Not all obese people are disabled by their weight, so labeling them as such would be discriminatory.

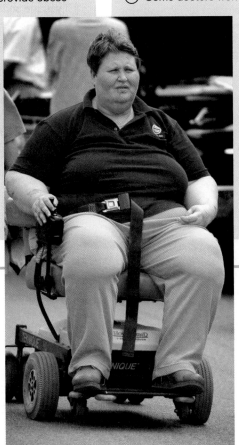

Where Do You Stand?

◯ What positive results might come from classifying overweight or obese individuals as disabled?

◯ What negative consequences might result?

◯ How would you determine whether an individual is disabled because of his or her weight?

◯ Are there legitimate situations where a person who is overweight or obese should be labeled as disabled?

◯ Do you think labeling obesity as a disability would alter the way our society perceives and behaves toward overweight and obese individuals? If so, in what way?

Aftercare for gastric surgery patients often includes counseling to help them cope with the urge to eat after the ability to eat normal portions has been removed, as well as other adjustment problems. Even after undergoing surgery, people must learn to eat healthy foods and exercise. Otherwise, they can gain weight all over again.

Unlike restrictive and malabsorption surgeries, which facilitate overall weight loss, *liposuction* is a surgical procedure in which fat cells are removed from specific areas of the body. Generally, liposuction is considered cosmetic surgery rather than weight-loss surgery and is used for spot reducing and body contouring. Liposuction is by no means risk free, as infections, severe scarring, and even death have resulted. In many cases, people who have liposuction regain fat in those areas or require multiple surgeries to repair lumpy, irregular surfaces from which the fat was removed.

Trying to Gain Weight

For some people, trying to gain weight is a challenge for a variety of metabolic, hereditary, psychological, and other reasons. If you are one of these individuals, the first priority is to determine why you cannot gain weight. Perhaps you're an athlete and you burn more calories than you manage to eat. Perhaps you're stressed out and skipping meals to increase study time. Among older adults, the senses of taste and smell may decline, which makes food taste different and therefore less pleasurable to eat. Visual problems and other disabilities may make meals more difficult to prepare, and dental problems may make eating more difficult. See the **Skills for Behavior Change** box for several weight-gaining strategies. People who are too thin need to take the same steps as those who are overweight or obese to find out what their healthy weight is and attain that weight.

Tips for Gaining Weight

❭ Eat more frequently, spend more time eating, eat high-calorie foods first if you fill up fast, and always start with the main course.

❭ Put extra spreads such as peanut butter, cream cheese, or cheese on your foods. Make your sandwiches with extra-thick slices of bread and add more filling. Take seconds whenever possible, and eat high-calorie, nutrient-dense snacks such as nuts, cheese, whole-grain tortilla chips, and guacamole during the day.

❭ Add high-calorie drinks that have a healthy balance of nutrients, such as whole milk.

❭ Try to eat with people you are comfortable with. Avoid people who you feel are analyzing what you eat or make you feel as if you should eat less.

❭ If you are sedentary, be aware that exercise can increase appetite. If you are exercising, or exercising to extremes, moderate your activities until you've gained some weight.

❭ Avoid diuretics, laxatives, and other medications that cause you to lose body fluids and nutrients.

❭ Relax. Many people who are underweight operate at high gear most of the time. Slow down, get more rest, and control stress.

Assess yourself

Are You Ready to Jump Start Your Weight Loss?

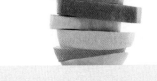

Live It! Assess Yourself
An interactive version of this assessment is available online in MasteringHealth™

If you are overweight or obese, complete each of the following questions by circling the response(s) that best represents your situation or attitudes, then total your points for each section. Section 1 indicates the factors that may predispose you to excess weight and make weight loss more challenging. Section 2 assesses how ready you are to begin losing weight right now.

Section 1 Family, Weight, and Diet History

1. How many people in your immediate family (parents or siblings) are overweight or obese?

   a. No one is overweight or obese (0 points)

   b. One person (1 point)

   c. Two people (2 points)

   d. Three or more people (3 points)

2. During which periods of your life were you overweight or obese? (Circle all that apply.)

   a. Birth through age 5 (1 point)

   b. Ages 6 to 11 (1 point)

   c. Ages 12 to 13 (1 point))

   d. Ages 14 to 18 (2 points)

   e. Ages 19 to present (2 points)

3. How many times in the last year have you made an effort to lose weight but have had little or no success?

   a. None. I've never thought about it. (0 points)

   b. I've thought about it, but I've never tried hard to lose weight. (1 point)

   c. I have tried 2 to 3 times. (1 point)

   d. I have tried at least once a month. (2 points)

   e. I have tried so many times, I can't remember the number. (3 points)

   Total points: _____

Scoring

A score higher than 3 suggests that you may have several challenges ahead as you begin a weight loss program. The higher your score, the greater the likelihood of challenges.

Your own weight problems may be related, at least in part, to the eating habits and preferences you learned at home, and it may take a conscious effort to change them. If in the past you tried repeatedly to lose weight but returned to your old behaviors, you may have to reframe your thinking.

Section 2 Readiness to Change

Attitudes and Beliefs About Weight Loss

1. What is/are your main reason(s) for wanting to lose weight? (Circle all that apply.)

   a. I want to please someone I know or attract a new person. (0 points)

   b. I want to look great and/or fit into smaller size clothes for an upcoming event (wedding, vacation, date, etc.). (1 point)

   c. Someone I know has had major health problems because of being overweight/obese. (1 point)

   d. I want to improve my health and/or have more energy. (2 points)

   e. I was diagnosed with a health problem (pre-diabetes, diabetes, high blood pressure, etc.) because of being overweight/obese. (2 points)

2. What do you think about your weight and body shape? (Circle all that apply.)

   a. I'm fine with being overweight, and if others don't like it, tough! (0 points)

   b. My weight hurts my energy levels and my performance and holds me back. (1 points)

   c. I feel good about myself, but think I will be happier if I lose some of my weight. (1 points)

   d. I'm self-conscious about my weight and uncomfortable in my skin. (1 point)

   e. I'm really worried that I will have a major health problem if I don't change my behaviors now. (2 points)

Daily Eating Patterns

3. Which of the following statements describes you? (Circle all that apply.)

   a. I think about food several times a day, even when I'm not hungry. (0 point)

   b. There are some foods or snacks that I can't stay away from, and I eat them even when I'm not hungry. (0 point)

   c. I tend to eat more meat and fatty foods and never get enough fruits and veggies. (0 points)

   d. I've thought about the weaknesses in my diet and have some ideas about what I need to do. (1 point)

   e. I haven't really tried to eat a "balanced" diet, but I know that I need to start now. (1 point)

4. When you binge or eat things you shouldn't or too much at one sitting, what are you likely to do? (Circle all that apply.)

   a. Not care and go off of my diet. (0 points)

   b. Feel guilty for a while, but then do it again the next time I am out. (0 points)

   c. Fast for the next day or two to help balance the high consumption day. (0 points)

   d. Plan ahead for next time and have options in mind so that I do not continue to overeat. (1 point)

   e. Acknowledge that I have made a slip and get back on my program the next day. (1 point)

5. On a typical day, what are your eating patterns? (Circle all that apply.)

   a. I skip breakfast and save my calories for lunch and dinner. (0 point)

   b. I never really sit down for a meal. I am a "grazer" and eat whatever I find that is readily available. (0 point)

   c. I try to eat at least five servings of fruits and veggies and restrict saturated fats in my diet. (1 points)

   d. I eat several small meals, trying to be balanced in my portions and getting foods from different food groups. (1 points)

Commitment to Weight Loss and Exercise

6. How would you describe your current support system for helping you lose weight? (Circle all that apply.)

   a. I believe I can do this best by doing it on my own. (0 points)

   b. I am not aware of any sources that can help me. (0 points)

   c. I have two to three friends or family members I can count on to help me. (1 point)

   d. There are counselors on campus with whom I can meet to plan a successful approach to weight loss. (1 point)

   e. I have the resources to join Weight Watchers or other community or online weight loss programs. (1 point)

7. How committed are you to exercising? (Circle all that apply.)

   a. Exercise is uncomfortable, embarrassing, and/or I don't enjoy it. (0 points)

   b. I don't have time to exercise. (0 points)

   c. I'd like to exercise, but I'm not sure how to get started. (1 point)

   d. I've visited my campus recreation center or local gym to explore my options for exercise. (2 points)

   e. There are specific sports or physical activities I do already, and I can plan to do more of them. (2 points)

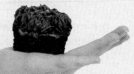

8. What statement best describes your motivation to start a weight loss/lifestyle change program?

    a. I don't want to start losing weight. (0 points)

    b. I am thinking about it sometime in the distant future. (0 points)

    c. I am considering starting within the next few weeks; I just need to make a plan. (1 point)

    d. I'd like to start in the next few weeks, and I'm working on a plan. (2 points)

    e. I already have a plan in place, and I'm ready to begin tomorrow. (3 points)

Total points: _____

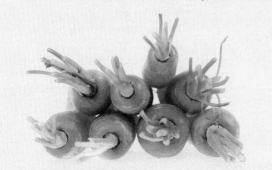

Scoring

A score higher than 8 indicates that you may be ready to change; the higher your score above 8, the more successful you may be. If you scored lower than 8, consider the following:

One of the first steps in making a plan to lose weight is to recognize your strengths and weaknesses and be ready to anticipate challenges. Think about the stages of change model (discussed in Chapter 1) to determine if your current thoughts and attitudes about weight loss reflect a good foundation for beginning a successful weight loss program. Which long-term motivations will you need to successfully lose weight? Which benefits of losing weight motivate you most strongly? Which behavioral changes are you ready to make to address your weight issues?

In order to lose weight, you will need to change your daily eating habits. Overeating (or eating poorly) may be a response to your food attitudes rather than to physical hunger. Poor eating may also reflect your emotional responses toward food, and/or unhealthy dietary choices. To increase your commitment to weight loss and exercise, think of friends or family who can support your efforts to stick to your plan. Also consider the wealth of available resources and where you can go for help. Having a plan and sticking to it will be crucial as you begin your weight loss journey!

YOUR PLAN FOR CHANGE

The **Assessyourself** identifies six areas of importance in determining your readiness for weight loss. If you wish to lose weight to improve your health, understanding your attitudes about food and exercise will help you succeed in your plan.

Today, you can:

○ Set "SMART" goals for weight loss and give them a reality check: Are they specific, measurable, achievable, relevant, and time-oriented? For example, rather than aiming to lose 15 pounds this month (which probably wouldn't be healthy or achievable), set a comfortable goal to lose 5 pounds. Realistic goals will encourage weight-loss success by boosting your confidence in your ability to make lifelong healthy changes.

○ Begin keeping a food log and identifying the triggers that influence your eating habits. Think about what you can do to eliminate or reduce the influence of your two most common food triggers.

Within the next 2 weeks, you can:

○ Get in the habit of incorporating more fruits, vegetables, and whole grains in your diet and eating less fat. The next time you make dinner, look at the proportions on your plate. If vegetables and whole grains do not take up most of the space, substitute 1 cup of the meat, pasta, or cheese in your meal with 1 cup of legumes, salad greens, or a favorite vegetable. You'll reduce the number of calories while eating the same amount of food!

○ Aim to incorporate more exercise into your daily routine. Visit your campus rec center or a local gym, and familiarize yourself with the equipment and facilities that are available. Try a new machine or sports activity, and experiment until you find a form of exercise you really enjoy.

By the end of the semester, you can:

○ Get in the habit of grocery shopping every week and buying healthy, nutritious foods while avoiding high-fat, high-sugar, or overly processed foods. As you make healthy foods more available and unhealthy foods less available, you'll find it easier to eat better.

○ Chart your progress and reward yourself as you meet your goals. If your goal is to lose weight and you successfully take off 10 pounds, reward yourself with a new pair of jeans or other article of clothing (which will likely fit better than before!).

MasteringHealth™

Build your knowledge—and health!—in the Study Area of MasteringHealth with a variety of study tools.

Summary

✱ Overweight, obesity, and weight-related health problems have reached epidemic levels. *Globesity*, or global rates of obesity, threatens the health of many countries. Obesogenic behaviors in an obesogenic environment are key reasons for our weight-related problems.

✱ Societal costs from obesity include increased health care costs, higher rates of diabetes and other diseases, and obesity-related discrimination. Individual health risks from overweight and obesity include a variety of disabling and deadly chronic diseases, increased risks for certain infectious diseases, and low self-esteem, depression, and stress.

✱ It is important to consider environmental, cultural, and socioeconomic factors when working to prevent obesity. Aside from key genes, metabolism, hormones, and excess fat cells, consider environmental factors, such as poverty, education level, and lack of access to nutritious food; lifestyle factors such as lack of physical activity; and others.

✱ Body composition is a reliable indicator for levels of overweight and obesity. There are many different methods of assessing body composition. Body mass index (BMI) is one of the most commonly accepted measures of weight based on height. *Overweight* is most commonly defined as a BMI of 25 to 29.9, and *obesity* as a BMI of 30 or greater. Waist circumference, or the amount of fat in the belly region, is believed to be related to the risk for several chronic diseases, particularly type 2 diabetes.

✱ Exercise, dieting, diet pills, surgery, and other strategies are used to maintain or lose weight. However, sensible eating behavior, aerobic exercise, and exercise that builds muscle mass offer the best options for weight loss and maintenance.

Pop Quiz

1. The rate at which your body consumes energy at complete rest in a neutral environment is your
   a. basal metabolic rate.
   b. resting metabolic rate.
   c. body mass index.
   d. set point.

2. All of the following statements are true *except* which?
   a. A slowing basal metabolic rate may contribute to weight gain after age 30.
   b. Hormones are increasingly implicated in hunger impulses and eating behavior.
   c. The more muscles you have, the fewer calories you will burn.
   d. Yo-yo dieting can make weight loss more difficult.

3. All of the following statements about BMI are true *except* which?
   a. BMI is based on height and weight measurements.
   b. BMI is accurate for everyone, including athletes with high amounts of muscle mass.
   c. Very low and very high BMI scores are associated with greater risk of mortality.
   d. BMI stands for *body mass index*.

4. Which of the following BMI ratings is considered overweight?
   a. 20
   b. 25
   c. 30
   d. 35

5. Which of the following body circumferences is most strongly associated with risk of heart disease and diabetes?
   a. Hip circumference
   b. Chest circumference
   c. Waist circumference
   d. Thigh circumference

6. The proportion of your total weight made up of fat is called
   a. body composition.
   b. lean mass.
   c. percentage of body fat.
   d. BMI.

7. One pound of additional body fat is created through consuming how many extra calories?
   a. 1,500 calories
   b. 3,500 calories
   c. 5,000 calories
   d. 7,000 calories

8. To lose weight, you must consume
   a. fewer calories than you expend.
   b. the same amount of calories as you spend.
   c. more calories than you expend.
   d. calories only from protein.

9. Successful weight maintainers are most likely to do which of the following?
   a. Eat two large meals a day before 1 P.M.
   b. Skip meals
   c. Eat only certain foods
   d. Make short- and long-term plans

10. Successful, healthy weight loss is characterized by
    a. a lifelong pattern of healthful eating and exercise.
    b. cutting out all fats and carbohydrates and eating a lean, mean, high-protein diet.
    c. never eating foods that are considered bad for you and rigidly adhering to a plan.
    d. a pattern of repeatedly losing and regaining weight.

Answers to these questions can be found on page A-1.

Think about It!

1. Discuss the pressures, if any, you feel to change your body's shape. Do these pressures come from media, family, friends, and other external sources, or from concern for your personal health?
2. Are you satisfied with your body weight right now? Why or why not? Are other members of your family suffering from weight-related health problems? How much do you worry that you will have a similar problem in the next 10 years? 20 years?
3. Which measurement would you choose to assess your fat levels? Why?
4. List the risk factors for your being overweight or obese right now. Which seem most likely to determine whether you will be obese in middle age?
5. Why do you think that obesity rates are rising in both developed and less-developed regions of the world? What strategies can we take collectively and individually to reduce risks of obesity?

Accessing Your Health on the Internet

The following websites explore further topics and issues related to personal health. For links to the websites below, visit the Study Area in MasteringHealth.

1. *Academy of Nutrition and Dietetics.* This site includes recommended dietary guidelines and other current information about weight control. www.eatright.org
2. *F as in Fat: How Obesity Threatens America's Future, 2011.* This report provides an excellent summary of the current status of obesity, obesity policies, and programs in the United States, as well as suggestions for new strategies and policies to reduce risks. http://healthyamericans .org/report/88
3. *Weight Control Information Network.* This is an excellent resource for diet and weight-control information. http://win.niddk.nih.gov/index.htm
4. *The Rudd Center for Food Policy and Obesity.* This website provides excellent information on the latest in obesity research, public policy, and ways we can stop the obesity epidemic at the community level. www.yaleruddcenter.org

Enhancing Your Body Image

LEARNING OUTCOMES

* Define what body image is, list the factors that influence it, and identify the elements of the body image continuum.

* Describe four myths about body image and the difference between being dissatisfied with your appearance and body image disorders.

* Describe the signs and symptoms of disordered eating, as well as the physical effects and treatment options for anorexia nervosa, bulimia nervosa, and binge-eating disorder.

* List the criteria, symptoms, and treatment for exercise disorders such as muscle dysmorphia and female athlete triad.

319
How does the media affect my body image?

322
What are people with extreme looks saying about their bodies?

325
How severe are the risks of eating disorders?

326
How can I talk to a friend about an eating disorder?

When you look in the mirror, do you like what you see? If you feel disappointed, frustrated, or even angry, you're not alone. A majority of adults are dissatisfied with their bodies. In a UK study, 93 percent of the women reported that they had had negative thoughts about their appearance during the past week.[1] Approximately 79 percent of the women in the study also reported that they would like to lose weight, despite the fact that the majority of the women sampled were actually within the underweight or "normal" weight ranges. A recent study found that female and male participants became increasingly dissatisfied with their bodies as their body mass index increased during the transition from middle school to high school and again from high school to young adulthood. For female participants, body dissatisfaction was notably high at the transition from high school to early young adulthood.[2] Tragically, negative feelings about one's body can contribute to behaviors that can threaten your health and your life. Having a healthy body image is a key indicator of self-esteem and can contribute to reduced stress, an increased sense of personal empowerment, and more joyful living.

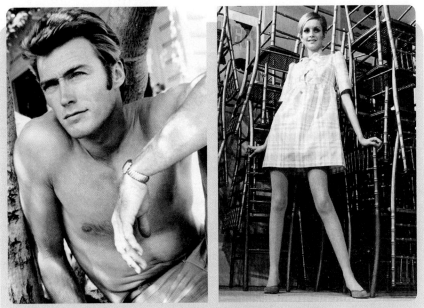

How does the media affect my body image?

Unrealistic images of male and female celebrities are nothing new. In the 1960s, brawny film stars such as Clint Eastwood and ultrathin models such as Twiggy dominated the media.

Dissatisfaction with one's appearance and shape is an all-too-common feeling in today's society that can foster unhealthy attitudes and thought patterns, as well as disordered eating and exercising behaviors.

What Is Body Image?

Body image refers to what you believe or emotionally feel about your body's shape, weight, and general appearance. The term involves more than what you see in the mirror, including the following:

- How you see yourself in your mind
- What you believe about your own appearance (including your real perceptions about your body)

- How comfortable you feel about your body, including your height, shape, and weight

A *negative body image* is defined as either a distorted perception of your shape or feelings of discomfort, shame, or anxiety about your body. You may be convinced that only other people are attractive and that your own body is a sign of personal failure. In contrast, a *positive body image* is a true perception of your appearance: You see yourself as you really are. You understand that everyone is different, and you celebrate your uniqueness—including your "flaws," which you know have nothing to do with your value as a person.

Is your body image negative or positive—or is it somewhere in between? The body image continuum in **Figure 1** on page 320 may help you decide.

80% of adult American women report dissatisfaction with their appearance.

Many Factors Influence Body Image

You're not born with a body image, but you begin to develop one at an early age as you compare yourself against images you see in the world around you and interpret the responses of family members and peers to your appearance.

The Media and Popular Culture
Images and celebrities in the media set the standard for what we find attractive, leading some people to go to dangerous extremes to have the biggest biceps or fit into size zero jeans. This obsession with appearance has long been part of American culture. During the early twentieth century, while men idolized the hearty outdoorsman President Teddy Roosevelt, women pulled their corsets ever tighter to achieve unrealistically tiny waists. In the 1920s and 1930s, men emulated the burly cops and robbers in gangster films, and women dieted and bound

---

body image How you see yourself in your mind, what you believe about your appearance, and how you feel about your body.

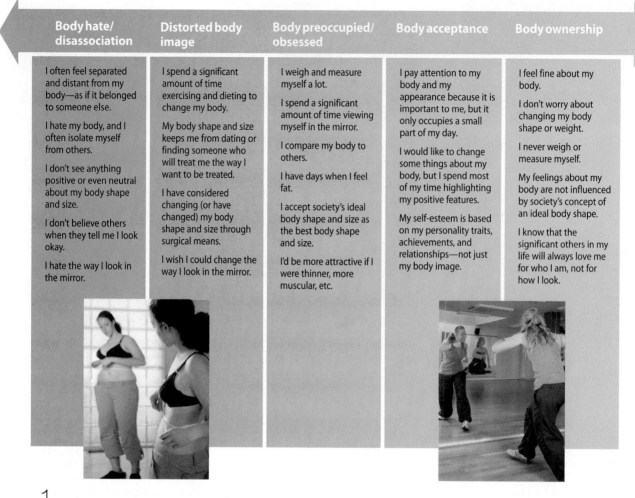

Body hate/ disassociation	Distorted body image	Body preoccupied/ obsessed	Body acceptance	Body ownership
I often feel separated and distant from my body—as if it belonged to someone else.	I spend a significant amount of time exercising and dieting to change my body.	I weigh and measure myself a lot.	I pay attention to my body and my appearance because it is important to me, but it only occupies a small part of my day.	I feel fine about my body.
I hate my body, and I often isolate myself from others.	My body shape and size keeps me from dating or finding someone who will treat me the way I want to be treated.	I spend a significant amount of time viewing myself in the mirror.	I would like to change some things about my body, but I spend most of my time highlighting my positive features.	I don't worry about changing my body shape or weight.
I don't see anything positive or even neutral about my body shape and size.	I have considered changing (or have changed) my body shape and size through surgical means.	I compare my body to others.	My self-esteem is based on my personality traits, achievements, and relationships—not just my body image.	I never weigh or measure myself.
I don't believe others when they tell me I look okay.	I wish I could change the way I look in the mirror.	I have days when I feel fat.		My feelings about my body are not influenced by society's concept of an ideal body shape.
I hate the way I look in the mirror.		I accept society's ideal body shape and size as the best body shape and size.		I know that the significant others in my life will always love me for who I am, not for how I look.
		I'd be more attractive if I were thinner, more muscular, etc.		

FIGURE 1 Eating Issues and Body Image Continuum

This continuum shows a range of attitudes and behaviors toward body image. Functioning at either extreme—not caring at all or being obsessed—leads to problems, whereas functioning in the "body acceptance" area means you are taking care of your body and emotions.

Source: Adapted from Smiley/King/Avey, "Eating Issues and Body Image Continuum," Campus Health Service, 1996. Copyright © 1997 Arizona Board of Regents for the University of Arizona.

Video Tutor: Body Image Continuum

their breasts to achieve the boyish "flapper" look. After World War II, both men and women strove for a healthy, wholesome appearance, but by the 1960s, tough guys were the male ideal, whereas rail-thin models embodied the nation's standard of female beauty. It is similar in today's society, with an obsession around appearance and idolizing thin celebrities such as David Beckham and Angelina Jolie.

Today, more than 68 percent of Americans are overweight or obese. Thus, a significant disconnect exists between the media's idealized images and the typical American body.[3] At the same time, the media is a more powerful and pervasive presence than ever before, bombarding us with messages telling us that we just don't measure up. In fact, one study with more than 7,400 participants from 26 countries concluded that exposure specifically to Western media was significantly associated with body weight ideals and body dissatisfaction.[4]

Family, Community, and Cultural Groups The people with whom we most often interact—our family members, friends, and others—strongly influence the way we see ourselves. Parents are especially influential in body image development. For instance, it's common and natural for fathers of adolescent girls to experience feelings of discomfort related to their daughters' changing bodies. If they are able to navigate these feelings successfully and validate the acceptability of their daughters' appearance throughout puberty, it's likely that they'll help their daughters maintain a positive body image. In contrast, if they verbalize or indicate even subtle judgments about their daughters' changing bodies, girls may begin to question how members of the opposite sex view their bodies in general. In addition, mothers who model body acceptance or body ownership may be more likely to foster a similar positive body image in their daughters, whereas mothers who are frustrated with or ashamed of their bodies may have a greater chance of fostering these negative attitudes in their daughters.

Interactions with siblings and other relatives, peers, teachers, coworkers, and others can also influence body image development. For instance, peer harassment (teasing and bullying) is widely acknowledged to contribute to a negative body image. Associations within one's cultural group also appear to influence body image. Studies have found that European American females experience the highest rates of body dissatisfaction, and as a minority group becomes more acculturated into the mainstream of Western society, the body dissatisfaction levels of women in that group increase.[5]

Physiological and Psychological Factors Recent neurological research suggests that people who have been diagnosed with a body image disorder show differences in the brain's ability to regulate *neurotransmitters* linked to mood.[6] Poor regulation of neurotransmitters is also involved in depression and in anxiety disorders, including obsessive-compulsive disorder. One recent study linked distortions in body image to a malfunctioning in the brain's visual processing region that was revealed by MRI scanning.[7]

How Can I Build a More Positive Body Image?

If you want to develop a more positive body image, your first step might be to challenge some commonly held attitudes in contemporary society. Have you been accepting these four myths?[8]

Myth 1: How you look is more important than who you are. Do you think your weight is important in defining who you are? How much does it matter

to you to have friends who are thin and attractive? How important do you think being thin is in trying to attract your ideal partner?

Myth 2: Anyone can be slender and attractive if they have willpower. When you see someone who is extremely thin, overweight, or obese, what assumptions do you make about that person? Have you ever berated yourself for not having the willpower to change some aspect of your body?

Myth 3: Extreme dieting is an effective weight-loss strategy. Do you believe in trying fad diets or quick-weight-loss products? How far would you be willing to go to attain the "perfect" body?

Myth 4: Appearance is more important than health. How do you evaluate whether a person is healthy? Do you believe it's possible for overweight people to be healthy? Is your desire to change some aspect of your body motivated by health reasons or by concerns about appearance?

To learn ways to bust these toxic myths and attitudes, and to build a more positive body image, check out the **Skills for Behavior Change** box on the following page.

Some People Develop Body Image Disorders

Although most Americans are dissatisfied with some aspect of their appearance, very few have a true body image disorder. However, several diagnosable body image disorders affect a small percentage of the population. Let's look at two of the most common.

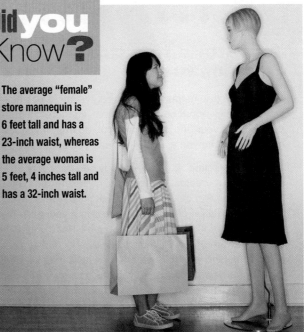

Sources: R. Duyff, *American Dietetic Association Complete Food and Nutrition Guide*, 4th ed. (Hoboken, NJ: John Wiley & Sons, Inc., 2012), 50; C. Fryar, Q. Gu, and C. Ogden, "Anthropometric Reference Data for Children and Adults: United States, 2007–2010," National Center for Health Statistics, Vital and Health Statistics series 11, no. 252 (2012), Available at www.cdc.gov

Body Dysmorphic Disorder (BDD) Approximately 1 percent of people in the United States suffer from **body dysmorphic disorder (BDD)**.[9] Persons with BDD are obsessively concerned with their appearance and have a distorted view of their own body shape, body size, weight, perceived lack of muscles, facial blemishes, size of body parts, and so on. Although the precise cause of the disorder isn't known, an anxiety disorder such as obsessive-compulsive disorder is often present as well. Contributing factors may include genetic susceptibility, childhood teasing, physical or sexual abuse, low self-esteem, and rigid sociocultural expectations of beauty.[10]

People with BDD may try to fix their perceived flaws through abuse of steroids, excessive bodybuilding, repeated cosmetic surgeries, extreme tattooing, or other appearance-altering behaviors. It is estimated that 10 percent of people seeking dermatology or cosmetic treatments have BDD.[11]

body dysmorphic disorder (BDD) Psychological disorder characterized by an obsession with one's appearance and a distorted view of one's body or with a minor or imagined flaw in appearance.

Ten Steps to a Positive Body Image

How do you turn negative body thoughts into a positive body image? One way is to think about new ways of looking more healthfully and happily at yourself and your body. The more you do that, the more likely you are to feel good about who you are and the body you naturally have.

Step 1. Appreciate all that your body can do. Every day your body carries you closer to your dreams. Celebrate all of the amazing things your body does for you—running, dancing, breathing, laughing, dreaming.

Step 2. Keep a list of things you like about yourself—things that aren't related to how much you weigh or how you look. Read your list often. Add to it as you become aware of more things to like about yourself.

Step 3. Remind yourself that true beauty is not skin deep. When you feel good about yourself and who you are, you carry yourself with a sense of confidence, self-acceptance, and openness that makes you beautiful. Beauty is a state of mind, not a state of your body.

Step 4. Look at yourself as a whole person. When you see yourself in a mirror or in your mind, choose not to focus on specific body parts. See yourself as others see you—as a whole person.

Step 5. Surround yourself with positive people. It is easier to feel good about yourself and your body when you are around others who are supportive and who recognize the importance of liking yourself just as you naturally are.

Step 6. Shut down those voices in your head that tell you your body is not "right" or that you are a "bad" person. You can overpower those negative thoughts with positive ones.

Step 7. Wear clothes that are comfortable and that make you feel good about your body. Work with your body, not against it.

Step 8. Become a critical viewer of social and media messages. Pay attention to images, slogans, or attitudes that make you feel bad about yourself or your body. Protest these messages: Write a letter to the advertiser or talk back to the image or message.

Step 9. Do something nice for yourself—something that lets your body know you appreciate it. Take a bubble bath, make time for a nap, or find a peaceful place outside to relax.

Step 10. Use the time and energy that you might have spent worrying about food, calories, and your weight to do something to help others. Sometimes reaching out to other people can help you feel better about yourself and can make a positive change in our world.

Source: "10 Steps to Positive Body Image" from National Eating Disorders Association Website, April 22, 2013. Copyright © 2013 National Eating Disorders Association. Reprinted with permission. For more information visit www.NationalEatingDisorders.org or call NEDA's helpline 1-800-931-2237.

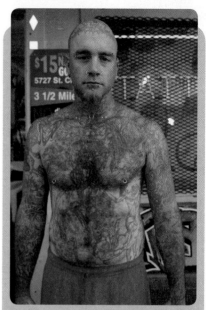

What are people with extreme looks saying about their bodies?

It's not always easy to spot people who are highly dissatisfied with their bodies, as they don't necessarily stick out in a crowd. For instance, people who cover their bodies with tattoos may have a strong sense of self-esteem. On the other hand, extreme tattooing can be an outward sign of a severe body image disturbance known as *body dysmorphic disorder*.

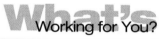

Working for You?

Which of these behaviors that contribute to a positive body image is true for you?

☐ I surround myself with people who are supportive of me and help to build me up, rather than be critical of me or others.

☐ I wear clothes that are comfortable and make me feel good.

☐ I remind myself that beauty is not just outer appearance.

Social Physique Anxiety An emerging problem, seen in both young men and women, is **social physique anxiety (SPA).** The desire to "look good" becomes so strong that it has a destructive and sometimes disabling effect on the person's ability to function effectively in relationships and interactions with others. People suffering from SPA spend a disproportionate amount of time fixating on their bodies, working out, and performing tasks that are ego centered and self-directed, rather than focusing on interpersonal relationships and general tasks.[12] Experts speculate that this anxiety may contribute to disordered eating behaviors.

social physique anxiety (SPA) A desire to look good that has a destructive effect on a person's ability to function well in social interactions and relationships.

What Is Disordered Eating?

People with a negative body image can fixate on a wide range of physical "flaws," from thinning hair to flat feet.

Eating disordered	Disruptive eating patterns	Food preoccupied/ obsessed	Concerned in a healthy way	Food is not an issue
I worry about what I will eat or when I will exercise all the time.	My food and exercise concerns are starting to interfere with my school and social life.	I think about food a lot.	I pay attention to what I eat in order to maintain a healthy body.	I am not concerned about what or how much I eat.
I follow a very rigid eating plan and know precisely how many calories, fat grams, or carbohydrates I eat every day.	I use food to comfort myself.	I'm obsessed with reading books and magazines about dieting, fitness, and weight control.	Food and exercise are important parts of my life, but they only occupy a small part of my time.	I feel no guilt or shame no matter what I eat or how much I eat.
I feel incredible guilt, shame, and anxiety when I break my diet.	I have tried diet pills, laxatives, vomiting, or extra time exercising in order to lose or maintain my weight.	I sometimes miss school, work, and social events because of my diet or exercise schedule.	I enjoy eating, and I balance my pleasure with my concern for a healthy body.	Exercise is not really important to me. I choose foods based on cost, taste, and convenience, with little regard to health.
I regularly stuff myself and then exercise, vomit, or use laxatives to get rid of the food.	I have fasted or avoided eating for long periods of time in order to lose or maintain my weight.	I divide food into "good" and "bad" categories.	I usually eat three balanced meals daily, plus snacks, to fuel my body with adequate energy.	My eating is very sporadic and irregular.
My friends and family tell me I am too thin, but I feel fat.	If I cannot exercise to burn off calories, I panic.	I feel guilty when I eat "bad" foods or when I eat more than what I feel I should be eating.	I am moderate and flexible in my goals for eating well and being physically active.	I don't worry about meals; I just eat whatever I can, whenever I can.
I am out of control when I eat.	I feel strong when I can restrict how much I eat.	I am afraid of getting fat.	Sometimes I eat more (or less) than I really need, but most of the time I listen to my body.	I enjoy stuffing myself with lots of tasty food at restaurants, holiday meals, and social events.
I am afraid to eat in front of others.	I feel out of control when I eat more than I wanted to.	I wish I could change how much I want to eat and what I am hungry for.		
I prefer to eat alone.				

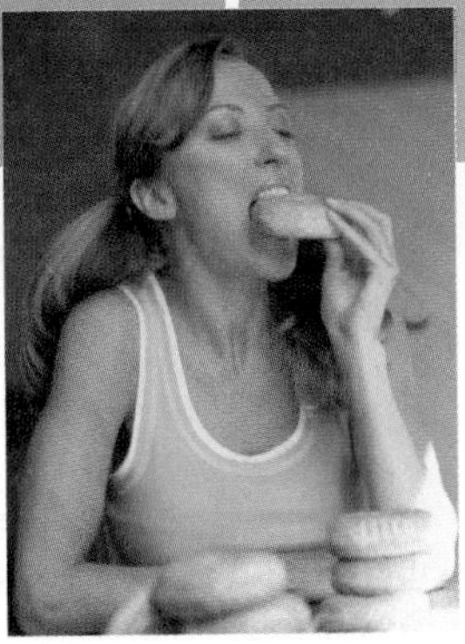

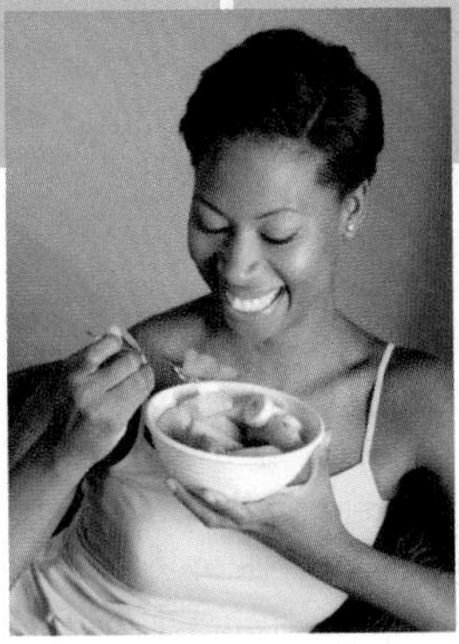

FIGURE 2 **Eating Issues Continuum**
This continuum shows progression from normal eating to eating disorders. Being concerned in a healthy way is the goal.
Source: Adapted from Smiley/King/Avey, "Eating Issues and Body Image Continuum," Campus Health Service, 1996. Copyright © 1997 Arizona Board of Regents for the University of Arizona.

Still, the "flaw" that causes distress to the majority of people with negative body image is overweight.

Check out the eating issues continuum in Figure 2: The column labeled "concerned in a healthy way" indicates a healthy acceptance of your body whereas the far left identifies a pattern of thoughts and behaviors associated with **disordered eating.** These behaviors can include chronic dieting, rigid eating patterns, abuse of diet pills and laxatives, self-induced vomiting, and many others.

Some People Develop Eating Disorders

Only some people who exhibit disordered eating patterns progress to a clinical **eating disorder.** The eating disorders defined by the American Psychiatric Association (APA) in *Diagnostic and Statistical Manual of Mental Disorders,* Fifth Edition, (DSM-5) are *anorexia nervosa, bulimia nervosa, binge-eating disorder,* and a cluster of less distinct conditions collectively referred to as *eating disorders not otherwise specified* (*EDNOS*).

At any given time, 10 percent or more of late adolescent and adult women in the United States report symptoms of eating disorders.[13] Although anorexia nervosa and bulimia nervosa affect people primarily in their

disordered eating A pattern of atypical eating behaviors that is used to achieve or maintain a lower body weight.

eating disorder A psychiatric disorder characterized by severe disturbances in body image and eating behaviors.

anorexia nervosa Eating disorder characterized by deliberate food restriction, self-starvation or extreme exercising to achieve weight loss, and an extremely distorted body image.

bulimia nervosa Eating disorder characterized by binge eating followed by inappropriate purging measures or compensatory behavior, such as vomiting or excessive exercise, to prevent weight gain.

teens and twenties, increasing numbers of children as young as 7 have been diagnosed, as have women as old as 80.[14] In 2012, 1.9 percent of college students reported that they were dealing with either anorexia or bulimia.[15] Disordered eating and eating disorders are also common among ballet dancers and athletes, particularly athletes in sports with an aesthetic component (e.g., figure skating or gymnastics) or that are tied to a weight class (e.g., tae kwon do, judo, or wrestling).[16]

Eating disorders are on the rise among men, who currently represent up to 25 percent of anorexia and bulimia patients.[17] Many men suffering from eating disorders fail to seek treatment because these illnesses are traditionally thought of as being a woman's problem.

What factors put individuals at risk? Eating disorders are very complex, and despite scientific research to try to understand them, their biological, behavioral, and social underpinnings remain elusive. Many people with these disorders feel disempowered in other aspects of their lives and try to gain a sense of control through food. Many are clinically depressed, suffer from obsessive-compulsive disorder, or have other psychiatric problems. In addition, studies have shown that individuals with low self-esteem, negative body image, and a high tendency for perfectionism are at risk.[18]

Anorexia Nervosa

Anorexia nervosa is a persistent, chronic eating disorder characterized by deliberate food restriction and severe, life-threatening weight loss. It involves self-starvation motivated by an intense fear of gaining weight, along with an extremely distorted body image. Anorexics eventually progress to restricting their intake of almost all foods. The little they do eat, they

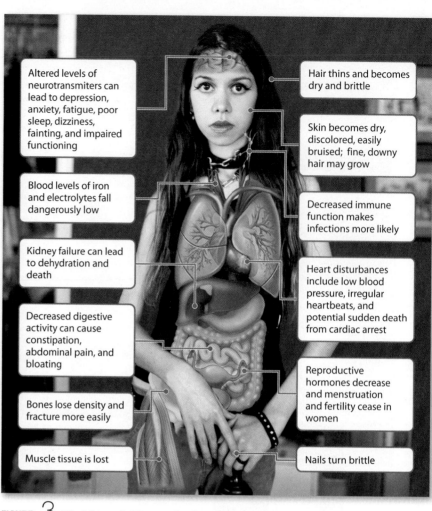

FIGURE 3 What Anorexia Nervosa Can Do to the Body

Altered levels of neurotransmiters can lead to depression, anxiety, fatigue, poor sleep, dizziness, fainting, and impaired functioning

Blood levels of iron and electrolytes fall dangerously low

Kidney failure can lead to dehydration and death

Decreased digestive activity can cause constipation, abdominal pain, and bloating

Bones lose density and fracture more easily

Muscle tissue is lost

Hair thins and becomes dry and brittle

Skin becomes dry, discolored, easily bruised; fine, downy hair may grow

Decreased immune function makes infections more likely

Heart disturbances include low blood pressure, irregular heartbeats, and potential sudden death from cardiac arrest

Reproductive hormones decrease and menstruation and fertility cease in women

Nails turn brittle

may purge through vomiting or using laxatives. Although they lose weight, people with anorexia nervosa never seem to feel thin enough and constantly identify body parts that are "too fat."

It is estimated that 0.3 percent of females suffer from anorexia nervosa in their lifetime.[19] The revised *DSM-5* criteria for anorexia nervosa are as follows:[20]

- Refusal to maintain body weight at or above a minimally normal weight for age and height
- Intense fear of gaining weight or becoming fat, even though considered underweight by all medical criteria
- Disturbance in the way in which one's body weight or shape is experienced, undue influence of body weight or shape on self-evaluation, or denial of the seriousness of the current low body weight

Physical symptoms and negative health consequences associated with anorexia nervosa are illustrated in Figure 3. Because it involves starvation and can lead to heart attacks and seizures, anorexia nervosa has the highest death rate (20%) of any psychological illness.[21]

The causes of anorexia nervosa are complex and variable. Many people with anorexia have other coexisting psychiatric problems, including low self-esteem, depression, an anxiety disorder, and substance abuse. Physical factors are thought to include an imbalance of neurotransmitters and genetic susceptibility.[22]

Bulimia Nervosa

Individuals with **bulimia nervosa** often binge on huge amounts of food and then engage in some kind of purging or compensatory behavior, such as vomiting, taking laxatives, or exercising excessively, to lose the calories they have just consumed. People with bulimia are obsessed with their bodies, weight gain, and appearance, but unlike those with anorexia, their problem is often hidden from the public eye because their weight may fall within a normal range or they may be overweight.

Up to 3 percent of adolescents and young women are bulimic; rates among men are about 10 percent of the rate among women.[23] The revised *DSM-5* diagnostic criteria for bulimia nervosa are as follows:[24]

● Recurrent episodes of binge eating (defined as eating, in a discrete period of time, an amount of food that is larger than most people would eat during a similar period of time and under similar circumstances, and experiencing a sense of lack of control over eating during the episode)
● Recurrent inappropriate compensatory behavior to prevent weight gain, such as self-induced vomiting; misuse of laxatives, diuretics, or other medications; fasting; or excessive exercise
● Binge eating and inappropriate compensatory behavior occurs on average at least once a week for 3 months
● Body shape and weight unduly influence self-evaluation
● The disturbance does not occur exclusively during episodes of anorexia nervosa

Physical symptoms and negative health consequences associated with bulimia nervosa are shown in **Figure 4**. One of the more common symptoms of bulimia is tooth erosion, which results from the excessive vomiting associated with this disorder. Bulimics who vomit are also at risk for electrolyte imbalances and dehydration, both of which can contribute to a heart attack and sudden death.

A combination of genetic and environmental factors is thought to cause bulimia nervosa.[25] A family history of obesity, an underlying anxiety disorder, and an imbalance in neurotransmitters are all possible contributing factors.

Binge-Eating Disorder Individuals with **binge-eating disorder** gorge like their bulimic counterparts but do not take excessive measures to lose the weight that they gain. Thus, they are often clinically obese. As in bulimia, binge-eating episodes are typically characterized by eating large amounts of food rapidly, even when not feeling hungry, and feeling guilty or depressed after overeating.[26]

binge-eating disorder A type of eating disorder characterized by gorging on food once a week or more, but not typically followed by a purge.

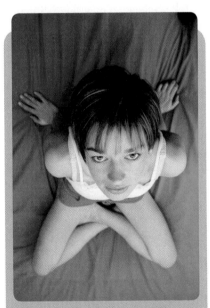

How severe are the risks of eating disorders?

People with anorexia nervosa put themselves at risk of starving to death. In addition, they may die from sudden cardiac arrest caused by electrolyte imbalances; this is also a risk for people with bulimia nervosa.

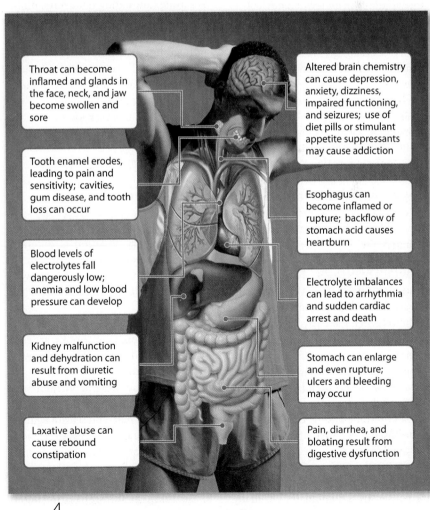

Throat can become inflamed and glands in the face, neck, and jaw become swollen and sore

Tooth enamel erodes, leading to pain and sensitivity; cavities, gum disease, and tooth loss can occur

Blood levels of electrolytes fall dangerously low; anemia and low blood pressure can develop

Kidney malfunction and dehydration can result from diuretic abuse and vomiting

Laxative abuse can cause rebound constipation

Altered brain chemistry can cause depression, anxiety, dizziness, impaired functioning, and seizures; use of diet pills or stimulant appetite suppressants may cause addiction

Esophagus can become inflamed or rupture; backflow of stomach acid causes heartburn

Electrolyte imbalances can lead to arrhythmia and sudden cardiac arrest and death

Stomach can enlarge and even rupture; ulcers and bleeding may occur

Pain, diarrhea, and bloating result from digestive dysfunction

FIGURE 4 **What Bulimia Nervosa Can Do to the Body**

A national survey reported that a lifetime prevalence of binge-eating disorder in the study participants was 1.4 percent.[27] The revised *DSM-5* criteria for binge-eating disorder are as follows:[28]

- Recurrent episodes of binge eating (defined as eating, in a discrete period of time, an amount of food that is larger than most people would eat during a similar period of time and under similar circumstances, and experiencing a sense of lack of control over eating during the episode)
- The binge-eating episodes are associated with three (or more) of the following: (1) eating much more rapidly than normal; (2) eating until feeling uncomfortably full; (3) eating large amounts of food when not feeling physically hungry; (4) eating alone because of embarrassment over how much one is eating; (5) feeling disgusted with oneself, depressed, or very guilty after overeating
- Experiencing marked distress regarding binge eating
- The binge eating occurs, on average, at least once a week for 3 months
- The binge eating is not associated with the recurrent use of inappropriate compensatory behavior (i.e., purging) and does not occur exclusively during the course of bulimia nervosa or anorexia nervosa

Eating Disorders Not Otherwise Specified The APA recognizes that some patterns of disordered eating qualify as a legitimate psychiatric illness but don't fit into the strict diagnostic criteria for anorexia, bulimia, or binge-eating disorder. Called **eating disorders not otherwise specified (EDNOS),** this group of disorders can include night eating syndrome and recurrent purging in the absence of binge eating.

Treatment for Eating Disorders Because eating disorders are caused by a combination of many factors, there are no quick or simple solutions. Without treatment, approximately 20 percent of people with a serious eating disorder will die from it. With treatment, long-term full recovery rates range from 44 to 76 percent for anorexia nervosa and from 50 to 70 percent for bulimia nervosa.[29]

Treatment often focuses first on reducing the threat to life. Once the patient is stabilized, long-term therapy focuses on the psychological, social, environmental, and physiological factors that led to the problem. Through therapy, the patient works on adopting new eating behaviors, building self-confidence, and finding other ways to deal with life's problems. Support groups can help the family and the individual learn to foster positive actions and interactions. Treatment of an underlying anxiety disorder or depression may also be a focus.

How Can You Help Someone with Disordered Eating?

Although every situation is different, there are several things you can do if you suspect someone you know is struggling with disordered eating:[30]

- **Learn** as much as you can about disordered eating through books, articles, brochures, and trustworthy websites.
- **Know the differences** between facts and myths about weight, nutrition, and exercise. Being armed with this information can help you reason against any inaccurate ideas that your friend may be using as excuses.
- **Be honest.** Talk openly and honestly about your concerns.
- **Be caring, but be firm.** Caring about your friend does not mean allowing

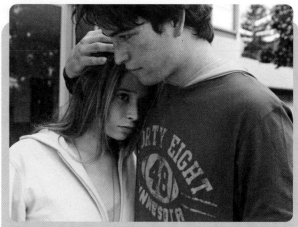

How can I talk to a friend about an eating disorder?

When talking to a friend about an eating disorder or disordered eating patterns, avoid casting blame, preaching, or offering unsolicited advice. Instead, be a good listener, let the person know that you care, and offer your support.

him or her to manipulate you. Avoid making rules or promises that you cannot or will not uphold.
- **Compliment** your friend's personality, successes, or accomplishments.
- **Be a good role model** for healthy eating, exercise, and self-acceptance.
- **Tell someone.** It may seem difficult to know when, if at all, to tell someone else about your concerns. Your friend needs as much support as possible, the sooner the better. Addressing disordered eating patterns in their beginning stages offers your friend the best chance for working through these issues and becoming healthy again.

Can Exercise Be Unhealthy?

Although exercise is generally beneficial to health, in excess it can be a problem.

See It! Videos

How do you treat the most common but least well known eating disorder? Watch **EDNOS: Most Dangerous, Unheard of Eating Disorder** in the Study Area of **MasteringHealth™**

Some People Develop Exercise Disorders

In a recent study, researchers showed that participants used excessive exercise or **compulsive exercise** as a way to regulate their emotions.[31] Also called *anorexia athletica,* compulsive exercise is characterized not by a *desire* to exercise but a *compulsion* to do so. That is, the person struggles with guilt and anxiety if he or she doesn't work out. Compulsive exercisers, like people with eating disorders, often define their self-worth externally. They over-exercise in order to feel more in control of their lives. Disordered eating or an eating disorder is often part of the picture.

Compulsive exercise can contribute to a variety of injuries. It can also put significant stress on the heart, especially if combined with disordered eating.

Muscle Dysmorphia

Muscle dysmorphia is a form of body image disturbance and exercise disorder in which a man believes that his body is insufficiently lean or muscular.[32] It appears to be a relatively new disorder. Men with muscle dysmorphia believe that they look "puny," when in reality they look normal or may even be unusually muscular. As a result of their adherence to a meticulous diet, their time-consuming workout schedule, and their shame over their perceived appearance flaws, they may neglect important social or occupational activities. Other behaviors characteristic of muscle dysmorphia include comparing oneself unfavorably to others, checking one's appearance in the mirror, and camouflaging one's appearance. Men with muscle dysmorphia also are likely to abuse anabolic steroids and dietary supplements.[33]

The Female Athlete Triad

Female athletes in competitive sports often strive for perfection. In an effort to be the best, they may put themselves at risk for developing a syndrome called the **female athlete triad.** *Triad* means "three," and the three interrelated problems are low energy intake, typically prompted by disordered eating behaviors; menstrual dysfunction such as amenorrhea; and poor bone density (Figure 5).[34]

How does the female athlete triad develop, and what makes it so dangerous? First, a chronic pattern of low energy intake and intensive exercise alters normal body functions. For example, when an athlete restricts her eating, she can deplete her body stores of nutrients essential to health. At the same time, her body will begin to burn its stores of fat tissue for energy. Adequate body fat is essential to maintaining healthy levels of the female reproductive hormone *estrogen*; when an athlete isn't getting enough food, estrogen levels decline. This can manifest as amenorrhea: The body is using all calories to keep the athlete alive, and nonessential body functions such as menstruation cease. In addition, fat-soluble vitamins, calcium, and estrogen are all essential for dense, healthy bones, so their depletion weakens the athlete's bones.

Not all athletes are equally prone to the female athlete triad: It is particularly prevalent in women who participate in highly competitive individual sports or activities that emphasize leanness and require wearing body-contouring clothing. Gymnasts, figure skaters, cross-country runners, and ballet dancers are among those at highest risk for the female athlete triad.

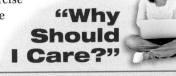

"Why Should I Care?"

Although exercising is generally beneficial to your health, doing it compulsively can lead to broken bones, joint injuries, and even depression. Remember that moderation is essential and taking rest days is important to your health.

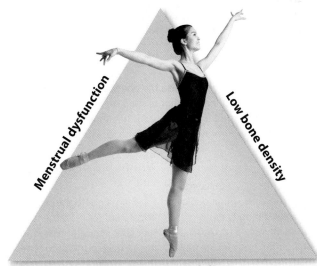

compulsive exercise Disorder characterized by a compulsion to engage in excessive amounts of exercise, and feelings of guilt and anxiety if the level of exercise is perceived as inadequate.

muscle dysmorphia Body image disorder in which men believe that their body is insufficiently lean or muscular.

female athlete triad A syndrome of three interrelated health problems seen in some female athletes: disordered eating, amenorrhea, and poor bone density.

See It! Videos

Can you go too far with extreme exercise? Watch **Young Boys Exercising to Extremes** in the Study Area of MasteringHealth™

FIGURE 5 **The Female Athlete Triad**
The female athlete triad is a cluster of three interrelated health problems.

(Triangle labels: Menstrual dysfunction, Low bone density, Low energy availability)

Assess **Yourself**

Are Your Efforts to Be Thin Sensible— Or Spinning Out of Control?

On one hand, just because you weigh yourself, count calories, or work out every day, don't jump to the conclusion that you have any of the health concerns discussed in this chapter. On the other hand, efforts to lose a few pounds can spiral out of control. To find out whether your efforts to be thin are harmful to you, take the following quiz from the National Eating Disorders Association (NEDA).

1. I constantly calculate numbers of fat grams and calories.   T   F
2. I weigh myself often and find myself obsessed with the number on the scale.   T   F
3. I exercise to burn calories and not for health or enjoyment.   T   F
4. I sometimes feel out of control while eating.   T   F
5. I often go on extreme diets.   T   F
6. I engage in rituals to get me through mealtimes and/or secretively binge.   T   F
7. Weight loss, dieting, and controlling my food intake have become my major concerns.   T   F
8. I feel ashamed, disgusted, or guilty after eating.   T   F
9. I constantly worry about the weight, shape, and/or size of my body.   T   F
10. I feel my identity and value are based on how I look or how much I weigh.   T   F

If any of these statements is true for you, you could be dealing with disordered eating. If so, talk about it! Tell a friend, parent, teacher, coach, youth group leader, doctor, counselor, or nutritionist what you're going through. Check out the NEDA's Sharing with EEEase handout at www.nationaleatingdisorders.org/sharing-eeease for help planning what to say the first time you talk to someone about your eating and exercise habits.

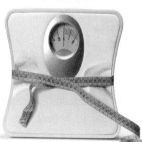

Source: Adapted from "NEDA Screening for Eating Disorders" by the National Eating Disorders Association (NEDA) and Screening for Mental Health, Inc. (SMH), from NEDA website. Copyright © 2013 NEDA and SMH. Reprinted with permission.

YOUR PLAN FOR CHANGE

The **Assess Yourself** activity gave you the chance to evaluate your feelings about your body and to determine whether or not you might be engaging in eating or exercise behaviors that could undermine your health and happiness. Below are some steps you can take to improve your body image, starting today.

Today, you can:

○ Talk back to the media. Write letters to advertisers and magazines that depict unhealthy and unrealistic body types. Boycott their products or start a blog commenting on harmful body image messages in the media.

○ Just for today, eat the recommended number of servings from every food group at every meal (see Chapter 9). And don't count calories!

Within the next 2 weeks, you can:

○ Find a photograph of a person you admire *not* for his or her appearance, but for his or her contribution to humanity. Put it next to your mirror to remind yourself that true beauty comes from within and benefits others.

○ Start a journal. Each day, record one thing you are grateful for that has nothing to do with your appearance. At the end of each day, record one small thing you did to make someone's world a little brighter.

By the end of the semester, you can:

○ Establish a group of friends who support you for who you are, not what you look like, and who get the same support from you. Form a group on a favorite social-networking site, and keep in touch, especially when you start to feel troubled by self-defeating thoughts or have the urge to engage in unhealthy eating or exercise behaviors.

○ Borrow from the library or purchase one of the many books on body image now available, and read it!

Improving Your Personal Fitness

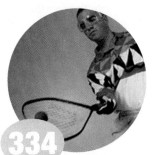

11

LEARNING OUTCOMES

* Describe the health benefits of being physically active.

* Distinguish between the physical activity required for health, physical fitness, and performance.

* Identify the motivating factors for becoming physically fit, including the benefits, goals, and challenges to manage.

* Understand and be able to use the FITT (frequency, intensity, time, and type) principles for the health-related components of physical fitness.

* Design a training program that works for you, incorporating the key components of a personal physical fitness program.

* Summarize ways to prevent and treat common injuries related to physical activity.

334
Can physical activity really reduce stress?

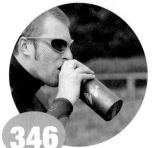

336
How can I motivate myself to be more physically active?

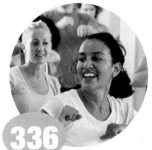

346
How much do I need to drink before, during, and after physical activity?

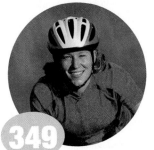

349
What can I do to avoid injury when I am physically active?

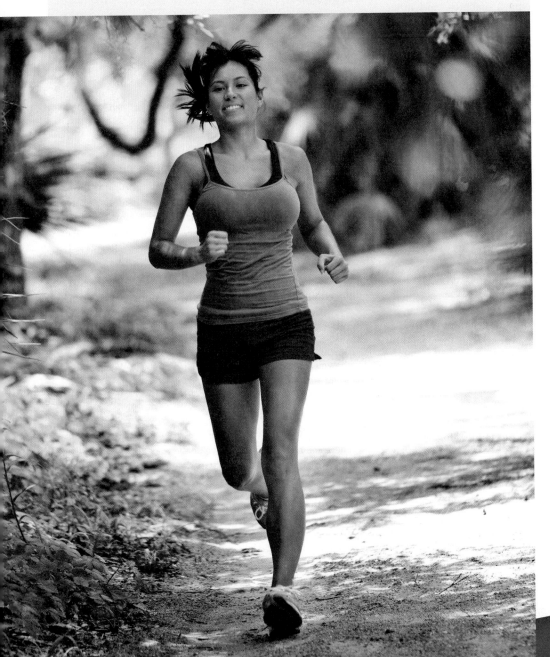

Most Americans are aware of the wide range of physical, social, and mental health benefits of physical activity and know that they should be more physically active. The physiological changes in the body that result from regular physical activity reduce the likelihood of coronary artery disease, high blood pressure, type 2 diabetes, obesity, and other chronic diseases. Furthermore, engaging in physical activity regularly helps to control stress, increases self-esteem, and contributes to that "feel-good" feeling.

Despite the fact that they know the importance of physical activity for their health and wellness, most people are not sufficiently active to obtain these optimal health benefits. Recent statistics indicate that 26.2 percent of American adults do not engage in any leisure-time physical activity, or activity done during one's "down" time.[1] The growing percentage of Americans who live physically inactive lives (that is, perform no physical activity or engage in less than 10 minutes total per week of moderate or vigorous intensity lifestyle activities) has been linked to the current high incidences of obesity, type 2 diabetes, and other chronic and mental health diseases.[2]

In general, college students are more physically active than older adults, but a recent survey indicated that 43.8 percent of college women and 51.9 percent of college men do not meet recommended guidelines for engaging in moderate or vigorous physical activities.[3]

Physical Activity for Health

Physical activity refers to all body movements produced by skeletal muscles that result in substantial increases in energy expenditure. Walking, swimming, strength training, dancing, and doing yoga are examples of physical activity. Physical activities can vary by light, moderate, or vigorous intensity. For example, walking on a flat surface at a casual pace requires little effort (light), whereas walking uphill is more intense and harder to do (moderate). Jogging and running are examples of vigorous intensity physical activities. There are three general categories of physical activity defined by the purpose for which they are done: leisure-time physical activity, occupational physical activity, and lifestyle physical activity.

physical activity Refers to all body movements produced by skeletal muscles resulting in substantial increases in energy expenditure.

exercise Planned, structured, and repetitive bodily movement done to improve or maintain one or more components of physical fitness.

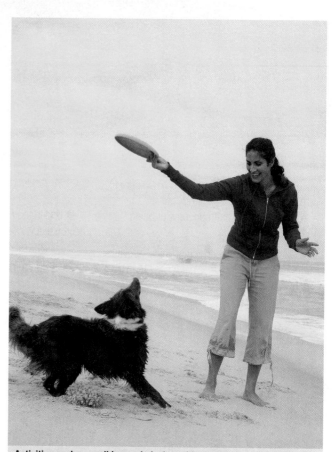

Activities such as walking and playing with your dog count toward your recommended daily physical activity.

Exercise refers to a particular kind of physical activity that fits into the leisure-time category. Although all exercise is physical activity, not all physical activity would be considered exercise. For example, walking from your car to class is physical activity, whereas going for a brisk 30-minute walk or jog is considered exercise. **Exercise** is defined as planned, structured, and repetitive bodily movements done most often to improve or maintain one or more components of physical fitness, such as cardiorespiratory endurance, muscular strength or endurance, or flexibility.

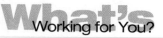

What's Working for You?

Maybe you are already engaging in physical activity. Which of the following are you already incorporating into your life?

☐ I go for a run several times a week.

☐ I walk to my classes.

☐ I participate in an intercollegiate or intramural sport.

☐ I do something physically active on the weekends.

☐ I lift weights at the gym several times a week.

From a major review of research on physical activity and health, researchers concluded that "there is irrefutable evidence of the effectiveness of regular physical activity in the primary and secondary prevention of several chronic diseases (e.g., cardiovascular disease, diabetes, cancer, hypertension, obesity, depression, and osteoporosis)."[4] Adding more physical activity to your day, like walking or cycling to school, can benefit your health. In fact, if all Americans followed the 2008 Physical Activity Guidelines (see Table 11.1), it is estimated that about one third of deaths related to coronary heart disease; one quarter of deaths related to stroke and osteoporosis; one fifth of deaths related to colon cancer, high blood pressure, and type 2 diabetes; and one seventh of deaths related to breast cancer could be prevented.[5]

Regular participation in physical activity improves more than 50 different physiological, metabolic, and psychological aspects of human life. Figure 11.1 on the following page summarizes some of these major health-related benefits.

Reduced Risk of Cardiovascular Diseases

Aerobic exercise is good for the heart and lungs and reduces the risk for heart-related diseases. It improves blood flow and eases the perfor-

mance of everyday tasks. Regular exercise makes the cardiovascular and respiratory systems more efficient by strengthening the heart muscle, enabling more blood to be pumped with each stroke, and increasing the number of *capillaries* (small blood vessels that allow gas exchange between blood and surrounding tissues) in trained skeletal muscles, which supply more blood to working muscles. Exercise also improves the respiratory system by increasing the amount of oxygen that is inhaled with each breath and distributed to body tissues.[6]

Regular physical activity can reduce hypertension, or chronic high blood pressure, a cardiovascular disease itself and a significant risk factor for other coronary heart diseases and stroke (see Chapter 12).[7] Regular aerobic exercise also improves the blood lipid profile. It typically increases high-density lipoproteins (HDLs, or "good" cholesterol), which are associated with lower risk for coronary artery disease because of their role in removing plaque built up in the arteries.[8] Triglycerides (a blood fat) typically decrease with aerobic exercise. Low-density lipoproteins (LDLs, or "bad" cholesterol) and total cholesterol are often improved with exercise due to weight loss and the improvements in HDL and triglycerides.

"Why Should I Care?"

Being physically active reduces your risk for many chronic diseases. That may not seem like an immediate concern, but there are a lot more immediate benefits: Becoming physically fit can help improve your physical appearance and sense of self-esteem, boost your resistance to diseases like colds and flus, reduce your stress level, improve your sleep, and help you concentrate. All that, and it's fun, too!

TABLE 11.1 2008 Physical Activity Guidelines for Americans

	Key Guidelines for Health*	For Additional Fitness or Weight Loss Benefits*	Additional Exercises
Adults	150 min/week moderate-intensity physical activity **OR** 75 min/week of vigorous-intensity physical activity **OR** Equivalent combination of moderate- and vigorous-intensity physical activity (i.e., 100 min moderate intensity + 25 min vigorous intensity)	300 min/week moderate-intensity physical activity **OR** 150 min/week of vigorous-intensity physical activity **OR** Equivalent combination of moderate- and vigorous-intensity physical activity (i.e., 200 min moderate intensity + 50 min vigorous intensity) **OR** More than the previously described amounts	Muscle strengthening activities for **all** the major muscle groups at least 2 days/week
Older Adults	If unable to follow above guidelines, then as much physical activity as their condition allows	If unable to follow above guidelines, then as much physical activity as their condition allows	In addition to muscle strengthening activities, exercise to improve balance
Children and Youth	60 min or more of moderate- or vigorous-intensity physical activity at least 3 days/week	At least 60 min of moderate- or vigorous-intensity physical activity on every day of the week	Include muscle strengthening activities at least 3 days/week Include bone-strengthening activities at least 3 days/week

*Accumulate this physical activity in sessions of 10 minutes or more at one time.
Source: Office of Disease Prevention and Health Promotion, U.S. Department of Health and Human Services, *2008 Physical Activity Guidelines for Americans: Be Active, Healthy, and Happy!*, ODPHP Publication no. U0036 (Washington, DC: U.S. Department of Health and Human Services, 2008), www.health.gov

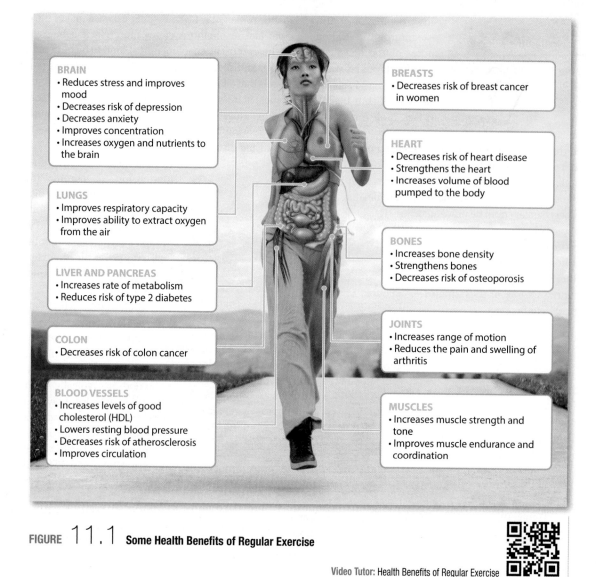

FIGURE 11.1 **Some Health Benefits of Regular Exercise**

Video Tutor: Health Benefits of Regular Exercise

Reduced Risk of Metabolic Syndrome and Type 2 Diabetes

Being regularly physically active reduces the risk of metabolic syndrome, a combination of risk factors that produces a synergistic increase in risk for heart disease and diabetes.[9] Metabolic syndrome includes high blood pressure, abdominal obesity, low levels of HDLs, high levels of triglycerides, and impaired glucose tolerance.[10] Regular participation in moderate-intensity physical activities reduces risk for each factor individually and collectively.[11]

Research indicates that a healthy dietary intake combined with sufficient physical activity could prevent many of the current cases of type 2 diabetes.[12] In a major national clinical trial, researchers found that exercising 150 minutes per week and eating fewer calories and less fat could prevent or delay the onset of type 2 diabetes.[13] (For more on diabetes prevention and management, see **Focus On: Minimizing Your Risk for Diabetes** on page 386.)

Reduced Cancer Risk

After decades of research, most cancer epidemiologists believe that the majority of cancers are preventable and can be avoided by healthier lifestyle and environmental choices.[14] In fact, a report released by the World Cancer Research Fund in conjunction with the American Institute for Cancer Research stated that two thirds of all cancers could be prevented based on lifestyle changes.[15] More specifically, one third of cancers could be prevented by being physically active and eating well. Regular physical activity appears to lower the risk for some specific cancers, particularly colon and rectal cancer.[16] Regular exercise is also associated with lower risk for breast cancer. Research on exercise and breast cancer risk has found that the earlier in life a woman starts to exercise, the lower her breast cancer risk.[17]

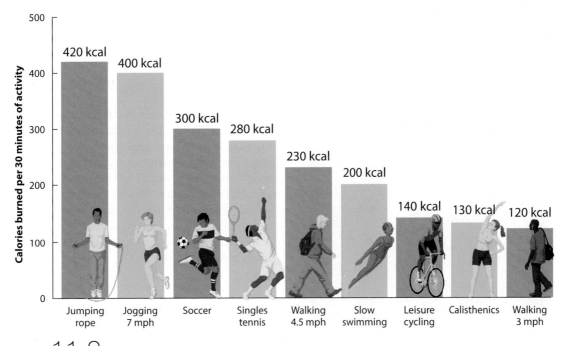

FIGURE 11.2 Calories Burned by Different Activities
The harder your physical activity, the more energy you expend. Estimated calories burned for various moderate and vigorous activities are listed for 30 minutes of activity. Note that the number of calories burned depends on body weight.

Improved Bone Mass and Reduced Risk of Osteoporosis

A common affliction for older people is *osteoporosis,* a disease characterized by low bone mass and deterioration of bone tissue, which increases fracture risk. Regular weight-bearing and strength-building physical activities are recommended to maintain bone health and prevent osteoporotic fractures. Although men and women are both negatively affected by osteoporosis, it is more common in women. Women (and men) have much to gain by remaining physically active and engaging in resistance training as they age—bone mass levels are significantly higher among active women than among sedentary women.[18] However, it appears that the full bone-related benefits of physical activity can only be achieved with sufficient hormone levels (estrogen in women, testosterone in men) and adequate calcium, vitamin D, and total caloric intakes.[19]

Improved Weight Management

For many people, the desire to lose or maintain weight is their main reason for physical activity.

On the most basic level, physical activity uses calories, and if calories expended exceed calories consumed over a span of time, the net result will be weight loss. The number of calories used depends on the intensity of the physical activity; **Figure 11.2** shows the caloric cost of various activities when done for 30 minutes.

In addition to the calories expended during physical activity, being regularly physically active has a direct positive effect on metabolic rate, keeping it elevated for several hours following vigorous physical activities (also see **Chapter 10**). An increased metabolic rate results in more calories being used and may contribute to fat loss, assuming dietary intake is not altered to compensate. Furthermore, regular physical activity may lead to body composition changes that favor weight management.[20]

Improved Immunity

Research shows that regular moderate-intensity physical activity reduces susceptibility to disease.[21] Just how regular physical activity positively influences immunity is not well understood. We know that moderate-intensity physical activity temporarily increases the number of white blood cells, which are responsible for fighting

If you want to lose weight, you need to move more and often!

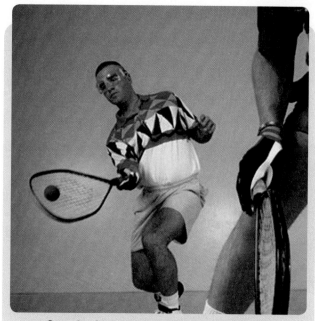

Can physical activity really reduce stress?

You bet it can! Although physical activity actually stimulates the stress response, a physically fit body adapts efficiently to the eustress of it, and as a result is better able to tolerate and effectively manage distress of all kinds.

infection.[22] However, while susceptibility to illness decreases with moderate activity, it increases as you move to more extreme levels of physical activity or exercise or if you continue to exercise without adequate recovery time and/or adequate dietary intake.[23] Athletes engaging in marathon-type events or very intense physical training programs have been shown to be at greater risk for upper respiratory tract infections in the first 8 hours after an intense exercise session.[24]

Improved Mental Health and Stress Management

Most people who engage in regular physical activity are likely to notice the psychological benefits, such as feeling better about oneself and an overall sense of well-being. Although these mental health benefits are difficult to quantify, they are frequently mentioned as reasons for continuing to be physically active. Learning new skills, developing increased ability and capacity in recreational activities, and sticking with a physical activity plan also improve self-esteem.

Regular aerobic physical activity can provide a break from stressors. It can improve the way the body handles stress by its effect on neurotransmitters associated with mood enhancement. Physical activity might also help the body recover from the stress response more quickly as fitness increases.[25]

Longer Life Span

Experts have long debated the relationship between physical activity and longevity. Several studies indicate significant decreases in long-term health risk and increases in years lived, particularly among those who have several risk factors for cardiovascular disease and who use physical activity as a means of risk reduction. Results from a study of nearly a million subjects showed that the largest benefits from physical activity occur in sedentary individuals who add a little physical activity to their lives, with additional benefits as physical activity levels increase.[26]

Physical Activity for Fitness and Performance

Physical fitness refers to a set of attributes that are either health or skill related. The health-related attributes—cardiorespiratory fitness, muscular strength and endurance, flexibility, and body composition—allow you to perform moderate- to vigorous-intensity physical activities on a regular basis without getting too tired and with energy left over to handle physical or mental emergencies. **Figure 11.3** on the following page identifies the major health related components of physical fitness.

30 minutes of physical activity a day—all at one time or in three 10-minute sessions—provides substantial health benefits.

Health-Related Components of Physical Fitness

Cardiorespiratory Fitness **Cardiorespiratory fitness** refers to the ability of the heart, lungs, and blood vessels to function efficiently. The primary category of physical activity known to improve cardiorespiratory fitness is **aerobic exercise.** The word *aerobic* means "with oxygen" and describes any type of exercise that requires oxygen to make energy for prolonged activity. Aerobic activities such as swimming, cycling, and jogging are excellent exercises for improving or maintaining cardiorespiratory fitness.

physical fitness Refers to a set of attributes that allow you to perform moderate- to vigorous-intensity physical activities on a regular basis without getting too tired and with energy left over to handle physical or mental emergencies.

cardiorespiratory fitness The ability of the heart, lungs, and blood vessels to supply oxygen to skeletal muscles during sustained physical activity.

aerobic exercise Any activity that requires oxygen to make energy.

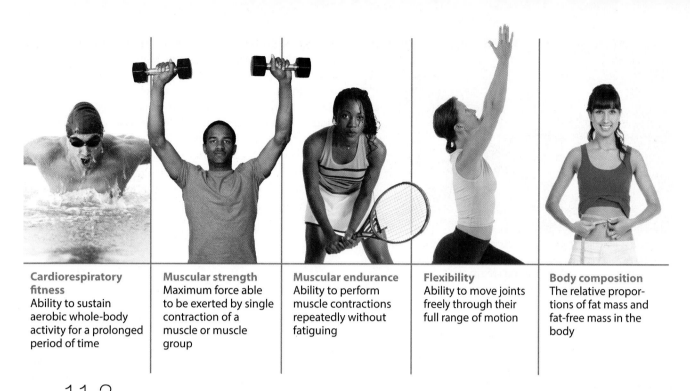

| **Cardiorespiratory fitness** Ability to sustain aerobic whole-body activity for a prolonged period of time | **Muscular strength** Maximum force able to be exerted by single contraction of a muscle or muscle group | **Muscular endurance** Ability to perform muscle contractions repeatedly without fatiguing | **Flexibility** Ability to move joints freely through their full range of motion | **Body composition** The relative proportions of fat mass and fat-free mass in the body |

FIGURE 11.3 Components of Physical Fitness

Cardiorespiratory fitness is measured by determining **aerobic capacity (power),** the volume of oxygen the muscles consume during exercise. Maximal aerobic power (commonly written as VO_{2max}) is defined as the maximal volume of oxygen that the muscles consume during exercise. Aerobic capacity is most often determined from a walk or run test on a treadmill. For greatest accuracy, this is done in a lab and requires special equipment and technicians to measure the precise amount of oxygen entering and exiting the body. Indirect or field tests can also be used to get a general sense of one's cardiorespiratory fitness; one such test, the 1.5-mile run test, is described in the **Assess Yourself** box on page 350.

Muscular Strength

Muscular strength refers to the amount of force a muscle or group of muscles can generate in one contraction. The most common way to assess the strength of a particular muscle or muscle group is to measure the maximum amount of weight you can move one time (and no more) or your one repetition maximum (1 RM).

Muscular Endurance

Muscular endurance is the ability of a muscle or group of muscles to exert force repeatedly without fatigue or the ability to sustain a muscular contraction. The more repetitions you can perform successfully (e.g., push-ups) or the longer you can hold a certain position (e.g., flexed arm hang), the greater your muscular endurance. General muscular endurance is most often measured from the number of curl-ups or push-ups an individual can do; the curl-up test is described in the **Assess Yourself** box.

Flexibility

Flexibility refers to the range of motion, or the amount of movement possible, at a particular joint or series of joints: the greater the range of motion, the greater the flexibility. Various tests measure the flexibility of the body's joints, including range of motion tests for specific joints. One of the most common measures of general flexibility is the sit-and-reach test, described in the **Assess Yourself** box.

Body Composition

Body composition is the fifth and final health-related component of physical fitness. Body composition describes the relative proportions and distribution of fat and fat-free (muscle, bone, water, organs) tissues in the body. (For more details on body composition, including its measurement, see Chapter 10.)

Skill-Related Components of Physical Fitness

In addition to the five health-related components of physical fitness, physical fitness for athletes involves attributes that improve their ability to perform athletic tasks. These attributes, called the *skill-related components* of physical fitness, also help recreational athletes and general exercisers increase fitness levels and their ability to perform daily tasks. The skill-related components of physical fitness (also called sport skills)

aerobic capacity (power) The functional status of the cardiorespiratory system; refers specifically to the volume of oxygen the muscles consume during exercise.

muscular strength The amount of force that a muscle is capable of exerting in one contraction.

muscular endurance A muscle's ability to exert force repeatedly without fatiguing or the ability to sustain a muscular contraction for a length of time.

flexibility The range of motion, or the amount of movement possible, at a particular joint or series of joints.

body composition Describes the relative proportions of fat and fat-free (muscle, bone, water, organs) tissues in the body.

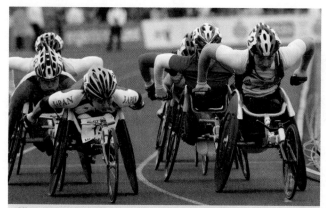

All people, including those with disabilities, can develop optimal levels of physical fitness and participate in physical activities they enjoy—including competitive sports.

moving each day. Take the stairs instead of the elevator, walk farther from your car to the store, and plan for organized movement each day, such as a 10- to 15-minute walk. In addition, you can start your muscle fitness program with simple body weight exercises, emphasizing proper technique and body alignment before adding any resistance.

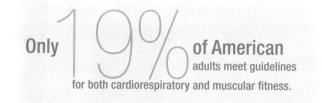

Only 19% of American adults meet guidelines for both cardiorespiratory and muscular fitness.

Overcoming Common Obstacles to Physical Activity

People have real and perceived barriers that prevent regular physical activity, ranging from personal ("I do not have time") to environmental ("I do not have a safe place to be

are *agility, balance, coordination, power, speed,* and *reaction time.* Note that some of the skill-related fitness components can impact health. For example, consider the importance of balance and coordination for older adults who are at increased risk for falls.

Athletes undertake specific exercises to increase their sport skills, and regular training results in significant improvements. Improving your sport skills can be as easy as participating regularly in any sport or activity. Playing football will increase reaction time and power, while dancing will increase balance, agility, and coordination. Another way to increase sport skills is to perform drills that mimic a sport-specific skill or work specifically on any of the skill-related components of fitness. You can practice drills in group exercise classes that incorporate sport skills, or you can work with a personal trainer.

Getting Motivated and Committing to Your Physical Fitness

To succeed at incorporating physical fitness into your life, you need to design a fitness program that takes obstacles into account and that is founded on the activities you enjoy most.

What If I Have Been Inactive for a While?

If you have been physically inactive for the past few months or longer, first make sure that your physician clears you for exercise. Consider consulting a personal trainer or fitness instructor to help you get started. In this phase of a fitness program, known as *the initial conditioning stage,* you may begin at levels lower than those recommended for physical fitness. Starting slowly will ease you into a workout regime with a minimum of soreness. For example, you might start your cardiorespiratory program by simply getting

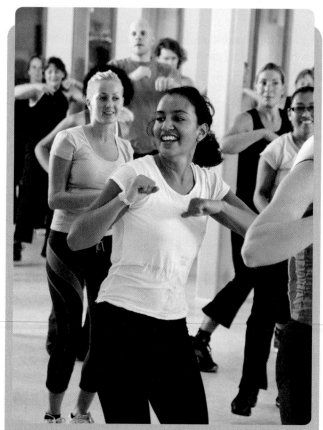

How can I motivate myself to be more physically active?

One great way to motivate yourself is to sign up for an exercise class. Find something that interests you—dance, yoga, aerobics, martial arts, acrobatics—and get involved. The structure, schedule, social interaction, and challenge of learning a new skill can be the motivation you need to get moving!

active"). Some people may be reluctant if they are over-weight, feel they are not fit enough to work out with their more fit friends, or feel they lack the knowledge and skills required.

Think about what stops you from being physically active and write these things down. Review Table 11.2 for suggestions on overcoming your hurdles or barriers to physical activity.

Incorporating Physical Activity in Your Life

When designing your program, you can boost your chances of achieving your physical fitness goals by considering several factors. First, choose activities that you genuinely like doing, are convenient or easy for you to do, and are appropriate for you. For example, choose jogging because you like to run and there are beautiful trails nearby rather than swimming when you do not like the water and the pool is difficult to get to. Likewise, choose physical activities that you are capable of doing. If you are overweight or obese and have been inactive for months, do not sign up for advanced aerobics classes. Start slow, plan enjoyable activities, and progress to more strenuous or vigorous physical activities as your physical fitness improves. You may choose to walk more to achieve the recommended goal of 10,000 steps per day; keep track with a pedometer (or step counter). Try to make physical activity a part of your routine by fitting it in when you already have to move—such as getting to class or work. See the **Be Healthy, Be Green** box on the following page for more on this topic.

Creating Your Own Fitness Program

The first step in creating a personal physical fitness program is identifying your goals. Take time to reflect on your personal circumstances and desires regarding physical fitness. Do you want to be better at sports or feel better about your

TABLE
11.2 Overcoming Obstacles to Physical Activity

Obstacle	Possible Solution
Lack of time	• Look at your schedule. Where can you find 30-minute time slots? Perhaps you need to focus on shorter times; so long as you accumulate your physical activity in 10-minute bouts, it counts toward the total time recommended. • Multitask. Read while riding an exercise bike or listen to lecture tapes while walking. • Be physically active during your lunch and study breaks as well as between classes. Skip rope or throw a Frisbee with a friend. • Select activities that require less time, such as brisk walking or jogging. • Ride your bike to class, or park (or get off the bus) farther from your destination.
Social influence	• Invite family and friends to be active with you. • Join an exercise class to meet new people. • Explain the importance of physical activity and your commitment to it to people who may not support your efforts. • Find a role model to support your efforts. • Plan for physically active dates—go for a walk, dancing, or bowling.
Lack of motivation, willpower, or energy	• Schedule your physical activity time just as you would any other important commitment. • Enlist the help of a friend or family member to make you accountable for getting to your physical activity. • Give yourself an incentive—but not food or inactivity. • Schedule your workouts when you feel most energetic. • Remind yourself that physical activity gives you more energy. • Get things ready; for example, if you choose to walk in the morning, set out your clothes and shoes the night before.
Lack of resources	• Select an activity that requires minimal equipment, such as walking, jogging, jumping rope, or calisthenics. • Identify inexpensive resources on campus or in the community. • Use active forms of transportation. • Take advantage of no-cost opportunities, such as playing catch in the park or green space on campus.

Source: Adapted from National Center for Chronic Disease Prevention and Health Promotion, "How Can I Overcome Barriers to Physical Activity?," Updated May 2011, www.cdc.gov

BE HEALTHY, BE GREEN

TRANSPORT YOURSELF!

Before we became a car culture, much of our transportation was human powered. Historically, bicycling and walking were important means of transportation and recreation in the United States. Even in the first few decades after the automobile started to be popular, people continued to get around under their own power.

The more we use our cars to get around, the more congested our roads, the more polluted our air, and the more sedentary our lives become. That is why many people are now embracing a movement toward more active transportation. *Active transportation* means getting out of your car and using your own power to travel from place to place—whether walking, riding a bike, skateboarding, or rollerskating. The following are just a few of the many reasons to make active transportation a bigger part of your life:

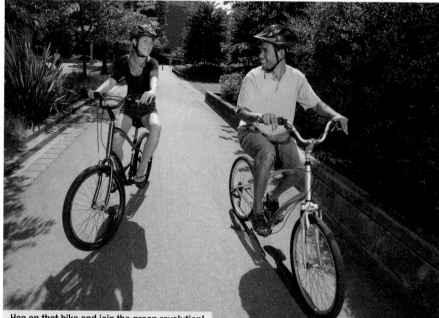

Hop on that bike and join the green revolution!

* You will be adding more physical activity into your daily routine. People who walk, bike, or use other active forms of transportation to complete errands are more likely to meet the physical activity guidelines.

* Walking or biking can save you money. With rising gas prices and parking fees, in addition to increasing car maintenance and insurance costs, active transportation could add up to considerable savings. During the course of a year, regular bicycle commuters who ride 5 miles to work can save about $500 on fuel and more than $1,000 on other expenses related to driving.

* Walking or biking may save you time! Cycling is usually the fastest mode of travel door to door for distances up to 5 or 6

miles in city centers. Walking is simpler and faster for distances of about a mile or two.

* You will enjoy being outdoors. Research is emerging on the physical and mental health benefits of nature and being outdoors. So much of what we do is inside, with recirculated air and artificial lighting, that our bodies are deficient in fresh air and sunlight.

* You will be making a significant contribution to the reduction of air pollution. Driving less means fewer pollutants emitted into the air. Leaving your car at home just 2 days a week will reduce greenhouse gas emissions by an average of 1,600 pounds per year.

* You will contribute to global environmental health. Annually, personal

transportation accounts for the consumption of approximately 136 billion gallons of gasoline, or the production of 1.2 billion tons of carbon dioxide. Reducing vehicle trips will help reduce overall greenhouse gas emissions and reduce the need to source more fossil fuel.

Sources: T. Gotschi and K. Mills, *Active Transportation for America: The Case for Increased Federal Investment in Bicycling and Walking* (Washington, DC: Rails to Trails Conservancy, 2008); D. Shinkle and A. Teigens, *Encouraging Bicycling and Walking: The State Legislative Role* (Washington, DC: National Conference of State Legislatures, 2008), Updated April 2009, www.americantrails.org; U.S. Environmental Protection Agency, "Climate Change: What You Can Do—On the Road," Updated June 2012, www.epa.gov

body? Is your goal to manage stress, improve health, and reduce your risk of chronic diseases? Perhaps your most vital goal will be to commit to physical fitness for the long haul—to establish a realistic schedule of diverse physical activities that you can maintain and enjoy throughout your life. Your physical fitness goals and objectives should be both achievable for you and in line with what you truly want. Achievable,

truly desired goals increase motivation, and this, in turn, leads to a better chance of success.

To set successful goals, try using the *SMART* system. SMART goals are **s**pecific, **m**easurable, **a**ction-oriented, **r**ealistic, and **t**ime-oriented.

A vague goal would be "Improve fitness by exercising more." A SMART goal would be as follows:

- *Specific*: "Participate in a resistance training program that targets all of the major muscle groups 3 to 5 days per week."
- *Measurable*: "Improve fitness classification from average to good."
- *Action-oriented*: "I'll meet with a personal trainer to learn how to safely do resistance exercises and to plan a workout for the gym and home."
- *Realistic*: "I'll increase the weight I can lift by 20 percent (not 200 percent)."
- *Time-oriented*: "I'll try my new weight program for 8 weeks, then reassess."

Principles of Fitness Training: FITT

Assuming you intend to improve your health-related physical fitness (although the principles also apply to performance-related physical fitness), you should use the **FITT (Frequency, Intensity, Time,** and **Type)**[27] principle to define your exercise program. The FITT prescription **(Figure 11.4)** uses the following criteria:

- **Frequency** refers to the number of times per week you need to engage in particular exercises to achieve the desired level of physical fitness in a particular component.

- **Intensity** refers to how hard your workout must be to achieve the desired level of physical fitness.
- **Time**, or the *duration*, refers to how many minutes or repetitions of an exercise are required at a specified intensity during any one session to attain the desired level of physical fitness for each component.
- **Type** refers to what kind of exercises should be performed to improve the specific component of physical fitness.

The FITT Principle for Cardiorespiratory Fitness

The most effective aerobic exercises for building cardiorespiratory fitness are total body activities involving the large muscle groups of your body. Examples

FITT Acronym for frequency, intensity, time, and type; the terms that describe the essential components of a program or plan to improve a parameter of physical fitness.

frequency As part of the FITT prescription, refers to how many days per week a person should exercise to improve a parameter of physical fitness.

intensity As part of the FITT prescription, refers to how hard or how much effort is needed when a person exercises to improve a parameter of physical fitness.

time As part of the FITT prescription, refers to how long a person needs to exercise each time to improve a parameter of physical fitness.

type As part of the FITT prescription, refers to what kind of exercises a person needs to do to improve a parameter of physical fitness.

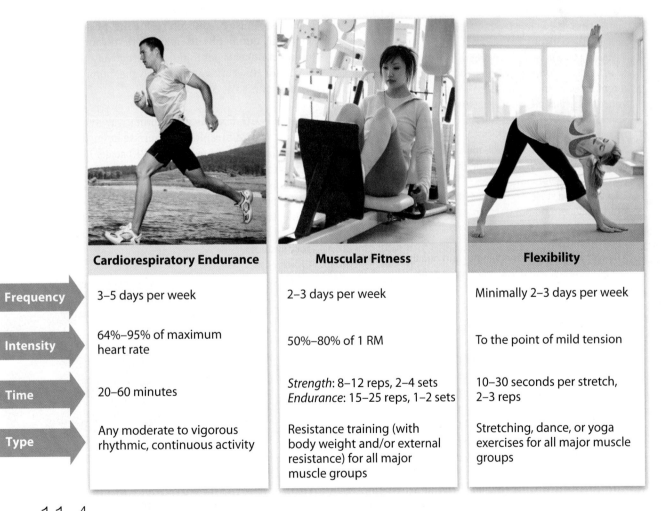

	Cardiorespiratory Endurance	**Muscular Fitness**	**Flexibility**
Frequency	3–5 days per week	2–3 days per week	Minimally 2–3 days per week
Intensity	64%–95% of maximum heart rate	50%–80% of 1 RM	To the point of mild tension
Time	20–60 minutes	*Strength*: 8–12 reps, 2–4 sets *Endurance*: 15–25 reps, 1–2 sets	10–30 seconds per stretch, 2–3 reps
Type	Any moderate to vigorous rhythmic, continuous activity	Resistance training (with body weight and/or external resistance) for all major muscle groups	Stretching, dance, or yoga exercises for all major muscle groups

FIGURE 11.4 **The FITT Principle Applied to Cardiorespiratory Fitness, Muscular Strength and Endurance, and Flexibility**

Plan It, Start It, Stick with It!

The most successful physical activity program is one that you enjoy and is realistic and appropriate for your skill level and needs.

❭ **Make it enjoyable.** Pick something you like to do so that you will make the effort and find the time to engage in physical activity.

❭ **Start slow.** If you have been physically inactive for a while, any type and amount of physical activity is a step in the right direction. Start slowly, letting your body adapt so there is not too much pain the next day. You will be able to increase the amount and intensity of your activity each week and will be on your way to meeting the physical activity recommendations and your personal goals!

❭ **Make only one lifestyle change at a time.** It is not realistic to change everything at once. Furthermore, success with one behavioral change will increase your belief in yourself and encourage you to make other positive changes.

❭ **Set SMART goals for your physical fitness program.** It takes several months to feel the benefits of your physical activity. Be patient.

❭ **Choose a time to be physically active and stick with it.** Learn to establish priorities and keep to a schedule. Try different times of the day to learn what works best for you. Yet, be flexible, so if something comes up that you cannot work around, you will still find time to do some physical activity.

❭ **Record your progress.** Include the intensity, time, and type of physical activities; your emotions; and your personal achievements.

❭ **Take lapses in stride.** Sometimes life gets in the way. Start again and do not despair; your commitment to physical fitness has ebbs and flows like most everything else in life.

❭ **Reward yourself.** Find meaningful and healthy ways to reward yourself when you reach your goals.

at least 75 minutes per week for vigorous intensity. Approximately 1,000 calories per week is associated with 150 minutes of moderate intensity exercise.

But how do you know whether you are doing moderate or vigorous exercise intensity? The most common methods used to determine the intensity of cardiorespiratory endurance exercises are target heart rate, rating of perceived exertion, and the talk test.

Target Heart Rate The exercise intensity required to improve cardiorespiratory endurance is a heart rate between 64 and 95 percent of your maximum heart rate. One way to calculate this **target heart rate** is to start by subtracting your age from 220 to get your predicted maximum heart rate. Your target heart rate would be 64 to 95 percent of that predicted maximum heart rate. For example, if you are a 20-year-old male, your estimated maximum heart rate is 200 ($220 - 20 = 200$). Your target heart rate would be somewhere between 128 ($200 \times 0.64 = 128$) and 190 ($200 \times 0.95 = 190$) beats per minute.

Take your pulse during your workout to determine how close you are to your target heart rate. Lightly place your index and middle fingers over one of the major arteries in your neck or on the artery on the inside of your wrist (Figure 11.5). Start counting your pulse immediately after you stop exercising, as your heart rate decreases rapidly. Using a watch or a clock, take your pulse for 6 seconds (the first pulse is "0") and multiply this number by 10 (add a zero to your count) to get the number of beats per minute. Alternatively, you can take your pulse for 10 seconds and multiply that number by 6; first pulse is still counted as "0."

Perceived Exertion Another way to determine the intensity of cardiorespiratory exercise intensity is to use Borg's rating of perceived exertion (RPE) scale. Perceived exertion refers to how hard you feel you are working, which you might base on your heart rate, breathing rate, amount that you are sweating, and level of fatigue. This scale uses a rating from 6 (no exertion at all) to 20 (maximal exertion). An RPE of 12 to 16 is generally recommended for training the cardiorespiratory system.

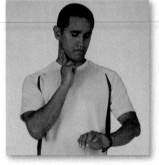
ⓐ Carotid pulse

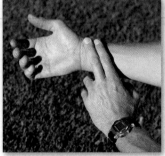
ⓑ Radial pulse

FIGURE 11.5 **Taking a Pulse**
Palpation of the carotid (neck) or radial (wrist) artery is a simple way of determining heart rate.

include walking briskly, cycling, jogging, fitness classes, and swimming.

To improve cardiorespiratory fitness, the American College of Sports Medicine (ACSM) recommends 3 to 5 days per week of moderate to vigorous, rhythmic, continuous activity, at 64 to 95 percent of your maximum heart rate, for 20 to 60 minutes at a time, depending on level of intensity; 20 minutes is fine for vigorous intensity, but moderate-intensity workouts should be at least 30 minutes.[28] The recommended amount of aerobic exercise is at least 150 minutes per week for moderate intensity and

target heart rate The heart rate range of aerobic exercise that leads to improved cardiorespiratory fitness (i.e., 40% to 90% of heart rate reserve).

The Talk Test The easiest method of measuring cardiorespiratory exercise intensity is the talk test. A moderate level of exercise (heart rate at 64 to 75 percent of maximum) is a conversational level of exercise. At this level you are able to talk while exercising. If you can talk, but only in short fragments and not sentences, you are at a vigorous level of exercise (heart rate at 76 to 95 percent of maximum). If you are breathing so hard that speaking at all is difficult, the intensity of your exercise may be too high. Conversely, if you are able to sing or laugh heartily while exercising, the intensity of your exercise is light and may be insufficient for maintaining or improving cardiorespiratory fitness.

The FITT Principle for Muscular Strength and Endurance

The FITT principle for muscular strength and endurance includes 2 to 3 days per week of exercises that train the major muscle groups, using enough sets and repetitions and sufficient resistance to improve muscular strength and endurance.[29] One of the important principles of strength training is the idea of *reversibility*. Reversibility means that if you stop exercising, your body responds by deconditioning (reverting back to its untrained state).

To improve muscular strength or endurance, resistance training using either your own body weight or devices that provide a fixed, variable, or accommodating load or resistance is most often recommended (see Table 11.3). For general health benefits, two to four sets with 8 to 12 repetitions per set is recommended.

TABLE 11.3 | **Methods of Providing Exercise Resistance**

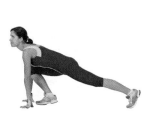

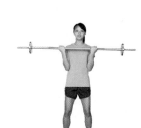

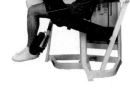

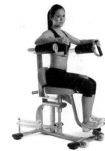

Body Weight Resistance (Calisthenics)	Fixed Resistance	Variable Resistance	Accommodating Resistance
• Uses your own body weight to develop muscular strength and endurance. • Improves overall muscular fitness and, in particular, core body strength and overall muscle tone.	• Provides a constant resistance throughout the full range of movement. • Requires balance and coordination; promotes development of core body strength.	• Resistance is altered so that the muscle's effort is consistent throughout the full range of motion. • Provides more controlled motion and isolates certain muscle groups.	• Sometimes called isokinetic machines; they maintain a constant speed throughout the range of motion. • Requires a maximal effort as the machine controls the speed of exercise. • Often used for rehabilitation after injury.
Examples: Push-ups, pull-ups, curl-ups, dips, leg raises, chair sits, etc.	**Examples:** Free weights, such as barbells and dumbbells.	**Examples:** Weight machines in gyms and homes (Nautilus or Bowflex).	**Examples:** Specific machines in rehabilitation facilities and gyms.

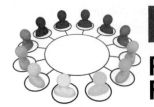

PHYSICAL ACTIVITY AND EXERCISE FOR SPECIAL POPULATIONS

In some cases, modifications to the FITT prescription may be suggested for people with the special considerations mentioned below. It is recommended that all individuals, but particularly those with health conditions, consult with a physician before beginning any exercise program.

ASTHMA

Regular physical activity provides benefits for individuals with asthma. It strengthens the respiratory muscles, making it easier to breathe; improves immune system functioning; and helps maintain weight.

Before engaging in exercise, ensure that your asthma is under control. Ask about adjusting your medications; for example, your doctor may recommend you use your inhaler 15 minutes prior to exercise. Keep your inhaler nearby. Warm up and cool down properly; it is particularly important that you allow your lungs and breathing rate to adjust slowly. Protect yourself from your asthma triggers when exercising. If you have symptoms while exercising, stop and use your inhaler; if an asthma attack persists, call 9-1-1.

OBESITY

Obese individuals may have limitations such as heat intolerance, shortness of breath during physical activity, lack of flexibility, frequent musculoskeletal injuries, and difficulty with balance. Programs should emphasize physical activities that can be sustained for longer periods of time such as walking, swimming, or bicycling. Use caution when performing these

Athletes like Brandon Morrow, a Major League Baseball pitcher with type 1 diabetes, are living proof that chronic conditions needn't prevent you from achieving your physical activity goals.

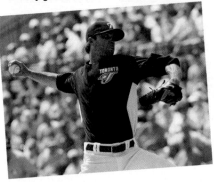

activities in hot or humid environments. Although it is recommended to start slowly (5 to 10 minutes of activity) and at a lower intensity (55% to 65% of maximal heart rate), the ultimate goal is to perform at least 30 minutes of exercise per session, resulting in over 250 minutes per week, to enhance weight loss and prevent weight re-gain. Regardless of weight loss, evidence suggests that individuals who are obese improve their health with cardiorespiratory and resistance training activities.

CORONARY HEART DISEASE

Although regular physical activity reduces risk of coronary heart disease, vigorous-intensity activity acutely increases risk of sudden cardiac death and myocardial infarction (heart attack). Individuals with coronary heart disease must consult their physicians.

HYPERTENSION

Using the FITT prescription, individuals who are hypertensive should engage in physical activity on most, if not all, days of the week, at a moderate intensity (12 to 13 on the Borg RPE scale), for 30 minutes or more.

DIABETES

Physical activity benefits individuals with diabetes in many ways. It controls blood glucose (for individuals with type 2 diabetes) by improving transport into the cells, controls body weight, and reduces risk for heart disease.

Before people with type 1 diabetes engage in physical activity, they must learn how to manage their resting blood glucose levels. Individuals should have an exercise partner; eat 1 to 3 hours prior to the activity; eat complex carbohydrates after the activity; avoid late-evening exercise; and monitor their blood glucose before, during, and after activity.

One of the most important factors for individuals with type 2 diabetes is the duration of their physical activity. Because a critical objective of the management of type 2 diabetes is to reduce body fat (obesity), the recommendations for duration are longer—reaching 60 minutes per session. For sessions of this length, it is prudent to reduce the intensity of the activity to a target heart rate range of 40 to 60 percent of maximal heart rate.

Source: P. Williamson, *Exercise for Special Populations* (Philadelphia: Lippincott Williams & Wilkins, 2011).

To determine the intensity of exercise needed to improve muscular strength and endurance, you need to know the maximum amount of weight you can lift (or move) in one contraction. This value is called your **one repetition maximum (1 RM).** It can be individually determined or predicted from a 10 RM test. Once your 1 RM is determined, it is used as the basis

one repetition maximum (1 RM)
The amount of weight or resistance that can be lifted or moved only once.

for intensity recommendations to improve muscular strength and endurance. Muscular strength is improved when resistance loads are greater than 60 percent of your 1 RM, whereas muscular endurance is improved using loads less than 50 percent of your 1 RM.

The time recommended for muscular strength and endurance exercises is measured in repetitions and sets rather than in minutes of exercise.

Repetitions and Sets To increase muscular strength, you need higher intensity and fewer repetitions and sets: Use a resistance of 60 percent or greater of your 1 RM (or at least 40 percent if you are new to resistance training), and perform 8 to 12 repetitions per set, with two to four sets performed overall. The recommendations for improving muscular endurance are to perform one or two sets of 15 to 25 repetitions using a resistance that is less than 50 percent of your 1 RM.

Rest Periods Resting between exercises can reduce fatigue and help with performance and safety in subsequent sets. A rest period of 2 to 3 minutes is recommended when using the guidelines for general health benefits. However, the rest period when working to develop strength or endurance will vary. Note that this rest period refers specifically to the muscle group being exercised, and it is possible to alternate muscle groups, thus taking advantage of your time available to train. For example, you can alternate a set of push-ups with curl-ups so that the muscle groups worked in one set can rest while you are working the other muscle groups.

Specificity, Exercise Selection, and Exercise Order When selecting the type of strength-training exercises to do, the *specificity principle* must be considered. According to this principle, the effects of resistance training are specific to the muscles exercised. To improve total body strength, you must include exercises for all the major muscle groups, which can typically be accomplished with 8 to 10 exercises. You must also ensure that your *overload* is sufficient to increase strength and endurance, that is, you are creating a degree of tension in your muscles that is greater than what they are accustomed to.

Another important concept to consider is *exercise selection*. The exercises you choose should be specific for the muscles and muscle groups you are targeting.

Finally, for optimal resistance training effects, it is important to pay attention to *exercise order*. When training all major muscle groups in a single workout, complete large muscle, multijoint muscle group exercises (e.g., the bench press or leg press) before small muscle, single joint exercises (e.g., biceps curls, triceps extension); also complete high-intensity exercises before lower-intensity exercises.

The FITT Principle for Flexibility

Improving flexibility not only enhances the efficiency of your movements, but also enhances your sense of well-being and helps you manage stress effectively. Furthermore, inflexible muscles are susceptible to injury. Flexibility training is effective in reducing the incidence and severity of lower back problems and muscle or tendon injuries that can occur during sports and everyday physical activities.[30] Improved flexibility also means less tension and pressure on joints, resulting in less joint pain and joint deterioration.[31]

The most effective exercises for improving flexibility involve stretching of the major muscle groups of your body when the body is already warm, as it is after cardiorespira-tory activities. The most common exercises for improving flexibility involve **static stretching.** Static stretching techniques slowly and gradually lengthen a muscle or group of muscles and their tendons. The primary strategy is to decrease the resistance to stretch (tension) within a tight muscle targeted for increased range of motion.[32] To do this, you repeatedly stretch the muscle and its tendons of attachment to elongate them. With each repetition of a static stretch, your range of motion improves temporarily due to the slightly lessened sensitivity of tension receptors in the stretched muscles, and when done regularly, range of motion increases.[33] **Figure 11.6** on the following page illustrates some basic stretching exercises to increase flexibility.

The FITT principle calls for a minimum of 2 to 3 days per week for flexibility training; however, daily training produces the most benefits. Perform or hold static stretching positions at the "point of tension"—a tension or mild discomfort, but not pain, in the muscle(s) you are stretching.[34] You should hold the stretch at the point of tension for 10 to 30 seconds and repeat two or three times in relatively close succession.[35] The recommendation for general health benefits is 60 seconds per exercise.

Implementing Your Fitness Program

Develop a Progressive Plan

As your physical fitness improves, you need to adjust the frequency, intensity, time, and type of your exercise to maintain or continue to improve your level of physical fitness. Experts recommend that you begin an exercise regimen by gradually increasing the frequency or time of your workouts, then make gradual increases in exercise intensity. Exercise frequency depends on time and intensity, but the goal is to reach 5 days per week (or 150 minutes total) for moderate intensity exercise. Intensity should also be increased gradually, by no more than 10 percent each week. For beginners, increase the time 5 to 10 minutes every 1 to 2 weeks for the first 4 to 6 weeks until the target time is met. Choosing different types of activities can produce a higher level of physical fitness (because different muscle groups are used) and also to keep you motivated and interested enough to continue training regularly.

Design Your Exercise Session

A well-designed exercise program should improve or maintain cardiorespiratory fitness, muscular strength and endurance, flexibility, and body composition. But what should you do when you begin your exercise routine? A comprehensive workout should include a warm-up, cardiorespiratory and/or

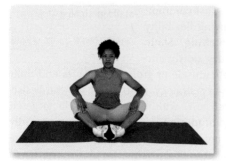

(a) Stretching the inside of the thighs

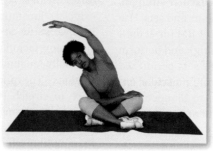

(b) Stretching the upper arm and the side of the trunk

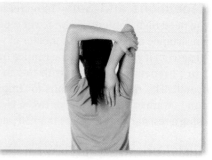

(c) Stretching the triceps

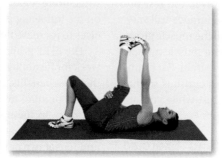

(d) Stretching the trunk and the hip

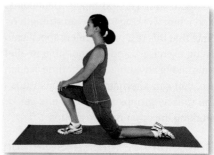

(e) Stretching the hip, back of the thigh, and the calf

(f) Stretching the front of the thigh and the hip flexor

FIGURE 11.6 **Stretching Exercises to Improve Flexibility and Prevent Injury**
Use these stretches as part of your warm-up and cool-down. Hold each stretch for 10 to 30 seconds, and repeat two to three times for each limb.

resistance training, and then a cool-down to finish the session. Each of these is described in more detail below.

Warm-Up The primary purpose of the warm-up is to prepare the body physically and mentally for the cardiorespiratory and/or resistance training that is to follow. Generally, a warm-up involves large body movements, followed by light stretching of the muscle groups to be used. Usually 5 to 15 minutes long, a warm-up is shorter when you are geared up and ready to go and longer when you are struggling with your motivation to get moving or your muscles are cold or feel tight. The important thing is to listen to your body and take the time needed to prepare it for more intense activity. The warm-up provides a transition from rest to physical activity by slowly increasing heart rate, blood pressure, breathing rate, and body temperature. These gradual changes improve joint lubrication, increase muscles' and tendons' elasticity and flexibility, and facilitate performance during the next stage of the workout.

Cardiorespiratory and/or Resistance Training The next stage of your workout, immediately following the warm-up, may involve cardiorespiratory training, resistance training, or a little of both. If you are in a fitness center, you may choose to use one or more of the aerobic training devices for the recommended time. (The **Money & Health** box on the following page offers suggestions on choosing a fitness center.) Before or after cardiorespiratory training, you may choose to follow your prescribed program for strength and endurance training. Regardless of what you choose, the bulk of the workout occurs in this stage and will last at least 20 to 30 minutes.

Resistance training to improve muscular strength and endurance can be done with free weights, machines, or even your own body weight.

Money&Health

INVESTING IN YOUR PHYSICAL HEALTH!
HOW TO SHOP FOR A FITNESS FACILITY

Do you really need to belong to a gym to meet your physical fitness goals? The short answer is no. You can achieve your personal goals without spending lots of money joining a fitness center. All you need is your own body to use as resistance and a safe place for activity. However, you may enjoy the experience of going to a fitness center or using exercise equipment. The following tips will help guide you through the process of finding a place to exercise.

✱ Visit several facilities before making a decision, if possible during the time when you intend to use them (so you can see how busy or crowded they are at that time).
✱ Determine whether the location and hours of operation are convenient for you.
✱ Consider the exercise classes offered. What is the schedule? Can you try a class for free?
✱ Evaluate the equipment. Is it sufficient to cover your training needs (i.e., aerobic exercise machines; resistance-training equipment, including both free weights and machines; mats; and other items to assist with stretching)? Is it kept clean and in good condition? Do they offer instruction in how to use the equipment?
✱ Consider the personnel (including training in first aid and CPR), options for working with a personal trainer, and how friendly and approachable they are.

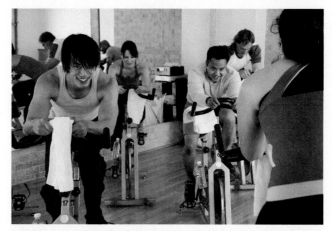

Before you sign on the dotted line, check out the classes, equipment, and personnel a fitness center offers.

✱ Consider the financial implications. What membership benefits, student rates, or other discounts are available? Steer clear of clubs that pressure you for a long-term commitment and do not offer trial memberships or grace periods that allow you to get a refund.

Cool-down and Stretching Just as you ease into a workout with a warm-up, you should slowly transition from physical activity to rest. The cool-down lasts 10 to 15 minutes and should gradually reduce your heart rate, blood pressure, and body temperature to preexercising levels. The cool-down reduces the risk of blood pooling in the extremities and facilitates quicker recovery between exercise sessions. Generally, the cool-down starts with 5 to 10 minutes of moderate- to low-intensity activity followed by 5 to 10 minutes of stretching exercises. Because of the body's increased temperature, the cool-down is an excellent time to stretch to improve flexibility.

Explore Activities That Develop Multiple Components of Fitness

Some forms of activity have the potential to improve several components of physical fitness and thus improve your everyday functioning ("functional" exercises). For example, core strength training improves posture and can prevent back pain. In addition, yoga, tai chi, and Pilates improve flexibility,

muscular strength and endurance, balance, coordination, and agility. They also develop the mind-body connection through concentration on breathing and body position. Some people see these activities as strongly connected to their spiritual health as well, particularly when time is spent relaxing, breathing deeply, and trying to clear the mind.

Among America's 207 million active people, fitness sports such as yoga, boot camp-style training, and other fitness classes are the most popular physical activities.

Core Strength Training The body's core muscles include the deep back, abdominal, and hip muscles that attach to the spine and pelvis. The contraction of these core muscles provides the basis of support for movements of the upper and lower body and powerful movements of the extremities. A weak core can result in poor posture, low

traumatic injuries Injuries that are accidental and occur suddenly.

overuse injuries Injuries that result from the cumulative effects of day-after-day stresses placed on tendons, muscles, and joints.

back pain, and muscle injuries. You can develop core strength by doing various exercises, including calisthenics, yoga, or Pilates. Holding yourself in a front or reverse plank (an up and reverse of the push-up position) and holding or doing abdominal curl-ups are examples of exercises that increase core strength. Increased core strength does not happen from one single exercise, but rather from a structured regime of postures and exercises. The use of instability devices (stability ball, wobble boards, etc.) and exercises to train the core have become popular.[36] Although research suggests instability training is effective for improving core strength and reducing back pain, it should not replace traditional programs completely; it should rather be used in conjunction with and become part of the FITT prescription.[37]

Yoga Yoga, based on ancient Indian practices, blends the mental and physical aspects of exercise—a union of mind and body that participants often find relaxing and satisfying. If done regularly, yoga improves flexibility, vitality, posture, agility, balance, coordination, and muscular strength and endurance. Many people report an improved sense of general well-being, too.

The practice of yoga focuses attention on controlled breathing as well as physical exercise and incorporates a complex array of static stretching and strengthening exercises expressed as postures (*asanas*). During a session, participants move to different asanas and hold them for 30 seconds or longer. Asanas, singly or in combination, can be changed and adapted for young and old, to accommodate physical limitations or disabilities, or to provide well-conditioned athletes with a challenging workout.

Tai Chi Tai chi is an ancient Chinese form of exercise that combines stretching, balance, muscular endurance, coordination, and meditation. It increases range of motion and flexibility while reducing muscular tension. It involves a series of positions called *forms* that are performed continuously. Tai chi is often described as "meditation in motion" because it promotes serenity through gentle movements that connect the mind and body.

Pilates Pilates was developed by Joseph Pilates in 1926 as an exercise style that combines stretching with movement against resistance, frequently aided by devices such as tension springs or heavy rubber bands. It teaches body awareness, good posture, and easy, graceful body movements while improving flexibility, coordination, core strength, muscle tone, and economy of motion.

Preventing and Treating Fitness-Related Injuries

Eager to improve their fitness quickly, beginners often injure themselves by doing too much too soon. Two basic types of injuries stem from fitness-related activities: traumatic injuries and overuse injuries. **Traumatic injuries** occur suddenly and usually by accident. Typical traumatic injuries are broken bones, torn ligaments and muscles, contusions, and lacerations. If a traumatic injury causes a noticeable loss of function and immediate pain or pain that does not go away after 30 minutes, consult a physician.

Overuse injuries result from the cumulative effects of day-after-day stresses placed on tendons, muscles, and joints during exercise. These injuries occur most often in repetitive activities such as swimming, running, bicycling, and step aerobics. The forces that occur normally during physical activity are not enough to cause a ligament sprain or muscle strain as in a traumatic injury, but when these forces are applied daily for weeks or months, they can result in an overuse injury.

The three most common overuse injuries are runner's knee, shin splints, and plantar fasciitis. Runner's knee is a general term describing a series of problems involving the muscles, tendons, and ligaments around the knee. S*hin splints* is a general term used for any pain that occurs below the knee and above the ankle in the shin. Plantar fasciitis is an inflammation of the plantar fascia, a broad band of dense, inelastic tissue in the foot. Rest, variation of routine, and stretching are the first lines of treatment for any of these overuse injuries. If pain continues, a physician visit is recommended.

In addition to injuries, beginners can be susceptible to marketers, friends, teammates, or other acquaintances pushing performance-enhancing drugs or other supplements with promises

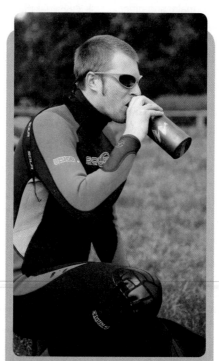

How much do I need to drink before, during, and after physical activity?

The American College of Sports Medicine and the National Athletic Trainers' Association recommend consuming 14 to 22 ounces of fluid several hours prior to and about 6 to 12 ounces per 15 to 20 minutes during physical activity—assuming you are sweating.

Men	Excellent	Very Good	Good	Fair	Needs Improvement		Women	Excellent	Very Good	Good	Fair	Needs Improvement
Ages 20–29	≥ 40 cm	34–39 cm	30–33 cm	25–29 cm	≤ 24 cm		Ages 20–29	≥ 41 cm	37–40 cm	33–36 cm	28–32 cm	≤ 27 cm
Ages 30–39	≥ 38 cm	33–37 cm	28–32 cm	23–27 cm	≤ 22 cm		Ages 30–39	≥ 41 cm	36–40 cm	32–35 cm	27–31 cm	≤ 26 cm
Ages 40–49	≥ 35 cm	29–34 cm	24–28 cm	18–23 cm	≤ 17 cm		Ages 40–49	≥ 38 cm	34–37 cm	30–33 cm	25–29 cm	≤ 24 cm
Ages 50–59	≥ 35 cm	28–34 cm	24–27 cm	16–23 cm	≤ 15 cm		Ages 50–59	≥ 39 cm	33–38 cm	30–32 cm	25–29 cm	≤ 24 cm
Ages 60–69	≥ 33 cm	25–32 cm	20–24 cm	15–19 cm	≤ 14 cm		Ages 60–69	≥ 35 cm	31–34 cm	27–30 cm	23–26 cm	≤ 22 cm

*Note: These norms are based on a sit-and-reach box in which the zero point is set at 26 cm. When using a box in which the zero point is set at 23 cm, subtract 3 cm from each value in this table.

Source: From *Canadian Physical Activity, Fitness & Lifestyle Approach: CSEP-Health & Fitness Program's Appraisal and Counselling Strategy*, 3rd edition, © 2003. Reprinted with permission from the Canadian Society for Exercise Physiology.

3 Evaluating Your Cardiorespiratory Endurance (The 1.5-Mile Run Test)

This test assesses your cardiorespiratory endurance level.

Procedure

Find a local track, typically one-quarter mile per lap, to perform your test. Run 1.5 miles; use a stopwatch to measure how long it takes to reach that distance. If you become extremely fatigued during the test, slow your pace or walk—do not overstress yourself! If you feel faint or nauseated or experience any unusual pains in your upper body, stop and notify your instructor. Use the chart below to estimate your cardiorespiratory fitness level based on your age and sex. Note that women have lower standards for each fitness category because they have higher levels of essential fat than men do.

Men	**Excellent**	**Good**	**Fair**	**Poor**		**Women**	**Excellent**	**Good**	**Fair**	**Poor**	
20–29 yrs	< 10:10	10:10–11:29	11:30–12:38	> 12:38		20–29 yrs	< 11:59	11:59–13:24	13:25–14:50	> 14:50	
30–39 yrs	< 10:47	10:47–11:54	11:55–12:58	> 12:58		30–39 yrs	< 12:25	12:25–14:08	14:09–15:43	> 15:43	
40–49 yrs	< 11:16	11:16–12:24	12:25–13:50	> 13:50		40–49 yrs	< 13:24	13:24–14:53	14:54–16:31	> 16:31	
50–59 yrs	< 12:09	12:09–13:35	13:36–15:06	> 15:06		50–59 yrs	< 14:35	14:35–16:35	16:36–18:18	> 18:18	
60–69 yrs	< 13:24	13:24–15:04	15:05–16:46	> 16:46		60–69 yrs	< 16:34	16:34–18:27	18:28–20:16	> 20:16	

Fitness Categories for 1.5-Mile Run Test

Source: The Cooper Institute, *Physical Fitness Assessments and Norms for Adults and Law Enforcement*, Dallas, Texas. Copyright © 2007 by The Cooper Institute. Reprinted with permission.

YOUR PLAN FOR CHANGE

The **Assessyourself** activity helped you determine your current level of physical fitness. Based on your results, you may decide that you should take steps to improve one or more components of your physical fitness.

Today, you can:

○ Visit your campus fitness facility and familiarize yourself with the equipment and resources. Find out what classes they offer, and take home a copy of the schedule.

○ Walk between your classes; make an extra effort to take the long way to get from building to building. Use the stairs instead of the elevator or escalator.

○ Take a stretch break. Spend 5 to 10 minutes between homework projects or just before bed doing some type of physical activity to relax.

Within the next 2 weeks, you can:

○ Shop for comfortable workout clothes and appropriate footwear.

○ Look into group activities that you might enjoy on your campus or in your community.

○ Ask a friend to join you in your workout once a week. Agree on a date and time in advance so you both will be committed to following through.

○ Plan for a physically active outing—dancing, bowling, or shooting hoops—with a friend or date. Use active transportation (i.e., walk or cycle) to get to a movie or go out for dinner.

By the end of the semester, you can:

○ Establish a regular routine (3 to 5 days per week) of physical activity or exercise. Mark your exercise times on your calendar and keep a log to track your progress.

○ Take your workouts to the next level. If you have been working out at home, try going to a gym or participating in an exercise class. If you are walking, perhaps try intermittent jogging or sign up for a fitness event such as a charity 5K run.

MasteringHealth™

Build your knowledge—and health!—in the Study Area of MasteringHealth with a variety of study tools.

Summary

* Benefits of regular physical activity include reduced risk of cardiovascular diseases, metabolic syndrome and type 2 diabetes, and cancer, as well as improved blood lipoproteins, bone mass, weight control, immunity to disease, mental health, stress management, and life span.

* Planning to improve your physical fitness involves setting SMART goals and designing a program using the FITT principle.

* For general health benefits, every adult should participate in moderate-intensity activities for 30 minutes a day at least 5 days a week.

* To improve cardiorespiratory fitness, you should engage in moderate to vigorous, continuous, and rhythmic activities 3 to 5 days per week at an exercise intensity of 64 to 95 percent of your maximum heart rate for 20 to 60 minutes at a time.

* Muscular strength is improved by engaging in resistance training exercises two to three times per week, using an intensity of greater than 60 percent of 1 RM and completing two to four sets of 8 to 12 reps. Muscular endurance is improved by engaging in resistance training exercises two to three times per week, using an intensity of less than 50 percent of 1 RM and completing one or two sets of 15 to 25 reps.

* Flexibility is improved by engaging in two to three repetitions of static stretching exercises at least 2 to 3 days a week (and preferably daily), where each stretch is held for 10 to 30 seconds.

* A comprehensive workout repeated regularly will increase physical fitness and should include an overall warm-up, aerobic activities, strength-development exercises, and a cool-down period with an emphasis on stretching exercises.

* The popular exercise forms of yoga, tai chi, and Pilates all develop multiple components of physical fitness, including flexibility, strength, and endurance.

* Physical activity–related injuries are generally caused by overuse or trauma. The most common overuse injuries are plantar fasciitis, shin splints, and runner's knee. Proper footwear and protective equipment help to prevent injuries. Treatment for all fitness related injuries begins with RICE: rest, ice, compression, and elevation. Exercise in the heat or cold requires special precautions, especially maintaining hydration.

Pop Quiz

1. What is physical fitness?
   a. It can be health-related or performance-related.
   b. It means having enough reserves after working out to cope with a sudden challenge.
   c. It involves cardiorespiratory fitness, muscular strength and endurance, flexibility, and body composition.
   d. All of the above

2. The maximum volume of oxygen consumed by the muscles during exercise defines
   a. target heart rate.
   b. muscular strength.
   c. aerobic capacity.
   d. muscular endurance.

3. Flexibility is the range of motion around
   a. specific bones.
   b. a joint or series of joints.
   c. the tendons.
   d. the muscles.

4. Theresa wants to lower her ratio of fat to her total body weight. She wants to work on her
   a. flexibility.
   b. muscular endurance.
   c. muscular strength.
   d. body composition.

5. Type 2 diabetes can be prevented by
   a. completely eliminating sugar from your diet.
   b. getting your blood sugar level tested.
   c. engaging in daily physical activity.
   d. It cannot be prevented.

6. Janice has been lifting 95 pounds while doing three sets of six leg curls. To become stronger, she began lifting 105 pounds while doing leg curls. What principle of strength development does this represent?
   a. Reversibility
   b. Overload
   c. Flexibility
   d. Specificity of training

7. An example of aerobic exercise is
   a. brisk walking.
   b. bench-pressing weights.
   c. stretching exercises.
   d. holding yoga poses.

8. Miguel is a cross-country runner and is therefore able to sustain moderate-intensity, whole-body activity for extended periods of time. This ability relates to what component of physical fitness?
   a. Flexibility
   b. Body composition
   c. Cardiorespiratory fitness
   d. Muscular strength and endurance

9. The "talk test" measures
   a. exercise intensity.
   b. exercise time.
   c. exercise frequency.
   d. exercise type.

10. Overuse injuries can be prevented by
    a. monitoring the quantity and quality of your workouts.
    b. engaging in only one type of aerobic training.
    c. working out daily.
    d. working out with a friend.

Answers to these questions can be found on page A-1.

Think about It!

1. How do you define *physical fitness*? What are the key components of a physical fitness program? What should you consider when planning and starting a physical fitness program?
2. What do you do to motivate yourself to engage in physical activity on a regular basis? What and who helps you to be physically active?
3. Describe the FITT prescription for cardiorespiratory fitness, muscular strength and endurance, and flexibility training.

4. What precautions do you need to take when exercising outdoors in the heat and in the cold?
5. Your roommate decided to start running to improve his or her cardiorespiratory fitness. What advice would you give to make sure he or she gets off to a good start, does not get injured, and continues the program throughout the year?
6. Identify at least four physiological and psychological benefits of physical activity. How would you promote these benefits to nonexercisers?

Accessing Your Health on the Internet

The following websites explore further topics and issues related to personal health. For links to the websites below, visit the Study Area in MasteringHealth.

1. *American College of Sports Medicine.* This site is the link to the American College of Sports Medicine and all its resources. www.acsm.org
2. *American Council on Exercise.* Information is found here on exercise and disease prevention. www.acefitness.org
3. *Centers for Disease Control and Prevention, National Center for Chronic Disease Prevention and Health Promotion, Division of Nutrition, Physical Activity, and Obesity.* This site is a great resource for current information on exercise and health. www.cdc.gov/nccdphp/dnpao
4. *National Strength and Conditioning Association.* This site is a resource for personal trainers and others interested in conditioning and fitness. www.nsca-lift.org
5. *The President's Council on Fitness, Sports, and Nutrition.* Look here for information on fitness programs. www.fitness.gov

12 Reducing Your Risk of Cardiovascular Disease and Cancer

LEARNING OUTCOMES

✳ Describe the anatomy and physiology of the heart and circulatory system and the importance of healthy heart function.

✳ Discuss the incidence, prevalence, and outcomes of cardiovascular disease in the United States, including its impact on society.

✳ Review major types of cardiovascular disease, modifiable and nonmodifiable risk factors, prevention methods, and current strategies for diagnosis and treatment.

✳ Discuss heart disease prevention methods, and current strategies for diagnosis and treatment.

✳ Define cancer.

✳ Identify common causes of and risk factors for cancer.

✳ Characterize the impact of cancer on people of the United States and the globe.

✳ Describe the different types of cancer, including the risks they pose to people at different ages and stages of life.

✳ Outline strategies and recommendations for cancer prevention, screening, and treatment.

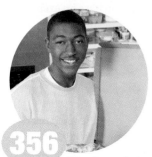

356

Is there anything I can do to improve my cholesterol level?

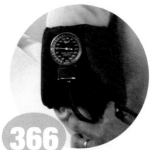

366

Are cardiovascular diseases hereditary?

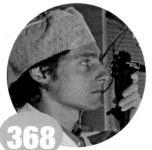

368

What does it mean for a tumor to be malignant?

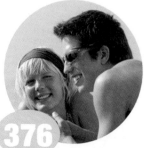

376

Is there any safe way to tan?

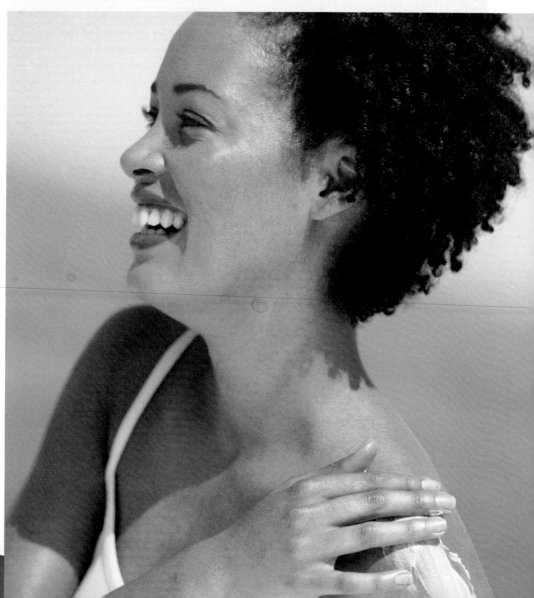

The two groups of chronic diseases that contribute to the greatest global burden of death, illness, and disability are *cardiovascular diseases* and *cancer*. (Diabetes, another major cause of global health problems, is discussed in **Focus On: Minimizing Your Risk for Diabetes** beginning on page 386.) Cardiovascular disease (CVD) is the number one cause of death globally: Ischemic heart disease (also known as coronary artery disease) kills over 7.3 million people each year, whereas stroke and cerebrovascular diseases kill another 6.2 million—nearly 30 percent of all deaths in the world. With soaring rates of obesity and diabetes internationally, CVD rates are also likely to increase in future decades.[1] Like CVD, cancer exacts a heavy toll, causing significant disability and accounting for nearly 13 percent of all deaths—primarily from cancer of the lung, stomach, liver, colon, and female breasts. Increasingly, the less developed regions of the world are among those hardest hit by these chronic diseases.[2]

What do we mean when we say a disease is chronic? Essentially, **chronic diseases** are defined as illnesses that are prolonged, do not resolve spontaneously, and are rarely cured completely. As such, they are responsible for significant rates of disability, lost productivity, pain, and suffering among the global population, not to mention soaring health care costs. Cardiovascular diseases, in particular, and cancer, to a lesser extent, are closely related to lifestyle factors such as obesity, sedentary behavior, poor nutrition, stress, lack of sleep, tobacco use, and excessive alcohol use. The good news is that in many cases, these lifestyle factors can be changed or modified to decrease disease risks.

Cardiovascular Disease: An Overview

Early in 2013, the American Heart Association (AHA) reported that death rates from cardiovascular disease had declined by nearly 33 percent in the last decade. Sounds great, doesn't it? In spite of this promising decline, nearly 84 million Americans—more than 1 out of every 3 adults—suffer from one or more types of **cardiovascular disease (CVD),** the broad term used to include diseases of the heart and blood vessels such as high blood pressure, coronary heart disease (CHD), heart failure, stroke, and congenital cardiovascular defects.[3] Much of the improvement in death rates is due to improved diagnosis, early intervention and treatment, and a multi-billion dollar market in pharmaceuticals designed to keep the heart and circulatory system ticking along. We've also made improvements in knowledge about risks and selected behavioral areas, yet CVD continues to be a threat regardless of age, socioeconomic status, or gender **(Figure 12.1)**.[4] How do CVD death rates compare to other chronic diseases? Nearly one third of all deaths in the United States have CVD as an underlying cause—more than cancer, chronic lower respiratory diseases, and accidental deaths combined.[5] In fact, CVD has been the leading killer of both men and women in the United States every year since 1900, with the exception of 1918, when a pandemic flu killed more people.[6] Recognizing that selected risk factors were key to changing the future course of CVD, the American Heart Association is aiming, by 2020, to improve Americans' cardiovascular health by 20 percent and to reduce death from CVDs and stroke by 20 percent.[7] As part of this strategy, the AHA has begun to focus more on **ideal cardiovascular health (ICH)** rather than mortality rates and the disease process. ICH is defined as the absence of clinical indicators of CVD and the simultaneous presence of the following seven behavioral and health factor metrics.[8]

Behaviors:
- Not smoking
- Sufficient physical activity
- A healthy diet pattern
- An appropriate energy balance and normal body weight

Health Factors:
- Having optimal total cholesterol without medication
- Having optimal blood pressure without medication
- Having optimal fasting blood glucose without medication[9]

chronic disease An illness that is prolonged, does not resolve spontaneously, and is rarely cured.

cardiovascular disease (CVD) Disease of the heart and blood vessels.

ideal cardiovascular health (ICH) The absence of clinical indicators of CVD and the presence of certain behavioral and health factor metrics.

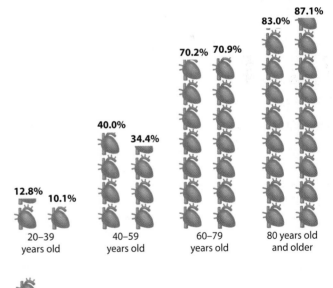

Men with CVD; each heart = 10% of the population

Women with CVD; each heart = 10% of the population

FIGURE 12.1 Prevalence of Cardiovascular Diseases (CVDs) in Adults Aged 20 and Older by Age and Sex
Source: Data from A. S. Go et al., "Heart Disease and Stroke Statistics—2013 Update: A Report from the American Heart Association," *Circulation* 127 (2013): e6-e245.

How are we doing with respect to these ideal healthy heart measures today? In short, not so hot. Less than 1 percent of the total population meets all of the ideal heart health measures, whereas just over 17 percent met two to three of the indicators. Nearly 83 percent had poor ideal cardiovascular health. The young in America tend to be most likely to meet the ideal healthy heart measures.[10]

Clearly, the best defense against CVD is to reduce your risks and prevent it from developing in the first place. Understanding how your cardiovascular system works and the factors that can impair its functioning will help you understand your risk and how to reduce it.

Understanding the Cardiovascular System

The **cardiovascular system** is the network of organs and vessels through which blood flows as it carries oxygen and nutrients to all parts of the body. It includes the *heart, arteries, arterioles* (small arteries), *veins, venules* (small veins), and *capillaries* (minute blood vessels).

cardiovascular system Organ system, consisting of the heart and blood vessels, that transports nutrients, oxygen, hormones, metabolic wastes, and enzymes throughout the body.

atria (singular: atrium) The heart's two upper chambers, which receive blood.

ventricles The heart's two lower chambers, which pump blood through the blood vessels.

arteries Vessels that carry blood away from the heart to other regions of the body.

arterioles Branches of the arteries.

capillaries Minute blood vessels that branch out from the arterioles and venules; their thin walls permit exchange of oxygen, carbon dioxide, nutrients, and waste products among body cells.

veins Vessels that carry blood back to the heart from other regions of the body.

venules Branches of the veins.

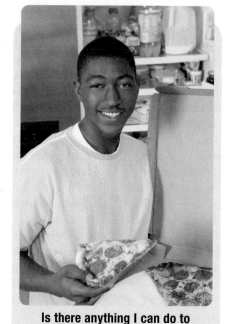

Is there anything I can do to improve my cholesterol level?

About 25 percent of your blood cholesterol level comes from foods you eat, and this is where you can make real improvements.

The Heart: A Mighty Machine

The heart is a muscular, four-chambered pump, roughly the size of your fist. It is a highly efficient, extremely flexible organ that contracts 100,000 times each day and pumps the equivalent of 2,000 gallons of blood through the body. In a 70-year lifetime, an average human heart beats 2.5 billion times.

Under normal circumstances, the human body contains approximately 6 quarts of blood, which transports nutrients, oxygen, waste products, hormones, and enzymes throughout the body. Blood also aids in regulating body temperature, cellular water levels, and acidity levels of body components, and it helps defend the body against toxins and harmful microorganisms. An adequate blood supply is essential to health and well-being.

The heart has four chambers that work together to circulate blood constantly throughout the body. The two upper chambers of the heart, called **atria,** are large collecting chambers that receive blood from the rest of the body. The two lower chambers, known as **ventricles,** pump the blood out again. Small valves regulate the steady, rhythmic flow of blood between chambers and prevent leakage or backflow between them.

Heart Function Heart activity depends on a complex interaction of biochemical, physical, and neurological signals. Here are the four basic steps involved in heart function (see Figure 12.2 on the following page):

1. Deoxygenated blood enters the right atrium after having been circulated through the body.

2. From the right atrium, blood moves to the right ventricle and is pumped through the pulmonary artery to the lungs, where it receives oxygen.

3. Oxygenated blood from the lungs then returns to the left atrium of the heart.

4. Blood from the left atrium moves into the left ventricle. The left ventricle pumps blood through the aorta to all body parts.

Various types of blood vessels are required for different parts of this process. **Arteries** carry blood away from the heart; all arteries carry oxygenated blood, *except* for pulmonary arteries, which carry deoxygenated blood to the lungs, where the blood picks up oxygen and gives off carbon dioxide. As the arteries branch off from the heart, they branch into smaller blood vessels called **arterioles,** and then into even smaller blood vessels known as **capillaries.** Capillaries have thin walls that permit the exchange of oxygen, carbon dioxide, nutrients, and waste products with body cells. Carbon dioxide and other waste products are transported to the lungs and kidneys through **veins** and **venules** (small veins).

For the heart to function properly, the four chambers must beat in an organized manner. Your heartbeat is governed by an electrical impulse that directs the heart muscle to move when the impulse travels across it, resulting in a sequential contraction of the four chambers. This signal starts in a small bundle of highly specialized cells, the **sinoatrial node (SA**

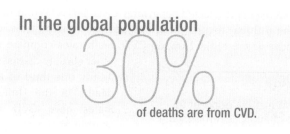

In the global population

30%

of deaths are from CVD.

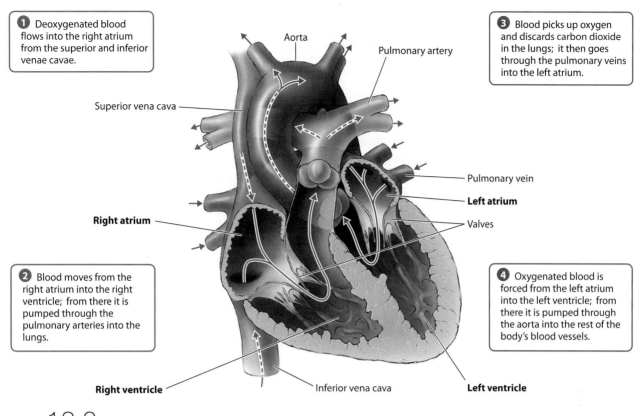

① Deoxygenated blood flows into the right atrium from the superior and inferior venae cavae.

③ Blood picks up oxygen and discards carbon dioxide in the lungs; it then goes through the pulmonary veins into the left atrium.

Aorta

Pulmonary artery

Superior vena cava

Pulmonary vein

Left atrium

Right atrium

Valves

② Blood moves from the right atrium into the right ventricle; from there it is pumped through the pulmonary arteries into the lungs.

④ Oxygenated blood is forced from the left atrium into the left ventricle; from there it is pumped through the aorta into the rest of the body's blood vessels.

Right ventricle

Inferior vena cava

Left ventricle

FIGURE 12.2 **Blood Flow within the Heart**

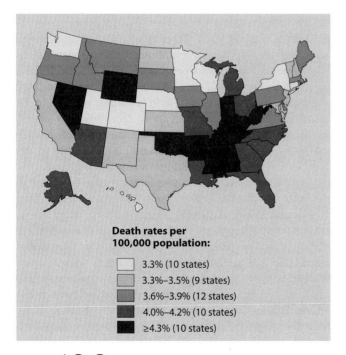

FIGURE 12.3 **Prevalence of Heart Attack Deaths among U.S. Adults**

The 2009 prevalence of acute myocardial infarction (heart attack) deaths among U.S. adults (18+).

Source: Division for Heart Disease and Stroke Prevention: Data Trends & Maps website. U.S. Department of Health and Human Services, Centers for Disease Control and Prevention (CDC), National Center for Chronic Disease Prevention and Health Promotion, Atlanta, GA, 2010. Available at www.cdc.gov

Death rates per 100,000 population:

- 3.3% (10 states)
- 3.3%–3.5% (9 states)
- 3.6%–3.9% (12 states)
- 4.0%–4.2% (10 states)
- ≥4.3% (10 states)

node), located in the right atrium. The SA node serves as a natural pacemaker for the heart. People with a damaged SA node must often have a mechanical pacemaker implanted to ensure the smooth passage of blood through the sequential phases of the heartbeat.

At rest, the average adult heart beats 70 to 80 times per minute, although a well-conditioned heart may beat only 50 to 60 times per minute to achieve the same results. If your resting heart rate is routinely in the high 80s or 90s, it may indicate that you are out of shape or suffering from some underlying illness. When overly stressed, a heart may beat more than 200 times per minute. A healthy heart functions more efficiently and is less likely to suffer damage from overwork.

sinoatrial node (SA node) Cluster of electric pulse–generating cells that serves as a natural pacemaker for the heart.

Cardiovascular Disease

What are the major cardiovascular diseases that we should be worried about today? And how are we doing now in terms of achieving *ideal CVD health status*? Although there are several types of CVD and derivatives thereof, the key ones we will consider are hypertension, atherosclerosis, peripheral arterial disease (PAD), coronary heart disease (CHD), angina pectoris, arrhythmia, congestive heart failure, and stroke. Many forms of CVD are potentially fatal, and **Figure 12.3** presents prevalence of heart attack deaths among adults in the United States.

Hypertension

Blood pressure measures how hard blood pushes against the walls of vessels as your heart pumps. Sustained high blood pressure is called **hypertension**. It is known as the "silent killer" because it has few overt symptoms. Untreated hypertension damages blood vessels and increases your chance of angina, heart failure, peripheral artery disease, stroke, and heart attack. Hypertension can also cause kidney damage and contribute to vision loss, erectile dysfunction, and memory problems.[11]

The prevalence of hypertension in the United States increased almost 10 percent between 2005 and 2009. Today, more than one in three adults in America have high blood pressure, but there are large disparities in self-reported hypertension by race/ethnicity, age, sex, level of education, and state. At nearly 44 percent, African Americans have the highest rate of high blood pressure in the United States or even worldwide. Rates are also much higher among the elderly, men, and those who don't have a high school education.[12] Although awareness of hypertension has increased and most diagnosed individuals are using hypertension medications, only 53 percent of those on meds have their hypertension under control.[13] Women who take oral contraceptives are two to three times more likely to have high blood pressure than women who do not.[14]

Blood pressure is measured by two numbers, for example, 110/80 mm Hg, stated as "110 over 80 millimeters of mercury." The top number, **systolic blood pressure,** refers to the pressure of blood in the arteries when the heart muscle contracts, sending blood to the rest of the body. The bottom number, **diastolic blood pressure,** refers to the pressure of blood on the arteries when the heart muscle relaxes, as blood is re-entering the heart chambers. Normal blood pressure varies depending on age, weight, and physical condition, and high blood pressure is usually diagnosed when systolic pressure is 140 or above (see Table 12.1). When only systolic pressure is high, the condition is known as *isolated systolic hypertension* (*ISH*), the most common form of high blood pressure in older Americans.

Systolic blood pressure tends to increase with age, whereas diastolic blood pressure typically increases until age 55 and then declines. Men under the age of 45 are at nearly twice the risk of becoming hypertensive as their female counterparts; however women tend to have higher rates of hypertension after age 65.[15] A key indicator of a growing threat from hypertension is the fact that more and more people (over 30 percent of the population) are considered to be **prehypertensive,** meaning that their blood pressure is above normal, but not yet in the hypertensive range. These individuals have a significantly greater risk of becoming hypertensive.[16]

hypertension Sustained elevated blood pressure.

systolic blood pressure The upper number in the fraction that measures blood pressure, indicating pressure on the walls of the arteries when the heart contracts.

diastolic blood pressure The lower number in the fraction that measures blood pressure, indicating pressure on the walls of the arteries during the relaxation phase of heart activity.

prehypertensive Blood pressure is above normal, but not yet in the hypertensive range.

arteriosclerosis A general term for thickening and hardening of the arteries.

atherosclerosis Condition characterized by deposits of fatty substances (plaque) on the inner lining of an artery.

plaque Buildup of deposits in the arteries.

TABLE 12.1 | Blood Pressure Classifications

Classification	Systolic Reading (mm Hg)		Diastolic Reading (mm Hg)
Normal	Less than 120	and	Less than 80
Prehypertension	120–139	or	80–89
Hypertension			
Stage 1	140–159	or	90–99
Stage 2	Greater than or equal to 160	or	Greater than or equal to 100

Note: If systolic and diastolic readings fall into different categories, treatment is determined by the highest category. Readings are based on the average of two or more properly measured, seated readings on each of two or more health care provider visits.

Source: National Heart, Lung, and Blood Institute, *The Seventh Report of the Joint National Committee on Prevention, Detection, Evaluation, and Treatment of High Blood Pressure,* NIH Publication no. 03-5233 (Bethesda, MD: National Institutes of Health, 2003).

Atherosclerosis

Arteriosclerosis, thickening and hardening of arteries, is a condition that underlies many cardiovascular health problems and is believed to be the biggest contributor to disease burden globally. **Atherosclerosis** is a type of arteriosclerosis and is characterized by deposits of fatty substances, cholesterol, cellular waste products, calcium, and fibrin (a clotting material in the blood) in the inner lining of an artery. *Hyperlipidemia* (abnormally high blood levels of *lipids,* which are non-water-soluble molecules, such as fats and cholesterol) is a key factor in this process, and the resulting buildup is referred to as **plaque.**

As plaque accumulates, these fatty substances adhere to the inner lining of the blood vessels. The vessel walls become narrow and may eventually block blood flow or rupture. This is similar to putting your thumb over the end of a hose while water is running through it. Pressure builds within arteries just as pressure builds in the hose. If vessels are weakened and pressure persists, the artery may become weak and eventually burst. Fluctuation in the blood pressure levels within arteries may actually damage their internal walls, making it even more likely that plaque will accumulate.

45% of adults aged 20 and over have cholesterol levels at or above 200 mg/dL.

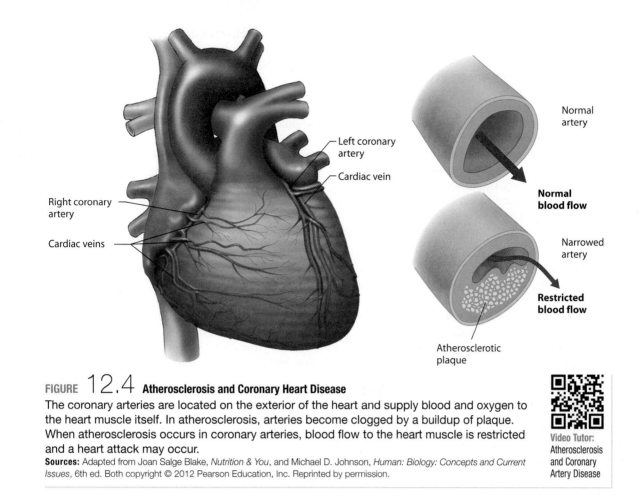

FIGURE 12.4 **Atherosclerosis and Coronary Heart Disease**
The coronary arteries are located on the exterior of the heart and supply blood and oxygen to the heart muscle itself. In atherosclerosis, arteries become clogged by a buildup of plaque. When atherosclerosis occurs in coronary arteries, blood flow to the heart muscle is restricted and a heart attack may occur.
Sources: Adapted from Joan Salge Blake, *Nutrition & You*, and Michael D. Johnson, *Human: Biology: Concepts and Current Issues*, 6th ed. Both copyright © 2012 Pearson Education, Inc. Reprinted by permission.

Video Tutor:
Atherosclerosis
and Coronary
Artery Disease

Atherosclerosis is the most common form of *coronary artery disease (CAD).* It occurs as plaques are deposited in vessel walls and restrict blood flow and oxygen to the body's main coronary arteries on the outer surface of the heart, often eventually resulting in a heart attack (see Figure 12.4). When circulation is impaired and blood flow to the heart is limited, the heart may become starved for oxygen—a condition commonly referred to as **ischemia.** Sometimes coronary artery disease is referred to as ischemic heart disease.

greater risk for stroke and heart attack compared to those without the condition.[19] Sometimes PAD in the arms can be caused by trauma, certain diseases, radiation therapy, or repetitive motion syndrome, or the combined risks of these factors and atherosclerosis. According to current thinking, four factors discussed later in this chapter are responsible for this damage: inflammation, elevated levels of cholesterol and triglycerides in the blood, high blood pressure, and tobacco use.

Peripheral Artery Disease (PAD)

When atherosclerosis occurs in the upper or lower extremities, such as in the arms, feet, calves, or legs, and causes narrowing or complete blockage of arteries, it is often called **peripheral artery disease (PAD).** As many as 20 percent of adults 65 and older in the United States have symptoms, and many are not receiving treatment.[17] Most often characterized by pain and aching in the legs, calves, or feet upon walking/exercise, and relieved by rest (known as *intermittent claudication*), PAD is a leading cause of disability in people over the age of 50. While it strikes both men and women, men and smokers tend to develop it more frequently.[18] In recent years, increased attention has been drawn to PAD's role in subsequent blood clots and resultant heart attacks. People with PAD are thought to have two or three times

Coronary Heart Disease (CHD)

Of all the major cardiovascular diseases, **coronary heart disease (CHD)** is the greatest killer, accounting for nearly 1 in 6 deaths in the United States. Over one million new and recurrent heart attacks occur in the United States each year.[20] A **myocardial infarction (MI),** or **heart attack,** involves an area of the heart that suffers permanent damage because its normal blood supply has been blocked. This condition is often brought on by a blood clot in a coronary artery or an atherosclerotic narrowing that

ischemia Reduced oxygen supply to a body part or organ.

peripheral artery disease (PAD) Atherosclerosis occurring in the lower extremities, such as in the feet, calves, or legs, or in the arms.

coronary heart disease (CHD) A narrowing of the small blood vessels that supply blood to the heart.

myocardial infarction (MI; heart attack) A blockage of normal blood supply to an area in the heart.

What to Do in the Event of a Heart Attack

Chest pain—which can feel like uncomfortable pressure, squeezing, or pain, or even like heartburn or indigestion, and can last for a few minutes and then go away—is the most common symptom of a heart attack, but many people, especially women, experience different symptoms. Recognizing them and acting quickly can mean the difference between life and death. Other typical heart attack symptoms can include the following:

1. Intense pain in the left arm
2. A cold, clammy sweat
3. Feeling of weakness or lightheadedness, including actual fainting
4. Pain or discomfort in the jaw, neck, back, arms, or shoulders, or even the upper part of the stomach—but not below the belly button. This symptom is more common in women.
5. Shortness of breath, which can occur with minimal physical activity or even at rest. Sometimes, this is a patient's only heart attack symptom.
6. Nausea, vomiting, or indigestion, especially for women; also, a burning sensation in the throat.
7. Impending sense of doom.

If you experience any of these symptoms without a plausible explanation, or if you are with someone who is experiencing them, don't wait more than 5 minutes to call 9-1-1. Do not try to drive yourself or a family member who may be having a heart attack. If you are with someone who may be having a heart attack, you may also try cardiopulmonary resuscitation (CPR), following guidelines by the American Heart Association at www.heart.org.

Sources: Centers for Disease Control and Prevention, "Act Fast during Heart Attacks," 2009, www.cdc.gov; U.S. Department of Health and Human Services, Office on Women's Health, "Heart Attack Symptoms," 2011, www.womenshealth.gov; Mayo Clinic, "Heart Attack," 2012, www.mayoclinic.com

ble to adapt on its own, and outside lifesaving support is critical. See the **Skills for Behavior Change** box to learn what to do in case of a heart attack.

Angina Pectoris

Angina pectoris occurs when there is not enough oxygen to supply heart muscle, resulting in chest pain or pressure. Approximately 2 percent of the U.S. population between the ages of 25 and 45 experience angina pectoris, with over 13 percent of men and nearly 11 percent of women experiencing mild to moderate symptoms by the age of 65.[21] Generally, the more serious the oxygen deprivation, the more severe the pain. Although angina pectoris is not a heart attack, it does indicate underlying heart disease.

Currently, there are several methods of treating angina. Mild cases may be treated simply with rest. Drugs such as *nitroglycerin* can dilate veins and provide pain relief. Other medications such as *calcium channel blockers* can relieve cardiac spasms and arrhythmias, lower blood pressure, and slow heart rate. *Beta-blockers,* the other major type of drugs used to treat angina, control potential overactivity of the heart muscle.

Arrhythmias

Over the course of a lifetime, most people experience some type of **arrhythmia,** an irregularity in heart rhythm that occurs when the electrical impulses in your heart that coordinate heartbeat don't work properly. Often described as a heart "fluttering" or racing, these irregularities send many people to the emergency room, only to find that they are fine. A racing heart in the absence of exercise or anxiety may be experiencing *tachycardia,* the medical term for abnormally fast heartbeat. On the other end of the continuum is *bradycardia,* or abnormally slow heartbeat. When a heart goes into **fibrillation,** it beats in a sporadic, quivering pattern, resulting in extreme inefficiency in moving blood through the cardiovascular system. If untreated, fibrillation may be fatal.

Not all arrhythmias are life-threatening. In many instances, excessive caffeine or nicotine consumption can trigger an arrhythmia episode. However, severe cases may require drug therapy or external electrical stimulus to prevent serious complications. When in doubt, it is always best to check with your doctor.

Heart Failure

When the heart muscle is damaged or overworked and lacks the strength to keep blood circulating normally through the body, blood and fluids begin to back up into the lungs and other body tissues. As this buildup continues, there is often fluid accumulation in the feet, ankles, and legs, along with shortness of breath and tiredness. Known as heart failure or **congestive heart failure,** this condition is increasingly common, particularly among those with a history of other heart problems. Currently nearly 6.6 million adults have heart failure in the United States, with cases estimated to rise to nearly 10 million by 2030.[22]

blocks an artery. When blood does not flow readily, there is a corresponding decrease in oxygen flow. If the blockage is extremely minor, an otherwise healthy heart will adapt over time by enlarging existing blood vessels and growing new ones to reroute blood through other areas. Some populations, particularly women, seem to fare worse upon having a heart attack than do others. For a variety of reasons, women are more likely to die after a first heart attack than men are.

When heart blockage is more severe, however, the body is una-

angina pectoris Chest pain occurring as a result of reduced oxygen flow to the heart.

arrhythmia An irregularity in heartbeat.

fibrillation A sporadic, quivering pattern of heartbeat that results in extreme inefficiency in moving blood through the cardiovascular system.

congestive heart failure (CHF) An abnormal cardiovascular condition that reflects impaired cardiac pumping and blood flow; pooling blood leads to congestion in body tissues.

Underlying causes of heart failure may include heart injury from a number of CVD risks, including uncontrolled high blood pressure, rheumatic fever, pneumonia, heart attack, or other cardiovascular problems. Certain prescription drugs such as NSAIDS and diabetes medications also increase risks, as do chronic drug and alcohol abuse. In some cases, the damage is due to radiation or chemotherapy treatments for cancer. When heart failure occurs, weakened muscles respond poorly, impairing blood flow out of the heart through the arteries. The return flow of blood through the veins begins to back up, causing congestion in body tissues. Untreated, heart failure can be fatal. However, most cases respond well to treatment that includes *diuretics* ("water pills") to relieve fluid accumulation; drugs, such as *digitalis,* that increase the pumping action of the heart; and drugs called *vasodilators,* which expand blood vessels and decrease resistance, allowing blood to flow more freely and making the heart's work easier. Prevention of underlying CVD risks is the best means of reducing your risks of heart failure.

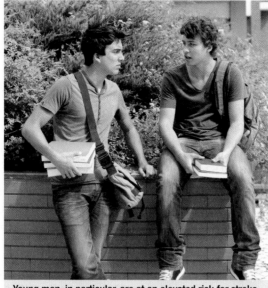
Young men, in particular, are at an elevated risk for stroke.

Stroke

Like heart muscle, brain cells must have a continuous adequate supply of oxygen in order to survive. A **stroke** (also called a *cerebrovascular accident*) occurs when the blood supply to the brain is interrupted. Strokes may be either *ischemic* (caused by plaque formation that narrows blood flow or a clot that obstructs a blood vessel) or *hemorrhagic* (due to a weakening of a blood vessel that causes it to bulge or rupture). An **aneurysm** (a widening or bulge in a blood vessel that may become hemorrhagic) is the most well-known of the hemorrhagic strokes. When any of these events occurs, oxygen deprivation kills brain cells.

Some strokes are mild and cause only temporary dizziness or slight weakness or numbness. More serious interruptions in blood flow may impair speech, memory, or motor control. Other strokes affect parts of the brain that regulate heart and lung function and kill within minutes. According to the American Heart Association's latest statistics, nearly 7 million Americans suffer a stroke every year, and almost 129,000 people die as a result. Strokes cause countless levels of disability and suffering and account for 1 in 19 deaths each year, surpassed only by CHD, cancer, and chronic

lower respiratory diseases.[23] Even scarier, it is thought that more young people are having strokes than ever before, possibly due to increased obesity and hypertension among that age group.[24] Many strokes are preceded days, weeks, or months earlier by **transient ischemic attacks (TIAs),** brief interruptions of the blood supply to the brain that cause only temporary impairment.[25] Symptoms of TIAs include dizziness, particularly when first rising in the morning, weakness, temporary paralysis or numbness in the face or other regions, temporary memory loss, blurred vision, nausea, headache, slurred speech, or other unusual physiological reactions. Some people may experience unexpected falls or have blackouts; however, others may have no obvious symptoms. TIAs often indicate an impending major stroke. The earlier a stroke is recognized and treatment started (best results are seen if treatment begins within the first 1–2 hours), the more effective that treatment will be. See the **Skills for Behavior Change** box for tips on recognizing a possible stroke.

stroke A condition occurring when the brain is damaged by disrupted blood supply; also called cerebrovascular accident.

aneurysm A weakened blood vessel that may bulge under pressure and, in severe cases, burst.

transient ischemic attacks (TIAs) Brief interruption of the blood supply to the brain that causes only temporary impairment; often an indicator of impending major stroke.

See It! Videos

See how two young women have regained their lives after experiencing a stroke. Watch **Stroke in Young Adults** in the Study Area of MasteringHealth™

One of the greatest U.S. medical successes in recent years has been the decline in the fatality rate from strokes, which has dropped by one third since the 1980s and continues to fall.[26] Greater awareness of stroke symptoms, improvements in emergency medicine protocols and medicines, and a greater emphasis on fast rehabilitation and therapy after a stroke have helped many survive. Unfortunately, like many victims of other forms of CVD, stroke survivors do not always make a full recovery. Problems with speech, memory, swallowing, and daily life activities can persist, even with therapies and medications. Depression is also an issue for many recovering from stroke and CHD.

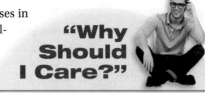

"Why Should I Care?"

The cost of medical care for heart disease in the United States is expected to triple over the next 20 years, rising from an estimated $273 billion in 2010 to $818 billion in 2030. The cost of lost productivity is expected to rise from $172 billion in 2010 to $276 billion in 2030. These projections will exact a tremendous toll on our country, with individuals forced to carry more and more of the burden of these costs.

and nearly 52 percent of those over the age of 60 meet the criteria for MetS.[30] Although different professional organizations have slightly different criteria for MetS, the National Cholesterol Education Program's Adult Treatment Panel (NCEP/ATP III) is the one commonly used. According to these criteria, for a diagnosis of metabolic syndrome a person would have three or more of the following risks:[31]

- Abdominal obesity (waist measurement of more than 40 inches in men or 35 inches in women)
- Elevated blood fat (triglycerides greater than 150)
- Low levels of HDL ("good") cholesterol (less than 40 in men and less than 50 in women)
- Elevated blood pressure greater than 135/85
- Elevated fasting glucose greater than 100 mg/dL (a sign of insulin resistance or glucose intolerance)

The use of the metabolic syndrome classification and other, similar terms has been important in highlighting the relationship between the number of risks a person possesses and that person's likelihood of developing CVD and diabetes. Groups such as the AHA and others are giving increased attention to focusing on multiple risks and emphasizing cardiovascular health in lifestyle interventions.

Reducing Your Risks

Research has shown strong associations between CVD problems and obesity, exposure to smoking, lack of physical activity, high cholesterol, diabetes, high blood pressure, and genetics. Newer research indicates that for people aged 12–39, smoking, high body fat, and high blood glucose increase the chances of dying from CVD-related complications before age 60.[27] As mentioned previously, hypertension doesn't just wreak havoc with your heart and circulatory system; it may eventually lead to slowing of cognitive function and increase your risks for Alzheimer's disease.[28] Typical CVD risk factors also increase risks for insulin resistance and type 2 diabetes.[29] **Cardiometabolic risks** are the combined risks that indicate physical and biochemical changes that can lead to these major diseases. Some of these risks result from choices and behaviors, and so are modifiable, whereas others are inherited or intrinsic (such as your age and gender) and cannot be modified.

Metabolic Syndrome: Quick Risk Profile

Over the past decade, different health professionals have attempted to establish diagnostic cutoff points for a cluster of combined cardiometabolic risks, variably labeled as *syndrome X, insulin resistance syndrome,* and, most recently,

cardiometabolic risks Risk factors that impact both the cardiovascular system and the body's biochemical metabolic processes.

metabolic syndrome (MetS) A group of metabolic conditions occurring together that increases a person's risk of heart disease, stroke, and diabetes.

metabolic syndrome (MetS). Historically, metabolic syndrome is believed to increase the risk for atherosclerotic heart disease by as much as three times the normal rates. It has captured international attention, since over 20 percent of people aged 20–39, 41 percent of people age 40–59,

Modifiable Risks

It may surprise you to realize that younger adults are not invulnerable to CVD risks. The reality is that from the first moments of your life, you begin to accumulate increasing numbers of risks. Your past and future lifestyle choices may haunt you as you enter your middle and later years of life. Behaviors you choose today and over the coming decades can actively reduce or promote your risk for CVD.

Avoid Tobacco Although smoking rates declined by over 50 percent between 1965 and 2007, these dramatic declines have come to a virtual standstill in the last 5 years. Today, approximately 21 percent of U.S. adults age 18 and over are regular smokers.[32] In spite of massive campaigns to educate us about the dangers of smoking, and in spite of increasing numbers of states and municipalities enacting policies to go "smoke free," cigarette smoking remains the leading cause of preventable death in the United States, accounting for approximately 1 of every 5 deaths. Just how great a risk is smoking when it comes to CVD? Consider these statistics:[33]

- Cigarette smokers are two to four times more likely to develop CHD than nonsmokers.
- Cigarette smoking doubles a person's risk of stroke.
- Smokers are more than 10 times more likely than nonsmokers to develop peripheral vascular diseases.

How does smoking damage the heart? There are two plausible explanations. One is that nicotine increases heart rate, heart output, blood pressure, and oxygen use by heart muscles. The heart is forced to work harder to obtain sufficient oxygen. The other explanation is that chemicals in smoke damage and inflame the lining of the coronary arteries, allowing cholesterol and plaque to accumulate more easily, increasing blood pressure and forcing the heart to work harder.

The good news is that if you stop smoking, your heart begins to mend itself. After 1 year, a former smoker's risk of heart disease drops by 50 percent. Between 5 to 15 years after quitting, the risk of stroke and CHD becomes similar to that of nonsmokers. Younger, college-age students take note: studies have shown that those who quit smoking at age 30 reduce their chance of dying prematurely from smoking-related diseases by more than 90 percent.[34] Those diagnosed with early stage lung cancer more than double their 5-year survival chances (63–70%) if they quit smoking versus people who keep smoking (29–33%).[35] Younger smokers (under age 45) who quit a year before diagnosis are significantly more likely to survive for 2 years than are those who continue smoking.[36]

Cut Back on Saturated Fat and Cholesterol Cholesterol is a fatty, waxy substance found in the bloodstream and in your body cells. Although we tend to hear only bad things about it, in truth, cholesterol plays an important role in the production of cell membranes and hormones and in other body functions. However, when blood levels of it get too high, risks for CVD escalate.

Cholesterol comes from two primary sources: your body (which involves genetic predisposition) and food. Much of your cholesterol level is predetermined: 75 percent of blood cholesterol is produced by your liver and other cells, and the other 25 percent comes from the foods you eat. The good news is that changing your diet can make real improvements in your overall cholesterol level, even if yours is naturally high.

Diets high in saturated fat and *trans* fats are known to raise cholesterol levels, send the body's blood-clotting system into high gear, and make the blood more viscous in just a few hours, increasing the risk of heart attack or stroke. Increased blood levels of cholesterol also contribute to atherosclerosis. Total cholesterol level isn't the only level to be concerned about; the type of cholesterol also matters. The two major types of blood cholesterol are *low-density lipoprotein (LDL)* and *high-density lipoprotein (HDL)*. Low-density lipoprotein, often referred to as "bad" cholesterol, is believed to build up on artery walls. In contrast, high-density lipoprotein, or "good" cholesterol, appears to remove cholesterol from artery walls, thus serving as a protector. In theory, if LDL levels get too high or HDL levels too low, cholesterol will accumulate inside arteries and lead to cardiovascular problems.

Triglycerides are also gaining increasing attention as a key factor in CVD risk. When you consume extra calories, the body converts the extra to triglycerides, which are stored in fat cells. High levels of blood triglycerides are often found in people who have high cholesterol levels, heart problems, diabetes, or who are overweight. As people get older, heavier, or both, their triglyceride and cholesterol levels tend to rise. It is recommended that a baseline cholesterol test (known as a lipid panel or lipid profile) be taken at age 20, with follow-ups every 5 years. This test, which measures triglyceride levels as well as HDL, LDL, and total cholesterol levels, requires that you fast for 12 hours prior to the test, are well hydrated, and avoid coffee and tea prior to testing. Men over the age of 35 and women over the age of 45 should have their lipid profile checked annually, with more frequent tests for those at high risk. See Table 12.2 on the following page for recommended levels of cholesterol and triglycerides.

In general, LDL (or "bad" cholesterol) is more closely associated with cardiovascular risk than is total cholesterol. Until recently, most authorities agreed that looking only at LDL ignored the positive effects of "good" cholesterol (HDL) and that raising HDL was an important goal. There has been general agreement that the best method of evaluating risk is to examine the ratio of HDL to total cholesterol, or the percentage of HDL in total cholesterol. If the level of HDL is lower than 35 mg/dL, cardiovascular risk increases dramatically. To reduce risk, the goal has been to manage the ratio of HDL to total cholesterol by lowering LDL levels, raising HDL, or both. New research indicates that trying to raise HDL as a means of preventing negative CVD outcomes may not be as beneficial as once thought.[37] Drugs that were effective in raising HDL levels had little or no effect on CVD risks or mortality. Regular exercise and a healthy diet low in saturated fat continue to be the best methods for maintaining healthy

See It! Videos
What habits can you change now to improve your heart health? Watch **Importance of Heart Health in Your Youth** in the Study Area of MasteringHealth™

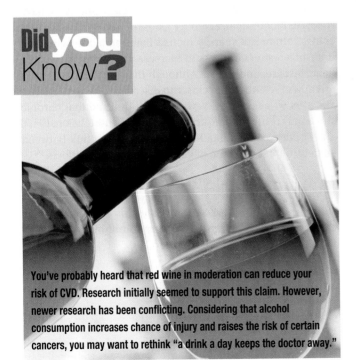

Did you Know?
You've probably heard that red wine in moderation can reduce your risk of CVD. Research initially seemed to support this claim. However, newer research has been conflicting. Considering that alcohol consumption increases chance of injury and raises the risk of certain cancers, you may want to rethink "a drink a day keeps the doctor away."

TABLE

12.2

Recommended Cholesterol Levels for Lower/Moderate Risk Adults

Total Cholesterol Level (lower numbers are better)	
Less than 200 mg/dL	Desirable
200–239 mg/dL	Borderline high
240 mg/dL and above	High

HDL Cholesterol Level (higher numbers are better)	
Less than 40 mg/dL (for men)	Low
60 mg/dL and above	Desirable

LDL Cholesterol Level (lower numbers are better)	
Less than 100 mg/dL	Optimal
100–129 mg/dL	Near or above optimal
130–159 mg/dL	Borderline high
160–189 mg/dL	High
190 mg/dL and above	Very high

Triglyceride Level (lower numbers are better)	
Less than 150 mg/dL	Normal
150–199 mg/dL	Borderline high
200–499 mg/dL	High
500 mg/dL and above	Very high

Source: Adapted from National Heart, Lung, and Blood Institute, National Institutes of Health, *ATP III Guidelines At-A-Glance Quick Desk Reference*, NIH Publication No. 01-3305, Update on Cholesterol Guidelines, 2004. Available from www.nhlbi.nih.gov

ratios. See the **Health Headlines** box on the following page for information about foods and dietary practices that can help maintain healthy cholesterol levels.

In spite of encouraging declines in high LDL levels through drug-based treatments, Americans continue to have higher-than-recommended overall cholesterol levels. About 45 percent of adults aged 20 and over have cholesterol levels at or above 200 mg/dL, and another 16 percent have levels in excess of 240 mg/dL.[38] Over half of all men aged 65 and over and nearly 40 percent of all women aged 65 or older are taking anti-hyperlipidemia prescription drugs and other medications to reduce blood fats.[39]

Maintain a Healthy Weight No question about it—body weight plays a role in CVD. Researchers are not sure whether high-fat, high-sugar, high-calorie diets are a direct risk for CVD or whether they invite risk by causing obesity, which strains the heart, forcing it to push blood through the many miles of capillaries that supply each pound of fat. A heart that has to continuously move blood through an over-abundance of vessels may become damaged. Overweight people are more likely to develop heart disease and stroke even if they have no other risk factors. This is especially true if you're an "apple" (thicker around your upper body and waist) rather than a "pear" (thicker around your hips and thighs).

Exercise Regularly Inactivity is a clear risk factor for CVD.[40] The good news is that you do not have to be an exercise fanatic to reduce your risk. Even modest levels of low-intensity physical activity—walking, gardening, housework, dancing—are beneficial if done regularly and over the long term. Exercise can increase HDL, lower triglycerides, and reduce coronary risks in several ways.

Control Diabetes Heart disease death rates among adults with diabetes are two to four times higher than the rates for adults without diabetes. At least 65 percent of people with diabetes die of some form of heart disease or stroke.[41] Because overweight people have a higher risk for diabetes, distinguishing between the effects of the two conditions is difficult. People with diabetes also tend to have elevated blood fat levels, increased atherosclerosis, and a tendency toward deterioration of small blood vessels, particularly in the eyes and extremities. However, through a prescribed regimen of diet, exercise, and medication, they can control much of their increased risk for CVD. (See **Focus On: Minimizing Your Risk for Diabetes** starting on page 386 for more on preventing and controlling diabetes.)

Control Your Blood Pressure In general, the higher your blood pressure, the greater is your risk for CVD. Key factors in increasing blood pressure include obesity, lack of exercise, atherosclerosis, kidney damage from diabetes complications, and other factors.[42] Treatment of hypertension can involve dietary changes (avoiding high sodium, processed foods and cutting calories when appropriate),[43] medication, regular exercise, controlling stress, and getting enough sleep.

Manage Stress People under stress may suffer from a variety of health-related problems. They may start smoking, smoke more than they otherwise would, or suffer extreme anxiety reactions. They may also anger more easily, have difficulty sleeping, experience gastrointestinal difficulties, have spikes in blood sugar, and have a host of negative health outcomes.[44] In recent years, scientists have tended to agree that unresolved stress appears to increase risk for hypertension, heart disease, and stroke. Although the exact mechanism is unknown, scientists are closer to discovering why stress can affect us so negatively. Newer studies indicate that chronic stress may result in three times the risk of hypertension, CHD, and sudden cardiac death and that there is a link between anxiety, depression, and negative cardiovascular effects.[45]

Nonmodifiable Risks

Unfortunately there are some risk factors for CVD that we cannot prevent or control. The most important include the following:

● **Race and ethnicity.** Although Caucasians tend to have more heart disease, African Americans are 40 percent more likely to have hypertension and also have a higher risk of stroke.

HEART-HEALTHY SUPER FOODS

The foods you eat play a major role in your CVD risk. While many foods can increase your risk, several have been shown to reduce the chances that cholesterol will be absorbed in the cells, reduce levels of LDL cholesterol, or enhance the protective effects of HDL cholesterol. To protect your heart, include the following in your diet:

✳ **Fish high in omega-3 fatty acids.** Consumption of fish such as salmon, sardines, and herring has been believed to reduce risks of CVD. New research raises questions about this research.

✳ **Olive oil.** Using any of a number of monounsaturated fats in cooking, particularly extra virgin olive oil, helps lower total cholesterol and raise your HDL levels. Canola oil; margarine labeled "*trans* fat free"; and cholesterol-lowering margarines such as Benecol, Promise Activ, or Smart Balance are also excellent choices.

✳ **Whole grains and fiber.** Getting enough fiber each day in the form of 100 percent whole wheat, steel cut oats, oat bran, flax-seed, fruits, and vegetables helps lower LDL or "bad" cholesterol. Soluble fiber, in particular, seems to keep cholesterol from being absorbed in the intestines.

✳ **Plant sterols and stanols.** These are essential components of plant membranes and are found naturally in vegetables, fruits, and legumes. In addition, many food products, including juices and yogurt, are now fortified with them. These compounds are believed to benefit your heart health by blocking cholesterol absorption in the bloodstream, thus reducing LDL levels.

✳ **Nuts.** Long maligned for being high in calories, walnuts, almonds, and other nuts are naturally high in omega-3 fatty acids, which are important in lowering cholesterol and good for the blood vessels themselves.

✳ **Chocolate and green tea.** Could it really be true? Are dark chocolate and green teas really protecting us from cardiovascular diseases? Over the past decade, several major studies have indicated that dark chocolate appears to significantly reduce blood pressure, whereas green tea seems to reduce LDL cholesterol. The flavonoids in chocolate and green tea act as powerful antioxidants that protect the cells of the heart and blood vessels. Research also suggests that the cocoa flavonols in dark chocolate my reduce the risk of blood clots and improve blood flow in the brain.

Much more research on all of these foods must be done to say definitively how beneficial they might be, and what dosage is recommended.

Sources: A. Mente et al., "A Systematic Review of the Evidence Supporting a Causal Link between Dietary Factors and Coronary Heart Disease," *Archives of Internal Medicine* 169, no. 7 (2009): 659–669; R. M. van Dam, L. Naidoo, and R. Landberg, "Dietary Flavonoids and the Development of Type 2 Diabetes and Cardiovascular Disease: Review of Recent Findings," *Current Opinion in Lipidology* 24, no. 1 (2013): 25–33, doi: 10.1097/MOL.0b013e32835bcdff; L. Hooper et al., "Effects of Chocolate, Cocoa, and Flavan-3-ols on Cardiovascular Health: A Systematic Review and Meta-analysis of Randomized Trials," *American Journal of Clinical Nutrition* 95, no. 3 (2012): 740-–751, doi: 10.3945/ajcn.111.023457

The rate of high blood pressure in African Americans is among the highest in the world. CVD risks are also higher among Hispanic/Latino Americans. Importantly, racial and ethnic minorities have a significantly greater risk of dying from CVD-related diseases.[46]

● **Heredity.** A tendency toward heart disease seems to be, at least in part, hereditary.[47] The amount of cholesterol you produce, tendencies to form plaque, and a host of other factors have genetic links. If you have close relatives with CVD, your risk may be double that of others. The younger these relatives are, and the closer their relationship to you (parents or siblings, in particular), the greater your risk will be. The difficulty comes in sorting out genetic influences from the multiple confounders common among family members that may also influence risk, including environment, stress, learned dietary habits, and so on. Newer research has focused on studying the interactions between nutrition and genes (nutrigenetics) and the role that diet may play in increasing or decreasing risks among certain genetic profiles.[48]

● **Age.** Although cardiovascular disease can affect people of any age, 82 percent of all heart attacks occur in people over age 65.[49] The rate of CVD increases with age for both sexes.

● **Gender.** Men are at greater risk for CVD until about age 60. Women under age 35 have a fairly low risk unless they have high blood pressure, kidney problems, or diabetes. Using oral contraceptives and smoking also increase the risk. Women also have poorer health outcomes and higher death rates than do men when they have a heart attack.[50]

Other Risk Factors Being Studied

Several other factors and indicators have been linked to CVD risk, including inflammation and homocysteine levels.

Inflammation and C-Reactive Protein Recent research has prompted many experts to believe that inflammation may play a major role in atherosclerosis development. Inflammation occurs when tissues are injured by bacteria, trauma, toxins, or heat, among other things. Injured vessel walls are more prone to plaque formation. To date, several factors, including cigarette smoke, high blood pressure, high LDL cholesterol, diabetes mellitus, certain forms of arthritis, and exposure to toxic substances, have all been linked to increased risk of inflammation. However, the greatest risk appears to be from certain infectious disease pathogens, most notably *Chlamydia pneumoniae*, a common cause of respiratory infections; *Helicobacter pylori* (a bacterium that causes ulcers); herpes simplex virus (a virus that most of us have been exposed to); and *Cytomegalovirus* (another herpes virus infecting most Americans before the age of 40). During an inflammatory reaction, **C-reactive proteins** tend to be present at high levels. A recent meta-analysis of over 38 studies with nearly 170,000 subjects has shown a strong association between C-reactive proteins in the blood and increased risks for atherosclerosis and CVD.[51] Blood tests can test these proteins using a highly sensitive assay called *hs-CRP* (high-sensitivity C-reactive protein); if levels are high, action could be taken to reduce inflammation.

C-reactive protein (CRP) A protein whose blood levels rise in response to inflammation.

homocysteine An amino acid normally present in the blood that, when found at high levels, may be related to higher risk of cardiovascular disease.

Fish oil, flax, and other foods high in omega-3 have been recommended by the AHA and other groups for their anti-inflammatory properties, but new research analyzing over 20 studies found little benefit in reducing risk for cardiovascular disease.[52] While initial studies cast doubt on omega-3's benefits, more research is necessary to determine the actual role that inflammation plays in increased risk of CVD or if there is something unique about inflammation that omega-3 may work to counter.[53]

Homocysteine In the last decade, an increasing amount of attention has been given to the role of **homocysteine**—an amino acid normally present in the blood—in increased risk for CVD. When present at high levels, homocysteine may be related to higher risk of coronary heart disease, stroke, and peripheral artery disease. Although research is still in its infancy in this area, scientists hypothesize that homocysteine works in much the same way as c-reactive proteins—inflaming the inner lining of the arterial walls, promoting fat deposits on the damaged walls, and encouraging the development of blood clots.[54] When early studies indicated that folic acid and other B

Tomatoes, citrus fruit, vegetables, and fortified grain products are good sources of folic acid, which may play a role in reducing homocysteine and CVD risk, though new research has called some of this potential benefit into question.

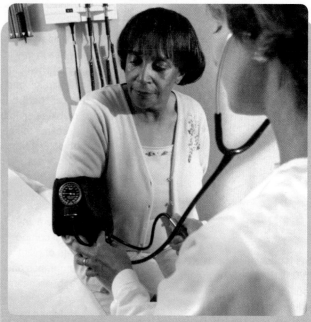

Are cardiovascular diseases hereditary?

Many behavioral and environmental factors contribute to a person's risk for cardiovascular diseases, but research suggests that there are hereditary aspects as well. If there is a history of CVD in your family, or your racial or ethnic background indicates a propensity for CVD, it is all the more important for you to find out your family history of CVD and have regular blood pressure and blood cholesterol screenings, as well as avoid lifestyle risks.

vitamins may help break down homocysteine in the body, food manufacturers responded by adding folic acids to a number of foods and touting the CVD benefits. A recent large meta-analysis indicates that folic acid neither increases nor decreases the risk of cancer at doses much higher than are present in flours and other fortified products.[55] With conflicting research, the jury is still out on the role of folic acid in CVD risk reduction. In fact, professional groups such as the American Heart Association do not currently recommend taking folic acid supplements to lower homocysteine levels and prevent CVD.[56] For now, a healthy diet is the best preventive action.

Weapons against Cardiovascular Disease

Today, CVD patients have many diagnostic, treatment, prevention, and rehabilitation options that were not available a generation ago. Medications can strengthen heartbeat, control arrhythmias, remove fluids (in the case of congestive heart failure), reduce blood pressure, improve heart function, and reduce pain. Among the most common groups of drugs are the following: *statins*, chemicals used to lower blood cholesterol levels; *ACE inhibitors*, which cause the muscles surrounding blood vessels to contract, thereby lowering blood pressure; and *beta-blockers*, which reduce blood pressure by blocking the effects of the hormone epinephrine. New treatment procedures and techniques are saving countless lives. Even long-standing methods of cardiopulmonary resuscitation (CPR) have been changed recently to focus primarily on chest compressions rather than mouth-to-mouth breathing. The thinking behind this is that people will be more likely to do CPR if the risk for exchange of body fluids is reduced—and any effort to save a person in trouble is better than inaction.

Techniques for Diagnosing Cardiovascular Disease

Several techniques are used to diagnose CVD, including electrocardiogram, angiography, and positron emission tomography scans. An **electrocardiogram (ECG)** is a record of the electrical activity of the heart. Patients may undergo a *stress test*—standard exercise on a stationary bike or treadmill with an electrocardiogram and no injections—or a *nuclear stress test,* which involves injecting a radioactive dye and taking images of the heart to reveal problems with blood flow. While these tests provide a good indicator of potential heart blockage or blood flow abnormalities, a more accurate method of testing for heart disease is **angiography** (often referred to as *cardiac catheterization*). In this procedure, a needle-thin tube called a *catheter* is threaded through heart arteries, a dye is injected, and an X-ray image is taken to discover which areas are blocked. A more recent and even more effective method of measuring heart activity is *positron emission tomography (PET),* which produces three-dimensional images of the heart as blood flows through it. Other tests include the following:

- **Magnetic resonance imaging (MRI).** This test uses powerful magnets to look inside the body. Computer-generated pictures can show the heart muscle and help physicians identify damage from a heart attack and evaluate disease of larger blood vessels such as the aorta.
- **Ultrafast computed tomography (CT).** This is an especially fast form of X-ray imaging of the heart designed to evaluate bypass grafts, diagnose ventricular function, and measure calcium deposits.
- **Cardiac calcium score.** This test measures the amount of calcium-containing plaque in the coronary arteries, a marker for overall atherosclerotic buildup. The greater amount of calcium, the higher your calcium score and the greater your risk of heart attack. Concerns have been raised over higher than average exposure to radiation from these tests.

Bypass Surgery, Angioplasty, and Stents

Coronary bypass surgery has helped many patients who suffered coronary blockages or heart attacks. In a coronary artery bypass graft (CABG), referred to as a "cabbage," a blood vessel is taken from another site in the patient's body (usually the saphenous vein in the leg or the internal thoracic artery in the chest) and implanted to bypass blocked coronary arteries and transport blood to heart tissue.

Another procedure, **angioplasty** (sometimes called *balloon angioplasty*), carries fewer risks and may be more effective than bypass surgery in selected cases. As in angiography, a thin catheter is threaded through blocked heart arteries. The catheter has a balloon at the tip, which is inflated to flatten fatty deposits against the artery walls, allowing blood to flow more freely. A stent (a mesh-like stainless steel tube) may be inserted to prop open the artery. Although highly effective, stents can lead to inflammation and tissue growth in the area that can actually lead to more blockage and problems. In about 30 percent of patients, the treated arteries become clogged again within 6 months. Newer stents are usually medicated to reduce this risk. Nonetheless, some surgeons argue that given this high rate of recurrence, bypass may be a more effective treatment. Today, newer forms of laser angioplasty and *atherectomy*, a procedure that removes plaque, are being done in several clinics.

Aspirin and Other Drug Therapies

Although aspirin has been touted for its blood-thinning qualities and possibly reducing risks for future heart attacks among those who already have had MI events, the benefits of an aspirin regimen for otherwise healthy adults remains in question. New research seems to indicate an increased risk of gastrointestinal bleeding and stroke in those who take it daily.[57] Furthermore, once a patient has taken aspirin regularly for possible protection against CHD, stopping this regimen may, in fact, increase his or her risk.[58]

If a victim reaches an emergency room and is diagnosed fast enough, a form of clot-busting therapy called **thrombolysis** can be performed. Thrombolysis involves injecting an agent such as *tissue plasminogen activator (tPA)* to dissolve the clot and restore some blood flow to the heart, thereby reducing the amount of tissue that dies from ischemia.[59] These drugs must be administered within 1 to 3 hours after a heart attack for best results.

Cancer: An Overview

Cancer is exceeded only by heart disease as the greatest killer in the United States.[60] Although there were over 580,000 deaths in 2013, the **5-year survival rates** (the relative

electrocardiogram (ECG) A record of the electrical activity of the heart; may be measured during a stress test.

angiography A technique for examining blockages in heart arteries.

coronary bypass surgery A surgical technique whereby a blood vessel taken from another part of the body is implanted to bypass a clogged coronary artery.

angioplasty A technique in which a catheter with a balloon at the tip is inserted into a clogged artery; the balloon is inflated to flatten fatty deposits against artery walls and a stent is typically inserted to keep the artery open.

thrombolysis Injection of an agent to dissolve clots and restore some blood flow, thereby reducing the amount of tissue that dies from ischemia.

5-year survival rates The percentage of people in a study or treatment group who are alive 5 years after they were diagnosed with or treated for cancer.

remission A temporary or permanent period when cancer is responding to treatment and under control. This often leads to the disappearance of the signs and symptoms of cancer.

cancer A large group of diseases characterized by the uncontrolled growth and spread of abnormal cells.

neoplasm A new growth of tissue that serves no physiological function and results from uncontrolled, abnormal cellular development.

tumor A neoplasmic mass that grows more rapidly than surrounding tissue.

malignant Very dangerous or harmful; refers to a cancerous tumor.

benign Harmless; refers to a noncancerous tumor.

biopsy Microscopic examination of tissue to determine whether a cancer is present.

metastasis Process by which cancer spreads from one area to different areas of the body.

rates for survival in persons who are living 5 years after diagnosis) are up dramatically from the virtual death sentences of many cancers in the early 1900s. Today, of the approximately 1.7 million people diagnosed each year, about 68 percent will still be alive 5 years from now—an increase of nearly 20 percent since the 1970s—and survival rates for people diagnosed with many cancers in early stages approach 100 percent.[61] For some, their cancer will be in **remission,** which means the cancer is responding to treatment and under control. Others will be considered "cured," meaning that they have no subsequent cancer in their bodies and can expect to live a long and productive life. Lifestyle, follow-up by health care providers, preventive treatments, environmental conditions, immune system functioning, and several other factors can influence the course of any cancer.

Although treatments and survival statistics have improved, nearly half of all American males and one third of American females will still develop cancer at some point in their lives.[62] In the following sections, we provide an overview of factors that increase risk of cancer and discuss ways to reduce them.

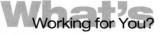

You may already be taking actions to lessen your CVD and cancer risks. Which of the following are true for you?

☐ I don't smoke or I have committed to quitting and joined a group to do it.

☐ I apply sunscreen every day, do regular self-exams, and eat a balanced diet.

☐ I know my family history for CVD and cancer.

tumor is malignant is through **biopsy,** or microscopic examination of cell development.

Benign and malignant tumors differ in several key ways. Benign tumors generally consist of ordinary-looking cells enclosed in a fibrous shell or capsule that prevents their spreading to other body areas. Malignant tumors are usually not enclosed in a protective capsule and can therefore spread to other organs (Figure 12.5 on the following page). This process, known as **metastasis,** makes some forms of cancer particularly aggressive in their ability to overcome bodily defenses. By the time they are diagnosed, malignant tumors have frequently metastasized throughout the body, making treatment extremely difficult. Unlike benign tumors, which merely expand to take over a given space, malignant cells invade surrounding tissue, emitting clawlike protrusions that disturb the RNA and DNA within normal cells. Disrupting these substances, which control cellular metabolism and

What Is Cancer?

Cancer is the general term for a large group of diseases characterized by the uncontrolled growth and spread of abnormal cells. If these cells aren't stopped, they can impair vital functions of the body and lead to death. When something interrupts normal cell function, uncontrolled growth and abnormal cellular development result in a **neoplasm,** a new growth of tissue serving no physiological function. This neoplasmic mass often forms a clumping of cells known as a **tumor.**

Not all tumors are **malignant** (cancerous); in fact, most are **benign** (noncancerous). Benign tumors are generally harmless unless they grow to obstruct or crowd out normal tissues. A benign tumor of the brain, for instance, is life threatening when it grows enough to restrict blood flow and cause a stroke. The only way to determine whether a

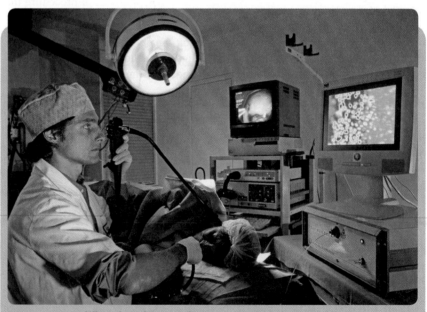

What does it mean for a tumor to be malignant?

A malignant tumor is cancerous. Malignant tumors are generally more dangerous than benign tumors because cancer cells divide quickly and can spread, or metastasize, to other parts of the body. Physicians usually order biopsies of tumors, in which sample cells are taken from the tumor and studied under a microscope to determine whether they are cancerous. Newer techniques, like the minimally invasive "optical biopsy" shown here, allow for the microscopic examination of tissue without doing a physical biopsy.

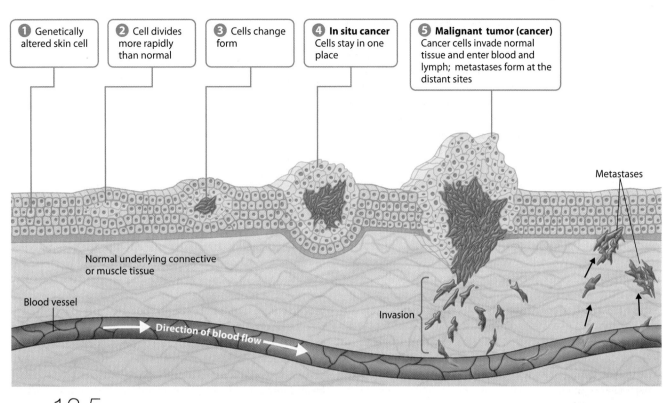

Labels on figure:

1 Genetically altered skin cell

2 Cell divides more rapidly than normal

3 Cells change form

4 **In situ cancer** Cells stay in one place

5 **Malignant tumor (cancer)** Cancer cells invade normal tissue and enter blood and lymph; metastases form at the distant sites

Metastases

Normal underlying connective or muscle tissue

Blood vessel

Direction of blood flow

Invasion

FIGURE 12.5 Metastasis
A mutation to the genetic material of a skin cell triggers abnormal cell division and changes cell formation, resulting in a cancerous tumor. If the tumor remains localized, it is considered in situ cancer. If the tumor spreads, it is considered a malignant cancer.

Video Tutor: Metastasis

reproduction, produces **mutant cells** that differ in form, quality, and function from normal cells.

Cancer staging is a classification system that describes how much a cancer has spread at the time it is diagnosed; it helps doctors and patients decide on appropriate treatments and estimate a person's life expectancy. Cancers are typically staged based on the size of a tumor, how deeply it has penetrated, the number of lymph nodes that are affected, and the degree of metastasis or spread, known as the *TNM* (for *tumor, node,* and *metastasis*) system. The most commonly known staging system assigns the numbers zero to four to the disease (see Table 12.3). In addition to staging, many tumors are assigned a grade based on the degree of abnormality of the cancer cells. Lower grade tumors tend to be closest to normal, whereas higher grade tumors may appear as highly abnormal. Typically, the lower the stage and grade, the better the prognosis.[63]

What Causes Cancer?

Causes of cancer are generally divided into two categories of risk factors: *hereditary* and *acquired* (environmental). Where hereditary factors cannot be modified, environmental factors are potentially modifiable. Specific examples include tobacco use; poor nutrition; physical inactivity; obesity; inflammation; certain infectious agents; certain medical treatments; drug

TABLE 12.3 Cancer Stages

Stage	Definition
0	Early cancer, when abnormal cells remain only in the place they originated.
I	Higher numbers indicate more extensive disease: Larger tumor size and/or spread of the cancer
II	beyond the organ in which it first developed to nearby lymph nodes and/or organs adjacent to the
III	location of the primary tumor.
IV	Cancer has spread to other organs.

and alcohol consumption; excessive sun exposure; and exposures to **carcinogens** (cancer-causing agents) in food, the air we breathe, the water we drink, and our homes and workplaces. Hereditary and environmental factors may interact to make cancer more likely, accelerate cancer progression, or increase individual susceptibility during certain periods of life, but the mechanisms are not fully understood. We do not know why some people have malignant cells in their body and never develop cancer, whereas others develop the disease.

mutant cells Cells that differ in form, quality, or function from normal cells.

cancer staging A classification system that describes how far a person's disease has advanced.

carcinogens Cancer-causing agents.

Lifestyle Risks

Anyone can develop cancer; however, most cases affect adults beginning in middle age. In fact, nearly 77 percent of cancers are diagnosed at age 55 and above.[64] Cancer researchers refer to one's cancer risk when they assess risk factors. *Lifetime risk* refers to the probability that an individual, over the course of a lifetime, will develop cancer or die from it. In the United States, men have a lifetime risk of about 1 in 2; women have a lower risk, at 1 in 3.[65]

Relative risk is a measure of the strength of the relationship between risk factors and a particular cancer. Basically, relative risk compares your risk if you engage in certain known risk behaviors with that of someone who does not engage in such behaviors. For example, if you are a man and smoke, your relative risk of getting lung cancer is about 23 times greater than that of a male nonsmoker.[66]

Over the years, researchers have found that diet, a sedentary lifestyle (and resultant obesity), overconsumption of alcohol, tobacco use, stress, and other lifestyle factors play a role in the incidence of cancer. Keep in mind that a high relative risk does not guarantee cause and effect, but it does indicate the likelihood of a particular risk factor being related to a particular outcome.

Tobacco Use
Of all the potential risk factors for cancer, smoking is among the greatest. In the United States, tobacco is responsible for nearly 1 in 5 deaths annually, accounting for at least 30 percent of all cancer deaths and 80 percent of all lung cancer deaths.[67] In fact, by all accounts, smoking is the leading cause of preventable death in the United States and around the world today.[68] Smoking is associated with increased risk of at least 15 different cancers, including those of the nasopharynx, nasal cavity, paranasal sinuses, lip, oral cavity, pharynx, larynx, lung, esophagus, pancreas, uterine cervix, kidney, bladder, and stomach, and acute myeloid leukemia.

Poor Nutrition, Physical Inactivity, and Obesity
Mounting scientific evidence suggests that about one-third of the cancer deaths that occur in the United States each year may be due to lifestyle factors such as overweight or obesity, physical inactivity, and poor nutrition.[69] Dietary choices—particularly high-calorie, high-fat and high-animal-protein diets—and physical activity are the most important modifiable determinants of cancer risk (besides not smoking). Several studies indicate a relationship between a high body mass index (BMI) and death rates from cancers of the esophagus, colon, rectum, liver, stomach, kidney, and pancreas, and others.[70]

Just how great is the risk for someone with a high BMI? Women who gain 55 pounds or more after age 18 have almost a 50 percent greater risk of breast cancer compared to those who maintain their weight.[71] The relative risk of colon cancer in men is 40 percent higher for obese men than it is for nonobese men. The relative risks of gallbladder and endometrial cancers are five times higher in obese individuals than they are in individuals of healthy weight. Numerous other studies support the link between various forms of cancer and obesity.[72]

Stress and Psychosocial Risks
Although stress has been implicated in increased susceptibility to several types of cancers, most reports of cancer being caused by stress are observational in nature, meaning that people note that they get cancer after being highly stressed. Many of these studies lack scientific rigor or are simply too small to show definitive results. A recent large meta-analytic study of work stress and cancer risk found no relationship between job strain and risk for colorectal, lung, breast, or prostate cancer.[73] That said, people who are under chronic, severe stress or who suffer from depression or other persistent emotional problems do show higher rates of cancer than do their healthy counterparts. The exact mechanisms for how stress may increase risk of cancer development, or contribute to poorer health outcomes once cancer has developed, remains unclear. Chronic sleep deprivation, unhealthy diet, and emotional or physical trauma may weaken the immune system and increase cancer susceptibility. More research is necessary to confirm the underlying mechanisms of a connection between stress and cancer.

Genetic and Physiological Risks

If your parents, aunts and uncles, siblings, or other close family members develop cancer, does it mean that you have a genetic predisposition toward it? Although there is still much uncertainty about this, scientists believe that about 5 percent of all cancers are strongly hereditary in that some people may be more predisposed to the malfunctioning of genes that ultimately cause cancer.[74]

Suspected cancer-causing genes are called **oncogenes.** While these genes are typically dormant, certain conditions such as age, stress, and exposure to carcinogens, viruses, and radiation may activate them. Once activated, they cause cells to grow and reproduce uncontrollably. Scientists are uncertain whether only people who develop cancer have oncogenes or whether we all have genes that can become oncogenes under certain conditions.

Certain cancers, particularly those of the breast, stomach, colon, prostate, uterus, ovaries, and lungs, appear to run in families. For example, a woman runs a much higher risk of breast cancer and/or ovarian cancer if her mother or sisters (primary relatives) have had the disease or if she inherits the breast cancer susceptibility genes (BRCA1 or BRCA2).

oncogenes Suspected cancer-causing genes.

Hodgkin's disease and certain leukemias show similar familial patterns. The complex interaction of hereditary predisposition, lifestyle, and environment on the development of cancer makes it a challenge to determine a single cause. Even among those predisposed to genetic mutations, avoiding risks may decrease chances of cancer development.

Reproductive and Hormonal Factors The effects of reproductive factors on breast and cervical cancers have been well documented. Increased numbers of fertile or menstrual cycle years (early menarche, late menopause), not having children or having them later in life, recent use of birth control pills or hormone replacement therapy, and opting not to breast-feed, all appear to increase risks of breast cancer.[75] However, while the above factors appear to play a significant role in increased risk for non-Hispanic white women, they do not appear to have as strong an influence on Hispanic women.[76]

Studies also suggest that women on hormone supplements or hormone replacement therapy have a slightly increased risk of lung cancer.[77]

Alcohol and Cancer Risks

Numerous studies have implicated alcohol consumption with increased risk of cancers, and even low levels of alcohol (three drinks per week) are associated with increased risk of oral, esophagus, and breast cancer in women. With heavy drinking, incidence rises dramatically for cancers of the oral cavity and esophagus, stomach, colon, liver, and pancreas.[78]

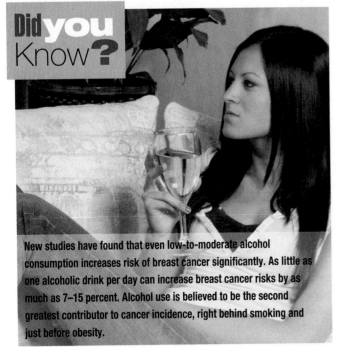

Did you Know?

New studies have found that even low-to-moderate alcohol consumption increases risk of breast cancer significantly. As little as one alcoholic drink per day can increase breast cancer risks by as much as 7–15 percent. Alcohol use is believed to be the second greatest contributor to cancer incidence, right behind smoking and just before obesity.

Source: W. Chen et al., "Moderate Alcohol Consumption during Adult Life: Drinking Patterns and Breast Cancer Risk," *The Journal of the American Medical Association* 306, no. 17 (2011): 1884–1890K.

Inflammation and Cancer Risks

As with CVD, an emerging theory in cancer research is that inflammatory processes in the body play a significant role in the development of cancer—from initiation and promoting cancer cells to paving the way for them to invade, spread, and weaken the immune response.[79] According to some researchers, the vast majority of cancers (90%) are caused by cellular mutations and environmental factors that occur as a result of inflammation. These same researchers believe that up to 20 percent of cancers are the result of chronic infections, 30 percent are the result of tobacco smoking and inhaled particulates such as asbestos, and 35 percent are due to dietary factors.[80] The common denominator in these threats is inflammation that primes the system for cancer to gain a foothold and spread.[81] If inflammation is indeed a key factor, reducing inflammation via stress reduction, sleep, dietary supplements, low-dose aspirin, and other behaviors may prove beneficial in reducing cancer risks.

Occupational and Environmental Risks

Overall, workplace hazards account for only a small percentage of all cancers. However, various substances are known to cause cancer when exposure levels are high or prolonged. One is asbestos, a fibrous material once widely used in the construction, insulation, and automobile industries. Nickel, chromate, and chemicals such as benzene, arsenic, and vinyl chloride have been shown definitively to be carcinogens for humans. People who routinely work with certain dyes and radioactive substances may also have increased risks for cancer. Working with coal tars, as in the mining profession, or with inhalants, as in the auto-painting business, is hazardous. So is working with herbicides and pesticides, although evidence is inconclusive for low-dose exposures. Several federal and state agencies are responsible for monitoring such exposures and ensuring that businesses comply with standards designed to protect workers.

You don't have to work in one of these industries to come in contact with environmental carcinogens. See the **Be Healthy, Be Green** box on the following page to explore some ways you can avoid carcinogens in the products you buy and use every day.

Radiation Ionizing radiation (IR)—radiation from X-rays, radon, cosmic rays, and ultraviolet radiation (primarily ultraviolet B, or UVB, radiation)—is the only form of radiation proven to cause human cancer. Evidence that high-dose IR causes cancer comes from studies of atomic bomb survivors, patients receiving radiotherapy, and certain occupational groups (e.g., uranium miners). Virtually any part of the body can be affected by IR, but bone marrow and the thyroid are particularly susceptible. Radon exposure in homes can increase lung cancer risk, especially in cigarette smokers. To reduce the risk of harmful effects, diagnostic medical and dental X-rays are set at the lowest dose levels possible.

BE HEALTHY, BE GREEN

GO GREEN AGAINST CANCER

There are many things you can do to help reduce the number of carcinogens in the environment and to limit your exposure to those that are present. The following are just a few ideas:

1. **Leave the car at home.** Try commuting by bicycle or by foot instead of driving. This will reduce your daily carbon emissions and your risk for cancer by increasing your physical activity.

Don't risk your health for beauty! Read the labels on your cosmetics and avoid products containing potentially carcinogenic chemicals such as phthalates and parabens.

2. **Choose organic foods when possible.** Conventional produce is often sprayed with chemicals and pesticides. When we eat these chemicals, our risk for cancer can be elevated.

3. **When shopping for home furnishings, explore ecofriendly furniture, upholstery, and home textiles.** Many furnishings are manufactured with toxic chemicals that are released into the air. This can dramatically reduce indoor air quality and increase your risk for cancer. Select products that have not been treated with stain-resistant chemicals and look for ecofriendly flooring, carpets, and other products. Such ecofriendly products include bamboo, recycled glass or metal tiles, cork, and flooring made from reclaimed wood products.

4. **Use "green" paper.** By purchasing ecofriendly paper products that are bleach free, we reduce the amount of dioxins released into the atmosphere. Dioxins are carcinogenic, and fewer of them in the atmosphere will reduce everyone's risk for cancer.

5. **Buy ecofriendly hygiene products.** When purchasing personal hygiene products or cosmetics, select items that are environmentally responsible. Consider avoiding products containing the following chemicals, all of which are suspected or confirmed carcinogens:

* Diethanolamine (DEA)
* Formaldehyde (commonly found in eye shadows)
* Phthalates
* Parabens

6. **Avoid dry cleaning.** Conventional dry cleaning uses a chemical called *perchloroethylene* (PERC), an agent known to increase the risk for cancer and harm the environment. If dry cleaning is unavoidable, explore local dry cleaners using ecofriendly alternatives such as "wet cleaning," which includes biodegradable soaps or silicone-based solvents and special machinery to reduce shrinkage.

Nonionizing radiation produced by radio waves, cell phones, microwaves, computer screens, televisions, electric blankets, and other products has been a topic of great concern in recent years, but research has not proven excess risk to date. A wide range of studies has been conducted, and no consistent link between cell phone use and cancers of the brain, nerves, or other tissues of the head or neck has been shown. Additionally, most of the key policy-making and health organizations have indicated that the existing research does not support a cell phone/cancer link. Stay tuned, because major studies of adults from several countries and children are underway to help provide more insight.[82] (See **Chapter 15** for more on the potential environmental and health hazards of radiation.)

Chemicals in Foods

Much of the concern about chemicals in foods centers on the possible harm caused by pesticide and herbicide residues. Although some of these chemicals cause cancer at high doses in experimental animals, the very low concentrations found in some foods are well within established government safety levels. Continued research regarding pesticide and herbicide use is essential, and scientists and consumer groups stress the importance of a balance between chemical use and the production of high-quality food products. Prevention efforts should focus on policies to protect consumers, develop low-chemical pesticides and herbicides, and reduce environmental pollution.

Infectious Diseases and Cancer

According to experts, over 10 percent of all malignancies in the United States are caused by viruses, bacteria, and parasites.[83] Worldwide, approximately 20 percent of human cancers have been traced to infectious agents, primarily viruses.[84] Infections are thought to influence cancer development in several ways, most commonly through chronic inflammation, suppression of the immune system, or chronic stimulation.

Hepatitis B, Hepatitis C, and Liver Cancer

Viruses such as hepatitis B (HBV) and C (HCV) are believed to stimulate the growth of cancer cells in the liver because they are chronic diseases that inflame liver tissue—potentially priming the liver for cancer or making it more hospitable for cancer development. Global increases in hepatitis B and C rates and concurrent rises in liver cancer rates seem to provide evidence of such an association.

Human Papillomavirus and Cervical Cancer Nearly 100 percent of women with cervical cancer have evidence of human papillomavirus (HPV) infection—a virus believed to be a major cause of cervical cancer. Fortunately, only a small percentage of HPV cases progress to cervical cancer.[85] Today, a vaccine is available to help protect young women from becoming infected with HPV and developing cervical cancer. (For more on the HPV vaccine, see the discussion in **Chapter 13.**)

Types of Cancers

Cancers are grouped into four broad categories based on the type of tissue from which each arise:

- **Carcinomas.** Epithelial tissues (tissues covering body surfaces and lining most body cavities) are the most common sites for cancers called *carcinomas*. These cancers affect the outer layer of the skin and mouth as well as the mucous membranes. They metastasize through the circulatory or lymphatic system initially and form solid tumors.
- **Sarcomas.** Sarcomas occur in the mesodermal, or middle, layers of tissue—for example, in bones, muscles, and general connective tissue. They metastasize primarily via the blood in the early stages of disease. These cancers are less common but generally more virulent than carcinomas. They also form solid tumors.
- **Lymphomas.** Lymphomas develop in the lymphatic system—the infection-fighting regions of the body—and metastasize through the lymphatic system. Hodgkin's disease is an example. Lymphomas also form solid tumors.
- **Leukemias.** Cancer of the blood-forming parts of the body, particularly the bone marrow and spleen, is called leukemia. A nonsolid tumor, leukemia is characterized by an abnormal increase in the number of white blood cells.

Figure 12.6 shows the most common sites of cancer and the estimated number of new cases and deaths from each type in 2013. A comprehensive discussion of the many different forms of cancer is beyond the scope of this book, but we will discuss the most common types in the next sections.

Lung Cancer

Lung cancer is the leading cause of cancer deaths for both men and women in the United States. Even as rates have decreased in recent decades, it still killed an estimated

Estimated New Cases of Cancer*		Estimated Deaths from Cancer*	
Female	Male	Female	Male
Breast 232,340 (29%)	Prostate 238,590 (28%)	Lung & bronchus 72,220 (26%)	Lung & bronchus 87,260 (28%)
Lung & bronchus 110,110 (14%)	Lung & bronchus 118,080 (14%)	Breast 39,620 (14%)	Prostate 29,720 (10%)
Colon & rectum 69,140 (9%)	Colon & rectum 73,680 (9%)	Colon & rectum 24,530 (9%)	Colon & rectum 26,300 (9%)
Uterine corpus 49,560 (6%)	Urinary bladder 54,610 (6%)	Pancreas 18,980 (7%)	Pancreas 19,480 (6%)
Thyroid 45,310 (6%)	Melanoma of the skin 45,060 (5%)	Ovary 14,030 (5%)	Liver & intrahepatic bile duct 14,890 (5%)
Non-Hodgkin lymphoma 31,630 (4%)	Kidney & renal pelvis 40,430 (5%)	Leukemia 10,060 (4%)	Leukemia 13,660 (4%)
Melanoma of the skin 31,630 (4%)	Non-Hodgkin lymphoma 37,600 (4%)	Non-Hodgkin lymphoma 8,430 (3%)	Esophagus 12,220 (4%)
Kidney & renal pelvis 24,720 (3%)	Oral cavity & pharynx 29,620 (3%)	Uterine corpus 8,190 (3%)	Urinary bladder 10,820 (4%)
Pancreas 22,480 (3%)	Leukemia 27,880 (3%)	Liver & intrahepatic bile duct 6,780 (2%)	Non-Hodgkin lymphoma 10,590 (3%)
Ovary 22,240 (3%)	Pancreas 22,740 (3%)	Brain & other nervous system 6,150 (2%)	Kidney & renal pelvis 8,780 (3%)
All Sites 805,500 (100%)	All Sites 854,790 (100%)	All Sites 273,430 (100%)	All Sites 306,920 (100%)

*Excludes basal and squamous cell skin cancers and in situ carcinoma except urinary bladder. Percentages may not total 100% due to rounding.

FIGURE 12.6 Leading Sites of New Cancer Cases and Deaths, 2013 Estimates
Source: Data from American Cancer Society, *Cancer Facts & Figures 2013* (Atlanta: American Cancer Society, Inc.), table on page 4. Note that percentages do not add up to 100 due to omissions of certain rare cancers as well as rounding of statistics.

228,190 Americans in 2013.[86] Since 1987, more women have died each year from lung cancer than from breast cancer, which over the previous 40 years had been the leading cause of cancer deaths in women. Although past reductions in smoking rates bode well for cancer and CVD statistics, there is growing concern about the number of youth, particularly young women and persons of low income and low educational level, who continue to pick up the habit. There is also concern about the increase in lung cancers among those who have never smoked—representing as many as 15 percent of all lung cancers. This type of lung cancer is believed to be related to exposure to secondhand smoke, radon gas, asbestos, wood-burning stoves, and aerosolized oils caused by cooking with oil and deep fat frying.[87] It also seems resistant to traditional lung cancer therapies, and prognosis is often bleak at diagnosis.[88]

90% of all lung cancers could be avoided if people did not smoke.

Detection, Symptoms, and Treatment Symptoms of lung cancer include a persistent cough, blood-streaked sputum, chest pain, and recurrent attacks of pneumonia or bronchitis. Treatment depends on the type and stage of the cancer. Surgery, radiation therapy, and chemotherapy are all options. If the cancer is localized, surgery is usually the treatment of choice. If it has spread, surgery is combined with radiation and chemotherapy. Despite advances in medical technology, survival rates 1 year after diagnosis are only 41 percent overall. The 5-year survival rate for all stages combined is only 16 percent.[89] Newer tests, such as low-dose CT scans, molecular markers in sputum, and improved biopsy techniques, have helped improve diagnosis, but we still have a long way to go.

Risk Factors and Prevention Smokers, especially those who have smoked for more than 20 years, and people who have been exposed to secondhand smoke and industrial substances such as arsenic and asbestos or to radiation are at the highest risk for lung cancer. Quitting smoking does reduce the risk,[90] but exposure to both secondhand cigarette smoke and radon gas is also believed to play an important role in lung cancer development.[91]

Breast Cancer

Women have about a 1 in 8 chance of developing breast cancer in their lifetime. For women from birth to age 39, the chance is about a 1 in 202, with significantly higher rates after menopause.[92] In 2013, approximately 232,340 women and 2,240 men in the United States were diagnosed with invasive breast cancer for the first time. In addition, 66,640 new cases of in situ breast cancer, a more localized cancer, were diagnosed. About 40,000 women (and 400 men) died, making breast cancer the second leading cause of cancer death for women.[93]

Detection, Symptoms, and Treatment The earliest signs of breast cancer are usually observable on mammograms, often before lumps can be felt. However, mammograms are not foolproof. Hence, regular breast self-examination (BSE) can be helpful (see **Student Health Today: Breast Awareness and Self-Exam** on the following page). Although mammograms detect between 80 and 90 percent of breast cancers in women without symptoms, a newer form of magnetic resonance imaging (MRI) appears to be more accurate, particularly in women with genetic risks for tumors.[94]

Once breast cancer has grown enough that it can be felt by palpating the area, many women will recognize the threat and seek medical care. Symptoms may include persistent breast changes, such as a lump in the breast or surrounding lymph nodes, thickening, dimpling, skin irritation, distortion, retraction or scaliness of the nipple, nipple discharge, or tenderness.

Treatments range from a lumpectomy to radical mastectomy to various combinations of radiation or chemotherapy. Among nonsurgical options, promising results have been noted among women using *selective estrogen-receptor modulators (SERMs)* such as tamoxifen and raloxifene, particularly women whose cancers appear to grow in response to estrogen. These drugs, as well as new *aromatase inhibitors,* work by blocking estrogen. The 5-year survival rate for people

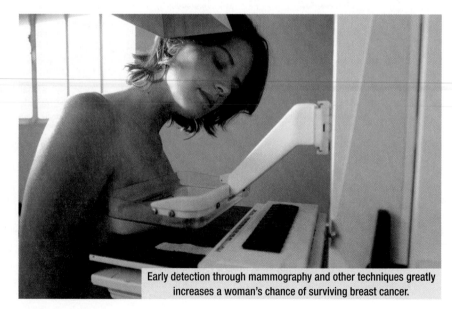

Early detection through mammography and other techniques greatly increases a woman's chance of surviving breast cancer.

BREAST AWARENESS AND SELF-EXAM

For the last two decades, breast self-exam has been recommended by major health organizations as a form of early breast cancer screening. However, a 2009 "study of studies" done by the U.S. Preventive Services Task Force determined that breast self-exams did not decrease suffering and death and, in fact, often lead to unnecessary worry, unnecessary tests, and increased health care costs. As a result of this research, several groups have downgraded the recommendation about breast self-exams from "do them and do them regularly" to "learn how to do them, and if you desire, do them to know your body and be able to recognize changes."

To do a breast self-exam, begin by standing in front of a mirror to inspect the breasts, looking for their usual symmetry. Some breasts are not symmetrical, and if this is not a change, it is okay. Raise and lower both arms while checking that the breasts move evenly and freely. Next, inspect the skin, looking for areas of redness, thickening, or dimpling, which might have the appearance of an orange peel. Look for any scaling on the nipple.

To feel for lumps, raise one arm above your head while either standing or lying. This will flatten out the breast, making

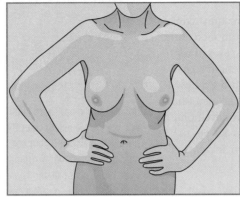

① Face a mirror and check for changes in symmetry.

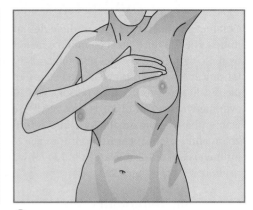

② Either standing or lying down, use the pads of the three middle fingers to check for lumps. Follow an up and down pattern on the breast to ensure all tissue gets inspected.

it easier to feel the tissue. Using the index, middle, and fourth fingers of your opposite hand, gently push down on the breast tissue and move the fingers in small circular motions, varying pressure from light to more firm. Start at one edge of the breast and move upward and then downward, working your way across the breast until all of the breast tissue has been covered. Often breast tissue will feel dense and irregular, and this is usually normal. It helps to do regular self-exams to become familiar with what your breast tissue feels like; then, if there is a change, you will notice. Cancers usually feel like a dense or firm little rock and are very different from the normal breast tissue.

Next, lower the arm and reach into the top of the underarm and pull downward with gentle pressure feeling for any enlarged lymph nodes. To complete the exam, squeeze the tissue around the nipple. If you notice discharge from the nipple and you have not recently been breastfeeding, consult your doctor. Likewise, if you notice any asymmetry, skin changes, scaling on the nipple, or new lumps in the breast, you should see your doctor for evaluation.

Source: Adapted from Breast Self-Exam Illustration Series, National Cancer Institute Visuals Online Collection, U.S. National Institutes of Health, 1984.

---

with localized breast cancer is 98 percent today; for higher stage cancer, the 5-year survival rate drops dramatically.[95] As with most cancers, the earlier it is diagnosed, the greater the chances for a full recovery.

Risk Factors and Prevention

The incidence of breast cancer increases with age. Although there are many possible risk factors, those that are well supported by research include family history of breast cancer, menstrual periods that started early and ended late in life, weight gain after the age of 18, obesity after menopause, recent use of oral contraceptives or postmenopausal hormone therapy, never having children or having a first child after age 30, consuming two or more alcoholic drinks per day, and physical inactivity. Women with dense breasts, high bone mineral density, and exposure to high dose radiation are also at increased risk.[96] Genes also appear to account for approximately 5 to 10 percent of all cases of breast cancer. Women who possess *BRCA1* and *BRCA2* gene mutations have a 60 to 80 percent risk of developing breast cancer by age 70, whereas women without the mutations have a 7 percent risk. Because these genes are rare, routine screening for them is not recommended unless there is a strong family history of breast cancer.[97]

International differences in breast cancer incidence correlate with variations in diet, especially fat intake, although a causal role for these dietary factors has not been firmly

See It! Videos

Could you have inherited breast cancer from a female relative? Watch **Breast Cancer Patients Getting Younger** in the Study Area of MasteringHealth™

Colon and Rectal Cancers

Colorectal cancers (cancers of the colon and rectum) continue to be the third most common cancer in both men and women, with 102,480 cases of colon and 40,340 cases of rectal cancer diagnosed in the United States in 2013 and 50,830 deaths. Most cases occur in persons age 50 and over; however, new cases can occur at any age.[100] Younger men and women have approximately a 1 in 1,200 risk of developing colon and rectal cancer from birth to age 39. At age 50, risk for men is about 1 in 106 and 1 in 134 for women, increasing to about 1 in 20 by age 70.

Detection, Symptoms, and Treatment Because colorectal cancer tends to spread slowly, the prognosis is quite good if it is caught in the early stages. While later stages may have symptoms such as stool changes, bleeding, cramping or pain in the lower abdomen, and unusual fatigue, colorectal cancers usually have no early symptoms. Regular screenings, such as colonoscopy or barium enemas, are recommended for those at high risk. Treatment often consists of radiation or surgery. Chemotherapy, although not used extensively in the past, is today a possibility.

Risk Factors and Prevention Anyone can get colorectal cancer, but people who are over age 50, who are obese, who have a family history of colon and rectal cancer, a personal or family history of polyps (benign growths) in the colon or rectum, or who have type 2 diabetes or inflammatory bowel problems such as colitis are at increased risk. Other possible risk factors include diets high in fat or low in fiber, smoking, sedentary lifestyle, heavy drinking, red or processed meat consumption, and low intake of fruits and vegetables.[101]

Regular exercise, a diet with lots of fruits and other plant foods, maintaining a healthy weight, and moderation in alcohol consumption appear to be among the most promising prevention strategies. Consumption of milk and calcium also appears to decrease risks. While new research suggests that non-steroidal anti-inflammatory drugs (NSAIDS), post-menopausal hormones, folic acid, calcium supplements, selenium, and vitamin E may also decrease risks,[102] drugs are not recommended as a preventive measure because risks associated with their use might outweigh any benefit.

malignant melanoma A virulent cancer of the melanocytes (pigment-producing cells) of the skin.

Skin Cancer

Skin cancer is the most common form of cancer in the United States today with about 3.5 million people diagnosed in 2013.[103] The two most common types of skin cancer—basal cell and squamous cell carcinomas—are highly curable.

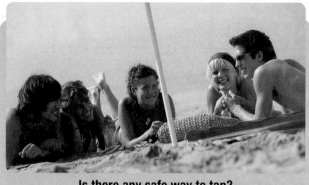

Is there any safe way to tan?

Unfortunately, no. There is no such thing as a "safe" tan, because a tan is visible evidence of UV-induced skin damage. Whether the UV rays causing your tan came from the sun or from a tanning bed, the damage, premature aging, and cancer risk are the same. Nor is an existing "base tan" protective against further damage. According to the American Cancer Society, tanned skin provides only about the equivalent of sun protection factor (SPF) 4 sunscreen—much too weak to be considered protective. Wearing sunscreen of SPF 15 or higher every day can prevent further damage and diminish the cumulative effects of sun exposure.

Malignant melanoma is a much more lethal form of skin cancer. An estimated 12,650 will die of skin cancer in 2013.[104]

Detection, Symptoms, and Treatment Many people do not know what to look for when examining themselves for skin cancer. Fortunately, potentially cancerous growths are often visible as abnormalities on the skin. Basal and squamous cell carcinomas can be a recurrent annoyance, showing up most commonly on the face, ears, neck, arms, hands, and legs as warty bumps, colored spots, or scaly patches. Bleeding, itchiness, pain, or oozing are other symptoms that warrant attention.[105] Surgery may be necessary to remove them, but they are seldom life threatening.

Melanoma, in contrast, is an invasive killer that may appear as a skin lesion that changes size, shape, or color and that spreads throughout organs of the body. While melanoma is less common than basal and squamous cell carcinomas, it is responsible for the majority of skin cancer deaths. This is one of the few cancers that develops frequently in younger people, and melanoma rates increase to 1 in 50 for males and 1 in 20 for females by age 70.[106] Figure 12.7 on the following page shows melanoma compared to basal cell and squamous cell carcinomas. A simple *ABCD* rule outlines the warning signs of melanoma:

- **Asymmetry.** One half of the mole or lesion does not match the other half.
- **Border irregularity.** The edges are uneven, notched, or scalloped.
- **Color.** Pigmentation is not uniform. Melanomas may vary in color from tan to deeper brown, reddish black, black, or deep bluish black.

established. Sudden weight gain has also been implicated. Research also shows that regular exercise, even some forms of recreational exercise, can reduce risk,[98] and so might increasing dietary fiber intake.[99]

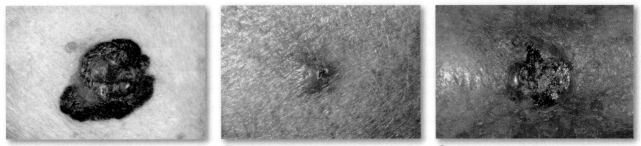

(a) Malignant melanoma   (b) Basal cell carcinoma   (c) Squamous cell carcinoma

FIGURE 12.7 **Types of Skin Cancers**
Preventing skin cancer includes keeping a careful watch for any new pigmented growths and for changes to any moles. The ABCD warning signs of melanoma (a) include *asymmetrical* shapes, irregular *borders*, *color* variation, and an increase in *diameter*. Basal cell carcinoma (b) and squamous cell carcinoma (c) should be brought to your physician's attention, but are not as deadly as melanoma.

- **Diameter.** The diameter is greater than 6 millimeters (about the size of a pea).

Treatment of skin cancer depends on its seriousness. Surgery is performed in 90 percent of all cases. Radiation therapy, *electrodesiccation* (tissue destruction by heat), and *cryosurgery* (tissue destruction by freezing) are also common forms of treatment. For melanoma, treatment may involve surgical removal of the regional lymph nodes, radiation, or chemotherapy.

Risk Factors and Prevention Anyone overexposed to ultraviolet radiation without adequate protection is at risk for skin cancer. The risk is greatest for people who fit the following categories:

- Have fair skin; blonde, red, or light brown hair; blue, green, or gray eyes
- Always burn before tanning or burn easily and peel readily
- Don't tan easily but spend lots of time outdoors
- Use no or low sun protection factor (SPF) sunscreens or old, expired suntan lotions
- Have previously been treated for skin cancer or have a family history of skin cancer
- Have experienced severe sunburns during childhood

Preventing skin cancer is a matter of limiting exposure to harmful UV rays found in sunlight. What happens when you expose yourself to sunlight? Biologically, the skin responds to photodamage by increasing its thickness and the number of pigment cells (melanocytes), which produce the "tan" look. The skin's cells that ward off infection are also prone to photodamage, lowering the normal immune protection of our skin and priming it for cancer. Photodamage also causes wrinkling by impairing the elastic substances (collagens) that keep skin soft and pliable. Stay safe in the sun by limiting sun exposure when its rays are strongest, between 10:00 A.M. and 4:00 P.M., and by applying an SPF 15 or higher sunscreen before going outside.

Despite the risk of skin cancer, many Americans are still "working on a tan," and many tanning salon patrons incorrectly believe that tanning booths are safer than sitting in the sun. The truth is that there is no such thing as a safe tan from *any* source! Every time you tan, whether in the sun or in a salon, you are exposing your skin to harmful UV light rays. All tanning lamps emit UVA rays, and most emit UVB rays as well; both types can cause long-term skin damage and contribute to cancer. Even worse, some salons do not calibrate the UV output of their tanning bulbs properly, which can cause more or less exposure than you paid for.

Prostate Cancer

Cancer of the prostate is the most frequently diagnosed cancer in American males today, excluding skin cancer, and is the second leading cause of cancer deaths in men after lung cancer. In 2013, about 239,000 new cases of prostate cancer were diagnosed in the United States. About 1 in 6 men will be diagnosed with prostate cancer during his lifetime, but only 1 in 36 will die of it.[107]

Detection, Symptoms, and Treatment The prostate is a muscular, walnut-sized gland that surrounds part of a man's urethra, the tube that transports urine and sperm out of the body. As part of the male reproductive system, its primary function is to produce seminal fluid. Symptoms of prostate cancer include weak or interrupted urine flow; difficulty starting or stopping urination; feeling the urge to urinate frequently; pain upon urination; blood in the urine; or pain in the low back, pelvis, or thighs. Many men have no symptoms in the early stages.

Men over the age of 40 should have an annual digital rectal prostate examination. Another screening method for prostate cancer is the **prostate-specific antigen (PSA)** test, which is a blood test that screens for an

prostate-specific antigen (PSA) An antigen found in prostate cancer patients.

See It! Videos
Is there such a thing as a 'safe' tan? Watch **Extreme Tanning** in the Study Area of MasteringHealth™

indicator of prostate cancer. However, in 2011, a governmental panel called the United States Preventive Services Task Force made the recommendation that healthy men no longer receive the PSA test because overall it does not save lives and may in fact lead to painful, unnecessary cancer treatments. If you have a family history or other symptoms, consult with your physician.

Fortunately, 90 percent of all prostate cancers are detected while they are still in the local or regional stages and tend to progress slowly. Over the past 20 years, the 5-year survival rate for all stages combined has increased from 67 percent to almost 99 percent, and the 15-year survival rate is over 76 percent.[108]

Risk Factors and Prevention Chances of developing prostate cancer increase dramatically with age. More than 60 percent of prostate cancers are diagnosed in men over the age of 65, and 97 percent occur in men 50 or older.[109] The disease is discovered because it has progressed to the point of displaying symptoms, or, more likely, men are seeing a doctor for other problems and get a screening test or PSA test.

Race is also a risk factor in prostate cancer. The highest prostate cancer incidence rates in the world are found in African American men and Jamaican men of African descent. They are also more likely to be diagnosed at more advanced stages than other racial groups.[110]

Having a father or brother with prostate cancer more than doubles a man's risk of getting prostate cancer himself. Interestingly, the risk is higher for men with an affected brother than it is for those with an affected father.[111]

Eating more fruits and vegetables, particularly those containing lycopene, a pigment found in tomatoes and other red fruits, may lower the risk of prostate cancer. The best advice is to follow the national dietary recommendations and maintain a healthy weight.

Ovarian Cancer

Ovarian cancer is the fifth leading cause of cancer deaths for women, with about 22,240 diagnoses in 2013 and just over 14,000 deaths.[112] Ovarian cancer causes more deaths than any other cancer of the reproductive system because women tend not to discover it until the cancer is at an advanced stage. Overall, 1-year survival rates are 75 percent, and 5-year survival rates are 44 percent.[113]

Ovarian cancer symptoms are often not obvious, and it is common for women to have no early symptoms at all. A woman may complain of feeling bloated, having pain in the pelvic area, feeling full quickly or feeling the need to urinate more frequently. Some may experience persistent digestive disturbances, while other symptoms include fatigue, pain during intercourse, unexplained weight loss, unexplained changes in bowel or bladder habits, and incontinence.

Primary relatives (mother, daughter, sister) of a woman who has had ovarian cancer are at increased risk, as are those with a family or personal history of breast or colon cancer. Women who have never been pregnant are more likely to develop ovarian cancer than those who have had a child, and the use of fertility drugs may also increase a woman's risk.

Research shows that using birth control pills, adhering to a low-fat diet, having multiple children, and breast-feeding can all reduce the risk of ovarian cancer. General prevention strategies such as focusing on a healthy diet, exercise, sleep, stress management, and weight control are good ideas to lower your risk for any of the diseases discussed in this chapter. Getting annual pelvic examinations is important, and women over the age of 40 should have a cancer-related checkup every year.

Cervical and Endometrial (Uterine) Cancer

Most uterine cancers develop in the body of the uterus, usually in the endometrium (lining). The rest develop in the cervix, located at the base of the uterus. In 2013, an estimated 12,340 new cases of cervical cancer and 49,560 cases of endometrial cancer were diagnosed in the United States.[114] Increased estrogen levels as a result of menopausal estrogen therapy, being overweight/obese, and never having children may dramatically increase risk for endometrial cancer. In addition, risks are increased by treatment with tamoxifen for breast cancer, metabolic syndrome, late menopause, a history of polyps in the uterus or ovaries, a history of other cancers, and race (white women are at higher risk). The overall incidence of cervical and uterine cancer has been declining steadily over the past decade. This decline may be due to more regular screenings of younger women using the **Pap test,** a procedure in which cells taken from the cervical region are examined for abnormal cellular activity. Although Pap tests are very effective for detecting early-stage cervical cancer, they are less effective for detecting cancers of the uterine lining. Early warning signs of uterine cancer include bleeding outside the normal menstrual period or after menopause or persistent unusual vaginal discharge. As of 2013, it is recommended women get a Pap test every 2 years beginning at age 21. Between ages 30 and 65, women should have an HPV and Pap test every 5 years and a Pap test alone every 3 years. Those with parents and/or siblings with breast cancer should talk with their doctor about having tests more frequently.

The primary cause of cervical cancer is infection with certain types of the human papillomavirus (HPV). Having sex at a young age and having multiple partners and unprotected sex can increase risks dramatically. Progression to cancer appears to be related to a weakened immune system, multiple births, cigarette smoking, and using oral contraceptives. Today, both young men and women have the option of getting vaccinated against HPV. Other sexually transmitted infections such as herpes may also increase risks.

Pap test A procedure in which cells taken from the cervical region are examined for abnormal activity.

Testicular Cancer

Testicular cancer is one of the most common types of solid tumors found in young adult men, affecting nearly 7,920 young men in 2013.[115] Those between the ages of 15 and 35 are at greatest risk. There has been a steady increase in testicular cancer frequency over the past several years in this age group.[116] However, with a 96 percent 5-year survival rate, it is one of the most curable forms of cancer. Although the cause of testicular cancer is unknown, several risk factors have been identified. Men with undescended testicles appear to be at greatest risk, and some studies indicate a genetic influence.

In general, testicular tumors first appear as an enlargement of one or both of the testis, a lump or thickening in testicular tissue. Some men report a heavy feeling, dull ache, or pain that extends to the lower abdomen or groin area. Testicular self-exams have long been recommended for young men to perform monthly as a means of detecting testicular cancer (Figure 12.8). However, recent studies discovered that findings from monthly self-exams result in testing for noncancerous conditions and thus are not cost-effective. For this reason, the U.S. Preventive Services Task Force stopped recommending self-exams. Regardless, most cases of testicular cancer are discovered through self-exam, and there is currently no other screening tests for the disease.

The testicular self-exam is best done after a hot shower, which relaxes the scrotum. Standing in front of a mirror, hold the testicle with one hand while gently rolling its surface between the thumb and fingers of your other hand. Feel underneath the scrotum for the tubes of the epididymis and blood vessels that sit close to the body. Repeat with the other testicle. Look for any lump, thickening, or pea-like nodules, paying attention to any areas that may be painful over the entire surface of the scrotum. When done, wash your hands with soap and water. Doing regular self-exams will help you to know what is normal for you and to note any irregularity. Consult a doctor if you note anything that is unusual.

Pancreatic Cancer: Deadly and on the Rise

Pancreatic cancer is one of the deadliest forms of cancer, with most patients dying within 1 year of diagnosis and only 6 percent surviving 5 years. Although most cases occur after age 50, there are increasing numbers of cases at earlier ages. Overall, rates are higher in African Americans and in populations with lower socioeconomic status and education levels. They are also about 30 percent higher in men than women.

Tobacco use appears to be a key risk factor, as is obesity, consumption of high levels of red meat, and high-fat diet. Fam-

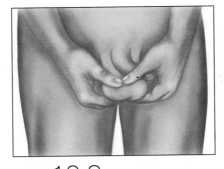

FIGURE 12.8 **Testicular Self-Exam**
Source: From Michael Johnson, *Human Biology: Concepts and Current Issues*. 3rd ed. Copyright © 2006. Reprinted with permission of Pearson Education, Inc.

ily history, possible genetic links, and a history of chronic inflammation of the pancreas over the years (*pancreatitis*), seem to increase risk. Also, there appears to be a greater risk among diabetics and those who have had infections with hepatitis B and C and the *Helicobacter* bacteria. Because pancreatic cancer has few early symptoms, there is no reliable test to detect it in its early stages. Often, by the time it is diagnosed via CT or MRI examinations, it is too advanced to treat effectively.

Facing Cancer

The earlier cancer is diagnosed, the better the prospect for survival. Make a realistic assessment of your own risk factors; avoid those behaviors that put you at risk; and increase healthy behaviors, such as improving your diet and exercise levels, reducing stress, and getting regular checkups. Even if you have significant risks, there are factors you can control. Do you have a family history of cancer? If so, what types? Make sure you know which symptoms to watch for, avoid known carcinogens—such as tobacco—and other environmental hazards, and follow the recommendations for self-exams and medical checkups outlined in Table 12.4 on page 380.

The use of several high-tech imaging systems to detect cancer has become standard. **Magnetic resonance imaging (MRI)** uses a huge electromagnet to detect hidden tumors by mapping the vibrations of the various atoms in the body on a computer screen. Another key weapon is the **computed tomography scan (CT scan),** which uses X-rays to examine parts of the body. In both of these painless, noninvasive procedures, cross-sectioned pictures can reveal a tumor's shape and location more accurately than can conventional X-ray images. Early in 2011, the FDA approved the first 3D mammogram machines, which offer significant improvements in imaging and breast cancer detection but deliver nearly double the radiation risk of conventional mammograms.

magnetic resonance imaging (MRI) A device that uses magnetic fields, radio waves, and computers to generate an image of internal tissues of the body for diagnostic purposes without the use of radiation.

computed tomography scan (CT scan) A scan by a machine that uses radiation to view internal organs not normally visible on X-ray images.

stereotactic radiosurgery A type of radiation therapy that can be used to zap tumors. Also known as gamma knife surgery.

Cancer Treatments

Cancer treatments vary according to the type of cancer and the stage in which it's detected. Surgery, in which the tumor and surrounding tissue are removed, is one common treatment. New **stereotactic radiosurgery**, also known as

Cancer Site	Screening Procedure	Age and Frequency of Test
Breast	Mammograms	The National Cancer Institute recommends that women in their forties and older have mammograms every 1 to 2 years. Women who are at higher-than-average risk of breast cancer should talk with their health care provider about whether to have mammograms before age 40 and how often to have them.
Cervix	Pap test (Pap smear)	Women should begin having Pap tests 3 years after they begin having sexual intercourse or when they reach age 21 (whichever comes first). Most women should have a Pap test at least once every 3 years.
Colon and rectum	*Fecal occult blood test:* Sometimes cancer or polyps bleed. This test can detect tiny amounts of blood in the stool. *Sigmoidoscopy:* Checks the rectum and lower part of the colon for polyps. *Colonoscopy:* Checks the rectum and entire colon for polyps and cancer.	People aged 50 and older should be screened. People who have a higher-than-average risk of cancer of the colon or rectum should talk with their doctor about whether to have screening tests before age 50 and how often to have them.
Prostate	Prostate-specific antigen (PSA) test	Some groups encourage yearly screening for men over age 50, and some advise men who are at a higher risk for prostate cancer to begin screening at age 40 or 45. Others caution against routine screening. Currently, Medicare provides coverage for an annual PSA test for all men age 50 and older.

Sources: National Cancer Institute, National Institutes of Health, "What You Need to Know About Cancer Screening," www.cancer.gov; National Cancer Institute, "Fact Sheet, Prostate-Specific Antigen (PSA) Test," www.cancer.gov

---

radiotherapy Use of radiation to kill cancerous cells.

chemotherapy Use of drugs to kill cancerous cells.

gamma knife surgery, uses a targeted dose of gamma radiation to zap tumors with pinpoint accuracy without any blood loss or ever using a scalpel. **Radiotherapy** (the use of radiation) or **chemotherapy** (the use of drugs) to kill cancerous cells are also used. When cancer has spread throughout the body, it is necessary to use some form of chemotherapy.

Whether used alone or in combination, virtually all cancer treatments have side effects, including nausea, nutritional deficiencies, hair loss, and general fatigue. The more aggressive the cancer, the more likely that there will be side effects from powerful drugs and invasive procedures. In the process of killing malignant cells, some healthy cells are also destroyed, and long-term damage to the cardiovascular system, kidneys, liver, and other body systems can be significant.

New ways of killing tumors and new chemotherapeutic drug cocktails are being developed regularly. Promising areas of research include *immunotherapy,* which enhances the body's own disease-fighting mechanisms, *cancer-fighting vaccines* to combat abnormal cells, *gene therapy* to increase the patient's immune response, and treatment with various substances that block cancer-causing events along the cancer pathway. Another promising avenue of potential treatment is *stem cell research,* although controversy around the use of stem cells continues to slow research. Because our knowledge of cancer treatment is constantly evolving, those who have been diagnosed with cancer and their loved ones should do their best to access information on the best cancer centers for specific types of cancer, new treatments being developed, and whether or not they are eligible for new clinical trials and experimental treatments that might be available for particularly aggressive cancers.

CVD and Cancer: What's Your Personal Risk?

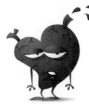

1 Evaluating Your CVD Risk

Complete each of the following questions and total your points in each section.

A: Your Family Risk for CVD

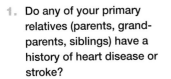

	Yes (1 point)	No (0 point)	Don't Know
1. Do any of your primary relatives (parents, grandparents, siblings) have a history of heart disease or stroke?	○	○	○
2. Do any of your primary relatives have diabetes?	○	○	○
3. Do any of your primary relatives have high blood pressure?	○	○	○
4. Do any of your primary relatives have a history of high cholesterol?	○	○	○
5. Would you say that your family consumed a high-fat diet (lots of red meat, whole dairy, butter/margarine) during your time spent at home?	○	○	○

Total points: _____

B: Your Lifestyle Risk for CVD

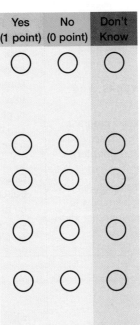

	Yes	No	Don't Know
1. Is your total cholesterol level higher than it should be?	○	○	○
2. Do you have high blood pressure?	○	○	○
3. Have you been diagnosed as pre-diabetic or diabetic?	○	○	○
4. Would you describe your life as being highly stressful?	○	○	○
5. Do you smoke?	○	○	○

Total points: _____

C: Your Additional Risks for CVD

1. How would you best describe your current weight?
   a. Lower than what it should be for my height and weight (0 points)
   b. About what it should be for my height and weight (0 points)
   c. Higher than it should be for my height and weight (1 point)
2. How would you describe the level of exercise that you get each day?
   a. Less than what I should be exercising each day (1 point)
   b. About what I should be exercising each day (0 points)
   c. More than what I should be exercising each day (0 points)
3. How would you describe your dietary behaviors?
   a. Eating only the recommended number of calories each day (0 points)
   b. Eating less than the recommended number of calories each day (0 points)
   c. Eating more than the recommended number of calories each day (1 point)
4. Which of the following best describes your typical dietary behavior?
   a. I eat from the major food groups, especially trying to get the recommended fruits and vegetables. (0 points)
   b. I eat too much red meat and consume too much saturated and *trans* fats from meat, dairy products, and processed foods each day. (1 point)
   c. Whenever possible, I try to substitute olive oil or canola oil for other forms of dietary fat. (0 points)

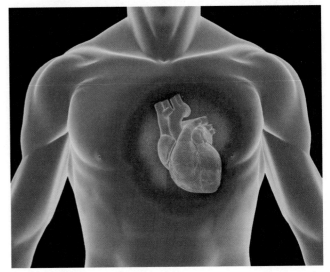

5. Which of the following (if any) describes you?
   a. I watch my sodium intake and try to reduce stress in my life. (0 points)
   b. I have a history of chlamydia infection. (1 point)
   c. I try to eat 5 to 10 mg of soluble fiber each day and try to substitute a non-animal source of protein (beans, nuts, soy) in my diet at least once each week. (0 points)

Total points: _____

Scoring Part 1

If you scored between 1 and 5 in any section, consider your risk. The higher the number, the greater your risk will be. If you answered Don't Know for any question, talk to your parents or other family members as soon as possible to find out if you have any unknown risks.

YOUR PLAN FOR CHANGE

The preceding **Assessyourself** activity evaluated your risk of heart disease. Based on your results and the advice of your physician, you may need to take steps to reduce your risk of CVD.

Today, you can:

○ Get up and move! Take a walk in the evening, use the stairs instead of the escalator, or ride your bike to class. Start thinking of ways you can incorporate more physical activity into your daily routine.

○ Begin improving your dietary habits by reading labels and making healthier choices with low-sodium foods, low-fat foods, and nutrient-dense fruits and vegetables. Replace the meat and processed foods you might normally eat with a serving of fresh fruit or bean/legume-based protein and green leafy vegetables. Eat more monounsaturated fat, foods with lower cholesterol counts, and watch your total calorie consumption.

Within the next 2 weeks, you can:

○ Begin a regular exercise program, even if you start slowly. Set small goals and try to meet them. (See **Chapter 11** for ideas.)

○ Practice a new stress management technique. For example, learn how to meditate. (See **Chapter 3** for other ideas for managing stress.)

○ Get enough rest. Make sure you get at least 8 hours of sleep per night.

By the end of the semester, you can:

○ Find out your hereditary risk for CVD. Call your parents and find out if your grandparents or aunts or uncles developed CVD. Get your blood pressure checked. Ask family members if they are on medications for their heart or blood pressure. Ask what their latest cholesterol LDL/HDL levels. Do you have a family history of diabetes?

○ Get a full lipid panel for yourself. Once you know your levels, you'll have a better sense of what risk factors to focus on as you work to reduce your levels. If your levels are high, talk to your doctor about how to reduce them.

2 Evaluating Your Cancer Risk

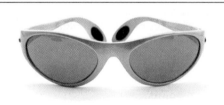

Read each question and circle the number corresponding to each Yes or No. Individual scores for specific questions should not be interpreted as a precise measure of relative risk, but the totals in each section give a general indication of risk.

A: Cancers in General

		Yes	No
1.	Do you smoke cigarettes on most days of the week?	2	1
2.	Do you consume a diet that is rich in fruits and vegetables?	1	2
3.	Are you obese, or do you lead a primarily sedentary lifestyle?	2	1
4.	Do you live in an area with high air pollution levels or work in a job where you are exposed to several chemicals on a regular basis?	2	1
5.	Are you careful about the amount of animal fat in your diet, substituting olive oil or canola oil for animal fat whenever possible?	1	2

		Yes	No
6.	Do you limit your overall consumption of alcohol?	1	2
7.	Do you eat foods rich in lycopenes (such as tomatoes) and antioxidants?	1	2
8.	Are you "body aware" and alert for changes in your body?	1	2
9.	Do you have a family history of ulcers or of colorectal, stomach, or other digestive system cancers?	2	1
10.	Do you avoid unnecessary exposure to radiation and microwave emissions?	1	2

Total points: _____

B: Skin Cancer

		Yes	No
1.	Do you spend a lot of time outdoors, either at work or at play?	2	1
2.	Do you use sunscreens with an SPF rating of 15 or more when you are in the sun?	1	2
3.	Do you use tanning beds or sun booths regularly to maintain a tan?	2	1
4.	Do you examine your skin once a month, checking any moles or other irregularities, particularly in hard-to-see areas such as your back, genitals, neck, and under your hair?	1	2
5.	Do you purchase and wear sunglasses that adequately filter out harmful sun rays?	1	2

Total points: _____

C: Breast Cancer

		Yes	No
1.	Do you check your breasts at least monthly using breast self-exam procedures?	1	2
2.	Do you look at your breasts in the mirror regularly, checking for any irregular indentations/lumps, discharge from the nipples, or other noticeable changes?	1	2
3.	Has your mother, sister, or daughter been diagnosed with breast cancer?	2	1
4.	Have you ever been pregnant?	1	2
5.	Have you had a history of lumps or cysts in your breasts or underarm?	2	1

Total points: _____

D: Cancers of the Reproductive System

Men

		Yes	No
1.	Do you examine your penis regularly for unusual bumps or growths?	1	2
2.	Do you perform regular testicular self-examinations?	1	2
3.	Do you have a family history of prostate or testicular cancer?	2	1
4.	Do you practice safe sex and wear condoms during every sexual encounter?	1	2
5.	Do you avoid exposure to harmful environmental hazards such as mercury, coal tars, benzene, chromate, and vinyl chloride?	1	2

Total points: _____

Women

		Yes	No
1.	Do you have regularly scheduled Pap tests?	1	2
2.	Have you been infected with HPV, Epstein-Barr virus, or other viruses believed to increase cancer risk?	2	1
3.	Has your mother, sister, or daughter been diagnosed with breast, cervical, endometrial, or ovarian cancer (particularly at a young age)?	2	1
4.	Do you practice safer sex and use condoms with every sexual encounter?	1	2
5.	Are you obese, taking estrogen, or consuming a diet that is very high in saturated fats?	2	1

Total points: _____

Scoring Part 2

Look carefully at each question for which you received a 2. Are there any areas in which you received mostly 2s? Did you receive total points of 11 or higher in A? Did you receive total points of 6 or higher in B through D? If so, you have at least one identifiable risk. The higher the score is, the more risks you may have.

YOUR PLAN FOR CHANGE

The preceding **Assess yourself** activity identified certain factors and behaviors that can contribute to increased cancer risks. If you engage in potentially risky behaviors, consider steps you can take to change these risks and improve your future health.

Today, you can:

○ Perform a breast or testicular self-exam (see pages 375 and 379, respectively, for instructions) and commit to doing one every month.

○ Take advantage of the healthy, low-calorie, low-fat, low-sodium items on the salad bar for lunch or dinner, and load up on greens, or prepare or order veggies such as steamed broccoli or sautéed spinach. Keep salad dressings, bacon, and ham to minimums.

Within the next 2 weeks, you can:

○ Buy a bottle of sunscreen (with SPF 15 or higher) and begin applying it as part of your daily routine. (Be sure to check the expiration date!)

○ Find out your family health history. Talk to your parents, grandparents, or an aunt or uncle to find out if family members have developed cancer. This will help you assess your own genetic risk.

By the end of the semester, you can:

○ Work toward achieving a healthy weight. If you aren't already engaged in a regular exercise program, begin one now. Maintaining a healthy body weight and exercising regularly will lower your risk for cancer.

○ Stop smoking, avoid secondhand smoke, and limit your alcohol intake.

MasteringHealth™

Build your knowledge—and health!—in the Study Area of MasteringHealth with a variety of study tools.

Summary

✳ The cardiovascular system consists of the heart and a network of vessels that supplies the body with nutrients and oxygen. Cardiovascular diseases (CVD) include atherosclerosis, peripheral artery disease (PAD), coronary heart disease (CHD), angina pectoris, arrhythmias, congestive heart failure (CHF), stroke, and hypertension.

✳ *Cardiometabolic risks* refer to combined factors that increase a person's chances of CVD and diabetes. *Metabolic syndrome* is a term for when a person possesses three or more cardiometabolic risk factors.

✳ Many risk factors for CVD can be controlled, such as tobacco use, high blood triglyceride or cholesterol levels, high sodium intake, and hypertension, inactivity, obesity, diabetes, and stress. Some risk factors, such as age, gender, race, and heredity, cannot be controlled. Other factors being studied include inflammation and homocysteine levels.

✳ Methods for treating heart blockages include coronary bypass surgery, angioplasty, and the use of stents. Drugs can reduce high blood pressure and treat other symptoms.

✳ Cancer is a group of diseases characterized by uncontrolled growth and spread of abnormal cells. These cells may create tumors. Malignant (cancerous) tumors can spread to other parts of the body through metastasis.

✳ Lifestyle factors for cancer risk include tobacco use, poor nutrition, inactivity, obesity, and possibly stress. Biological factors include genes, race, age, and gender. Carcinogens in the environment and infectious diseases may also lead to cancer.

✳ Each cancer has unique risks, causes, prevention strategies, and treatments. Being informed about your risks and taking action is a key to prevention.

✳ Early diagnosis improves cancer survival rate. New types of cancer treatments include combinations of radiotherapy, chemotherapy, and immunotherapy.

Pop Quiz

1. Atherosclerosis is characterized by:
   a. angina.
   b. heart attack.
   c. high blood pressure.
   d. plaque formation.

2. Which of the following is *not* correct?
   a. Lung cancer is the leading cause of cancer death in adults.
   b. CVD and CHD are the same thing.
   c. Women are more likely to die after having a first heart attack than are men.
   d. Some viruses can cause cancer.

3. Severe chest pain due to reduced oxygen flow to the heart is called
   a. angina pectoris.
   b. arrhythmias.
   c. peripheral artery disease.
   d. congestive heart failure.

4. A stroke results when
   a. a heart stops beating.
   b. the blood vessels of the legs are narrowed.
   c. blood supply to the brain has been blocked or severely restricted.
   d. the blood pressure rises.

5. The "bad" type of cholesterol found in the bloodstream is known as
   a. high-density lipoprotein.
   b. low-density lipoprotein.
   c. total cholesterol.
   d. triglyceride.

6. Which of the following is *not* a major cause of cancer?
   a. Diets high in animal proteins
   b. Environment and genetics
   c. Obesity
   d. High-carbohydrate foods

7. Suspected cancer-causing genes are
   a. epigenes.
   b. oncogenes.
   c. primogenes.
   d. metastogenes.

8. The greatest number of cancer deaths for both sexes is caused by
   a. colorectal cancer.
   b. leukemia.
   c. lung cancer.
   d. skin cancer.

9. The fecal occult blood test is the most basic screening test used for
   a. lung cancer.
   b. prostate cancer.
   c. cervical cancer.
   d. colorectal cancer.

10. The more serious, life-threatening type of skin cancer is
    a. basal cell carcinoma.
    b. squamous cell carcinoma.
    c. malignant melanoma.
    d. non-Hodgkin lymphoma.

Answers to these questions can be found on page A-1.

Think about It!

1. List the different types of CVD. Compare and contrast their symptoms, risk factors, prevention, and treatment.

2. Discuss the role that exercise, stress management, dietary

changes, medical checkups, and other factors can play in reducing risk for CVD. What role may chronic infections and inflammation play in CVD?

3. Describe some of the diagnostic and treatment alternatives for CVD. If you had a heart attack today, which treatment would you prefer?

4. List the likely causes of cancer. Do any of them put you personally at greater risk? What can you do to reduce your risk? What risk factors do you share with family members? With friends?

5. What can you do to reduce your risk of developing cancer or increase your chances of surviving it?

6. What are the pluses and minuses of breast and testicular self-exams?

Accessing Your Health on the Internet

The following websites explore further topics and issues related to personal health. For links to the websites below, visit the Study Area in MasteringHealth.

1. *American Heart Association.* Home page for the leading private organization dedicated to heart health. www.heart.org

2. *National Heart, Lung, and Blood Institute.* A valuable resource for information on all aspects of cardiovascular health and wellness. www.nhlbi.nih.gov

3. *American Cancer Society.* Provides information, statistics, and resources regarding cancer. www.cancer.org

4. *National Cancer Institute.* Valuable information on clinical trials and a comprehensive database of cancer treatment information. www.cancer.gov

5. *Oncolink.* A site that offers information on cancer support services, cancer causes, screening, and prevention. www.oncolink.org

6. *CancerCare.* Nonprofit source for information and support for cancer patients, survivors and their families. www.cancercare.org

Minimizing Your Risk for Diabetes

LEARNING OUTCOMES

* Differentiate among types of diabetes and identify common risk factors.

* Describe the main tests for, symptoms of, and complications associated with diabetes.

* Explain how diabetes can be prevented and treated.

390 Do college students really need to be concerned about diabetes?

392 What unique challenges do people with diabetes face?

394 People with diabetes can't eat sweets, right?

394 Do people with diabetes have to give themselves injections?

Like many Americans, Nora is overweight. She used to figure it was no big deal; she'd put herself on a strict diet and exercise program as soon as she graduated and started to live "a normal life." But last week her mom called and told Nora that she'd just found out that she has type 2 diabetes. Her voice sounded shaky as she told Nora about her own mother's death from kidney failure—a complication of diabetes—at age 52, a few months before Nora was born. Later, Nora searched online for information about her risk for diabetes. Her Hispanic ethnicity, family history, high stress level and lack of sleep, excessive weight, and sedentary lifestyle made her a prime candidate.

The next morning, Nora stopped off at the campus health center and made an appointment for a diabetes screening. She was instructed to fast the night before and was scheduled for an appointment first thing in the morning. At her visit, the nurse practitioner took a blood sample. A few days later, she called to tell Nora that she needed to make changes to her diet and lifestyle to reduce her risk for developing type 2 diabetes like her mom.

The Centers for Disease Control and Prevention (CDC) estimates that 25.8 million people—8.3 percent of the U.S.

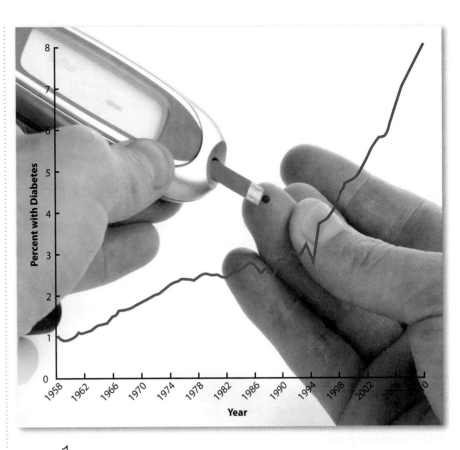

FIGURE 1 Percentage of U.S. Population with Diagnosed Diabetes, 1958–2010

Source: Data from the Centers for Disease Control and Prevention, "Increasing Prevalence of Diagnosed Diabetes—United States and Puerto Rico, 1995–2010," 2012, www.cdc.gov

---

population—have diabetes.[1] Up from less than 1 percent in 1958, diabetes is the fastest-growing chronic disease in American history (Figure 1). Diabetes is the seventh-leading killer in America today—responsible for nearly 225,000 deaths annually.[2] Diabetes rates increase as we age, and they aren't as high for college-age adults. The prevalence among Americans aged 20 to 44 is 3.7 percent, but rates are increasing across all age groups. Diabetes also seems to be increasing more dramatically among younger adults than among older Americans; over 215,000 people under the age of 20 have diabetes.[3] Currently, the direct and indirect costs of treating diabetes in the United States total $245 billion.[4] For an explanation of the personal financial toll that comes along with the body damage of diabetes, read the **Money & Health** box on the following page.

What Is Diabetes?

Diabetes mellitus is actually a group of diseases, each with its own mechanism, but all characterized by a persistently high level of sugar—technically, glucose—in the blood. A characteristic sign is the production of an unusually high volume of glucose-laden urine, a fact reflected in its name: *Diabetes* is derived from a Greek word meaning "to flow through," and *mellitus* is Latin for "sweet." The high blood glucose levels—or **hyperglycemia**—seen in diabetes can lead to a variety of serious health problems and even premature death. Before we describe what goes wrong to cause the different types of diabetes, let's look at how the body regulates blood glucose in a healthy person.

In Healthy People, Glucose Is Taken Up Efficiently by Body Cells

When you eat, carbohydrates are broken down into a monosaccharide called *glucose*—one of the main sources of energy for living organisms. Once the digestive system releases it into the bloodstream, glucose

diabetes mellitus A group of diseases characterized by elevated blood glucose levels.

hyperglycemia Elevated blood glucose level.

Money&Health

DIABETES: AT WHAT COST?

One in every 5 health care dollars is being spent on diabetes care today. Fees for doctor visits, testing supplies, laboratory results, and other necessities are often only partially covered, even for those who have insurance. If you are underinsured or uninsured, the *diabetes drain* on your bank account could be major.

To give you an idea of what it might cost someone who is diagnosed with type 2 diabetes and who doesn't have insurance, consider these very conservative monthly estimates:

Diabetic Health Care Need	Estimated Monthly Cost
Doctor visit for monitoring and testing	$200
Lab tests: A1C Glucose tolerance	$35–$75
Glucose meter test strips	$100
Lancets and lancing devices, alcohol wipes	$5–$10
Oral medications (metformin)	$13–$15. (Less for some generics; more for newer medications)

becomes available to all body cells—any of which use glucose to fuel metabolism, movement, and other activities. When there is more glucose available than required to meet your body's immediate needs, the excess is stored as glycogen in the liver and muscles for later use.

Glucose can't simply cross cell membranes on its own. Instead, cells have structures that transport it across in response to a signal generated by the **pancreas,** an organ located just beneath the stomach. Whenever a surge of glucose enters the bloodstream, the pancreas secretes a hormone called **insulin**, which stimulates cells to take up glucose from the bloodstream and use it for immediate energy. Conversion of glucose to glycogen for storage in the liver and muscles is also assisted by insulin. These actions lower the blood level of

glucose, and in response, the pancreas stops secreting insulin until the next influx of glucose arrives.

Type 1 Diabetes Is an Immune Disorder

The more serious and less prevalent form of diabetes, called **type 1 diabetes** (or insulin-dependent diabetes), is an autoimmune disease—the individual's immune system attacks and destroys normal body cells, in this case the insulin-making cells in the pancreas. Destruction of these cells causes a dramatic reduction, or total cessation, of insulin production. Without insulin, cells cannot take up glucose, and blood glucose levels become permanently elevated.

This form of diabetes used to be called *juvenile*

diabetes because it most often appears during childhood or adolescence; however, it can begin at any age. European

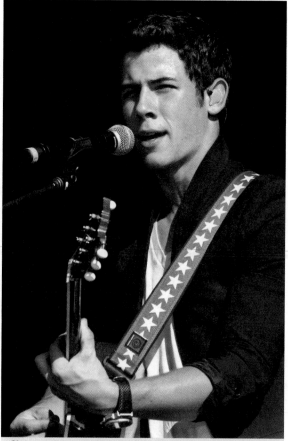

Singer and pop star Nick Jonas is one of the 5 to 10 percent of diabetics diagnosed with type 1.

pancreas Organ that secretes digestive enzymes into the small intestine and hormones, including insulin, into the bloodstream.

insulin Hormone secreted by the pancreas and required by body cells for the uptake and storage of glucose.

type 1 diabetes Form of diabetes mellitus in which the pancreas is not able to make insulin and therefore blood glucose cannot enter the cells to be used for energy.

In 2009, when a new strain of the "Spanish" flu that killed over 50 million people in 1918 became a modern day global threat known as *"swine flu"* or *"H1N1,"* people reacted with great fear. This new version—*"novel H1N1"*—was notably different from past strains in that it mainly killed young, otherwise healthy adults. Schools closed, churches cancelled services, and people feared the slightest cough or sneeze from others. Although exact numbers vary, there may have been over 575,000 *novel H1N1* deaths globally.[1]

After many "germ attacks" played out in the media, people wore masks in public, avoided handshakes, and did more hand-washing than ever before. Grocery stores gave out wipes to counteract reports of a myriad of pathogens found on shopping cart handles, and elementary teachers began wiping the hands of every child as the child came in from recess. Was all that worry warranted? What can we do to protect ourselves from real and imagined threats?

The truth is, **pathogens**—disease-causing agents—are everywhere. We inhale them, swallow them, rub them in our eyes, and are constantly in a hidden, high-stakes battle with them. Although many pathogens have existed as long as there has been life on the planet, new varieties seem to emerge daily. Historically, infectious diseases have wiped out whole groups of people through **epidemics** such as the Black Death, or bubonic plague, which killed up to one-third of the population of Europe in the 1300s. **Pandemics,** or global epidemics, continue to cause premature death throughout the world.

Despite constant bombardment by pathogens, our immune systems are usually adept at protecting us. Millions of microorganisms live in and on our bodies all the time, usually in a symbiotic, peaceful coexistence, and exposure to invading microorganisms helps us build resistance to various pathogens. Generally harmless to someone in good health, these organisms can cause serious health problems in those with weakened immune systems.

When pathogens gain entry into the body, they are apt to produce an infection or illness. The more easily these pathogens can gain a foothold in the body and sustain themselves, the more **virulent,** or aggressive, they may be in causing disease. By keeping your immune system strong, you increase your ability to resist and fight off even the most virulent pathogen.

The Process of Infection

Most diseases are *multifactorial:* They are caused by the interaction of several factors inside and outside the person. For a disease to occur, the person, or *host,* must be *susceptible,* which means that the immune system must be in a weakened condition (**immunocompromised**); an *agent* capable of *transmitting* a disease must be present; and the *environment* must be *hospitable* to the pathogen in terms of temperature, light, moisture, and other requirements. Although all pathogens pose a

threat if they gain entry and begin to grow in your body, the chances that they will do harm are actually quite small.

Routes of Transmission

Pathogens may enter the body by *direct contact* between infected persons, or by *indirect contact,* like touching an object an infected person has touched. **Table 13.1** lists common routes of transmission. You may also **autoinoculate** yourself, or transmit a pathogen from one part of your body to another—for example, by touching a herpes sore on your lip and then touching your eye.

Your best friend may be the source of *animalborne (zoonotic) infections.* Dogs, cats, livestock, and wild animals can spread numerous diseases through bites and feces or by carrying infected insects into living areas. Although *interspecies transmission* of diseases—transmission between humans and animals—is rare, it does occur.

pathogen A disease-causing agent.

epidemic Disease outbreak that affects many people in a community or region at the same time.

pandemic Global epidemic of a disease.

virulent Strong enough to overcome host resistance and cause disease.

immunocompromised Having an immune system that is impaired.

autoinoculate Transmit a pathogen from one part of your body to another part.

Risk Factors You Can Control

Surrounded by pathogens, how can you be sure you don't get sick? Too much stress, inadequate nutrition, a low fitness level, lack of sleep, misuse or abuse of drugs, poor personal hygiene, and high-risk behavior significantly

TABLE 13.1	Routes of Disease Transmission
Mode of Transmission	Aspects of Transmission
Contact	Either *direct* (e.g., skin or sexual contact) or *indirect* (e.g., infected blood or body fluid)
Foodborne or waterborne	Eating or coming in contact with contaminated food or water, or products passed through them
Airborne	Inhalation; droplet-spread as through sneezing, coughing, or talking
Vectorborne	Vector-transmitted via secretions, biting, egg laying, as done by mosquitoes, ticks, snails, or birds
Perinatal	Similar to contact infection; happens in the uterus or as the baby passes through the birth canal, or through breast-feeding

Reduce Your Risk of Infectious Disease

❭ **Limit exposure to pathogens.** Don't drag yourself to classes or work and infect others when you are seriously ill. Also, don't share utensils or drinking glasses, and keep your toothbrush away from those of others. Keep hands away from your mouth, nose, and eyes. Use disposable tissues rather than reusable handkerchiefs.

❭ **Exercise regularly.** Regular exercise raises core body temperature and kills pathogens, and sweat and oil make the skin a hostile environment for many bacteria.

❭ **Get enough sleep.** Sleep allows the body time to refresh itself, produce necessary cells, and reduce inflammation. Even a single night without sleep can increase inflammatory processes and delay wound healing.

❭ **Stress less.** Rest and relaxation, stress management practices, laughter, and calming music have all been shown to promote healthy cellular activity and bolster immune functioning.

❭ **Optimize eating.** Enjoy a healthy diet, including adequate amounts of water, fruits and vegetables, protein, and complex carbohydrates. Eat more omega-3 fatty acids to reduce inflammation, and restrict saturated fats.

drug resistance Occurs when microbes, such as bacteria, viruses or other pathogens grow and proliferate in the presence of chemicals that would normally kill them or slow their growth.

increase the risk for many diseases. In addition, college students are at higher risk because of the close living conditions; all these factors create higher risk for exposure to pathogens. The **Skills for Behavior Change** box lists some actions you can take to minimize risk of infection.

Hard to Control Risk Factors

Unfortunately, some risk factors for certain diseases are hard or impossible to control. The following are the most common:

● **Heredity.** Perhaps the single greatest factor influencing disease risk is genetics. It is often unclear whether hereditary diseases are due to inherited genetic traits or to inherited insufficiencies in the immune system. Some believe that we may inherit the quality of our immune system, thus some people are naturally more resistant to disease and infection.

● **Age.** Thinning of the skin, reduced sweating, and other physical changes can make people over 65 more vulnerable to disease. The very young also tend to be particularly vulnerable to infectious diseases.

● **Environmental conditions.** A growing body of research points to climate change as a major contributor to infectious diseases. As temperatures rise, insect populations may rise, potentially increasing cases of malaria. Dwindling water supplies are more likely to be contaminated since animals congregate more closely to them, spreading diseases among themselves.[2] In addition, natural disasters such as earthquakes and floods, as well as long-term exposure to toxic chemicals, can significantly contribute to increasing numbers of infectious diseases.[3]

● **Organism virulence and resistance.** Some organisms are particularly virulent, whereas other organisms have mutated and become resistant to the body's defenses and to medical treatments. **Drug resistance** occurs when pathogens grow and proliferate in the presences of chemicals that would normally slow growth or kill them. Carbapenem-resistant Enterobacteriaceae (CRE), for example, commonly spreads in hospital environments, develops from bacteria normally found in the gastrointestinal tract, and is resistant to virtually all current antibiotics. It is among the deadliest of the bacteria, with fatality rates as high as 50 percent in patients who get bloodstream infections.[4] See the **Be Healthy, Be Green** box on page 400 for more on drug resistance and superbugs.

Video Tutor: Chain of Infection

Your Body's Defenses against Infection

To gain entry into your body, pathogens must overcome barriers that prevent them from entering your body, mechanisms that weaken organisms, and substances that counteract the threat that these organisms pose. **Figure 13.1** on the following page summarizes some of the body's defenses against invasion and disease.

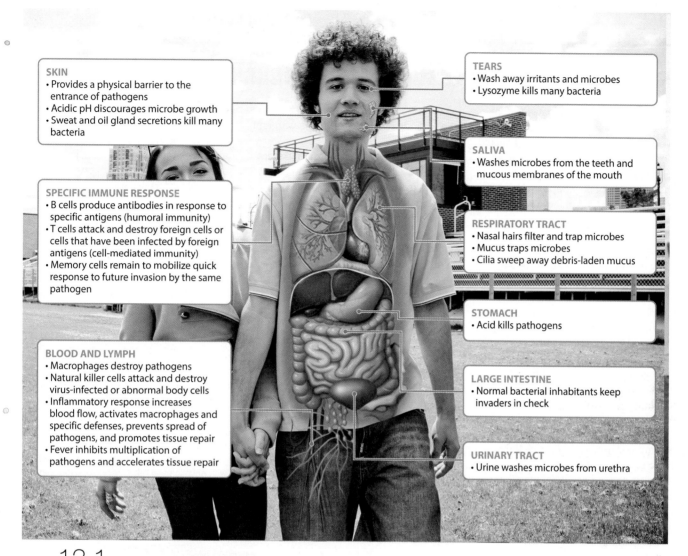

SKIN
- Provides a physical barrier to the entrance of pathogens
- Acidic pH discourages microbe growth
- Sweat and oil gland secretions kill many bacteria

SPECIFIC IMMUNE RESPONSE
- B cells produce antibodies in response to specific antigens (humoral immunity)
- T cells attack and destroy foreign cells or cells that have been infected by foreign antigens (cell-mediated immunity)
- Memory cells remain to mobilize quick response to future invasion by the same pathogen

BLOOD AND LYMPH
- Macrophages destroy pathogens
- Natural killer cells attack and destroy virus-infected or abnormal body cells
- Inflammatory response increases blood flow, activates macrophages and specific defenses, prevents spread of pathogens, and promotes tissue repair
- Fever inhibits multiplication of pathogens and accelerates tissue repair

TEARS
- Wash away irritants and microbes
- Lysozyme kills many bacteria

SALIVA
- Washes microbes from the teeth and mucous membranes of the mouth

RESPIRATORY TRACT
- Nasal hairs filter and trap microbes
- Mucus traps microbes
- Cilia sweep away debris-laden mucus

STOMACH
- Acid kills pathogens

LARGE INTESTINE
- Normal bacterial inhabitants keep invaders in check

URINARY TRACT
- Urine washes microbes from urethra

FIGURE 13.1 **The Body's Defenses against Disease-Causing Pathogens**
In addition to the defenses listed, many of the body's defensive secretions and fluids, such as earwax, tears, mucus, sweat, and blood, contain enzymes and other proteins that can kill some invading pathogens or prevent or slow their reproduction.

Physical and Chemical Defenses

Our most critical early defense system is the skin. Layered to provide an intricate web of barriers, the skin allows few pathogens to enter. Enzymes in body secretions such as sweat provide additional protection, destroying microorganisms on skin surfaces by producing inhospitable pH levels. Only through cracks or breaks in the skin can pathogens gain easy access to the body.

The internal linings, structures, and secretions of the body provide another layer of protection. Mucous membranes in the respiratory tract, for example, trap and engulf invading organisms. Cilia, hairlike projections in the lungs and respiratory tract, sweep invaders toward body openings, where they are expelled. Nose hairs trap airborne invaders with a sticky film. Tears, earwax, and other secretions contain enzymes that destroy or neutralize pathogens.

How the Immune System Works

Immunity is a condition of being able to resist a particular disease by counteracting the substance that produces the disease. Any substance capable of triggering an immune response—a virus, a bacterium, a fungus, a parasite, a toxin, or a tissue or cell from another organism—is called an **antigen.** The immune system has elaborate mechanisms for protecting you from invading microbes.

As soon as an antigen breaches the body's initial defenses, the body responds by forming **antibodies** specific to that antigen, much as a key is matched to a lock. The body analyzes the antigen, verifies that the antigen is not part of the body itself, and then produces a specific antibody to destroy or weaken the antigen.

antigen Substance capable of triggering an immune response.

antibodies Substances produced by the body that are individually matched to specific antigens.

ANTIBIOTIC RESISTANCE: BUGS VERSUS DRUGS

Bacteria and other microorganisms that cause infections and diseases evolve and develop ways to survive drugs that should kill or weaken them. This means that some microorganisms are becoming "super-bugs" that cannot be stopped with existing medications.

WHY IS ANTIBIOTIC RESISTANCE ON THE RISE?

✳ **Improper use of antibiotics and resulting growth of superbugs.** Don't take other people's unused antibiotics. They are prescribed for certain bacteria and may not even work for the infection you have. When used improperly, antibiotics kill only the weak bacteria and leave the strongest versions to thrive and replicate. Eventually, an entire colony of resistant bugs grows and passes on its resistance traits to new generations of bacteria.

If patients begin an antibiotic regimen and stop taking the drug before they finish the prescription or when they start to feel better, the hardiest bacteria are the survivors, and they are more resistant to drug treatments. Doctors also over-prescribe antibiotics: The Centers for Disease Control and Prevention (CDC) estimates that one-third of the 150 million prescriptions written each year are unnecessary, resulting in bacterial strains that are tougher than the drugs used to fight them.

✳ **Overuse of antibiotics in food production.** About 70 percent of antibiotic production today is used to treat sick animals or fish living in crowded feedlots or fish farms and to encourage growth in livestock, fish, and poultry. Farmed fish may be given antibiotics to fight off disease in controlled water areas. Although research in this area is only in its infancy, many believe that ingesting meats, animal products, and fish full of antibiotics may contribute to antibiotic resistance in humans. In addition, water runoff and sewage from feedlots can contaminate the water in rivers and streams with antibiotics.

✳ **Misuse and overuse of antibacterial soaps and other cleaning products.** Preying on the public's fear of germs and disease, the cleaning industry adds antibacterial ingredients to many soaps and household products. Just how much these products contribute to overall resistance is difficult to assess; as with antibiotics, the germs these products do not kill may become stronger than before.

WHAT CAN YOU DO?

✳ **Be responsible with medications.** Use antimicrobial drugs only for bacterial, not viral, infections. Take medications as prescribed and finish the full course. Consult with your health care provider if you feel it is necessary to stop your medication.

Don't dump unused drugs down the toilet or sink. If you don't know where to take them, talk to your local pharmacist or waste disposal company.

✳ **Use regular soap—not antibacterial soap—when washing your hands.** Research suggests that antibacterial agents contained in soaps actually may kill normal bacteria, thus creating an environment for resistant, mutated bacteria that are impervious to antibacterial cleaners and antibiotics.

✳ **Avoid food treated with antibiotics.** Know where your food comes from. Buy organic meat and poultry, particularly those that say that they have not been fed antibiotics or hormones. Look for farmed fish grown in U.S. coastal waters, where there is less likelihood of questionable fish feeding practice and less chance of contaminated water and antibiotics or growth hormones.

Sources: Association for Professionals in Infection Control and Epidemiology, "Responsible Use of Antibiotics" 2013, www.apic.org; Association for Professionals in Infection Control and Epidemiology, "Antibiotics, Preserving Them for the Future," 2012, www.apic.org; Centers for Disease Control and Prevention, National Center for Emerging and Zoonotic Infectious Diseases, Division of Healthcare Quality Promotion, "Diseases/Pathogens Associated with Antimicrobial Resistance," Updated January 2013, www.cdc.gov; Centers for Disease Control and Prevention, National Center for Immunization and Respiratory Diseases, Division of Bacterial Diseases, "Antibiotic Resistance Questions & Answers," Updated June 2009, www.cdc.gov

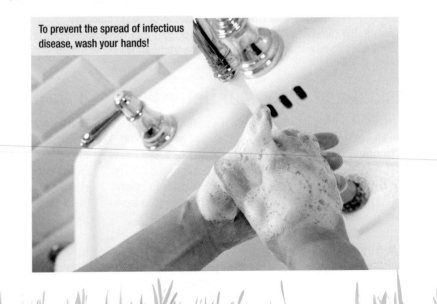

To prevent the spread of infectious disease, wash your hands!

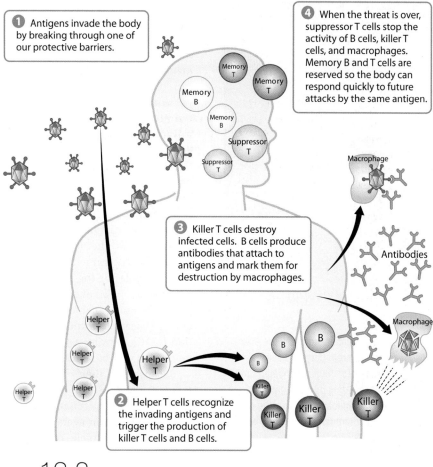

1 Antigens invade the body by breaking through one of our protective barriers.

2 Helper T cells recognize the invading antigens and trigger the production of killer T cells and B cells.

3 Killer T cells destroy infected cells. B cells produce antibodies that attach to antigens and mark them for destruction by macrophages.

4 When the threat is over, suppressor T cells stop the activity of B cells, killer T cells, and macrophages. Memory B and T cells are reserved so the body can respond quickly to future attacks by the same antigen.

FIGURE 13.2 **The Cell-Mediated Immune Response**

This process is part of a system called *humoral immune responses.* **Humoral immunity** is the body's major defense against many bacteria and the poisonous substances—**toxins**—they produce.

In **cell-mediated immunity,** specialized white blood cells called **lymphocytes** attack and destroy the foreign invader. Lymphocytes constitute the body's main defense against viruses, fungi, parasites, and some bacteria, and they are found in the blood, lymph nodes, bone marrow, and certain glands. Other key players in this immune response are **macrophages** (a type of phagocytic, or cell-eating, white blood cell).

Two forms of lymphocytes in particular, the *B lymphocytes* (B cells) and *T lymphocytes* (T cells), are involved in the immune response. *Helper T cells* are essential for activating B cells to produce antibodies. They also activate other T cells and macrophages. *Killer T cells* directly attack infected or malignant cells.

"Why Should I Care?"

An increasing number of chronic diseases are being linked to the inflammation that occurs when certain pathogens invade. Avoiding infections and their inflammatory side effects now has the added benefit that it may help you avoid certain chronic diseases later.

Suppressor T cells turn off or suppress the activity of B cells, killer T cells, and macrophages. After a successful attack on a pathogen, some attacker T and B cells are preserved as *memory T and B cells,* enabling the body to recognize and respond quickly to subsequent attacks by the same kind of organism. Once people have survived certain infectious diseases, they will likely not develop them again. **Figure 13.2** provides a summary of the cell-mediated immune response.

When the Immune System Misfires: Autoimmune Diseases Although immune response generally works in our favor, it sometimes targets its own tissue, builds up antibodies, and attempting to destroy that tissue. This is known as **autoimmune disease** (*auto* means "self"). Common autoimmune disorders include *rheumatoid arthritis, lupus, type 1 diabetes, celiac disease,* and *multiple sclerosis.*

Inflammatory Response, Pain, and Fever If an infection is localized, pus formation, redness, swelling, and irritation often occur. These symptoms are components of the body's inflammatory response and indicate that invading organisms are being fought systemically. The four cardinal signs of inflammation are *redness, swelling, pain, and heat.*

Pain is often one of the earliest signs that an injury or infection has occurred. Pathogens can kill or injure tissue at the site of infection, causing swelling that puts pressure on nerve endings in the area, causing pain. Although pain is unpleasant, it plays a valuable role in the body's response to injury or invasion by causing a person to avoid activity that may aggravate the injury and cause additional damage.

In addition to *inflammation,* another frequent indicator of infection is *fever,* or a body temperature above the average norm of 98.6°F. Caused by toxins secreted by pathogens that interfere with the

humoral immunity Aspect of immunity that is mediated by antibodies secreted by white blood cells.

toxins Poisonous substances produced by certain microorganisms that cause various diseases.

cell-mediated immunity Aspect of immunity that is mediated by specialized white blood cells that attack pathogens and antigens directly.

lymphocyte A type of white blood cell involved in the immune response.

macrophage A type of white blood cell that ingests foreign material.

autoimmune disease Disease caused by an overactive immune response against the body's own cells.

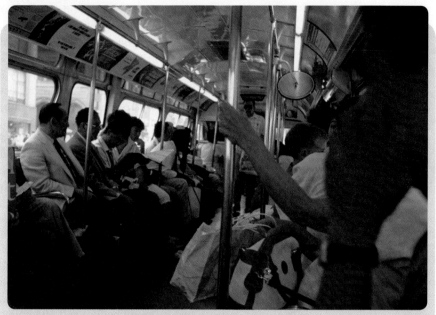

Why are vaccinations important?

Vaccinations can protect an individual from certain infectious diseases, and they are also important in controlling the prevalence of diseases in society at large. Certain diseases such as polio and diphtheria have become very rare as a result of immunizations, but until a disease is completely eradicated, it is important to keep vaccinating people against it. Otherwise, there is nothing to stop the disease from making a comeback and causing an epidemic. People who spend time in crowded places, such as commuters or frequent air travelers, and people at particular risk, such as hospital workers or college students who often live in close quarters, should be especially certain to stay up-to-date on their vaccinations.

control of body temperature, a fever also stimulates the body to produce more white blood cells. A mild fever is protective; raising body temperature by one or two degrees provides an environment that destroys some disease-causing organisms. As fevers increase beyond 101°F, risks to the patient outweigh any fever benefits and medical treatment should be obtained.

Vaccines Bolster Immunity

Vaccination is based on the principle that once people have been exposed to a specific pathogen, subsequent attacks will activate their memory T and B cells, thus giving them immunity.

A vaccine consists of killed or weakened versions of a disease-causing microorganism or an antigen that is similar to but less dangerous than the disease antigen. It is administered to stimulate the person's immune system to produce antibodies against future attacks—without actually causing the

vaccination Inoculation with killed or weakened pathogens or similar, less dangerous antigens, in order to prevent or lessen the effects of some disease.

disease (or by causing a very minor case of it). Vaccines typically are given orally or by injection, and this form of immunity is termed *artificially acquired active immunity*. Concern about the safety of vaccines has caused an increase in the number of parents who refuse to vaccinate their children (see the **Health Headlines** box on page 405).

Specific vaccination schedules have been established for various population groups. See Table 13.2 for recommended vaccines for teens and college students ages 19 to 26. Figure 13.3 on the following page shows the recommended vaccination schedule for the general adult population. Childhood vaccine schedules are available at the Centers for Disease Control and Prevention (CDC) website, as are requirements that vary by state.

Because of their close living quarters, high stress levels, and poor sleep habits, college students face a higher-than-average risk of infection from largely preventable diseases. Vaccines that should be a high priority among 20-somethings include *tetanus-diphtheria-pertussis vaccine (Tdap), meningococcal conjugate vaccine (MCV4), human papillomavirus (HPV)*, and the *influenza vaccine.*[5]

<table>
<tr><td>TABLE
13.2</td><td>**Recommended Vaccinations for Teens and College Students**</td></tr>
</table>

- Tetanus, diphtheria, pertussis vaccine (Td/Tdap)
- Meningococcal vaccine*
- HPV vaccine series
- Hepatitis B vaccine series
- Polio vaccine series
- Measles-mumps-rubella (MMR) vaccine series
- Varicella (chickenpox) vaccine series
- Influenza vaccine
- Pneumococcal polysaccharide (PPV) vaccine
- Hepatitis A vaccine series**

*Booster at age 16.
**For high-risk groups
Source: Centers for Disease Control and Prevention, "Recommendations and Guidelines: Vaccines Needed by Teens and College Students," May 2013, www.cdc.gov

Vaccine	Age group					
	19–21 years	22–26 years	27–49 years	50–59 years	60–64 years	≥65 years
Influenza*	1 dose annually					
Tetanus, diphtheria, pertussis (Td/Tdap)*	Substitute 1-time dose of Tdap for Td booster; then boost with Td every 10 yrs					
Varicella*	2 doses					
Human papillomavirus (HPV) Female*	3 doses					
Human papillomavirus (HPV) Male*	3 doses					
Zoster					1 dose	
Measles, mumps, rubella (MMR)*	1 or 2 doses					
Pneumococcal polysaccharide (PPSV23)	1 or 2 doses					1 dose
Pneumococcal 13-valent conjugate (PCV13)*	1 dose					
Meningococcal*	1 or more doses					
Hepatitis A*	2 doses					
Hepatitis B*	3 doses					

*Covered by the Vaccine Injury Compensation Program

For all persons in this category who meet the age requirements and who lack documentation of vaccination or have no evidence of previous infection; zoster vaccine recommended regardless of prior episode of zoster

Recommended if some other risk factor is present (e.g., on the basis of medical, occupational, lifestyle, or other indication)

No recommendation

FIGURE 13.3 Recommended Adult Immunization Schedule, by Vaccine and Age Group, 2013
Source: Centers for Disease Control and Prevention, "Recommended Adult Immunization Schedule—United States, 2012," *MMWR Weekly* 62, no. 1 (2013).
Note: Important explanations and additions to these recommendations should be checked by consulting the latest schedule at www.cdc.gov

Types of Pathogens and the Diseases They Cause

Pathogens fall into six categories: bacteria, viruses, fungi, protozoans, parasitic worms, and prions. Figure 13.4 (see page 404) shows several examples. Each has a particular route of transmission and characteristic elements that make it unique. In the following pages, we discuss each of these categories and give an overview of some diseases they cause that have a significant impact on public health.

Bacteria

Bacteria (singular: *bacterium*) are simple, single-celled organisms. There are three major types of bacteria, classified by shape: *cocci, bacilli,* and *spirilla.* Although there are several thousand known species of bacteria (and many more unknown), only just over 100 cause disease in humans. Often it is not the bacteria themselves that cause disease, but rather the toxins they produce.

Diseases caused by bacteria can be treated with **antibiotics**. However, today's arsenal of antibiotics is becoming less effective, as **antibiotic resistance** becomes more common—the percentages of resistant bacteria doubled between 2006 and 2008 and continue to increase.[6] "Superbugs" can result when successive generations of bacteria mutate to develop resistance to specific drugs. Refer back to the **Be Healthy, Be Green** box on page 400 for more about superbugs and antibiotic resistance.

bacteria (singular: *bacterium*) Simple, single-celled microscopic organisms; about 100 known species of bacteria cause disease in humans.

antibiotics Medicines used to kill microorganisms, such as bacteria.

antibiotic resistance The ability of bacteria or other microbes to withstand the effects of an antibiotic.

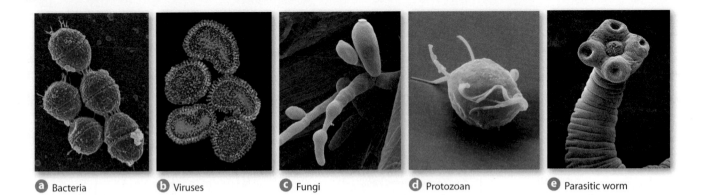

(a) Bacteria   (b) Viruses   (c) Fungi   (d) Protozoan   (e) Parasitic worm

FIGURE 13.4 Examples of Five Major Types of Pathogens
(a) Color-enhanced scanning electron micrograph (SEM) of *Streptococcus* bacteria, magnified 40,000×. (b) Colored transmission electron micrograph (TEM) of influenza (flu) viruses, magnified 32,000×. (c) Color SEM of *Candida albicans*, a yeast fungus, magnified 50,000×. (d) Color TEM of *Trichomonas vaginalis,* a protozoan, magnified 9,000×. (e) Color-enhanced SEM of a tapeworm, magnified 50×.

Staphylococcal Infections **Staphylococci** are present on the skin or in the nostrils of 20 to 30 percent of us at any given time, and usually cause no problems for otherwise healthy persons. The presence of bacteria on or in a person without infection is called **colonization.** A person can be colonized and then spread the infection to others, yet never develop the disease. For example, they can inadvertently touch their nose and spread those bacteria on a door handle, causing others who touch it to get sick. Likewise, when the pathogen is present and there is a cut or break in the skin, staphylococci may enter the system and cause an **infection.** If you have ever suffered from acne, boils, styes (infections of the eyelids), or infected wounds, you have probably had a "staph" infection. If you pick at pimples and don't wash your hands, you can transmit those same bacteria to your eyes or to other people.

One resistant form of staph, **methicillin-resistant Staphylococcus aureus (MRSA),** has come under intense international scrutiny as numerous cases have arisen around the world, especially in the United States.[7] Symptoms of MRSA infection often start with a rash or pimple-like skin irritation. Within hours, early symptoms may progress to redness, inflammation, pain, and deeper wounds. If untreated, MRSA may invade the blood, bones, joints, surgical wounds, heart valves, and lungs, and it can be fatal.[8]

Health care–associated or *health care–acquired MRSA (HA-MRSA)* arises in settings such as hospitals, nursing homes, and clinics, where invasive treatments, infectious pathogens, and weakened immune systems converge. While rates of HA-MRSA are on the decline, MRSA is on the rise in the home, workplace, and other communities. Known as *community-acquired MRSA,* this form is more difficult to isolate and prevent as there are so many possible ways of being infected.[9] Another type of MRSA appears to be spread among people who work closely with livestock in many regions of the world and is known as livestock-associated MRSA, or LA-MRSA.

Another form of resistant staph infection known as *linezolid-resistant S. aureus,* or LRSA, has emerged. Dubbed the "new MRSA," this resistant superbug has killed hundreds in Europe and is spreading rapidly in other countries. Because linezolid is one of the few treatments that still works in severe MRSA cases, many fear that the antibiotic "well" may be running dry.

Streptococcal Infections At least five types of the *Streptococcus* microorganism are known to cause bacterial infections. Group A streptococci (GAS) cause the most common diseases, such as streptococcal pharyngitis ("strep throat") and scarlet fever.[10] One particularly virulent group of GAS can lead to a rare but serious disease called *necrotizing fasciitis* ("flesh-eating strep").[11] Group B streptococci can cause illness in newborn babies, pregnant women, older adults, and adults with illnesses such as diabetes or liver disease. Since about 1 in 4 pregnant women have group B strep in their rectum or vagina, the CDC recommends testing for it in the last weeks of pregnancy. Expectant mothers who are group B positive can be treated with antibiotics to prevent problems in their newborn.[12]

The species *Streptococcus pneumoniae* is responsible for thousands of cases of bacterial meningitis and pneumonia each year and is the primary culprit in most ear infections. While antibiotic treatments are still effective, an increasing number of cases are becoming resistant.

staphylococci A group of round bacteria, usually found in clusters, that cause a variety of diseases in humans and other animals.

colonization The process of bacteria or some other infectious organisms establishing themselves in a host without causing infection.

infection The state of pathogens being established in or on a host and causing disease.

methicillin-resistant Staphylococcus aureus (MRSA) Highly resistant form of staph infection that is growing in international prevalence.

Streptococcus A round bacterium, usually found in chain formation.

See It! Videos
How can you protect yourself from a staph infection? Watch **Toxic Staph Outbreak** in MasteringHealth™

VACCINE BACKLASH: ARE THEY SAFE AND NECESSARY?

Immunizations are one of the greatest public health success stories of all time—so successful, in fact, that most people have never seen or heard of anyone having diseases like smallpox that once wiped out entire populations. Today, fear of the old "killer" diseases has waned and been replaced with distrust of the vaccines themselves, which some feel cause their own set of maladies.

In some communities, such as Ashland, Oregon, up to 25 percent of kindergartners' parents opt their children out of at least one vaccine. In other U.S. school districts and counties, these rates are even higher, and a general trend of avoiding vaccinations is growing. Undervaccination rates are particularly high in non-Hispanic, college-educated white families with incomes above $75,000 a year.

Some people object to mandatory vaccinations due to religious reasons, or because they consider them to be a government intrusion on individual rights. But the biggest single reason for anti-vaccination is a study published in 1998 in the journal *The Lancet*. The study claimed there was a link between measles, mumps, rubella (MMR) vaccines and development of autism. Ten years later *The Lancet* retracted the publication, saying the findings were false and that the research had not been not conducted in scientifically valid ways. It should be added that the lead author of the study was also fired from his research position and had his license to practice medicine revoked due to concerns that he had intentionally misled and misrepresented the truth.

Research is always ongoing, but the Centers for Disease Control and Prevention (CDC) in numerous studies has found no evidence that vaccines cause autism. Many large-scale European studies have also failed to find any link. Virtually all medical and public health organizations support vaccinations, pointing to stringent safety controls in the manufacturing and testing of vaccines, as well as ongoing safety monitoring, the long history

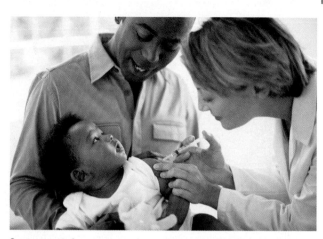

Some parents have expressed concern over the safety of vaccinations.

of vaccines in wiping out killer diseases across the globe, and the fact that risks from the diseases themselves are almost always much greater than those associated with a vaccine.

When large numbers of people avoid vaccinations, old killers are likely to reemerge. The reasons for vaccination far outweigh any arguments against them. Local rashes and reactions at injection sites, low-grade fever, discomfort, and even allergic reactions can occur. But the danger of major complications from getting vaccinations is extremely low, and generally pales in comparison to the effects of contracting the diseases that the vaccinations protect against.

Sources: Centers for Disease Control and Prevention, "Vaccine Safety," 2011, www.cdc; Centers for Disease Control and Prevention, "Concerns about Autism," 2011, www.cdc.gov; Centers for Disease Control and Prevention, "Vaccine Safety: Concerns about Autism," Modified January 2010, www.cdc.gov

Meningitis **Meningitis** is an infection and inflammation of the *meninges*—the membranes that surround the brain and spinal cord—of which bacterial meningitis is the most common form. Spread through contact with saliva, nasal discharge, feces, or respiratory and throat secretions, it is highly contagious. Fortunately, vaccines exist for *pneumococcal meningitis,* the most common form of bacterial meningitis, and *meningococcal meningitis,* a virulent form of bacterial meningitis prevalent on college campuses.[13] Students living in dormitories or high-density residences have a higher risk of contracting this disease than do those who live off campus or alone. The other vaccine-preventable form of bacterial meningitis is *Haemophilus influenzae* type b (Hib). Check your immunization table for information regarding who should get this vaccine.

Typical signs of many forms of meningitis are sudden fever, severe headache, and a stiff neck, particularly stiffness that causes difficulty touching your chin to your chest. Persons who are suspected of having meningitis should receive immediate, aggressive medical treatment. Talk to the medical or health education staff at your local student health center to see if they have the vaccine most likely to protect you in your area.

meningitis An infection of the meninges, the membranes that surround the brain and spinal cord.

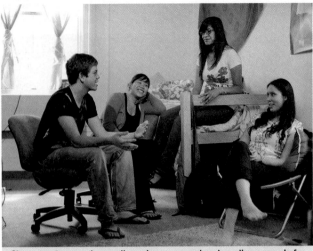

Close quarters, such as college dorms, are prime breeding grounds for some contagious diseases such as meningococcal meningitis.

include wasting/weight loss, fever, chronic cough and blood streaked sputum, fluid- and blood-filled lungs, and eventual spread throughout the body. The term is still used in some parts of the world today; however, TB is now widely recognized for these same symptoms. Airborne transmission via the respiratory tract is the primary mode of infection. Infected people can be contagious without showing symptoms and can transmit the disease while talking, coughing, sneezing, or singing.

The current recommended treatment for TB involves taking four drugs for 6 to 9 months; however, a new 12-dose regimen is available for high risk populations.[17] Medications may cause side effects ranging from minor stomach irritation to liver failure.[18] The lengthy, difficult treatment, along with barriers to obtaining drugs and care in many developing areas leads to missed doses and treatments that end before the cure and breeds drug-resistant bacteria. **Multidrug-resistant TB (MDR-TB)** is currently resistant to at least two of the best anti-TB drugs in use today, and **extensively drug-resistant TB (XDR-TB)**, is resistant to nearly all current TB drugs. These newer strains of tuberculosis are reaching epidemic proportions in over 58 countries.[19]

Tickborne Bacterial Diseases In the past few decades, certain tickborne diseases have become major health threats in the United States. The most noteworthy include two bacterially caused diseases. *Lyme disease* is present in many regions of the United States, particularly the upper Midwest. Symptoms of Lyme disease may range from none, to a rash or bull's-eye lesion and flu-like symptoms, to chronic arthritis, blindness, and long-term disability. *Ehrlichiosis,* another tickborne disease, has flu-like symptoms that may progress quickly to respiratory difficulties, and even death. Fortunately, antibiotics given early in the disease course are effective in preventing any serious threats from these diseases. The bottom line is, if you have flu-like symptoms in the typical non-flu months of the year, get it checked out.

Once believed to be closely related to viruses, **rickettsia** are now considered a small form of bacteria. They produce toxins and multiply within small blood vessels, causing vascular blockage and tissue death. Rickettsia require an insect vector (carrier) for transmission to humans. Two common forms of human rickettsial disease are *Rocky Mountain spotted fever* (*RMSF*), carried by a tick; and *typhus,* carried by a louse, flea, or tick. These diseases produce similar symptoms, including high fever, weakness, rash, and coma, and both can be life threatening.

For all insect-borne diseases, the best protection is to stay indoors at dusk and early morning to avoid hours of high insect activity. If you must go out, wear protective clothing or use bug sprays containing natural oils, pyrethrins, or DEET (diethyl toluamide), all products regarded as generally safe. If you are traveling in areas where insect-borne diseases are prevalent,

pneumonia Inflammatory disease of the lungs characterized by chronic cough, chest pain, chills, high fever, and fluid accumulation; may be caused by bacteria, viruses, fungi, chemicals, or other substances.

tuberculosis (TB) A disease caused by bacterial infiltration of the respiratory system.

multidrug-resistant TB (MDR-TB) Form of TB that is resistant to at least two of the best antibiotics available.

extensively drug-resistant TB (XDR-TB) Form of TB that is resistant to nearly all existing antibiotics.

rickettsia A small form of bacteria that live inside other living cells.

Pneumonia **Pneumonia** is a general term for a wide range of conditions that result in inflammation of the lungs and difficulty breathing. It is characterized by chronic cough, chest pain, chills, high fever, fluid accumulation, and eventual respiratory failure. Although bacterial and viral pathogens are the most common culprits, pneumonia can also be caused by fungi, occupational exposure, or trauma.

Bacterial pneumonia responds readily to antibiotic treatment in early stages, but can be deadly in more advanced stages. Forms of pneumonia caused by other organisms are more difficult to treat. Although medical advances have reduced the overall incidence of pneumonia, it continues to be a major threat in the United States and throughout the world.

Tuberculosis (TB) Only HIV/AIDS is a greater infectious agent killer than **tuberculosis** in the global population.[14] With about 9 million new cases in 2011, an astounding one-third of the world's population is infected with TB.[15] Although infection rates decreased dramatically in the United States since the 1950s, there were still over 10,000 cases in 2011.[16] TB is the number one infectious killer of women of reproductive age worldwide, as well as the leading cause of death among HIV-positive patients. Poverty and lack of access to treatment are also key risk factors.

Historically, people used the term *consumption* to refer to a bacterial respiratory disease with symptoms that

Ticks are a vector for several devastating bacterial diseases.

bed nets, routine "tick checks," and other protective measures may be necessary.

Viruses

Viruses are the smallest known pathogens, approximately 1/500th the size of bacteria, and hundreds of viruses are known to cause diseases in humans. Essentially, a virus consists of a protein structure that contains either *ribonucleic acid* (*RNA*) or *deoxyribonucleic acid* (*DNA*). Viruses are incapable of carrying out any life processes on their own. To reproduce, they must invade and inject their own DNA or RNA into a host cell and force it to make copies of themselves. The new viruses then erupt out of the host cell and seek other cells to invade.

Viral diseases can be difficult to treat because many viruses can withstand heat, formaldehyde, and large doses of radiation with little effect on their structure. Some viruses have **incubation periods** (the length of time required to develop fully and cause symptoms in their hosts) that last for years, which delays diagnosis. Drug treatment for viral infections is also limited. Drugs powerful enough to kill viruses generally kill the host cells, too, although some medications block stages in viral reproduction without damaging the host cells.

The Common Cold Some experts claim there may be over 200 different viruses responsible for the common cold. Any given cold's most likely cause is the rhinovirus, which causes 30 to 50 percent of all colds, followed by the coronavirus, responsible for 10 to 15 percent of all colds.[20] Colds are **endemic** (always present to some degree) throughout the world, with increasing prevalence in colder weather as people spend more time indoors. Otherwise healthy people carry cold viruses in their noses and throats most of the time, held in check until immune defenses are weakened. It is possible to "catch" a cold—through airborne transmission, touching skin-to-skin, or mucous membrane contact—and the hands are the greatest avenue for transmitting colds and other viruses. Obviously, then, covering your nose and mouth with a tissue, handkerchief, or even the crook of your elbow when sneezing is better than using your bare hand. Contrary to popular belief, you cannot catch a cold from getting a chill or being in the cold, but the chill may lower your immune system's resistance to a virus if one is present.

Influenza **Influenza,** or flu, is a contagious respiratory illness that includes fever and chills along with other cold symptoms. It is usually not life threatening except in persons who are over the age of 65, young children, or those with other underlying health conditions. Five to 20 percent of Americans get the flu each year, and of these, 200,000 will need hospitalization.[21] Once a person gets the flu, treatment is *palliative*—focused on relief of symptoms, rather than cure.

Since there are numerous and constantly mutating flu strains, vaccines are formulated for the few strains most likely to be prevalent in an upcoming season. If researchers

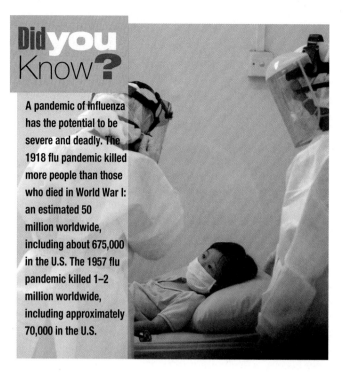

correctly predict strains, vaccines are thought to be 70 to 90 percent effective in healthy adults for about a year; if the prediction is off, a shot is less beneficial.[22] In spite of minor risks, the CDC now recommends everyone over the age of 6 months get the flu vaccine annually. Flu shots take 2 to 3 weeks to become effective, so it's best to get shots in the fall before the flu season begins.

Hepatitis One of the most highly publicized viral diseases is **hepatitis,** a virally caused inflammation of the liver. Hepatitis symptoms include fever, headache, nausea, loss of appetite, skin rashes, pain in the upper right abdomen, dark yellow (with brownish tinge) urine, and jaundice. Internationally, viral hepatitis is a major contributor to liver disease and accounts for high morbidity and mortality. Currently, there are several known forms (A, B, C, D, and E), with hepatitis A, B, and C having the highest rates of incidence.

viruses Minute microbes consisting of DNA or RNA that invade a host cell and use the cell's resources to reproduce themselves.

incubation period The time between exposure to a disease and the appearance of symptoms.

endemic Describing a disease that is always present to some degree.

influenza A common viral disease of the respiratory tract.

hepatitis A viral disease in which the liver becomes inflamed, producing symptoms such as fever, headache, and possibly jaundice.

Hepatitis A (HAV) is contracted by eating food or drinking water contaminated with human feces. Since vaccinations became available, HAV rates have declined by nearly 92 percent in the United States, but still more than 21,000 people are infected annually.[23] HAV is often spread through contaminated food, sexual contact with HAV-positive individuals, travel to regions where HAV is endemic, and use of contaminated needles. Fortunately, individuals infected with hepatitis A do not become chronic carriers, and vaccines for the disease are available. Many who contract HAV are asymptomatic (symptom-free).

Hepatitis B (HBV) is spread through body fluid exchange during unprotected sex, sharing needles when injecting drugs; through needlesticks on the job; or, in the case of a newborn baby, from an infected mother. Hepatitis B can lead to chronic liver disease or liver cancer. In spite of vaccine availability since 1982, there are currently over 1.2 million people in the United States who are chronically infected with HBV—over 35,000 new cases each year.[24] Needle exchange programs have helped reduce risks of HBV infection in some populations. Although global HBV infections have declined, they continue to be a major health problem, with over 350 million chronic carriers; the highest rates are in Asia and Africa.[25] Because the hepatitis B virus is considered 50 to 100 times more virulent than HIV, efforts to increase global vaccination rates have become a major priority.[26]

Hepatitis C (HCV) infections are on an epidemic rise in many regions of the world as resistant forms emerge. Some cases can be traced to blood transfusions or organ transplants. Currently, an estimated 17,000 new cases of HCV are diagnosed in the United States each year, with over 3.2 million people chronically infected.[27] Over 85 percent of those infected develop chronic infections; if the infection is left untreated, the person may develop cirrhosis of the liver, liver cancer, or liver failure. Liver failure resulting from chronic hepatitis C is the leading reason for liver transplants in the United States.[28] Although several vaccines are currently being tested and at least one is in early human trials, an actual vaccine is not yet available.

To prevent the spread of HBV and HCV use latex condoms correctly every time you have sex; don't share personal-care items that might have blood on them, such as razors or toothbrushes; get a blood test for HBV so you know your status; never share needles; and if you are having body art done, go only to reputable artists or piercers who follow established sterilization and infection-control protocols.

What's Working for You?

You probably already have habits or behaviors that help you avoid infection. Which of these habits do you have?

☐ I have soap for hand washing in the bathroom and kitchen and wash my hands regularly, particularly before preparing food and after using the bathroom.

☐ I make an effort to eat lots of fruits and vegetables and to exercise to help keep my immune system strong.

☐ I manage my stress and get enough sleep.

☐ When preparing food, I'm careful to make sure foods are cooked properly to avoid foodborne illnesses.

Other Pathogens

While bacteria and viruses account for many common diseases, other organisms can also infect people. Among these are fungi, protozoans, parasitic worms, and prions.

Fungi

Hundreds of species of **fungi** exist. While many of these multi- or unicellular organisms are beneficial—edible mushrooms, penicillin, and yeast used in bread—*candidiasis* (the cause of vaginal yeast infections, discussed later), athlete's foot, ringworm, jock itch, and toenail fungus are examples of common fungal diseases. With most fungal diseases, keeping the affected area clean and dry and treating it promptly with appropriate medications will generally bring relief. Fungal diseases typically transmit via physical contact, so avoid going barefoot in public showers, hotel rooms, and other areas where fungus may be present. *Valley Fever*—a potentially life-threatening respiratory disease common in the desert Southwest—and others may be spread to humans and pets via breathing in fungal spores.

Protozoans

Protozoans are single-celled organisms that cause diseases like malaria and African sleeping sickness and are largely controlled in the United States. A common waterborne protozoan disease in many regions of the country is *giardiasis*. Persons who drink contaminated water may be exposed to the *giardia* pathogen and will suffer intestinal pain and discomfort weeks after initial infection. Protection of water supplies is the key to prevention.

Parasitic Worms

Parasitic worms are the largest pathogens. Ranging in size from small pinworms typically found in children to large tapeworms that can take up large portions of the human intestines, most are more nuisance than threat. Of special note are the worm infestations associated with eating raw fish (as in some forms of sushi). You can prevent worm infestations by cooking fish and other foods to temperatures sufficient to kill the worms and their eggs. Other preventive measures you can take include getting your pets checked, being careful while swimming in international areas known for these infections, and wearing shoes in parks or places where animal feces are present.

Prions

A **prion** is a self-replicating, protein-based agent that can infect humans and other animals. One such prion is believed to be the underlying cause of spongiform diseases such as *bovine spongiform encephalopathy* (*BSE*, or "mad cow disease"). If humans eat contaminated meat from cattle with BSE, they may develop a mad cow–like disease known as *variant Creutzfeld-Jakob disease (vCJD)*. Symptoms of vCJD include loss of memory, tremors, and muscle spasms or "ticks." Over time, depression, difficulty walking, seizures, and severe dementia can ultimately lead to death in both cows and humans.[29] An increasing number of infected cattle have been found in the United States and globally; however, to date, there have been no confirmed human infections from U.S. beef.

Emerging and Resurgent Diseases

Although our immune systems are adept at responding to challenges, microbes and other pathogens constantly evolve and try to gain an edge. Within the past decade, rates for many infectious diseases have increased. This trend can be attributed to a combination of overpopulation, inadequate health care, increasing poverty, environmental changes, and drug resistance.[30] At the same time, world travel and trade of goods has become increasingly fast and easy, giving many pathogens ample opportunity to hitch a ride to new locations.

Measles and Mumps
The most well-known symptom of **mumps** is swelling of the salivary glands. In severe cases it can cause hearing loss or male sterility. In 2009 a U.S. mumps outbreak that sickened over 1,500 people was triggered by a single boy who contracted the disease while on a trip outside the United States.[31] **Measles**, known for its high fever and itchy red rash, is increasingly common—particularly on college campuses. Many young adults have not been vaccinated against measles or mumps because their parents may have thought the disease was long gone or had concerns about vaccination safety. Today, an increasing number of colleges and universities require verification of immunization with the MMR vaccination or a blood test that indicates immunity. (Refer back to the **Health Headlines** box on page 405 for more on vaccine backlash.)

West Nile Virus
Several thousand cases of West Nile Virus occur in the United States each year. Symptoms are flu-like and can include a form of encephalitis (inflammation of the brain). With hundreds of individuals disabled and 45 deaths from the infection annually, the elderly and those with impaired immune systems bear the brunt of the disease burden.[32] Today, only Alaska and Hawaii remain free of the disease in the United States. Spread by infected mosquitoes, the best way to avoid infection is through mosquito eradication programs, wearing mosquito repellant, and avoiding mosquito-infested areas altogether, especially at peak mosquito feeding times. There is no vaccine or specific treatment.

Avian (Bird) Flu
Avian influenza is an infectious disease of birds with strains capable of crossing the species barrier, causing severe illness in humans who come in contact with bird droppings or fluids. Bird flu appears to have originated in Asia and spread via migrating bird populations.[33] Although the virus has yet to mutate into a form highly infectious to humans, outbreaks in rural areas of the world (where people live in close proximity to poultry and other animals) have occurred. As of March, 2013, the WHO had recorded 468 cases of bird flu in humans, with 282 deaths.[34] Many health experts suggest that if the virus becomes easily transmissible between humans, it could become a major pandemic.[35]

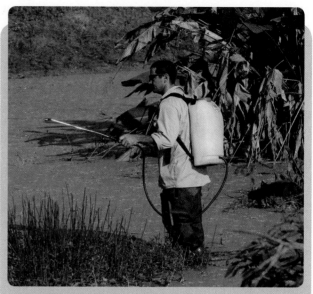

What can be done to prevent new diseases from emerging and spreading?

Poor control of pests, such as disease-spreading mosquitoes, is a symptom of larger problems such as infrastructure overload, pesticide misuse, lack of government funding, poverty, and environmental degradation. Attention to these issues is essential in preventing new and more virulent forms of disease from emerging and spreading.

Escherichia coli O157:H7
Escherichia coli O157:H7 is one of over 170 types of *E. coli* bacteria that can infect humans. Most *E. coli* organisms are harmless and live in the intestines of healthy animals and humans. *E. coli* O157:H7, however, produces a lethal toxin and can cause severe illness or death. You can get it from eating ground beef that is undercooked, drinking unpasteurized milk or juice, or swimming in sewage-contaminated water. Outbreaks in the United States have been caused by foods like frozen pizza and quesadillas, organic spinach and spring mix lettuce, raw clover sprouts, romaine lettuce, bologna, cheese, and poultry.

A symptom of infection is nonbloody diarrhea, usually 2 to 8 days after exposure; however, asymptomatic cases have been noted. Children, older adults, and people with weakened immune systems are particularly vulnerable to serious side effects such as kidney failure, intestinal damage, or death.

Strengthened regulations on chlorine levels in pools and the cooking of meat have helped reduce *E. coli* infections. Difficulties in isolating the source of infections have prompted a close examination of labeling and distribution of food products. The U.S. Department of Agriculture (USDA) as well as the Environmental Protection Agency (EPA), Food and Drug Administration, and others are all involved in developing food and transportation policies designed to keep the food supply safe.

mumps A once common viral disease that is controllable by vaccination.

measles A viral disease that produces symptoms such as an itchy rash and a high fever.

Sexually Transmitted Infections (STIs)

There are more than 20 known types of **sexually transmitted infections (STIs)**. Once referred to as *venereal diseases* and then *sexually transmitted diseases,* the current terminology is more reflective of the number and types of infections and of the fact that they are caused by pathogens. More virulent strains and antibiotic-resistant forms spell trouble in the days ahead.

Every year, there are at least 20 million new cases of STIs, only some of which are curable.[36] Sexually transmitted infections affect people of all backgrounds and socioeconomic levels, but they disproportionately affect women, minorities, and infants. STIs are also most prevalent in teens and young adults.[37]

Early symptoms of an STI are often mild and unrecognizable. Left untreated, some of these infections can have grave consequences, such as sterility, blindness, central nervous system destruction, disfigurement, and even death. Infants born to mothers carrying the organisms for these infections are at risk for a variety of health problems.

sexually transmitted infections (STIs) Infections transmitted through some form of intimate, usually sexual, contact.

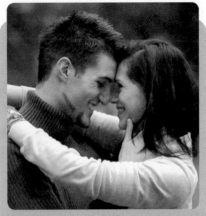

How can I tell if someone I'm dating has an STI?

You can't tell if someone has an STI just by looking at him or her, and many people with STIs are themselves unaware of the infection because it could be asymptomatic. The only way to know for sure is to go to a clinic and get tested. In addition, partners need to be open and honest with each other about their sexual histories and practice safer sex.

treatment. Unfortunately, they usually continue to be sexually active, thereby infecting unsuspecting partners. People who are uncomfortable discussing sexual issues may also be less likely to use and ask their partners to use condoms to protect against STIs and pregnancy. Another reason proposed for the STI epidemic is our casual attitude about sex. Evaluate your own attitude and beliefs about STIs by completing the **Assess Yourself** box on page 420.

Ignorance—about the infections, their symptoms, and the fact that someone can be asymptomatic but still infected—is also a factor. A person who is infected but asymptomatic can unknowingly spread an STI to others who also ignore or misinterpret symptoms. By the time anyone seeks medical help, he or she may have infected several others. In addition, many people mistakenly believe that certain sexual practices—oral sex, for example—carry no risk for STIs. In fact, oral sex practices among young adults may be responsible for increases in herpes and other infections. **Figure 13.5** shows the continuum of disease risk for various sexual behaviors, and the **Skills for Behavior Change** box on the following page offers tips for ways to practice safer sex.

What's Your Risk?

Generally, the more sexual partners a person has, the greater the risk for contracting an STI. Shame and embarrassment often keep infected people from seeking

Routes of Transmission

Sexually transmitted infections are generally spread through some form of intimate sexual contact. Less likely modes of transmission include mouth-to-mouth contact or contact with

High-risk behaviors	Moderate-risk behaviors	Low-risk behaviors	No-risk behaviors
Unprotected vaginal, anal, and oral sex—any activity that involves direct contact with bodily fluids, such as ejaculate, vaginal secretions, or blood—are high-risk behaviors.	Vaginal, anal, or oral sex with a latex or polyurethane condom and a water-based lubricant used properly and consistently can greatly reduce the risk of STI transmission. Dental dams used during oral sex can also greatly reduce the risk of STI transmission.	Mutual masturbation, if there are no cuts on the hand, penis, or vagina, is very low risk. Rubbing, kissing, and massaging carry low risk, but herpes can be spread by skin-to-skin contact from an infected partner.	Abstinence, phone sex, talking, and fantasy are all no-risk behaviors.

FIGURE 13.5 **Continuum of Disease Risk for Various Sexual Behaviors**
There are different levels of risk for various behaviors and various sexually transmitted infections (STIs); however, no matter what, any sexual activity involving direct contact with blood, semen, or vaginal secretions is high risk.

110 million

people are living with a STI in the United States.

fluids from body sores. Although each STI is a different infection caused by a different pathogen, all STI pathogens prefer dark, moist places, especially the mucous membranes lining reproductive organs. Most are susceptible to light, extreme temperature, and dryness, and many die quickly on exposure to air. Like other communicable infections, STIs have both pathogen-specific incubation periods and *periods of* communicability—times during which transmission is most likely.

Chlamydia

Chlamydia, an infection caused by the bacterium *Chlamydia trachomatis,* is the most commonly reported STI in the United States. Chlamydia infects an estimated 2.8 million Americans annually, the majority of them women, and often presents no symptoms.[38] Public health officials believe that this estimate could be higher, because many cases go unreported.

Signs and Symptoms
In men, early symptoms may include painful and difficult urination; frequent urination; and a watery, pus-like discharge from the penis. Symptoms in women may include a yellowish discharge, spotting between periods, and occasional spotting after intercourse. Women are especially likely to be asymptomatic; many do not realize they have the disease, which can put them at risk for secondary damage.[39]

Complications
Men can suffer injury to the prostate gland, seminal vesicles, and bulbourethral glands, as well as arthritis-like symptoms and inflammatory damage to the blood vessels and heart. Men can also experience epididymitis—inflammation of the area near the testicles. In women, chlamydia-related inflammation can injure the cervix or fallopian tubes, causing sterility, and it can damage the inner pelvic structure, leading to **pelvic inflammatory disease (PID)** (see the **Health in a Diverse World** box on page 412). If an infected woman becomes pregnant, she has a high risk for miscarriage and stillbirth. Women are at greater risks for urinary tract infections. Chlamydia may also be responsible for one type of *conjunctivitis,* an eye infection that affects not only

"Why Should I Care?"

Getting an STI can be painful, and you can infect your current partner with it. In the long term, it could affect the health of your children or your ability to have children.

adults but also infants, who can contract the disease from an infected mother during delivery. Untreated conjunctivitis can cause blindness.[40]

chlamydia Bacterially caused STI of the urogenital tract.

pelvic inflammatory disease (PID) Term used to describe various infections of the female reproductive tract.

Diagnosis and Treatment
A sample of urine or fluid from the vagina or penis is collected and tested to identify the presence of the bacteria. Unfortunately, chlamydia tests are not a routine part of many health clinics' testing procedures. If detected early, chlamydia is easily treatable with antibiotics such as tetracycline, doxycycline, or erythromycin.

COMPLICATIONS OF STIs: PID IN WOMEN, EPIDIDYMITIS IN MEN

If left untreated, many STIs can lead to serious complications for both men and women. Pelvic inflammatory disease (PID) can be caused by *Neisseria gonorrhoeae* or *Chlamydia trachomatis*. Pelvic inflammatory disease is a catchall term for a number of infections of the uterus, fallopian tubes, and ovaries that are complications resulting from an untreated STI.

Symptoms of PID vary but generally include lower abdominal pain, fever, unusual vaginal discharge, painful intercourse, painful urination, and irregular menstrual bleeding. The vague symptoms associated with chlamydial and gonococcal PID can cause a delay seeking medical care, thereby increasing the risk of permanent damage and scarring that can lead to infertility and other complications. In the United States, approximately 1 million women develop PID every year. It is estimated that 1 in 8 sexually active adolescent girls will develop PID before the age of 20.

Epididymitis is swelling (inflammation) of the epididymis, and it is most common among young men ages 19 to 35. Epididymitis is most commonly caused by the spread of *Neisseria gonorrhoeae*

or *Chlamydia trachomatis* from the urethra or the bladder. Symptoms can include blood in the semen, swollen groin area, discharge from the urethra, discomfort in the lower abdomen or pelvis, and pain during ejaculation or during urination. A physical examination along with other medical tests, including a testicular scan and tests for chlamydia and gonorrhea, can diagnose the condition. Treatment usually involves pain medications and anti-inflammatory medications.

The serious complications that can result from untreated STIs further illustrate the need for early diagnosis and treatment. Regular screening and testing is particularly important because many STIs are often asymptomatic, increasing the risk of complications such as PID and epididymitis.

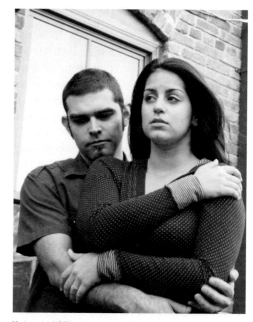

Untreated STIs can cause PID in women or epididymitis in men.

Sources: MedlinePlus, "Pelvic Inflammatory Disease (PID)," Updated 2011, www.nlm.nih.gov; Mayo Clinic Staff, "Urinary Tract Infection: Risk Factors," August 2012, www.mayoclinic.com; Centers for Disease Control and Prevention, Division of STD Prevention, National Center for HIV/AIDS, Viral Hepatitis, STD, and TB Prevention, "Sexually Transmitted Diseases Surveillance, 2011: STDs in Women and Infants," Updated 2012, www.cdc.gov; U. S. National Library of Medicine, "Epididymitis," Last review August 2012, www.ncbi.nlm.nih.gov; Centers for Disease Control and Prevention, "STD Treatment Guidelines 2010: Epididymitis," Updated January 2011, www.cdc.gov

Gonorrhea

Gonorrhea is surpassed only by chlamydia in number of cases. The CDC estimates that there are over 700,000 cases per year, plus numbers that go unreported.[41] Caused by the bacterial pathogen *Neisseria gonorrhoeae*, gonorrhea primarily infects the linings of the urethra, genital tract, pharynx, and rectum. It may spread to the eyes or other body regions by the hands or through body fluids, typically during vaginal, oral, or anal sex. It most frequently occurs in people in their early twenties.

gonorrhea Second most common bacterial STI in the United States; if untreated, may cause sterility.

Signs and Symptoms While some men are asymptomatic, a typical symptom is a white, milky discharge from the penis accompanied by painful, burning urination 2 to 9 days

after contact (**Figure 13.6** on the following page). Epididymitis can also occur as a symptom of infection.

Most women do not experience any symptoms, but others may have vaginal discharge or a burning sensation on urinating.[42] The organism can remain in the woman's vagina, cervix, uterus, or fallopian tubes for long periods with no apparent symptoms other than an occasional slight fever. Thus a woman can be unaware that she has been infected and that she is infecting her sexual partners.

Complications Gonorrhea may spread to the prostate, testicles, urinary tract, kidneys, and bladder in men, and scar tissue may cause sterility. In some cases, the penis develops a painful curvature during erection. If the infection goes undetected in a woman, it can spread to the fallopian tubes and ovaries, causing sterility or severe inflammation and PID. The bacteria can also spread up the reproductive tract, through

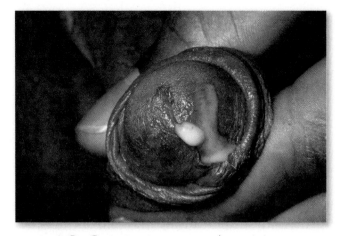

FIGURE 13.6 Gonorrhea

One common symptom of gonorrhea in men is a milky discharge from the penis, accompanied by burning sensations during urination. Whereas these symptoms will cause most men to seek diagnosis and treatment, women with gonorrhea are often asymptomatic, so they may not be aware they are infected.

the blood and infect the joints, heart valves, or brain. If an infected woman becomes pregnant, the infection can be transmitted to her baby during delivery, potentially causing blindness, joint infection, or a life-threatening blood infection.

Diagnosis and Treatment Diagnosis of gonorrhea requires a sample of either urine or fluid from the vagina or penis to detect the presence of the bacteria. In early stages gonorrhea is treatable with antibiotics, but it has begun to develop resistance. It is also important to recognize that chlamydia and gonorrhea often occur at the same time, but different antibiotics are needed to treat each infection separately.[43]

Syphilis

Syphilis is caused by a bacterium called *Treponema pallidum*. The incidence of syphilis is highest in adults aged 20 to 39 and is particularly high among African Americans and men who have sex with men. Because it is extremely delicate and dies readily on exposure to air, dryness, or cold, the organism is generally transferred only through direct sexual contact or from mother to fetus. The incidence of syphilis in newborns has continued to increase in the United States.[44]

Signs and Symptoms Syphilis is known as the "great imitator," because its symptoms resemble those of several other infections. It should be noted, however, that some people experience no symptoms at all. Syphilis can occur in four distinct stages:[45]

- **Primary syphilis.** The first stage of syphilis is often characterized by the development of a **chancre** (pronounced "shank-er"), a bacteria-oozing sore located at the infection site that usually appears about a month after initial infection (see **Figure 13.7**). In men, the site of the chancre tends to be

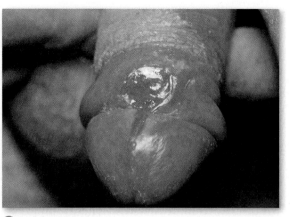

a Primary syphilis

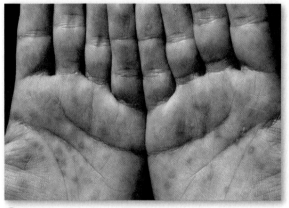

b Secondary syphilis

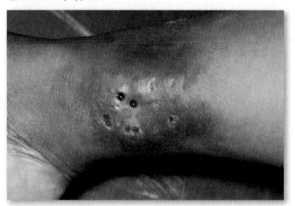

c Latent syphilis

FIGURE 13.7 Syphilis

A chancre on the site of the initial infection is a symptom of primary syphilis (a). A rash is characteristic of secondary syphilis (b). Lesions called *gummas* are often present in latent syphilis (c).

the penis or scrotum; in women, the site of infection is often internal, on the vaginal wall or high on the cervix where the chancre is not readily apparent, making the likelihood of detection small. In both men and women, the chancre will disappear in 3 to 6 weeks.

syphilis One of the most widespread bacterial STIs; characterized by distinct phases and potentially serious results.

chancre Sore often found at the site of syphilis infection.

- **Secondary syphilis.** If the infection is left untreated, a month to a year after the chancre disappears, secondary symptoms may appear, including a rash or white patches on the skin or on the mucous membranes of the mouth, throat, or genitals. Hair loss may occur, lymph nodes may enlarge, and the victim may develop a slight fever or headache. In rare cases, bacteria-containing sores develop around the mouth or genitals.
- **Latent syphilis.** After the secondary stage, if the infection is left untreated, the syphilis spirochetes begin to invade body organs, causing lesions called *gummas*. The infection now is rarely transmitted to others, except during pregnancy, when it can be passed to the fetus.
- **Tertiary/late syphilis.** Years after syphilis has entered the body, its effects become all too evident if still untreated. Late-stage syphilis indications include heart and central nervous system damage, blindness, deafness, paralysis, and dementia.

Complications Pregnant women with syphilis can experience premature births, miscarriages, stillbirths, or transmit the infection to her unborn child. An infected pregnant woman may transmit to her unborn child *congenital syphilis,* which can cause death; severe birth defects such as blindness, deafness, or disfigurement; developmental delays; seizures; and other health problems. Because in most cases the fetus does not become infected until after the first trimester, treatment of the mother during this time will usually prevent infection of the fetus.

Diagnosis and Treatment Syphilis can be diagnosed with a blood test or by collecting a sample from the chancre. It is easily treated with antibiotics, usually penicillin, for all stages except the late stage.

Herpes

Herpes is a general term for a family of infections characterized by sores or eruptions on the skin caused by the herpes simplex virus. While herpes can be transmitted by sexual contact, kissing or sharing eating utensils can also transmit the infection. Herpes infections range from mildly uncomfortable to extremely serious. **Genital herpes** affects approximately 16 percent of the population aged 14 to 49 in the United States.[46]

genital herpes STI caused by the herpes simplex virus.

There are two types of herpes simplex virus. Only about 1 in 6 Americans currently has HSV-2; however, about half of adults have HSV-1, usually appearing as cold sores on their mouths.[47] Both types can infect any area of the body **(Figure 13.8)**. Herpes simplex virus remains in certain nerve cells for life and can flare up when the body's ability to maintain itself is weakened.

Signs and Symptoms The precursor phase of a herpes infection is characterized by a burning sensation and redness at the site of infection. By the second phase, a blister filled with a clear fluid containing the virus forms. If you pick at this blister or otherwise touch the site, you can autoinoculate other body parts. Particularly dangerous is the possibility of spreading the infection to your eyes, as blindness can occur.

Over a period of days, the unsightly blister will crust over, dry up, and disappear, and the virus will travel to the base of an affected nerve supplying the area and become dormant. Only when the victim becomes overly stressed, when diet and sleep are inadequate, when the immune system is overworked, or when excessive exposure to sunlight or other stressors occur will the virus become reactivated (at the same site every time) and begin the blistering cycle all over again. Each time a sore develops, it casts off (sheds) viruses that can be highly infectious, but a herpes site can shed the virus even when no overt sore is present.

Complications Many physicians recommend cesarean deliveries for infected pregnant women, as herpes can be passed to the baby during birth. Additionally, women with a history of genital herpes appear to have a greater risk of developing cervical cancer.

Diagnosis and Treatment Diagnosis of herpes can be determined by collecting a sample from the suspected sore or by performing a blood test. Although there is no cure for herpes at present, certain prescription drugs like acyclovir, and over-the-counter medications like Abreva can be used to treat symptoms. Unfortunately, most only work if the infection is confirmed during the first few hours after contact. Other drugs, such as famciclovir (FAMVIR), may reduce viral shedding between outbreaks—potentially reducing risks to your sexual partners.[48]

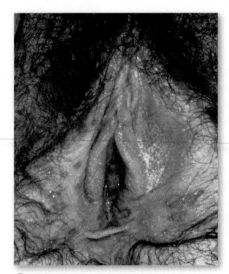

ⓐ Genital herpes is a highly contagious and incurable STI. It is characterized by recurring cycles of painful blisters on the genitalia.

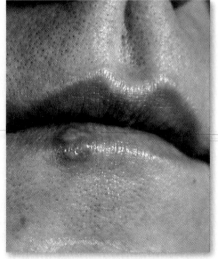

ⓑ Oral herpes, caused by the same type of virus as genital herpes, is extremely contagious and can cause painful sores and blisters around the mouth.

FIGURE 13.8 **Herpes**
Both genital and oral herpes can be caused by either herpes simplex virus type 1 or 2.

Human Papillomavirus (HPV) and Genital Warts

Genital warts (also known as *venereal warts* or *condylomas*) are caused by a group of viruses known as **human papillomavirus (HPV)**. There are over 100 different types of HPV; more than 40 types are sexually transmitted and are classified as either low risk or high risk. A person becomes infected when certain types of HPV penetrate the skin and mucous membranes of the genitals or anus. This is among the most common forms of STI, with 20 million Americans currently infected with genital HPV and approximately 6 million new cases each year.[49]

Signs and Symptoms The typical incubation period is 6 to 8 weeks after contact. People infected with low-risk types of HPV may develop genital warts, a series of bumps or growths on the genitals, ranging in size from small pinheads to large cauliflower-like growths (Figure 13.9).

Complications High-risk types of HPV (HPV-16 and -18) are responsible for an estimated 70 percent of cervical cancer cases.[50] Exactly how high-risk HPV infection leads to cervical cancer is uncertain, though it may lead to *dysplasia,* or changes in cells, that may lead to a precancerous condition. Six out of 10 cervical cancers occur in women who have never received a Pap test or who have not been tested for HPV in the past 5 years.[51]

In addition, HPV may pose a threat to a fetus during birth; cesarean deliveries may be considered in serious cases. New research has also implicated HPV as a possible risk factor for coronary artery disease, potentially causing an inflammatory response in the artery walls, leading to cholesterol and plaque buildup. (See **Chapter 12** for more on the effects of inflammation and plaque buildup on arteries.)

Diagnosis and Treatment Diagnosis of genital warts from low-risk types of HPV is determined through a visual examination. High-risk types can be diagnosed in women through microscopic analysis of cells from a Pap smear or by collecting a sample from the cervix to test for HPV DNA. There is currently no HPV DNA test for men.

Treatment is available only for the low-risk forms of HPV that cause genital warts. Most warts can be treated with topical medication or can be frozen with liquid nitrogen and then removed, but large warts may require surgical removal. There are currently two HPV vaccines that are licensed by the U.S. Food and Drug Administration (FDA) and recommended by the CDC. See the **Student Health Today** box on page 417 for more information about these vaccines.

genital warts Warts that appear in the genital area or the anus; caused by the human papillomavirus (HPV).

human papillomavirus (HPV) A group of viruses, many of which are transmitted sexually; some types of HPV can cause genital warts or cervical cancer.

candidiasis Yeastlike fungal infection often transmitted sexually; also called *moniliasis* or *yeast infection.*

trichomoniasis Protozoan STI characterized by foamy, yellowish discharge and unpleasant odor.

Candidiasis (Moniliasis)

Most STIs are caused by pathogens that come from outside the body; however, the yeast-like fungus *Candida albicans* is a normal inhabitant of the vaginal tract in most women. (See Figure 13.4c for a micrograph of this fungus.) Only when the normal chemical balance of the vagina is disturbed will these organisms multiply and cause the fungal disease **candidiasis,** also sometimes called *moniliasis* or a *yeast infection.*

Signs and Symptoms Symptoms of candidiasis include severe itching and burning of the vagina and vulva and a white, cheesy vaginal discharge.[52] When this microbe infects the mouth, whitish patches form, and the condition is referred to as *thrush.* Thrush infection can also occur in men and is easily transmitted between sexual partners. Symptoms of candidiasis can be aggravated by contact with soaps, douches, perfumed toilet paper, chlorinated water, and spermicides.

Diagnosis and Treatment Diagnosis of candidiasis is usually made by collecting a vaginal sample and analyzing it to identify the pathogen. Antifungal drugs applied on the surface or by suppository usually cure candidiasis in just a few days.

Trichomoniasis

Unlike many STIs, **trichomoniasis** is caused by a protozoan, *Trichomonas vaginalis.* (See Figure 13.4d for a micrograph of this organism.) The "trich" organism can be spread by sexual contact and by contact with items that have discharged fluids on them. An estimated 3.7 million new cases occur in the United States each year, although only about one third of

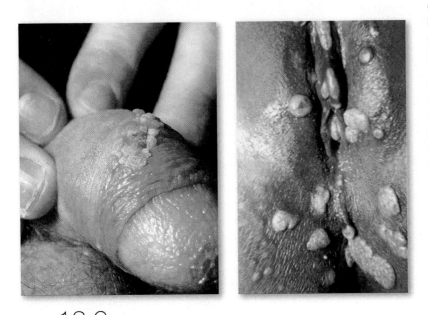

FIGURE 13.9 **Genital Warts**
Genital warts are caused by certain types of the human papillomavirus.

pubic lice Parasitic insects that can inhabit various body areas, especially the genitals.

acquired immunodeficiency syndrome (AIDS) A disease caused by a retrovirus, the human immunodeficiency virus (HIV), that attacks the immune system, reducing the number of helper T cells and leaving the victim vulnerable to infections, malignancies, and neurological disorders.

human immunodeficiency virus (HIV) The virus that causes AIDS by infecting helper T cells.

people who contract it experience symptoms.[53]

Signs and Symptoms Symptoms among women include a foamy, yellowish, unpleasant-smelling discharge accompanied by a burning sensation, itching, and painful urination. Most men with trichomoniasis do not have any symptoms, though some men experience irritation inside the penis, mild discharge, and a slight burning after urinating.[54]

Diagnosis and Treatment Diagnosis of trichomoniasis is determined by collecting fluid samples from the penis or vagina to test. Treatment includes oral metronidazole, usually given to both sexual partners to avoid the possible "ping-pong" effect of repeated cross-infection.

Pubic Lice

Pubic lice, often called "crabs," are small parasitic insects that are usually transmitted during sexual contact (Figure 13.10). More annoying than dangerous, they have an affinity for pubic hair and attach themselves to the base of these hairs, where they deposit their eggs (nits). One to 2 weeks later, these nits develop into adults that lay eggs and migrate to other body parts.

Signs and Symptoms Symptoms of pubic lice infestation include itchiness in the area covered by pubic hair, bluish-gray skin color in the pubic region, and sores in the genital area.

Diagnosis and Treatment Diagnosis of pubic lice involves an examination by a health care provider to identify

the eggs in the genital area. Treatment includes washing clothing, furniture, and linens that may harbor the eggs, and usually takes 2 to 3 weeks to kill all larval forms.

HIV/AIDS

Since **acquired immunodeficiency syndrome (AIDS)** was first recognized in the 1980s, approximately 65 million people worldwide have become infected with **human immunodeficiency virus (HIV),** the virus that causes AIDS. About 34 million people worldwide are living with HIV.[55] In the United States, there are over 1 million people infected with HIV and about 15,000 people died from HIV/AIDS in 2010, the last year for which data are available.[56] The vast majority of HIV-infected individuals (23.5 million) are in Sub-Saharan Africa and South and South East Asia (4 million). Globally, the numbers of people living with HIV have increased, even though the numbers of new infections have decreased in the last decade.[57]

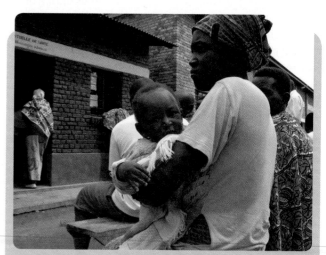

I don't hear much about HIV/AIDS anymore. Is it still a pandemic?

Yes! It may seem as if HIV/AIDS is no longer a problem; however, nothing could be further from the truth. In North America, 1.4 million people are living with HIV, and HIV and AIDS are still at pandemic levels, especially in developing nations. Sub-Saharan Africa has been hit hardest: 23.5 million people in the region are living with the disease. This mother and child are waiting for treatment outside an HIV clinic in Rwanda. HIV is spreading most rapidly in eastern Europe and central Asia, where 1.4 million people are currently HIV positive.

Source: UNAIDS, "UNAIDS World AIDS Day Report 2012," 2012, Available at www.unaids.org

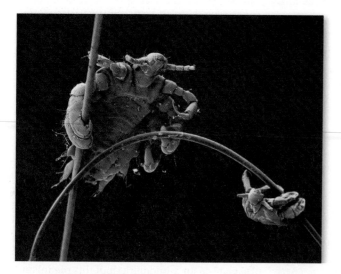

FIGURE 13.10 **Pubic Lice**
Pubic lice, also known as "crabs," are small, parasitic insects that attach themselves to pubic hair; they may also move and end up infesting other body hair, even as far away as eyebrows or the hair on the head.

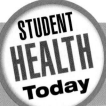

Q&A on HPV Vaccines

Most sexually active people will contract some form of human papillomavirus (HPV) at some time in their lives, though they may never even know it. There are about 40 types of sexually transmitted HPV, most of which cause no symptoms and go away on their own. Low-risk types can cause genital warts, but some high-risk types can cause cervical and other cancers. Every year in the United States, about 12,000 women are diagnosed with cervical cancer, and almost 4,000 die from this disease. There are currently two HPV vaccines that can help prevent women from becoming infected with HPV and subsequently developing cervical cancer.

● **Who should get the HPV vaccine?** There are two vaccines currently available—Cervarix and Gardasil. HPV vaccines are recommended for 11- and 12-year-old girls, but can be given to girls as young as 9 years old. It is also recommended for girls and women ages 13 through 26 who have not yet been vaccinated or completed the vaccine series. Ideally, females should get a vaccine before they become sexually active. Females who are sexually active may get less benefit from it because they may have already contracted an HPV type targeted by the vaccines.

One of the HPV vaccines, Gardasil, is also licensed, safe, and effective for males ages 9 through 26 years. The CDC recommends Gardasil for all boys 11 or 12 years old and for males ages 13 through

21 years who did not get any or all of the three recommended doses when they were younger. All men may receive the vaccine through the age of 26, but it is recommended that they should speak with their doctor to find out if getting vaccinated is right for them.

● **How are the two HPV vaccines, Cervarix and Gardasil, similar and different?** Both vaccines are very effective against high-risk HPV types 16 and 18, which cause 70 percent of cervical cancer cases. Both vaccines are given as shots and require three doses. But only Gardasil protects against low-risk HPV types 6 and 11. These HPV types cause 90 percent of cases of genital warts in females and males, so Gardasil is approved for use with males as well as females.

● **What do the two vaccines *not* protect against?** The vaccines do not protect against all types of HPV, so about 30 percent of cervical cancers will not be prevented by the vaccines. It will be important for women to continue getting screened for cervical cancer through regular Pap tests. Also, the vaccines do not prevent other sexually transmitted infections (STIs).

● **How safe are the HPV vaccines?** The vaccines are licensed by the FDA and approved by the CDC as safe and effective. They have been studied in thousands of females (ages 9 through 26) around the

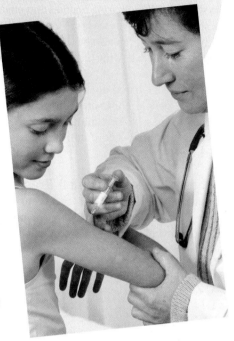

Many college campuses and state health departments offer free or low-cost vaccines for those whose insurance won't cover the cost.

world, and their safety continues to be monitored by the CDC and the FDA. Studies have found no serious side effects.

Sources: Centers for Disease Control and Prevention, "Vaccines and Preventable Diseases: HPV Vaccine—Questions & Answers," Reviewed January 2011, www.cdc.gov; American Cancer Society, "Human Papillomavirus (HPV), Cancer and HPV Vaccines—Frequently Asked Questions," Revised October 2010, www.cancer.org

How HIV Is Transmitted

HIV typically enters the body when another person's infected body fluids (e.g., semen, vaginal secretions, blood) gain entry through a breach in body defenses. If there is a break in mucous membranes of the genitals or anus (as can occur during sexual intercourse, particularly anal intercourse), the virus enters and begins to multiply, invading the bloodstream and cerebrospinal fluid. It progressively destroys helper T cells, weakening the body's resistance to disease.

HIV/AIDS is not highly contagious. It cannot reproduce outside a living host, except in a laboratory, and does not survive well in open air. As a result, HIV cannot be transmitted through casual contact, including sharing food utensils,

musical instruments, toilet seats, etc.[58] Research also provides overwhelming evidence that insect bites do not transmit HIV.[59]

Engaging in High-Risk Behaviors During the early days of the pandemic it appeared that HIV infected only homosexuals, but it quickly became apparent that the disease was related to certain high-risk behaviors rather than groups of people. **Figure 13.11** on page 418 shows the breakdown of sources of HIV infection among U.S. men and women.

The majority of HIV infections arise from the following:

● **Exchange of body fluids.** Substantial research indicates that blood, semen, and vaginal secretions are the major fluids of concern. Since the vaginal area is more susceptible to microtears, and because a woman is exposed to more semen than a man is to vaginal fluids, women are 4 to 10 times more likely than men to contract HIV through unprotected heterosexual intercourse.[60] In rare instances, the virus has been found in saliva, but most health officials state that saliva is a less significant risk than other shared body fluids.

- **Contaminated needles.** Although users of illicit drugs are the most obvious members of this category, people with diabetes who inject insulin or athletes who inject steroids may also share needles. Sharing needles and engaging in high-risk sexual activities increases risks dramatically. Tattooing and body piercing can also be risky (see the **Student Health Today** box on the following page).

Prior to 1985, blood donations were not checked for HIV, and some people contracted the virus from transfusions. Because of massive screening efforts, the risk of receiving HIV-infected blood is now almost nonexistent in developed countries.

Mother-to-Child (Perinatal) Transmission Mother-to-child transmission of HIV can occur during pregnancy, during labor and delivery, or through breast-feeding. Without antiretroviral treatment, approximately 25 percent of HIV-positive pregnant women will transmit the virus to their infant.[61]

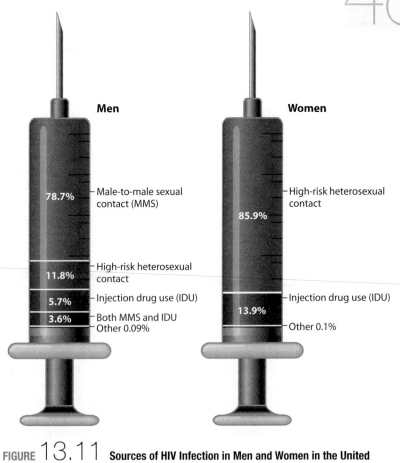

FIGURE 13.11 **Sources of HIV Infection in Men and Women in the United States, 2011**
Source: Data from Centers for Disease Control and Prevention, *HIV Surveillance Report, 2013,* vol. 23, www.cdc.gov

Signs and Symptoms of HIV/AIDS

A person may go for months or years after infection before any significant symptoms appear, and incubation time varies greatly from person to person. Without treatment, it takes an average of 8 to 10 years for the virus to cause the slow, degenerative changes in the immune system that are characteristic of AIDS. During this time, the person may experience *opportunistic infections* (infections that gain a foothold when the immune system is not functioning effectively). Colds, sore throats, fever, tiredness, nausea, night sweats, and other generally non–life-threatening conditions commonly appear and are described as pre-AIDS symptoms. Other symptoms of progressing HIV infection include wasting syndrome, swollen lymph nodes, and neurological problems. A diagnosis of AIDS, the final stage of HIV infection, is made when the infected person has either a dangerously low CD4 (helper T) cell count (below 200 cells per cubic milliliter of blood) or has contracted one or more opportunistic infections characteristic of the disease, such as Kaposi's sarcoma, tuberculosis, recurrent pneumonia, or invasive cervical cancer.

48% **of people** living with HIV and tuberculosis worldwide receive treatment.

Testing for HIV

Once antibodies have formed in reaction to HIV, a blood test known as the *ELISA* (enzyme-linked immunosorbent assay) may detect their presence. It can take 3 to 6 months after initial infection for enough antibodies to show a positive test result, and individuals with negative test results should be retested within 6 months. When a person who previously tested *negative* (no HIV antibodies present) has a subsequent test that is *positive,* seroconversion is said to have occurred. In such a situation, the person would typically take another ELISA test, followed by a more precise test known as the *Western blot,* to confirm the presence of HIV antibodies.

A polymerase chain reaction (PCR) test detects the genetic material of HIV instead of the antibodies to the virus and can identify HIV within the first few weeks of infection. It is often performed on babies born to mothers who are HIV positive. Rapid HIV tests using blood or oral fluids are also available and can produce results in 20 minutes. However, they require a confirmatory test with positive results, which may take up to several weeks. Home kits are also available, allowing

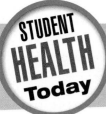
During body piercing or tattooing, the use of unsterile needles—which can transmit staph, HIV, hepatitis B and C, tetanus, and other diseases—poses a very real risk.

Laws and policies regulating body piercing and tattooing vary greatly by state. Because of the lack of universal regulatory standards and the potential for transmission of dangerous pathogens, anyone who receives a tattoo or body piercing cannot donate blood for 1 year.

If you opt for tattooing or body piercing, take the following safety precautions:

✳ Look for clean, well-lighted work areas, and inquire about sterilization procedures. Be wary of establishments that won't answer questions or show you their sterilization equipment.

✳ Packaged, sterilized needles should be used only once and then discarded. A

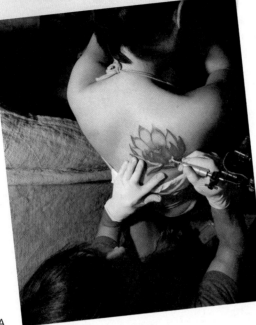

Like any activity that involves bodily fluids, tattooing carries some risk of disease transmission.

piercing gun should not be used, because it cannot be sterilized properly. Watch that the artist uses new needles and tubes from a sterile package before your procedure begins. Ask to see the sterile confirmation logo on the bag itself.

✳ Immediately before piercing or tattooing, the body area should be carefully sterilized. The artist should wash his or her hands and put on new latex gloves for each procedure. Make sure the artist changes those gloves if he or she needs to touch anything else, such as the telephone, while working.

✳ Leftover tattoo ink should be discarded after each procedure. Do not allow the artist to reuse ink that has been used for other customers. Used needles should be disposed of in a "sharps" container, a plastic container with the biohazard symbol clearly marked on it.

Source: Mayo Clinic Staff, "Tattoos: Understand Risks and Precautions," March 2012, www.mayoclinic.com

---

a person to take a blood or saliva sample and anonymously send it to a laboratory. The person then calls a number to find out their results, with professional counselors available to provide support.[62]

Health officials distinguish between *reported* and *actual* cases of HIV infection because it is believed that many HIV-positive people avoid being tested for fear of knowing the truth, or recrimination from employers, insurance companies, and medical staff. However, early detection and reporting are important because immediate treatment in early stages is critical.

what do you think?

Why is HIV testing important?

● Would you want any potential sexual partners to be tested for HIV or other STIs? How would you ask that person to get tested?

● How can you protect yourself from HIV?

New Hope and Treatments

New drugs have slowed the progression from HIV to AIDS and have prolonged life expectancies for most AIDS patients. Current treatments combine selected drugs, especially protease inhibitors and reverse transcriptase inhibitors. *Protease inhibitors* (e.g., amprenavir, ritonavir, and saquinavir) act to prevent the production of the virus in chronically infected cells that HIV has already invaded and seem to work best in combination with other therapies. Other drugs, such as AZT, ddI, ddC, d4T, and 3TC, inhibit the HIV enzyme *reverse transcriptase* before the virus has invaded the cell, thereby preventing the virus from infecting new cells. Combination treatments are still experimental, and no combination has proven effective for all people.

Preventing HIV Infection

The only way to prevent HIV infection is through the choices you make in sexual behaviors and drug use and by taking responsibility for your own health and the health of your loved ones. You can't determine the presence of HIV by looking at a person; you can't tell by questioning the person, unless he or she has been tested recently and is giving an honest answer. So what should you do?

Of course, the simplest answer is abstinence. If you do decide to be intimate, the next best option is to use a condom.

STIs: Do You Really Know What You Think You Know?

Live It! Assess Yourself

An interactive version of this assessment is available online in MasteringHealth™

The following quiz will help you evaluate whether your beliefs and attitudes about sexually transmitted infections (STIs) lead you to behaviors that increase your risk of infection. Indicate whether you believe the following items are true or false, then consult the answer key that follows.

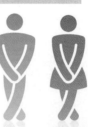

TRUE   **FALSE**

1. You can always tell when you've got an STI because the symptoms are so obvious. ○ ○

2. Some STIs can be passed on by skin-to-skin contact in the genital area. ○ ○

3. Herpes can be transmitted only when a person has visible sores on his or her genitals. ○ ○

4. Oral sex is safe sex. ○ ○

5. Condoms reduce your risk of both pregnancy and STIs. ○ ○

6. As long as you don't have anal intercourse, you can't get HIV. ○ ○

7. Sexually active females should have a regular Pap smear. ○ ○

8. Once genital warts have been removed, there is no risk of passing on the virus. ○ ○

9. You can get several STIs at one time. ○ ○

10. If the signs of an STI go away, you are cured. ○ ○

11. People who get an STI have a lot of sex partners. ○ ○

12. All STIs can be cured. ○ ○

13. You can get an STI more than once. ○ ○

Answer Key

1. **False.** The unfortunate fact is that many STIs show no symptoms. This has serious implications: (a) You can be passing on the infection without knowing it, and (b) the pathogen may be damaging your reproductive organs without you knowing it.

2. **True.** Some viruses are present on the skin around the genital area. Herpes and genital warts are the main culprits.

3. **False.** Herpes is most easily passed on when the sores and blisters are present because the fluid in the lesions carries the virus. But the virus is also found on the skin around the genital area. Most people contract herpes this way, unaware that the virus is present.

4. **False.** Oral sex is not safe sex. Herpes, genital warts, and chlamydia can all be passed on through oral sex. Condoms should be used on the penis. Dental dams should be placed over the female genitals during oral sex.

5. **True.** Condoms significantly reduce the risk of pregnancy when used correctly. They also reduce the risk of STIs. It is important to point out that abstinence is the only behavior that provides complete protection against pregnancy and STIs.

6. **False.** HIV is present in blood, semen, and vaginal fluid. Any activity that allows for the transfer of these fluids is risky. Anal intercourse is a high-risk activity, especially for the receptive (passive) partner, but other sexual activity is also a risk. When you don't know your partner's sexual history and you're not in a long-term monogamous relationship, condoms are a must.

7. **True.** A Pap smear is a simple procedure involving the scraping of a small amount of tissue from the surface of the cervix (at the upper end of the vagina). The sample is tested for abnormal cells that may indicate cancer. All sexually active women should have regular Pap smears.

8. **False.** Genital warts, which may be present on the penis, the anus, and inside and outside the vagina, can be

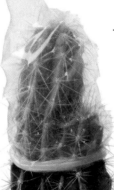

removed. However, the virus that caused the warts will always be present in the body and can be passed on to a sexual partner.

9. **True.** It is possible to have many STIs at one time. In fact, having one STI may make it more likely that a person will acquire more STIs. For example, the open sore from herpes creates a place for HIV to be transmitted.

10. **False.** The symptoms may go away, but your body is still infected. For example, syphilis is characterized by various stages. In the first stage, a painless sore called a *chancre* appears for about a week and then goes away.

11. **False.** If you have sex once with an infected partner, you are at risk for an STI.

12. **False.** Some STIs are viruses and therefore cannot be cured. There is no cure at present for herpes, HIV/AIDS, or genital warts. These STIs are treatable (to lessen the pain and irritation of symptoms), but not curable.

13. **True.** Experiencing one infection with an STI does not mean that you can never be infected again. A person can be reinfected many times with the same STI. This is especially true if a person does not get treated for the STI and thus keeps reinfecting his or her partner with the same STI.

Sources: Adapted from Jefferson County Public Health, "STD Quiz," modified January 2013, http://jeffco.us; Adapted from Family Planning Victoria, "Protection from Sexually Transmissible Infections," 2005, www.fpv.org.au

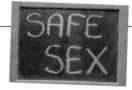

YOUR PLAN FOR CHANGE

The **Assess yourself** activity let you consider your beliefs and attitudes about STIs and identify possible risks you may be facing. Now that you have considered these results, you can begin to change behaviors that may be putting you at risk for STIs and for infection in general.

Today, you can:

◯ Put together an "emergency" supply of condoms. Outside of abstinence, condoms are your best protection against an STI. If you don't have a supply on hand, visit your local drugstore or health clinic. Remember that both men and women are responsible for preventing the transmission of STIs.

◯ To prevent infections in general, get in the habit of washing your hands regularly. After you cough, sneeze, blow your nose, use the bathroom, or prepare food, find

a sink, wet your hands with warm water, and lather up with soap. Scrub your hands for about 20 seconds (count to 20 or recite the alphabet), rinse well, and dry your hands.

Within the next 2 weeks, you can:

◯ Talk with your significant other honestly about your sexual history. Make appointments to get tested if either of you think you may have been exposed to an STI.

◯ Adjust your sleep schedule so that you're getting an adequate amount of rest every night. Being well rested is one key aspect of maintaining a healthy immune system.

By the end of the semester, you can:

◯ Check your immunization schedule and make sure you're current with all recommended vaccinations. Make an appointment with your health care provider if you need a booster or vaccine.

◯ If you are due for an annual pelvic exam, make an appointment. Ask your partner if he or she has had an annual exam and encourage him or her to make an appointment if not.

MasteringHealth™

Build your knowledge—and health!—in the Study Area of MasteringHealth with a variety of study tools.

Summary

* Your body uses several defense systems to keep pathogens from invading. The skin is the body's major protection, helped by enzymes and body secretions. The immune system creates antibodies to destroy antigens. Inflammation, fever, and pain play a role in defending the body. Vaccines bolster the body's immune system against specific diseases.

* The major classes of pathogens are bacteria, viruses, fungi, protozoans, parasitic worms, and prions. Bacterial infections include staphylococcal infections, streptococcal infections, meningitis, pneumonia, tuberculosis, and tickborne diseases. Major viral infections include the common cold, influenza, mononucleosis, and hepatitis.

* Emerging and resurgent diseases such as West Nile virus, avian flu, and *E. coli* O157:H7 pose significant threats for future generations. Many factors contribute to these risks.

* Sexually transmitted infections (STIs) are spread through vaginal intercourse, oral–genital contact, anal intercourse, hand–genital contact, and sometimes through mouth-to-mouth contact. Major STIs include chlamydia, gonorrhea, syphilis, herpes, human papillomavirus (HPV) and genital warts, candidiasis, trichomoniasis, and pubic lice.

* Acquired immunodeficiency syndrome (AIDS) is caused by the human immunodeficiency virus (HIV). HIV/AIDS is a global pandemic. Anyone can get HIV by engaging in unprotected sexual activities, by having received a blood transfusion before 1985, and by injecting drugs (or by having sex with someone who does).

Pop Quiz

1. Jennifer touched her viral herpes sore on her lip and then touched her eye. She ended up with the herpes virus in her eye as well. This is an example of
   a. acquired immunity.
   b. passive spread.
   c. autoinoculation.
   d. self-vaccination.

2. Which of the following do *not* assist the body in fighting disease?
   a. Antigens
   b. Antibodies
   c. Lymphocytes
   d. Macrophages

3. One of the best ways to prevent contagious viruses from spreading is to
   a. wash your hands frequently.
   b. cover your mouth when sneezing, and dispose of your tissues.
   c. keep your hands away from your mouth and eyes.
   d. All of the above

4. Which of the following is a *viral* disease?
   a. Hepatitis
   b. Pneumonia
   c. Malaria
   d. Streptococcal infection

5. Which of the following diseases is caused by a prion?
   a. Shingles
   b. Listeria
   c. Mad cow disease
   d. Trichomoniasis

6. The most commonly reported sexually transmitted bacterium is
   a. gonorrhea.
   b. chlamydia.
   c. syphilis.
   d. chancroid.

7. Pelvic inflammatory disease (PID) is
   a. a sexually transmitted infection.
   b. a type of urinary tract infection.
   c. an infection of a woman's fallopian tubes or uterus.
   d. a disease that both men and women can get.

8. Which of the following STIs cannot be treated with antibiotics?
   a. Chlamydia
   b. Gonorrhea
   c. Syphilis
   d. Herpes

9. Which of the following is *not* a true statement about HIV?
   a. You can tell if a potential sex partner has the virus by looking at him or her.
   b. The virus can be spread through semen or vaginal fluids.
   c. You cannot get HIV from a public restroom toilet seat.
   d. Unprotected anal sex increases risk of exposure to HIV.

10. After HIV/AIDS, which infectious disease kills more people than any other disease in the global population?
    a. Malaria
    b. Avian influenza
    c. Tuberculosis
    d. Hepatitis C

Answers to these questions can be found on page A-1.

Think about It!

1. What are three lifestyle changes you could make right now that would reduce your risk of developing an

infectious disease? What could you do to help protect your friends and family members? Your partner? How can you help reduce antibiotic resistance in the world today?

2. What is a pathogen? What are antigens? Antibodies? Discuss noncontrollable and controllable risk factors that can make you more or less susceptible to infectious pathogens in your immediate surroundings.

3. Explain why it is important to wash your hands often when you have a cold.

4. What is the difference between natural and acquired immunity? Discuss the importance of vaccinations in reducing societal risks for infectious diseases.

5. Identify five STIs and their symptoms. How are they transmitted? What are their potential long-term effects?

6. Why are women more susceptible to HIV infection than men? What implication does this have for prevention, treatment, and research?

Accessing Your Health on the Internet

The following websites explore further topics and issues related to personal health. For links to the websites below, visit the Study Area in MasteringHealth.

1. *Centers for Disease Control and Prevention (CDC).* This is the home page for the government agency dedicated to disease intervention and prevention, with links to all the latest data and publications put out by the CDC and access to the CDC research database, Wonder. www.cdc.gov

2. *Association for Professionals in Infection Control and Epidemiol-* ogy *(APIC).* Excellent resource for health professionals and consumers covering a wide range of infectious disease issues in health care, workplaces, schools, and in personal environment. www.apic.org

3. *American Sexual Health Association.* This site provides facts, support, and referrals about sexually transmitted infections and diseases. www.ashastd.org

4. *World Health Organization (WHO).* You'll gain access to the latest information on world health issues and direct access to publications and fact sheets at WHO's site. www.who.int

5. *AVERT.* This is an international site with information on HIV/AIDS, global STI statistics, interactive quizzes, and graphics displaying current statistics for vulnerable populations. www.avert.org

Reducing Risks and Coping with Chronic Diseases and Conditions

427 What causes asthma?

428 Why is my hay fever worse at certain times of the year?

429 What triggers a migraine headache?

431 What is the major cause of disability among young adults?

Typically, chronic diseases or conditions are those that take time to develop, cause progressive damage to the body, and are not easily cured. Most of the time, these chronic diseases are not caused by pathogens or transmitted by any form of personal contact. Genetics, the environment, lifestyle, and personal health habits are often implicated as underlying causes; however, the causes of many chronic diseases and conditions remain a mystery. Healthy changes in lifestyle; public health efforts aimed at research, prevention, and control; and an ever-growing arsenal of drugs that treat symptoms can minimize the effects of these diseases. Policies that protect the environment and keep us safe from chemicals can also make a difference. In this chapter we will highlight several chronic diseases, along with actions you can take to reduce your risks.

35 million

Americans live with chronic lung diseases such as asthma, emphysema, and bronchitis.

severe heat, or by years of inhaling the tar and chemicals in tobacco smoke. Occupational or home exposure to asbestos, silica dust, paint fumes and lacquers, pesticides, and a host of other environmental substances can cause lung deterioration. When the lungs are impaired, a condition known as **dyspnea,** or a choking type of breathlessness, can occur, even with mild exertion. As the lungs are oxygen deprived, the heart is forced to work harder and, over time, cardiovascular problems, suffocation, and death can occur.

Chronic Obstructive Pulmonary Disease

Chronic obstructive pulmonary disease (COPD) is a general term that refers to lower respiratory diseases where some form of obstruction interferes with a person's ability to breathe. Of the diseases, **chronic bronchitis** and **emphysema** cause the most disability and death, and their numbers are increasing. Because these conditions often occur together, the abbreviation *COPD* is often preferred by health professionals; COPD does not include other obstructive diseases such as asthma. Currently, 12 million people have diagnosed impaired lung function caused by COPD; however, these numbers are believed to grossly underestimate the over 24 million believed to have lung impairment.[3] The majority of COPD sufferers either smoke or smoked in the past. Other risks include a history of asthma, occupational exposure to certain industrial fumes or gases, and exposure to dusts, extreme temperatures, and other lung irritants.[4]

There is no cure for COPD, but much can be done to prevent it—chiefly quitting smoking or avoiding second hand smoke. Some occupations continue to pose risks, but major improvements in protecting workers have occurred in recent years. Today, most chemicals and products used in the home carry specific warning labels that suggest ways to avoid long-term exposure. The **Be Healthy, Be Green** box on the following page describes ways to minimize exposure to household chemicals.

Bronchitis

Bronchitis refers to inflammation and eventual scarring of the lining of the bronchial tubes. The bronchi connect the windpipe with the lungs; when they become inflamed or infected, less air flows from the lungs and heavy mucus forms. *Acute bronchitis* is the most common of the bronchial diseases, and symptoms often improve in a week or two.

When the symptoms of bronchitis last for at least 3 months of the year for 2 consecutive years, the condition is considered *chronic bronchitis*. In some cases, this chronic inflammation and irritation goes undiagnosed for years, particularly in smokers who feel it's a normal part of their lives. By the time many receive medical care, the damage is often already severe and may lead to heart and respiratory failure or to a chronic need to carry oxygen. Nearly 10 million Americans, the majority of whom are women, suffer from chronic bronchitis; 33 percent are under the age of 45. In 2011, non-Hispanic black Americans experienced more chronic bronchitis than non-Hispanic white Americans for the first time.[5]

---

dyspnea Shortness of breath, usually associated with disease of the heart or lungs.

chronic obstructive pulmonary diseases (COPDs) A collection of chronic lung diseases including emphysema and chronic bronchitis.

chronic bronchitis An inflammation and eventual scarring of the lining of the bronchial tubes.

emphysema Lung disease involving the gradual, irreversible destruction of the alveoli (tiny air sacs through which gas exchange occurs) of the lungs and difficulty in breathing.

> **Behaviors you pursue now can put you at a greater risk for chronic diseases. Do you know if you're putting yourself at greater risk?**

Chronic Lower Respiratory (Lung) Diseases

Chronic lower respiratory diseases (diseases of the lungs) are the third leading cause of death overall in the United States.[1] Today, more than 35 million Americans are living with chronic lung diseases such as asthma, emphysema, and bronchitis.[2]

Any disease or disorder that impairs lung function is considered a lung disease. The lungs can be damaged by a single exposure to a toxic chemical or

BE HEALTHY, BE GREEN

BE ECO-CLEAN AND ALLERGEN FREE

Exposure to household chemicals, dust, and pet dander may exacerbate asthma, allergies, and other respiratory problems. You can reduce exposure to noxious household chemicals and create a clean, comfortable home by using cleaning supplies and household products that are less toxic to the home environment. Because some companies may want you to believe their product is greener than it actually is, read the labels carefully and look for independent certifications such as the Green Seal and the Environmental Protection Agency's (EPA's) Design for the Environment program.

✳ For a handy glass and surface cleaner, mix 1/2 cup of white vinegar with 4 cups of water. Pour the solution into a spray bottle and keep the remainder for a quick and cheap refill. You can make another surface cleaner by combining 2 tablespoons of lemon juice with 4 cups of water.

✳ Baking soda is a great deodorizer and cleaner. Use it to remove carpet odors and to scour sinks, toilets, and bathtubs.
✳ Because chlorine can damage lungs, skin, and eyes, and chlorine production adds toxic chemicals such as carcinogenic dioxins to our environment, use a chlorine bleach alternative. For example, use 1/2 cup of hydrogen peroxide in your laundry or try oxygen-based bleaches.
✳ An all-purpose cleaner can be made of 1/2 cup of borax (found in the laundry aisle) and 1 gallon of hot water.
✳ For green air fresheners, use essential oils, such as lemon or lavender. Many store-bought air fresheners contain phthalates, often called "fragrance," that are related to respiratory problems and other noninfectious conditions. Place a few drops of essential oils on a piece of tissue paper, in a bowl of warm water, or in a store-bought diffuser.

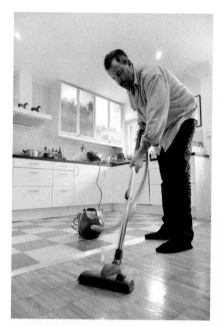

Making your own cleansers ensures that they are not harmful to your health.

Emphysema

Emphysema involves the gradual, irreversible destruction of the alveoli (tiny air sacs through which gas exchange occurs) of the lungs. Over 4.7 million Americans suffer from emphysema.[6] Over 90 percent of cases occur in people over the age of 45. Although emphysema was historically a "man's disease," today more women are diagnosed with emphysema than are men; in the last 5 years, emphysema rates have risen over 63 percent for women and declined 6 percent among men.[7] As the alveoli

extrinsic or allergic asthma A type of asthma associated with allergic triggers that tends to run in families and develops in childhood.

intrinsic or nonallergic asthma A type of asthma triggered by anything except an allergy.

are destroyed, the affected person finds it more and more difficult to exhale, struggling to take in a fresh supply of air before the air held in the lungs has been expended. The chest cavity gradually begins to expand, producing a barrel-shaped chest. (For more on emphysema and smoking, see **Chapter 8.**)

Asthma

Asthma is a long-term, chronic inflammatory disorder that blocks air flow into and out of the lungs. Asthma causes tiny airways in the lung to overreact with spasms in response to certain triggers. Symptoms include wheezing, difficulty breathing, shortness of breath, and coughing spasms. Although most asthma

attacks are mild and non–life-threatening, severe attacks can be so severe that, without rapid treatment, death may occur. Between attacks, most people have few symptoms (see **Figure 1** on the following page).

Asthma falls into two distinctly different types. The more common form of asthma, known as **extrinsic** or **allergic asthma,** is typically associated with allergic triggers; it tends to run in families and develop in childhood. Often by adulthood, a person has few episodes or the disorder completely goes away. **Intrinsic** or **nonallergic asthma** may be triggered by anything except an allergy.

Genetics may play a role in asthma development. Common asthma triggers vary from particular foods or medicines; to animal dander and other

14 Preparing for Aging, Death, and Dying

LEARNING OUTCOMES

✱ Define *aging*, and list the characteristics of successful aging.

✱ Explain how the growing population of older adults will affect society, including considerations of economics, health care, living arrangements, and ethical and moral issues.

✱ Discuss the biological and psychosocial theories of aging, and summarize major physiological changes that occur as a result of the normal aging process.

✱ Discuss unique health challenges faced by older adults, and describe strategies for

successful and healthy aging that can begin during young adulthood.

✱ Discuss death and the stages of the grieving process.

✱ Explore strategies for coping with death and loss.

✱ Explain the ethical concerns that arise from the concepts of the right to die and rational suicide.

✱ Review the decisions that need to be made when someone is dying or has died, including hospice care, funeral arrangements, wills, and organ donation.

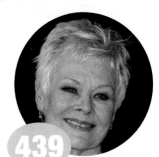

439
Is it really possible to "age gracefully"?

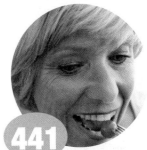

441
Is there any way to slow down the aging process?

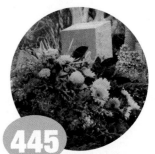

445
How can I help a friend who has just experienced a loss?

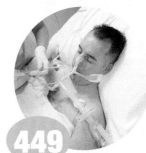

449
Why should I create a living will?

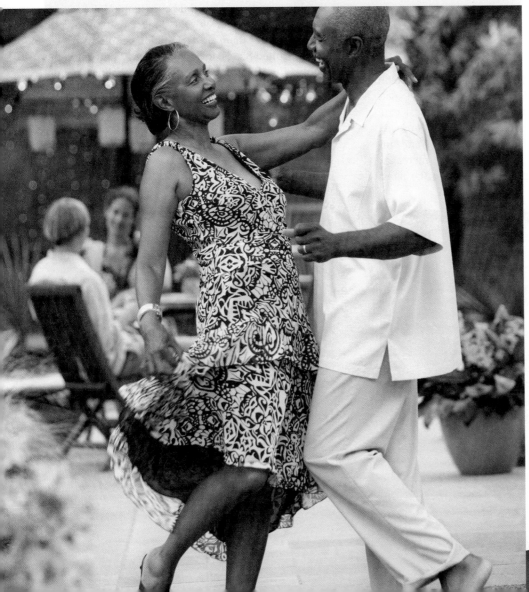

In a society that seems to worship youth, researchers have begun to offer good—even revolutionary—news about the aging process. Health promotion, disease prevention, and wellness-oriented activities can prolong vigor and productivity in older people, even among those who haven't always led model lifestyles or made healthful habits a priority. Numerous studies show that people who make even modest lifestyle changes can reap significant health benefits. In fact, getting older can mean getting better in many ways—particularly socially, psychologically, spiritually, and intellectually.

Aging

Aging has traditionally been described as the patterns of life changes that occur in members of all species as they grow older. Some believe that aging begins at the moment of conception. Others contend that it starts at birth. Still others believe that true aging does not begin until we reach our forties. The study of individual and collective aging processes, known as **gerontology**, explores the reasons for aging and the ways in which people cope with and adapt to this process. See the **Skills for Behavior Change** box for some characteristics shared among those who have aged well.

Older Adults: A Growing Population

The United States and much of the developed world are on the brink of a *longevity revolution,* one that will affect society in many ways. Medical care breakthroughs and improved understanding of fitness and nutrition have steadily increased life span. According to the latest statistics, life expectancy for a child born in the United States in 2012 is 78.9 years, over 30 years longer than for a child born in 1900.[1] Today there are 41.4 million people aged 65 or older in the United States, making up over 13 percent of the total population.[2] In comparison, a mere 3 million people were aged 65 and older in 1900 (see **Figure 14.1**).[3] Similar trends are true throughout the world, with the number of people over age 60 expected to double to 22 percent by 2050.

aging The patterns of life changes that occur in members of all species as they grow older.

gerontology The study of individual and collective aging processes.

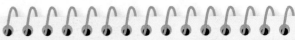

Aging Well

Many older Americans lead active, productive lives. The majority of adults over 65 continue to work, care for and help others, engage in social activities, and remain otherwise active.

The following characteristics, as indicated by older adults, can help with successful aging:

❭ Stay active through leisure activities and regular exercise.
❭ Maintain a normal weight range.
❭ Eat a healthy diet containing low levels of saturated fats, with plenty of fruits, vegetables, and whole grains.
❭ Participate in meaningful activities, like volunteering and other social activities.
❭ Don't smoke, and consume alcohol in moderation.

Sources: Federal Interagency Forum on Aging Related Statistics, "Older Americans 2012: Key Indicators of Well-Being," 2012, www.agingstats.gov; National Institute on Aging, "Healthy Aging: Lessons from the Baltimore Longitudinal Study of Aging," July 2010, www.nia.nih.gov

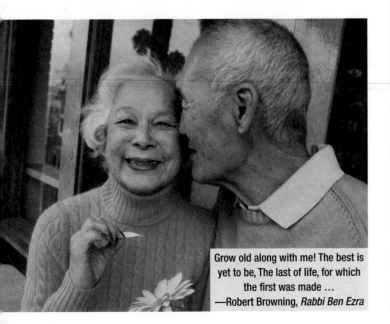

Grow old along with me! The best is yet to be, The last of life, for which the first was made …
—Robert Browning, *Rabbi Ben Ezra*

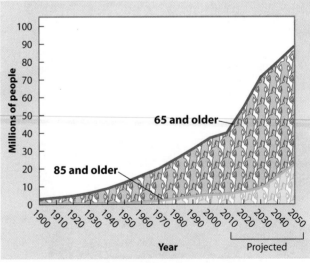

FIGURE 14.1 **Number of Americans 65 and Older (in millions), Years 1900–2008, and Projected 2013–2050**
Note: Data for 2010–2050 are projections of the population.
Source: Data from U.S. Census Bureau, Decennial Census, Population Estimates and Projections, www.census.gov

In addition to the method and details of body disposal, the type of memorial service, display of the body, and the site of burial or body disposition, loved ones must also consider the cost of funeral options, organ donation, and floral displays. Then, they usually have to contact friends and relatives, plan for the arrival of guests, choose markers, gather and submit obituary information to newspapers, and print memorial folders, in addition to many other details. The bereaved may experience undue stress, especially if the death is unexpected. People who make their own funeral arrangements ahead of time can save their loved ones from having to deal with unnecessary problems.

Wills

The issue of inheritance should be resolved before the person dies to reduce both conflict and needless expense. Unfortunately, many people are so intimidated by the thought of making a will that they never do so and die **intestate** (without a will). This is a mistake, especially because the procedure for establishing a legal will is relatively simple and inexpensive. If you don't make a will before you die, the courts (as directed by state laws) will make a will for you. Legal issues, rather than your wishes, will preside. Furthermore,

settling an estate takes longer when a person dies without a will.

intestate Dying without a will.

Organ Donation

Organ donation provides healthy organs and tissues that are transplanted from one person into another. A single donor may donate to nearly 50 people, and many organs are commonly donated. Most donations occur after death, but some things, such as a kidney, liver, or bone marrow, may be taken from a healthy living donor.[37]

The number of patients waiting for organ donations greatly outnumbers available organs. Although some people are opposed to organ transplants and tissue donation, others experience personal fulfillment from knowing that their organs may extend and improve someone else's life after their own death. The most important step on the road to being an organ donor is to enroll in your state's donor registry. Go to www.organdonor.gov to sign up under your state. It is also a good idea to indicate your decision on your driver's license, tell your family and physician, and include the donation in your will and living will. Uniform donor cards are available through the U.S. Department of Health and Human Services and through many health care foundations and nonprofit organizations.

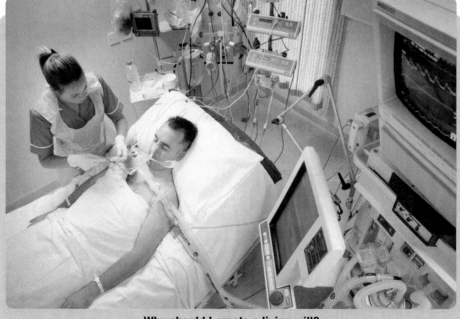

Why should I create a living will?

Today's sophisticated life-support technology can prolong a patient's life even in cases of terminal illness or mortal injury, yet not everyone would choose to have their life extended by such means. Unfortunately, by the time the situation arises, you may no longer be able to speak for yourself. Living wills, advance directives, and health care proxies can protect your wishes and aid your loved ones should you become incapacitated.

Are You Afraid of Death?

How anxious or accepting are you about the prospect of your death? Indicate how well each statement describes your attitude.

Not True at All = **0**   Mainly Not True = **1**   Not Sure = **2**

Somewhat True = **3**   Very True = **4**

1. I tend not to be very brave in times of crisis situations. **0 1 2 3 4**

2. I am something of a hypochondriac. **0 1 2 3 4**

3. I tend to be unusually frightened in airplanes at takeoff and landing. **0 1 2 3 4**

4. I would give a lot to be immortal in this body. **0 1 2 3 4**

5. I am superstitious that preparing for dying might hasten my death. **0 1 2 3 4**

6. My experience of friends and family dying has been wholly negative. **0 1 2 3 4**

7. I would feel easier being with a dying relative if he or she had not been told he or she was dying. **0 1 2 3 4**

8. I have fears of dying alone without friends around me. **0 1 2 3 4**

9. I have fears of dying slowly. **0 1 2 3 4**

10. I have fears of dying suddenly. **0 1 2 3 4**

11. I have fears of dying before my time or while my children are still young. **0 1 2 3 4**

12. I have fears of what could happen to my family after my death. **0 1 2 3 4**

13. I have fears of dying in a hospital or an institution. **0 1 2 3 4**

14. I have fears of not getting help with euthanasia. **0 1 2 3 4**

15. I have fears of dying without adequately having expressed my love to those I am close to. **0 1 2 3 4**

16. I have fears of being given unofficial and unwanted euthanasia. **0 1 2 3 4**

17. I have fears of getting insufficient pain control while dying. **0 1 2 3 4**

18. I have fears of being overmedicated and unconscious while dying. **0 1 2 3 4**

19. I have fears of being declared dead when not really dead or being buried alive. **0 1 2 3 4**

20. I have fears of what may happen to my body after death. **0 1 2 3 4**

Total points: _____

Interpreting Your Score

If you are extremely anxious (scoring 38 or more), you might consider counseling or therapy; if you are unusually anxious (scoring between 24 and 37), you might want to find a method of meditation, philosophy, or spiritual practice to help experience, explore, and accept your feelings about death. Average anxiety is a score under 24.

YOUR PLAN FOR CHANGE

The **Assess yourself** activity encouraged you to explore your death-related anxiety. Now that you have considered your results, you may want to take steps to lessen your fears about death and dying.

Today, you can:

○ Learn about advance directives. Visit a low-cost legal clinic for information and a sample. You can also locate samples online, including the "Five Wishes" document, which is available at www.agingwithdignity.org.

○ Fill out an organ donation card. Knowing that you may be able to prolong another person's life after your death can help you feel more at peace with your mortality.

Within the next 2 weeks, you can:

○ Write down a list of goals you want to attain by ages 30, 40, and 50. Think about the steps you need to take to attain these goals.

○ Talk to family members about their life goals. What have they achieved, and what do they wish they had done differently? What can you learn from their experiences?

By the end of the semester, you can:

○ Consider how you feel about various medical techniques that might be used in the event you become incapacitated. Do you feel comfortable being kept alive by a machine? Make your wishes on these matters known to family members and friends, and put them in writing.

○ Talk to your parents or grandparents about the arrangements they prefer in the event of their death. Do they want a burial or cremation? A full funeral or a small service? Making these decisions now will save you and your loved ones stress later.

MasteringHealth™

Build your knowledge—and health!—in the Study Area of MasteringHealth with a variety of study tools.

Summary

* Aging is the patterns of life changes that occur in members of all species as they grow older. The growing number of older adults (people aged 65 and older) has an increasing impact on society in terms of the economy, health care, housing, and ethical considerations.

* Biological explanations of aging include the wear-and-tear theory, the cellular theory, the genetic mutation theory, and the autoimmune theory.

* Aging changes the body and mind in many ways. Physical changes occur in the skin, bones and joints, head and face, urinary tract, heart and lungs, senses, sexual function, and intelligence and memory. Major physical concerns are osteoporosis, urinary incontinence, and changes in eyesight and hearing. Most older people maintain a high level of intelligence and memory. Potential mental problems include Alzheimer's disease.

* Lifestyle choices we make today will affect health status later in life. Choosing to exercise, eat a healthy diet, foster lasting relationships, and enrich your spiritual side will contribute to healthy aging.

* *Death* can be defined biologically in terms of brain death or the cessation of vital functions. Dying is a multifaceted emotional process, and individuals may experience emotional stages of dying such as denial, anger, bargaining, depression, and acceptance. Social death results when a person is no longer treated as living.

* Grief is the state of distress felt after loss. People differ in their responses to grief.

* The right to die by rational suicide involves ethical, moral, and legal issues. Choices of care for the terminally ill include hospice care. After death, making funeral arrangements adds to the pressures on survivors. Decisions should be made in advance of death through wills and organ donation cards.

Pop Quiz

1. Which biological theory of aging supports the concept that body cells are able to reproduce only so many times throughout life?
   a. Wear-and-tear theory
   b. Cellular theory
   c. Autoimmune theory
   d. Genetic mutation theory

2. The progressive breakdown of joint cartilage is known as
   a. osteoporosis.
   b. osteoarthritis.
   c. calcium loss.
   d. vitamin D deficiency.

3. Martha's ophthalmologist tells her that she has a condition that involves the breakdown of the light-sensitive area of the retina that is affecting her sharp, direct vision. What is this condition?
   a. Cataracts
   b. Glaucoma
   c. Macular degeneration
   d. Nearsightedness

4. What is the most common form of dementia in older adults?
   a. Alzheimer's disease
   b. Incontinence
   c. Depression
   d. Psychosis

5. The keys to successful aging include
   a. being physically active.
   b. eating a healthy diet.
   c. not smoking.
   d. All of the above

6. The study of death and dying is called
   a. thanatology.
   b. gerontology.
   c. biology.
   d. a living will.

7. The Kübler-Ross stage of dying in which the individual rejects death emotionally and feels a sense of shock and disbelief is known as
   a. acceptance.
   b. bargaining.
   c. denial.
   d. anger.

8. A culturally prescribed and accepted period of grief for someone who has died is known as
   a. bereavement.
   b. grief work.
   c. coping with loss.
   d. mourning.

9. Grief work is
   a. the process of integrating the reality of the loss with everyday life and learning to feel better.
   b. the total acceptance that a loved one has died.
   c. assigning feelings to the loss of a loved one.
   d. completing the cultural rituals required to express one's grief.

10. Kerri's elderly grandmother is terminally ill and wants to die without medical intervention. Her family has agreed to withhold treatment that may prolong her life. This is called
    a. rational suicide.
    b. health care proxy.
    c. passive euthanasia.
    d. active euthanasia.

Answers to these questions can be found on page A-1.

Think about It!

1. Discuss when you think people should start deciding whether to have an advance directive. What are some important considerations when preparing an advance directive?
2. As the older population grows, how will it affect your life? Would you be willing to pay higher taxes to support government social programs for older adults? Why or why not?
3. List the major physical and mental changes that occur with aging. Which of these, if any, can you change? Discuss actions you can start taking now to ensure a healthier aging process.
4. Discuss why so many of us deny death. How could death become a more acceptable topic to discuss?
5. Debate whether rational suicide should be legalized for the terminally ill. What restrictions would you include in a law?

Accessing Your Health on the Internet

The following websites explore further topics related to personal health. For links to the websites, visit the Study Area in MasteringHealth.

1. *Administration on Aging.* This is a link to the U.S. Department of Health and Human Services, dedicated to addressing the health needs of older adults. www.aoa.gov
2. *Alzheimer's Association.* This site includes media releases, position statements, fact sheets, and research on Alzheimer's disease. www.alz.org
3. *Grieving.com.* This forum site addresses all aspects of grief and loss, including terminal illness, non-death losses, and caregiving. http://forums.grieving.com
4. *National Hospice and Palliative Care Organization.* This site offers information on hospice care, including resources for finding a hospice, end-of-life issues, and advance directives. www.nhpco.org
5. *AARP.* This site includes comprehensive information on issues related to aging that include longevity and caregiving. www.aarp.org
6. *National Institute on Aging.* A site that provides information and research updates on aging related issues. www.nia.nih.gov

15 Promoting Environmental Health

LEARNING OUTCOMES

* Explain the environmental impact associated with global population growth.

* Discuss major causes of air pollution and the consequences of the accumulation of greenhouse gases and ozone depletion.

* Identify sources of water pollution and chemical contaminants often found in water.

* Distinguish municipal solid waste from hazardous waste and list strategies for reducing land pollution.

* Discuss the health concerns associated with ionizing and nonionizing radiation.

* Describe the physiological consequences of noise pollution and how to prevent or reduce its effects.

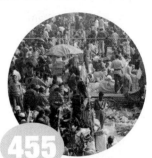

455

Why is population growth an environmental issue?

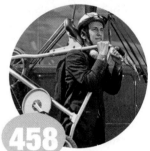

458

How can I reduce my carbon footprint?

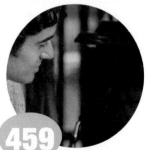

459

How can air pollution be a problem indoors?

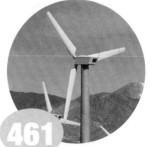

461

How can I help prevent global warming?

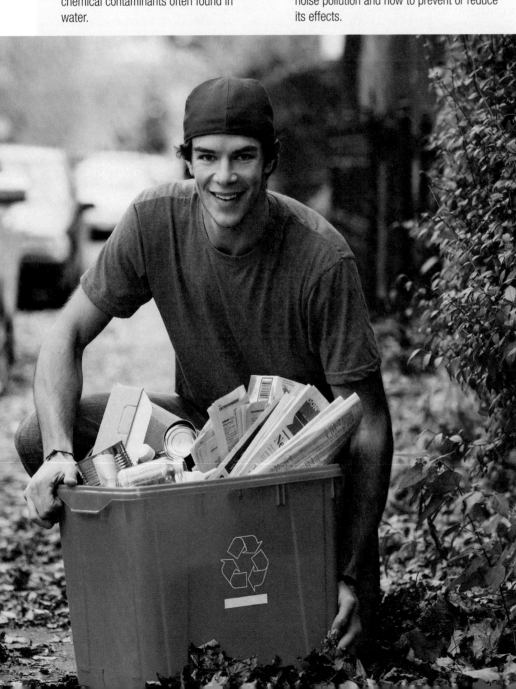

". . . the fact is, the 12 hottest years on record have all come in the last 15. Heat waves, droughts, wildfires, and floods—all are now more frequent and intense. We can choose to believe that Superstorm Sandy, and the most severe drought in decades, and the worst wildfires some states have ever seen were all just a freak coincidence. Or we can choose to believe in the overwhelming judgment of science—and act before it's too late."

Barack Obama, "2013 State of the Union Address," February 12, 2013.

We live in an especially dangerous time—for us and for future generations. The global population has grown more in the past 50 years than at any other time in human history, posing a potentially devastating threat to the natural resources we consume and our capacity to survive. Polar ice caps and glaciers are melting at rates that surpass even the most dire predictions of just a decade ago, and threats of rising sea levels loom large. One in four mammals is now threatened with extinction as humans destroy habitat, exacerbate drought and flooding due to climate change, voraciously consume precious resources, and pollute the environment. Clean water is becoming scarce, fossil fuels are being depleted at unprecedented rates, and massive amounts of solid and hazardous waste are threatening the future of all living things.

Individuals, communities, and political powers must take action now to make positive change. We must reduce consumption, waste less, be less selfish when it comes to personal comfort and perceived needs, and force governments to enact and enforce environmentally responsible legislation. Staying informed and becoming an advocate for a healthy environment are just two of the key things you can do to help.

The Threat of Overpopulation

The United Nations projects that the world population will grow from its current level of 7 billion to 9.3 billion by 2050 and over 10.1 billion by 2100[1] (Figure 15.1). Tomorrow's population will be more industrialized, consume more resources, and produce even more waste than did previous generations unless actions are taken to control population growth.[2]

carrying capacity of the earth The largest population that can be supported indefinitely given the resources available in the environment.

ecosystem Collection of physical (nonliving) and biological (living) components of an environment and the relationships between them.

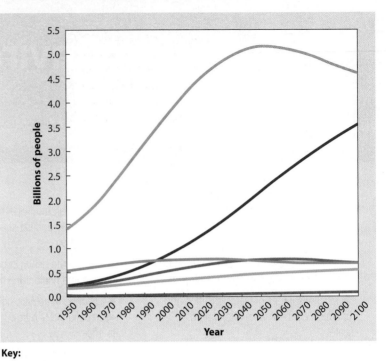

Key:
- Asia
- Africa
- Latin America and the Caribbean
- Europe
- Northern America
- Oceania

FIGURE 15.1 Estimated and Projected World Population Growth, 1950–2100

Source: United Nations, Department of Economic and Social Affairs, Population Division, "World Population Prospects: The 2010 Revision," http://esa.un.org, © 2011. Reprinted by permission.

Bursting with People: Measuring the Impact

Today, experts are analyzing the **carrying capacity of the earth**—the largest population that can be supported indefinitely, given the resources available in the environment. At what point will we be unable to restore the balance between humans and nature? Consider this: Since 1996, the demand for natural resources has doubled. One report indicates that it will take the resources of two planets to meet our growing demand by 2030. Simply put, we are running out of the natural resources necessary to sustain us, and the problem is growing at an unprecedented rate.[3] Evidence of the effects of unchecked population growth is everywhere:

- **Impact on other species.** Changes in the **ecosystem** are resulting in mass destruction of many species and their habitats.

97% of global growth in the next four decades will happen in Asia, Africa, Latin America, and the Caribbean.

Rain forests are being depleted, oceans are being polluted, and over half of the world's wetlands have been lost in the last century. The search for habitat to raise young grows more difficult for many species and many succumb to hazards produced by humans.[4] Twelve percent of birds are threatened with extinction. More than 100 mammal species are already extinct, and others, such as tigers, have seen populations decline by 95 percent in the last century. About one third of amphibians are already gone. Poaching of many species such as elephants and rhinos has decimated herds as people hunt for precious ivory.[5] Many of those that survive in areas where environmental contaminants threaten water and land have chemically induced ailments or genetic mutations that will hasten their demise.[6]

● **Impact on the food supply.** We are currently fishing the oceans at rates that are 250 percent more than they can regenerate, and scientists project a global collapse of all fish species by 2050.[7]

Aquatic ecosystems continue to be heavily exploited by chemical and human waste. Recent reports indicate that our oceans are 30 percent more acidic now than they were just 200 years ago, largely due to human-caused pollutants. Living coral reefs that support aquatic life have declined by over 50 percent in the last 27 years, with virtual dead zones stretching for miles on ocean floors.[8] Massive storms, earthquakes, radiation, invasive species, and other threats add to other contaminants, which hasten the demise of natural sea life and lead to increased aquaculture and fish farms rather than wild fish catches.

Today, our global quest for enough food means that increasing amounts of the earth's surface is used for agriculture. Because agriculture accounts for over 90 percent of our global water footprint, groundwater withdrawals have tripled in the last 50 years, which puts increased pressure on dwindling water reserves.[9] Drought and erosion make growing food increasingly difficult, and food shortages and famine are occurring in many regions of the world with increasing frequency.

● **Land degradation and contamination of drinking water.** The per capita availability of fresh water is declining rapidly, and contaminated water remains the greatest single environmental cause of human illness. Unsustainable land use and climate change are increasing land degradation, including erosion, toxic chemical infiltration, nutrient depletion, deforestation, and other problems that will inevitably affect human life.

● **Energy consumption.** "Use it *and* lose it" is an apt saying for our greedy use of nonrenewable **fossil fuels** (oil, coal, natural gas). Although we are seeing a shift toward renewable energy sources, such as hydropower, solar and wind power, and biomass power, the predominant energy sources are still fossil fuels. The United States is the largest consumer of liquid fossil fuels and natural gas, and among the top four consumers of nuclear power, coal, and hydroelectric power.[10] We live in bigger houses, drive more miles, consume more water, and waste more food than do most other nations. In many developing regions of the world, movement toward greater industrialization and more citizen affluence has also resulted in skyrocketing demand for limited fossil fuels.

fossil fuel Carbon-based material used for energy; includes oil, coal, and natural gas.

"Why Should I Care?"

Imagine waking up in the morning and finding that you have no water for a shower; that your lights can be used only a few hours each day or not at all; and gas is so expensive that you can't even think about driving your car. Such scenarios are not the imaginings of science fiction. Major difficulties loom unless we take action to change our current rate of population growth and our consumption of natural resources, and unless the global community acts together to enforce policies and programs to check rampant population growth.

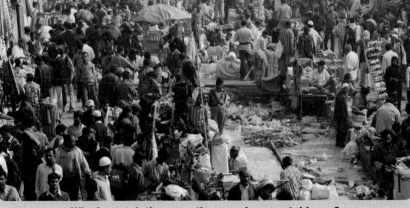

Why is population growth an environmental issue?

Every year the global population grows by 90 million, but Earth's resources are not expanding. Population increases are believed to be responsible for most of the current environmental stress.

Factors That Affect Population Growth

A number of factors have led to the world population's increase. Key indicators of growth patterns are fertility and mortality rates.

fertility rate Average number of births a female in a certain population has during her reproductive years.

pollutant Substance that contaminates some aspect of the environment and causes potential harm to living organisms.

Fertility rate refers to how many births a woman has by the end of her reproductive life. The global fertility rate in the world has declined to an average of 2.5 births per woman. While Europe, the United States, Mexico, China and others have shown consistent declines in recent years, other countries such as Niger (7 births per woman) and Somalia (6 births per woman) continue to have higher fertility rates. Today, the U.S. fertility rate is just over 2 births per woman—slightly more than "replacement" values necessary to sustain population growth. While some argue that lower fertility rates mean slowing population growth, current global projections (over 9.3 billion people by 2050) are actually based on continued declines (Table 15.1).[11] Historically, in countries where women have little education and little control over reproductive choices, and where birth control is either not available or frowned upon, pregnancy rates continue to rise. However, as women become more educated, obtain higher socioeconomic status, and have more control over reproduction—as birth control becomes more accessible—fertility rates decline. Recognizing that population control will be essential in the decades ahead, many countries have enacted strict population control measures or have encouraged their citizens to limit the size of their families. Proponents of *zero population growth* believe that each couple should produce only two offspring, allowing the population to stabilize.

Mortality rates from chronic and infectious diseases have declined as a result of improved public health infrastructure, increased availability of drugs and vaccines, better disaster preparedness, and other factors. As people live longer, they add more years of resource consumption and add to the overall human footprint on the environment.

Differing Growth Rates

The country projected to have the largest population increase in coming decades is India—adding another 600 million people by 2050—surpassing China as the most populous nation.[12] With a current population of over 316 million and a growth rate around 1 percent in 2012, the United States continues to lead most other industrialized nations in population growth rate.[13] It also has the largest "ecological footprint," exerting a greater impact on many of the planet's resources than any other nation.[14]

what do you think?

Should individuals get tax breaks for having fewer children?
● How would such policies compare to our current policies?
● Can you think of other policies that might be effective in encouraging population control and resource conservation in the United States?

TABLE 15.1 Selected Total Fertility Rates Worldwide—2013 Estimates

Country	Number of Children Born per Woman*	Rank
Niger	7.03	1
Mali	6.25	2
Somalia	6.16	3
Afghanistan	5.54	8
India	2.55	81
Mexico	2.25	99
Saudi Arabia	2.21	103
United States	2.06	121
Australia	1.77	162
Russia	1.61	178
Canada	1.59	180
China	1.55	184
Japan	1.39	208

*Indicates average number of children that would be born per woman if all women lived to the end of their childbearing years and bore children according to a given fertility rate at each age.
Source: Data from Central Intelligence Agency World Fact Book, "Total Fertility Rate (Children Born/Woman) 2013 Country Ranks, by Rank 2013," 2013, www.cia.gov

Air Pollution

The term *air pollution* refers to the presence of substances (suspended particles and vapors) not found in perfectly clean air. From the beginning of time, natural events, living creatures, and toxic byproducts have polluted the environment. Air pollution is not new, but the vast array of **pollutants** that now exist and their potential interactive effects are.

Air pollutants are either *naturally occurring* or *anthropogenic* (caused by humans). Naturally occurring air pollutants include *particulate matter*, such as ash from volcanic eruptions, soil, and dust. Anthropogenic sources include those caused by *stationary sources* (e.g., power plants, factories, and refineries) and *mobile sources* such as vehicles. Mobile sources include *on-road* vehicles (cars, trucks, and buses) or *off-road* sources (such as construction equipment). Planes, trains, and watercraft are considered *non-road* sources.[15] According to U.S. Environmental Protection Agency estimates, mobile sources are major contributors of air pollutants like carbon monoxide (CO), sulfur oxides (SO_x), and nitrogen oxides (NO_x). Motor vehicles alone contribute nearly 30 percent of all CO_2 emissions in the U.S.[16] For every gallon of gas you burn, 25 pounds of CO_2 and other gases are released—most of it from right out of your tailpipe.

15.2 Sources, Health Effects, and Welfare Effects for Major Air Pollutants

Pollutant	Description	Sources	Health Effects	Welfare Effects
Carbon monoxide (CO)	Colorless, odorless gas	Motor vehicle exhaust; indoor sources include kerosene and wood-burning stoves	Headaches, reduced mental alertness, heart attack, cardiovascular diseases, impaired fetal development, death	Contributes to the formation of smog
Sulfur dioxide (SO_2)	Colorless gas that dissolves in water vapor to form acid and interacts with other gases and particles in the air	Coal-fired power plants, petroleum refineries, manufacture of sulfuric acid, and smelting of ores containing sulfur	Eye irritation, wheezing, chest tightness, shortness of breath, lung damage	Contributes to the formation of acid rain, visibility impairment, plant and water damage, aesthetic damage
Nitrogen dioxide (NO_2)	Reddish brown, highly reactive gas	Motor vehicles, electric utilities, and other industrial, commercial, and residential sources that burn fuels	Susceptibility to respiratory infections, irritation of the lungs and respiratory symptoms (e.g., cough, chest pain, difficulty breathing)	Contributes to the formation of smog, acid rain, water quality deterioration, global warming, and visibility impairment
Ozone (O_3)	Gaseous pollutant when formed in the stratosphere	Vehicle exhaust and certain other fumes; formed from other air pollutants in the presence of sunlight	Eye and throat irritation, coughing, respiratory tract problems, asthma, lung damage	Plant and ecosystem damage, global warming
Lead (Pb)	Metallic element	Metal refineries, lead smelters, battery manufacturers, iron and steel producers	Anemia, high blood pressure, brain and kidney damage, neurological disorders, cancer, lowered IQ	Affects animals, plants, and the aquatic ecosystem
Particulate matter (PM)	Very small particles of soot, dust, or other matter, including tiny droplets of liquids	Diesel engines, power plants, industries, windblown dust, wood stoves, indoor cooking and heating	Eye irritation, asthma, bronchitis, lung damage, cancer, heavy metal poisoning, cardiovascular effects	Visibility impairment, atmospheric deposition, aesthetic damage

Source: U.S. Environmental Protection Agency, "Air and Radiation: Air Pollutants," 2012, www.epa.gov

Components of Air Pollution

Concern about air quality prompted Congress to pass the Clean Air Act in 1970 and to amend it several times since then. The act established standards for six of the most widespread air pollutants that seriously affect health: sulfur dioxide, particulates, carbon monoxide, nitrogen dioxide, ground-level ozone, and lead. See Table 15.2 for an overview of the sources and effects of these pollutants.

Photochemical Smog

Smog is a brownish haze produced by the photochemical reaction of sunlight with **hydrocarbons**, nitrogen compounds, and other gases in vehicle exhaust. It is sometimes called *ozone pollution* because ozone is a main component of smog. Smog tends to form in areas that experience a **temperature inversion**, in which a cool layer of air is trapped under a layer of warmer air, preventing the air from circulating. Smog is more likely to occur in valley areas surrounded by hills or mountains, as in Los Angeles or Phoenix.

The most noticeable adverse effects of smog are difficulty breathing, burning eyes, headaches, and nausea. Long-term exposure poses serious health risks, particularly for children, older adults, pregnant women, and people with chronic respiratory disorders.

Air Quality Index

The Air Quality Index (AQI) is a measure of how clean or polluted the air is on a given day. The AQI focuses on health effects that can happen within a few hours or days after breathing polluted air.

The AQI runs from 0 to 500: The higher the AQI value, the greater the level of air pollution and associated health risks. An AQI value of 100 generally corresponds to the national air quality standard for the pollutant, which is the level the EPA has set to protect public health. Air Quality Index values below 100 are generally considered satisfactory. When AQI

smog Brownish haze that is a form of pollution produced by the photochemical reaction of sunlight with hydrocarbons, nitrogen compounds, and other gases in vehicle exhaust.

hydrocarbons Chemical compounds containing carbon and hydrogen.

temperature inversion weather condition that occurs when a layer of cool air is trapped under a layer of warmer air.

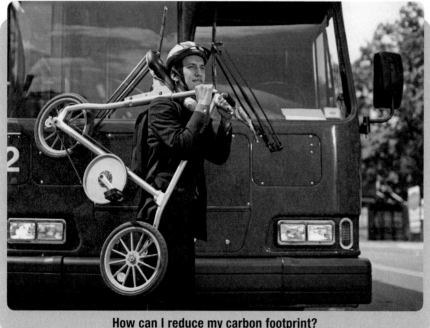

How can I reduce my carbon footprint?

Reducing our individual carbon footprint is a key goal in combating air pollution, global warming, and climate change. Making small changes such as driving less, riding your bike more, taking public transportation or carpooling, turning off lights, and recycling and composting can all help to reduce your carbon footprint.

values rise above 100, air quality is considered unhealthy—at certain levels for specific groups of people and at higher levels, for everyone.

As shown in **Figure 15.2**, the EPA has divided the AQI scale into six categories with corresponding color codes. National and local weather reports generally include information on the day's AQI.

Acid Deposition and Acid Rain

Acid deposition is replacing the term *acid rain* in scientific circles; it refers to the deposition of *wet* (rain, snow, sleet, fog, cloud water, and dew) and *dry* (acidifying particles and gases) acidic components that fall to the earth in dust or smoke.[17] Sulfur dioxide (SO_2) and nitrogen oxide (NO_x) cause damage to plants, aquatic animals, forests, and humans over time. Almost two thirds of all U.S. sulfur dioxide and one fourth of all U.S. nitrogen oxides come from burning fossil fuels to generate electricity.[18] When coal-powered plants, oil refineries, and other facilities burn these fuels, sulfur and nitrogen in the emissions combine with oxygen and sunlight to become sulfur dioxide and nitrogen oxide. Small acid particles are carried by the wind and combine with moisture to produce acidic rain or snow.[19]

Acid deposition gradually acidifies ponds, lakes, and other bodies of water. Once the acid content of the water reaches a certain level, plant and animal life cannot survive.[20] Ironically, acidified lakes

acid deposition Acidification process that occurs when pollutants are deposited by precipitation, clouds, or directly on the land.

leach To dissolve and filter through soil.

and ponds become a crystal-clear deep blue, giving the illusion of beauty and health even as they wreak destruction. Every year, acid deposition destroys millions of trees in Europe and North America. Sugar maples and other trees in the northeastern United States appear to be the newest victims of acid deposition because they are having difficulty regenerating seedlings destroyed by these deposits. Scientists have concluded that much of the world's forestlands are now experiencing damaging levels of acid deposition.[21]

Acid deposition aggravates and may even cause bronchitis, asthma, and other respiratory problems, and people with emphysema or heart disease may suffer from exposure.[22] It may also be hazardous to fetuses. Acid deposition can cause metals such as aluminum, cadmium, lead, and mercury to **leach** out of the soil. If these metals make their way into water or food supplies, they can cause cancer in humans.

Although there have been substantial reductions in SO_2 and NO_x emissions from power plants in the last decade, full recovery is still years away. Calls for increased production of coal and more refineries in the United States may result in significant increases in emissions in the next decades unless policies mandating "cleaner" coal technology are put into effect and monitored. Global pressure to reduce use and invest in technology to dramatically reduce coal emissions was a key aspect of 2012 global environmental meetings in Rio de Janeiro and in other parts of the world. Although coal is cleaner than

When the AQI is in this range:	... air quality conditions are	... as symbolized by this color:
0 to 50	Good	Green
51 to 100	Moderate	Yellow
101 to 150	Unhealthy for sensitive groups	Orange
151 to 200	Unhealthy	Red
201 to 300	Very unhealthy	Purple
301 to 500	Hazardous	Maroon

FIGURE 15.2 Air Quality Index

The EPA provides individual AQIs for ground-level ozone, particle pollution, carbon monoxide, sulfur dioxide, and nitrogen dioxide. All of the AQIs are presented using the general values, categories, and colors of this figure.

Source: U.S. Environmental Protection Agency, "Air Quality Index: A Guide to Air Quality and Your Health," Updated August 2011, www.airnow.gov

it was a decade ago from a production standpoint, the idea of clean coal is far from reality (even though a "clean coal" label suggests otherwise).[23]

Indoor Air Pollution

A growing body of scientific evidence indicates that the air within homes and other buildings can be 10 to 40 times more hazardous than outdoor air, even in the most industrialized cities. Potentially dangerous chemical compounds can increase risks of cancer, contribute to respiratory problems, reduce the immune system's ability to fight disease, and increase problems with allergies and allergic reactions.

Indoor air pollution comes primarily from cooking stoves and furnaces, woodstoves and space heaters, household cleaners and solvents, pesticides, passive cigarette smoke exposure, asbestos, formaldehyde, radon, and lead. An emerging source of indoor air pollution is mold. In addition, that "new car" smell we like is often related to potentially harmful chemicals found in interior fabrics, upholstery, and glues. Today, more and more manufacturers are offering green building products and furnishings, such as natural fiber fabrics, untreated wood for furniture and floors, low-VOC (volatile organic compound) paints, and many other products in an attempt to reduce potential pollutants. See the **Skills for Behavior Change** box for

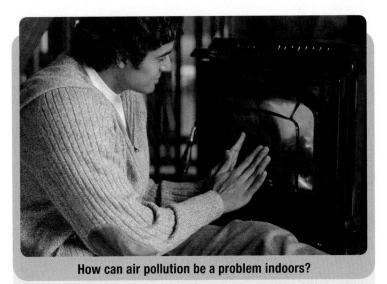

How can air pollution be a problem indoors?

Inside air can be 10 to 40 times more hazardous than outside air. Indoor air pollution comes from woodstoves, furnaces, cigarette smoke, asbestos, formaldehyde, radon, lead, mold, and household chemicals.

ideas on how to become a more environmentally conscious consumer of products for your home.

Multiple factors, including age, individual sensitivity, preexisting medical conditions, liver function, and the condition of the immune and respiratory systems contribute to a person's risk for being affected by indoor air pollution. Those with allergies may be particularly vulnerable. Health effects may develop over years of exposure or may occur in response to toxic levels of pollutants. Room temperature and humidity also play a role.

Preventing indoor air pollution should focus on three main areas: *source control* (eliminating or reducing contaminants), *ventilation improvements* (increasing the amount of outdoor air coming indoors), and *air cleaners* (removing particulates from the air).[24]

Environmental Tobacco Smoke
Perhaps the greatest source of indoor air pollution is *environmental tobacco smoke (ETS)*, also known as secondhand smoke, which contains carbon monoxide and cancer-causing particulates. The level of carbon monoxide in cigarette smoke in enclosed spaces has been found to be 4,000 times higher than that allowed in the clean air standard established by the EPA.[25]

Moreover, the U.S. Surgeon General has reported that there are more than 50 carcinogens in environmental tobacco smoke. Itchy eyes, breathing difficulties, headaches, nausea, and dizziness often occur in those with sensitivities. The only truly effective way to eliminate ETS in public places is to enact strict no-smoking policies. The Centers for Disease Control and Prevention (CDC) estimates that every U.S. state will have some form of smoking ban by 2020. Thirty-eight states currently have 100 percent smoking bans in restaurants, and 32 states have total bans in bars. In addition, many major cities and municipalities have banned indoor smoking. To date, as many as 82 percent of U.S. workers have some form of smoking ban in their workplace, and many cities have banned outdoor smoking in public places. To protect vulnerable children from smoking parents, bans on smoking in automobiles while children are present are on the increase.[26]

Home Heating

Woodstoves emit significant levels of particulates and carbon monoxide in addition to other pollutants, such as sulfur dioxide. If you rely on wood for heating, make sure that your stove is properly installed, vented, and maintained. Burning properly seasoned wood reduces particulates. People who rely on oil- or gas-fired furnaces also need to make sure that these appliances are properly installed, ventilated, and maintained.

asbestos Mineral compound that separates into stringy fibers and lodges in the lungs, where it can cause various diseases.

formaldehyde Colorless, strong-smelling gas released through outgassing; causes respiratory and other health problems.

radon Naturally occurring radioactive gas resulting from the decay of certain radioactive elements.

lead Highly toxic metal found in emissions from lead smelters and processing plants; also sometimes found in pipes or paint in older buildings.

Asbestos

Asbestos is a mineral compound that was once commonly used in insulating materials, but also found its way into vinyl flooring, shingles/roofing materials, heating pipe coverings, and many other products in buildings constructed before 1970. When bonded to other materials, asbestos is relatively harmless, but if its tiny fibers become loosened and airborne, they can embed themselves in the lungs. Their presence leads to cancer of the lungs, stomach, and chest lining and other life-threatening lung diseases called *mesothelioma* and *asbestosis*.

Formaldehyde

Formaldehyde is a colorless, strong-smelling gas present in some carpets, draperies, furniture, particleboard, plywood, wood paneling, countertops, and many adhesives. It is released into the air in a process called *outgassing*. Outgassing is highest in new products, but the process can continue for many years. Exposure to formaldehyde can cause respiratory problems, dizziness, fatigue, nausea, and rashes. Long-term exposure can lead to central nervous system disorders and cancer.

Radon

Radon, an odorless, colorless gas, penetrates homes through cracks, pipes, sump pits, and other openings in the basement or foundation. The U.S. Surgeon General warns that radon is the second leading cause of lung cancer, after smoking, each year.[27] The EPA estimates that as many as 8.1 million homes (1 out of every 15) throughout the country have elevated levels of radon.[28] Since 1988, the EPA and the Office of the Surgeon General have recommended that homes below the third floor be tested for radon and that Americans test their homes every 2 years or when they move into a new home. Low-cost radon test kits are available online, in hardware stores, and through other retail outlets.

Lead

Lead is a highly toxic metal common in paints used in many American homes before its banning in 1978. By some estimates, as many as 25 percent of U.S. homes still have lead-based paint hazards, and nearly 535,000 children aged 1 to 5 years old in the United States have blood lead levels that are high.[29] It is also found in batteries, soils, drinking water, older pipes, dishes, and other items. In recent years, toys produced in China and other regions of the world have been recalled owing to unsafe levels of lead. Low-income individuals living in older homes that may not be in compliance with newer recommended lead exposure are at higher risk. Risk in general appears to be greatest during home remodeling and for persons with occupations in fields such as construction, e-waste/recycling, and demolition.[30]

Lead affects the circulatory, reproductive, urinary tract, kidneys, and nervous systems, and it can accumulate in bone and other tissues. It is particularly detrimental to children and fetuses, and can cause birth defects, learning problems, behavioral abnormalities, and other health problems. To reduce unsafe exposure at home, use water filters, keep areas where children play clean and dust free, regularly wash the child's hands and toys, leave lead-based paint undisturbed if it is in good condition, or hire a professional contractor to remove it.

Mold

Molds are fungi that live both indoors and outdoors, producing tiny reproductive spores that waft through the air. When they land on a damp spot indoors, they may begin growing and digesting whatever they are on, including wood, paper, carpet, and food. In general, molds are harmless; however, exposure to molds may lead to nasal stuffiness, eye irritation, wheezing, skin irritation, fever, or shortness of breath for some people.[31] For ways to reduce your exposure to mold, see the **Skills for Behavior Change** box.

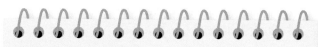

Skills for Behavior Change

Avoiding Mold

❱ Keep the humidity level between 40 and 60 percent.
❱ Be sure your living space has adequate ventilation, including exhaust fans in the kitchen and bathrooms.
❱ Add mold inhibitors to paints or buy paints with mold-resistant properties. If you notice a musty smell, call your landlord. If you see mold, call your landlord!
❱ Do not carpet bathrooms and basements.
❱ Use a dehumidifier in damp rooms.
❱ Wear masks and gloves when applying antimold products, and use them sparingly if at all.
❱ Get rid of mattresses and other furniture that may have been exposed to moisture or situations where slow drying may occur.
❱ Dry clothing thoroughly before folding and placing in drawers or closets.
❱ When buying or renting a house, have a mold inspection performed and check regularly.

Ozone Layer Depletion

The ozone layer is a stratum in the stratosphere—the highest level of Earth's atmosphere, located 12 to 30 miles above the surface—that protects our planet and its inhabitants from ultraviolet B (UVB) radiation, a primary cause of skin cancer. Such radiation damages DNA and weakens human and animal immune systems. In the 1970s, scientists began to warn of a breakdown in the ozone layer. Certain chemicals, especially refrigerants, solvents, and aerosols called **chlorofluorocarbons (CFCs)**, were contributing to the ozone layer's rapid depletion.

The U.S. government banned the use of CFCs, and the discovery of an ozone "hole" over Antarctica led to international treaties such as the Vienna Convention and Montreal Protocol, whereby the United States and other nations agreed to further reduce the use of CFCs and other ozone-depleting chemicals. Today, more than 197 United Nations countries have agreed to basic protocols designed to preserve and protect the ozone layer.[32] Although the ban on CFCs is believed to be responsible for slowing the depletion of the ozone layer, some CFC replacements may also cause damage by contributing to the enhanced greenhouse effect.

Climate Change

Climate change refers to a shift in typical weather patterns across the world. These changes can include fluctuations in seasonal temperatures, rain or snowfall amounts, and the occurrence of catastrophic storms. **Global warming** is a type of climate change where average temperatures increase. Over the last 100 years, the average temperature of the earth has increased by 1.5°F, with projections of another 2° to 11.5°F rise in the next 100 years.[33] Although there are questions surrounding changing weather patterns and increasing temperatures, there is widespread and growing consensus that humans are the biggest contributors to climate change. According to the National Aeronautics and Space Administration (NASA), the National Oceanic and Atmospheric Administration (NOAA), and the National Research Council, climate change poses major risks to live and excess **greenhouse gases** are a key culprit.[34]

The *greenhouse effect* is a natural phenomenon in which greenhouse gases such as **carbon dioxide (CO_2)** form a layer in the atmosphere, allowing solar heat to pass through and trapping some of the heat close to the surface, where it warms the planet. The natural greenhouse effect is important for keeping the planet warm enough for life, but human activities have increased greenhouse gases in the atmosphere, resulting in the **enhanced greenhouse effect**, raising the planet's temperature higher than normal by trapping excess heat (see **Figure 15.3** on the following page).

chlorofluorocarbons (CFCs) Chemicals that contribute to the depletion of the atmospheric ozone layer.

climate change A shift in typical weather patterns that includes fluctuations in seasonal temperatures, rain or snowfall amounts, and the occurrence of catastrophic storms.

global warming A type of climate change in which average temperatures increase.

greenhouse gases Gases that accumulate in the atmosphere where they contribute to global warming by trapping heat near the Earth's surface.

carbon dioxide (CO_2) Gas created by the combustion of fossil fuels, exhaled by humans and animals, and used by plants for photosynthesis; the primary greenhouse gas in the atmosphere.

enhanced greenhouse effect Warming of Earth's surface as a direct result of human activities that release greenhouse gases into the atmosphere, trapping more of the sun's radiation than is normal.

Scientific Evidence of Climate Change and Human-Caused Global Warming According to data from the National Oceanic and Atmospheric Administration (NOAA) and the National Aeronautics and Space Administration (NASA), climate responds to changes in greenhouse gases as well as solar output and the earth's orbit. Multiple reconstructions of the earth's climate history show that the amounts of greenhouse gases in the atmosphere went up dramatically around the time of the industrial revolution—when humans began burning fossil fuels on a large scale—and correlates very closely with temperature increases.[35] Studies also indicate that large changes in climate can occur in decades rather than centuries or thousands of years.[36] Changes in weather patterns are becoming more obvious.

Climate Change Challenges Direct results of climate change, such as rising sea levels, glacier retreat, drought, and increases in extreme weather events, have far-reaching impacts on humans. Because climate determines where many disease-spreading insects or other pathogens can reside, changes in climate may also mean increases in tropical diseases and changes in disease trends and patterns.

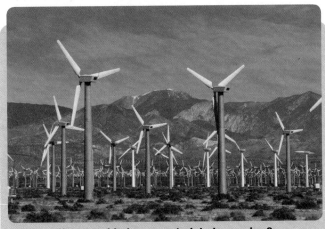

How can I help prevent global warming?

Global warming is a global problem. We need to work with other nations to ensure that everyone does their part. By reducing your use of fossil fuels; using high-efficiency vehicles; and supporting increased use of renewable resources such as solar, wind, and water power, you can help combat global warming.

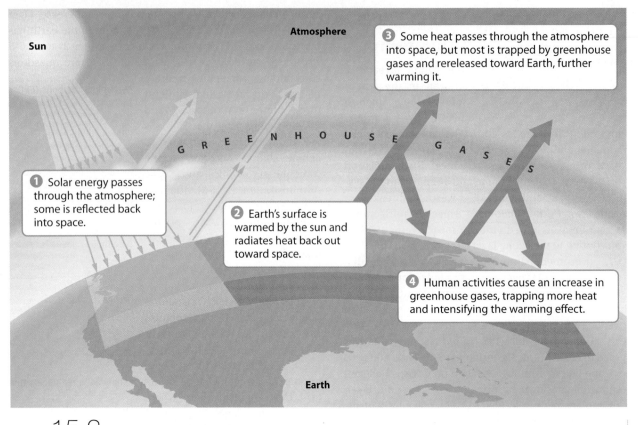

FIGURE 15.3 **The Enhanced Greenhouse Effect**
The natural greenhouse effect is responsible for making Earth habitable; it keeps the planet 33° degrees Celsius (60° Fahrenheit) warmer than it would be otherwise. An increase in greenhouse gases resulting from human activities is creating the enhanced greenhouse effect, trapping more heat and causing dangerous global climate change.

Video Tutor: Enhanced Greenhouse Effect

Reducing the Threat of Global Warming

Climate change problems are largely rooted in our energy, transportation, and industrial practices. Responsible for over 22 percent of all output (expected to increase by 43 percent by 2025), the United States is the greatest producer of greenhouse gases.[37] Rapid deforestation also contributes to the rise in greenhouse gases. Trees take in carbon dioxide, transform it, store the carbon for food, and release oxygen into the air. As we lose forests at the rate of hundreds of acres per hour, we lose the capacity to dissipate carbon dioxide.

Toward Sustainable Development

To slow climate change, most experts agree that reducing consumption of fossil fuels, shifting to alternative energy sources, and using mass transportation are all crucial, but clean energy, green factories, improved energy efficiency, and governmental regulation are also key. A major United Nations Conference on Sustainable Development and Environmental concerns (known as RIO+20) took place in 2012 in Rio de Janeiro and outlined a plan for protecting the environment (called "The World We Want") through **sustainable development**—development that meets the needs of the present without compromising the needs of future generations.[38] Unfortunately, some leaders of nations, including the United States, France, Germany, and the United Kingdom, opted not to attend, and the resulting paper contained only nonbinding objectives. Conferences in Kyoto and Copenhagen were similar in content and impact. By nearly every measure, sustainable development appears to be a challenge.

Although stricter laws on vehicular carbon emissions and the development of cars that operate on electricity, hydrogen, biodiesel, ethanol, or other alternative energy sources are promising, we have a long way to go to reduce fossil-fuel consumption. Meanwhile, many communities have created bicycle lanes and sponsor "bike to work" days. Scooters and other low-energy modes of transportation are becoming increasingly popular. Some college campuses have enacted policies allowing skateboard and rollerblade use on campus. Other campuses provide scooter and bike garages as protection from theft and vandalism and to encourage students

sustainable development Development that meets the needs of the present without compromising the ability of future generations to meet their own needs.

to use energy-efficient transportation. You can participate in this effort by finding ways to reduce your own **carbon footprint**, or the amount of CO_2 emissions you contribute to the atmosphere in your daily life.

Water Pollution and Shortages

Seventy-five percent of Earth is covered with water, and underneath the surface are reservoirs of groundwater. We draw our drinking water from this underground source and from fresh water on the surface; however, just 1 percent of the world's entire water supply is available for human use. The rest is too salty, too polluted, or locked away in polar ice caps.[39] Over half the global population faces a shortage of clean water. More than 2.6 billion people, about 40 percent of the planet's population, have no access to basic sanitation or adequate toilet facilities. More than 1 billion have no access to clean water, and more than 1.5 million deaths each year, mostly among children under 5 years of age, are attributed to illnesses caused by lack of safe water and sanitation.[40] Poor sanitation; overuse by agriculture, industry, and consumers; dwindling supplies; and population growth all contribute to the shortage, and annual global water requirements in the next few decades are estimated to outstrip current sustainable supplies by about 40 percent.[41] Between now and 2040, severe increases in global demand will affect economic growth and population health.[42] The **Skills for Behavior Change** box presents simple conservation measures you can adopt to save water where you live.

Water Contamination

Any substance that gets into the soil can potentially enter the water supply. Industrial pollutants and pesticides eventually work their way into the soil, then into groundwater. Underground storage tanks for gasoline may leak. U.S. Geological Survey researchers discovered the presence of low levels of many chemical compounds in a network of 139 targeted streams across the United States. Steroids, pharmaceuticals and personal care products, hormones, insect repellent, and wastewater compounds were all detected.[43]

Tap water in the United States is among the safest in the world. The Safe Drinking Water Act (SDWA) is the main federal law that ensures the quality of Americans' drinking water. Under SDWA, the EPA sets standards for drinking water quality and oversees the states, localities, and water suppliers who implement those standards. Cities and municipalities have policies and procedures governing water treatment, filtration, and disinfection to screen out pathogens and microorganisms. However, their ability to filter out increasing amounts of chemical by-products and other substances is in question. According to a recent Associated Press inquiry, a whole host of pharmaceuticals have been found in the drinking water of more than 41 million Americans.[44]

Congress has coined two terms, *point source* and *nonpoint source,* to describe general sources of water pollution. **Point source pollutants** enter a waterway at a specific location such as a pipe, ditch, culvert, or other conduit. The two major sources of point source pollution are sewage treatment plants and industrial facilities. **Nonpoint source pollutants**—commonly known as *runoff* and *sedimentation*—drain or seep into waterways from broad areas of land. Nonpoint source pollution results from a variety of land use practices and includes soil erosion and sedimentation, construction and engineering project waste, pesticide and fertilizer runoff, urban street runoff, acid mine drainage, septic tank

carbon footprint Amount of greenhouse gases produced, usually expressed in equivalent tons of carbon dioxide emissions.

point source pollutant Pollutant that enters waterways at a specific point.

nonpoint source pollutant Pollutant that runs off or seeps into waterways from broad areas of land.

Skills for Behavior Change

Waste Less Water!

IN THE KITCHEN
》 Turn off the tap while washing dishes. Shut water off after a quick rinse.
》 Repair leaky pipes and faucets. More than 3,000 gallons of water each year are lost to leaks.
》 Equip faucets with aerators to reduce water use by 4 percent.
》 Run dishwashers only when they are full, and use the energy-saving mode.

IN THE LAUNDRY ROOM
》 Wash only full loads or use a washing machine that adjusts to allow a reduced water level for smaller loads.
》 Upgrade to a high-efficiency washer to use 30 percent less water per load.

IN THE BATHROOM
》 A leaky toilet can waste about 200 gallons of water per day. Fix leaks.
》 Replace old toilets with high-efficiency models that use half the water per flush.
》 Take showers instead of baths, and limit showers to the time it takes to lather up and rinse off. Ideally, get wet, shut off water, lather up, and turn on water to rinse.
》 Replace old showerheads with efficient models that use 60 percent less water per minute.
》 Turn off the tap while brushing your teeth to save up to 8 gallons of water per day.

leakage, and sewage sludge. Among the pollutants causing the greatest potential harm are the following:

● **Gasoline and petroleum products.** More than 2 million underground storage tanks for gasoline and petroleum products are in the United States, most located at gasoline filling stations. Tank leaks allow petroleum to contaminate the ground and water.

● **Chemical contaminants.** *Organic solvents* are chemicals designed to dissolve grease and oil. These extremely toxic substances are used to clean clothing, painting equipment, plastics, and metal parts. Consumers often dump leftover products into the toilet or street drains. Industries pour leftovers into barrels, which are then buried. Eventually the chemicals eat through the barrels and leach into groundwater. For a description of one energy-harnessing process that poses groundwater risks, see the **Points of View** box on fracking on the following page.

● **Polychlorinated biphenyls.** Fire resistant and stable at high temperatures, **polychlorinated biphenyls (PCBs)** were used for many years as insulating materials in high-voltage electrical equipment such as transformers and older fluorescent lights. The human body does not excrete ingested PCBs but rather stores them in the liver and fatty tissues. PCB exposure is associated with birth defects, cancer, and skin problems. PCBs are no longer manufactured in the United States, but approximately 500 million pounds have been dumped into landfills and waterways, where they continue to pose an environmental threat.[45]

● **Dioxins.** **Dioxins** are found in herbicides (chemicals used to kill vegetation) and are produced during certain industrial processes. Dioxins have the ability to accumulate in the body and are much more toxic than PCBs. Long-term effects include possible immune system damage and increased risk of infections and cancer. Exposure to high concentrations of PCBs or dioxins for a short period of time can also have severe consequences, including nausea, vomiting, diarrhea, painful rashes and sores, and chloracne, an ailment in which the skin develops hard, black, painful pimples that may never go away.

● **Pesticides.** **Pesticides** are chemicals designed to kill insects, rodents, plants, and fungi. Americans use more than 5 billion pounds of pesticides each year, the majority of which settles on land and in our air and water.[46] Pesticides evaporate readily and are often carried out to sea or dispersed by winds over a large area. In tropical regions, many farmers use pesticides heavily, and the climate promotes their rapid release into the atmosphere. Pesticide residues cling to fruits and vegetables and can accumulate in the body. Potential hazards associated with pesticide exposure include birth defects, liver and kidney damage, and nervous system disorders.

polychlorinated biphenyls (PCBs) Toxic chemicals that were once used as insulating materials in high-voltage electrical equipment.

dioxins Highly toxic chlorinated hydrocarbons contained in herbicides and produced during certain industrial processes.

pesticides Chemicals that kill pests, such as insects or rodents.

municipal solid waste (MSW) Solid waste such as durable and nondurable goods; containers and packaging; food waste; yard waste; and miscellaneous waste from residential, commercial, institutional, and industrial sources.

Land Pollution

Much of the waste that ends up polluting water starts out polluting the land. Growing population creates more pressure on the land to accommodate increasing amounts of refuse, much of which is nonbiodegradable, and some of which is directly harmful to living organisms.

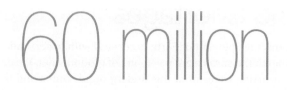

60 million

plastic bottles are added to American landfills each day.

Solid Waste

Each day, every person in the United States generates more than 4.4 pounds of **municipal solid waste (MSW)**, that is, trash, totaling about 250 million tons each year (**Figure 15.4**).[47] Approximately 2 percent, or 3.4 million tons, of the MSW is made up of electronic waste.[48] Several options for reducing electronic waste include recycling, electronic reuse programs, and donating used consumer electronics. (Find more information on locations for electronic waste recycling in your state and about ways to reduce electronic waste in your MSW at www.greenergadgets.org and www.ecyclingcentral.com). Although experts believe that up to 90 percent of our trash is

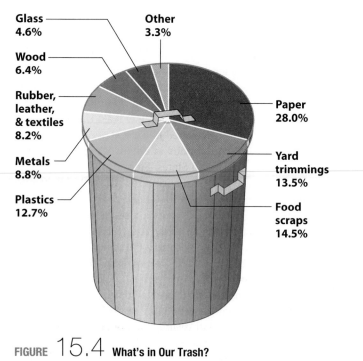

FIGURE 15.4 What's in Our Trash?
Source: Data from U.S. Environmental Protection Agency, *Municipal Solid Waste Generation, Recycling, and Disposal in the United States: Facts and Figures for 2011*, 2013, www.epa.gov

Fracking:
ENVIRONMENTAL THREAT OR ROAD TO ENERGY INDEPENDENCE?

Hydraulic fracturing of shale, more commonly known as *fracking,* is a new, less expensive method of extracting otherwise inaccessible natural gas from the ground. Some experts say fracking could provide the United States with enough natural gas to power the country for a century, helping us become energy independent. Questions about the environmental risks of the process remain unanswered.

In fracking, underground rock and dense soil crack open by pumping highly pressurized fluids into them. This creates fissures that allow oil or gas to flow to the surface for extraction. Much of the fracking liquid, a mixture of water, sand, ceramic beads, and other toxic chemicals, comes up with the gas or oil and is stored in pools for delivery to treatment plants. However, there is concern that a portion of this toxic, chemical-laden sludge can seep down and contaminate drinking water aquifers or surface water and groundwater sources. In addition to potential groundwater contamination, the EPA has noted that fracking causes airborne pollution from methane, sulfur oxide, benzene, and other pollutants, each of which pose significant risks to health and the environment. At present, fracking hazard regulations are not as well defined or monitored compared to other energy technologies. A recent rash of earthquakes in fracking areas has led to speculation that changing the internal pressures of the earth's surface may pose additional risks. To date, science is lacking information that definitively shows fracking to be either completely harmless or highly risky. In the meantime, the fracking industry is growing rapidly, with sand-mining production escalating daily in the upper Midwest in anticipation of a fracking boom that extends well beyond any underground rumbling.

Arguments for Fracking

◯ Fracking increases energy production and energy independence.
◯ Fracking increases the number of jobs and spurs economic growth.
◯ It increases profits for land owners, mineral rights owners, and large gas, oil, and supplying companies.
◯ Local business increases in communities where fracking operations occur.
◯ Fracking costs less than extraction of natural gas by other methods.

Arguments against Fracking

◯ Contamination of underground wells, surface waters, and aquifers is possible.
◯ Current groundwater contamination cleanup is difficult, if not impossible.
◯ Monitoring is difficult, and illegal violations occur.
◯ Regulation and oversight are as yet not clearly defined.
◯ Fracking may have far-reaching effects—air pollution, earthquakes, degradation of lands where sand is mined, transportation pollution, hazards to nearby lands/animals.

Hydraulic Fracturing (Fracking)
Source: Adapted from schematic found in "EPA Study of Hydraulic Fracturing and Drinking Water Safety; Initial Recommendations by Science Advisory Board," U.S. Environmental Protection Agency, 2010, www.epa.gov

Where Do You Stand?

◯ How would you prioritize the competing needs of jobs, energy production (that may cause pollution), and environmental destruction or danger?
◯ What criteria should be used to set rules for when or how fracking should take place?

Sources: EPA, "Natural Gas Extraction: Hydraulic Fracturing," 2012, www.epa.gov/hydraulicfracture/; U.S. Energy Information Administration (EIA), "What Is Shale Gas and Why Is It Important?", 2012, www.eia.gov/energy_in_brief/about_shale_gas.cfm

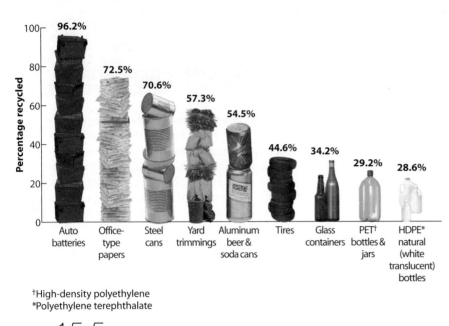

FIGURE 15.5 How Much Do We Recycle?

†High-density polyethylene
*Polyethylene terephthalate

Source: Data from U.S. Environmental Protection Agency, *Municipal Solid Waste Generation, Recycling, and Disposal in the United States: Facts and Figures for 2011*, 2013, www.epa.gov

plastic, and metals from the waste stream.

● *Composting* involves collecting organic waste, such as food scraps and yard trimmings, and allowing it to decompose with the help of microorganisms (mainly bacteria and fungi). This process produces a nutrient-rich substance used to fertilize gardens and for soil enhancement. Not all organic waste is composted. See the **Money & Health** box on the following page for more on the cost and prevalence of food waste.

● *Combustion with energy recovery* typically involves the use of boilers and industrial furnaces to incinerate waste and use the burning process to generate energy.

Hazardous Waste

hazardous waste Toxic waste that poses a hazard to humans or to the environment.

Superfund Fund established under the Comprehensive Environmental Response Compensation and Liability Act to be used for cleaning up toxic waste dumps.

recyclable, we still fall far short of this goal **(Figure 15.5)**. Currently, 34.7 percent of all MSW in the United States is recycled or composted, nearly 12 percent is burned at combustion facilities, and the remaining 54 percent is disposed of in landfills.[49]

The number of U.S. landfills has actually decreased in the past decade, but their sheer mass has increased. Many people worry that we are losing our ability to dispose of all of the waste we create. As communities run out of landfill space, it is becoming common to dump garbage at sea (contaminating ocean ecosystems) or ship it to landfills in developing countries (where it becomes someone else's problem). In today's throwaway society, we need to find more ways to recycle, reuse, and—most desirable of all—reduce what we consume.

Communities, businesses, and individuals can adopt strategies to reduce solid waste:

Hazardous waste has properties that make it capable of harming human health or the environment. The *Comprehensive Environmental Response and Liability Act* provides funds for cleaning up the most dangerous hazardous waste dump sites. This **Superfund** is financed through taxes on the chemical and petroleum industries (87%) and through federal tax revenues (13%). By the end of 2012, 68 percent

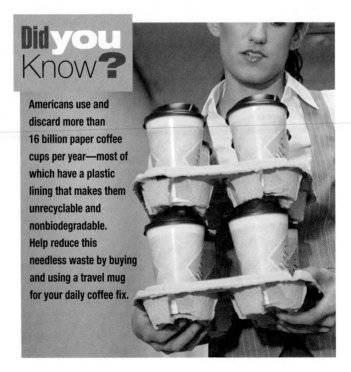

what do you think?

Do you know anyone who throws recyclable items away rather than recycling them?

● What do you think motivates their behavior?

● What might encourage them to recycle more than they do now?

● *Source reduction* (*waste prevention*) involves altering the design, manufacture, or use of products and materials to reduce the amount and toxicity of waste. The most effective waste-reducing strategy is preventing waste from being generated in the first place.

● *Recycling* involves sorting, collecting, and processing materials for reuse in new products and diverts items such as paper, cardboard, glass,

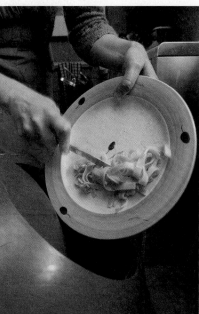

At a time when starvation, hunger, and food insecurity plague people throughout the world, a new study by Britain's Institute of Mechanical Engineers indicates that *up to half of the food produced worldwide never makes it into consumer's mouths*. Over 2 billion tons of food could feed millions, but it never reaches them.

Global consumer behaviors in more affluent nations are responsible for much of the waste. Big box stores that promote "bigger size is cheaper" entice people to buy more than they can eat before it spoils. Freezers in homes encourage waste as food dries up before it is eaten while other food sits on shelves until past the due date.

It isn't just our behaviors that contribute to the waste, however. When fresh produce is in surplus and demand is low, crops languish in fields. If weather or insects cause produce to be blemished, we reject it in stores and it is tossed in the trash. Americans are among the worst of the food wasters, wasting over 40 percent of all edible food. The average person in the United States dumps about 20 pounds of food each month, equivalent to between $28 and $43 per month. If we cut our food waste by just 15 percent, some estimate 26 million food-insecure people in the United States could be fed.

From an environmental perspective, when we waste food, we waste all of the time, effort, and resources that went into production and put unnecessary stress on the environment. By wasting less, we put less pressure on our vulnerable habitat.

What can you do?

✳ Be a better food planner. Make a list when shopping and only buy what you will use.
✳ Buy locally.
✳ Don't be picky. Buy fruit and vegetables even if they don't have a perfect shape, and eat them before they rot.
✳ Eat leftovers. Make a rule that you can't buy fast food or eat out when there is good food in your fridge.
✳ Eat lower on the food chain.
By eating more vegetables and nuts, legumes, and other food crops and reducing consumption of meat, dairy and other animals, you have a smaller footprint stomping on the planet.

Sources: Institute of Mechanical Engineers, "Global Food: Waste Not, Want Not," 2013, Available at www.imeche.org; J. Bloom, *American Wasteland* (Cambridge: DeCapo Press, 2010); National Resource Defense Council, "Food Facts: Your Scraps Add Up," March 2013, www.nrdc.org

---

of the Superfund sites on the National Priorities List (NPL) had been identified and controlled.[50] Massive cleanups are also beginning on some of most polluted waterways. Newer strategies and technologies for cleanup are being investigated, including nanotechnologies, that could drastically reduce costs.

The large number of U.S. hazardous waste dump sites indicates the severity of our toxic chemical problem. American manufacturers generate more than 1 ton of chemical waste per person per year (275 million tons annually).[51] Many wastes are now banned from land disposal or are being treated to reduce their toxicity before they become part of land disposal sites. The EPA has developed protective requirements for land disposal facilities, such as double liners, detection systems for substances that may leach into groundwater, and groundwater monitoring systems.

Radiation

Radiation is energy that travels in waves or particles. There are many different types of radiation, ranging from radio waves to gamma rays, all making up the electromagnetic spectrum. Exposure to radiation is an inescapable part of life on this planet, and only some of it poses a threat to human health.

nonionizing radiation Electromagnetic waves having relatively long wavelengths and enough energy to move atoms around or cause them to vibrate.

Nonionizing Radiation

Nonionizing radiation is radiation at the lower end of the electromagnetic spectrum. This radiation moves in relatively long wavelengths and has enough energy to move atoms around or to cause them to vibrate, but not enough to alter

ARE CELL PHONES HAZARDOUS TO YOUR HEALTH?

Cell phones emit radio frequency (RF) energy when turned on, and depending on how close the phone is to your head, as much as 60 percent of the energy penetrates your body. Could this harm you?

At high power levels, RF energy damages the body. In the United States, safety thresholds for cell phone radiation are set by the Federal Communications Commission. Currently, cell phones must emit levels no higher than less than half the safety threshold.

The U.S. Food and Drug Administration, the World Health Organization, and other major health agencies agree that research finds no link between cell phones and cancer or other disorders. They also suggest a need for more research since no long-term studies exist. A new European Cohort Study of Mobile phone use (COSMOS) will follow 250,000 people for the next 20 years to determine increased risks, and should provide much needed insight.

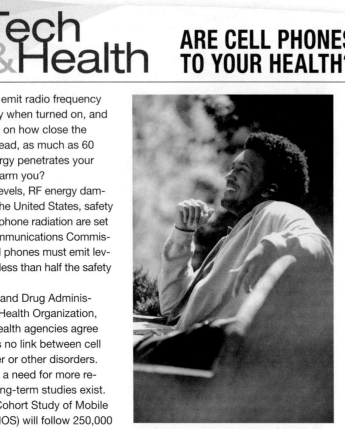

A hands-free device lets you keep your phone—and any radio-frequency energy it may emit—away from your head.

A few small changes in behavior can greatly reduce the amount of RF energy your body absorbs. First, limit the amount of time you spend talking on the phone. When you do make calls, use a hands-free device that keeps the phone away from your head. Because wireless earpieces also emit energy, only use them when you are actively engaged in a call. Finally, buy a phone that emits lower RF energy than others. Information on phone emissions is available from manufacturers in the form of specific absorption rate (SAR) charts, which are readily available on the Internet.

Sources: National Cancer Institute. Factsheet, "Cell Phones and Cancer Risk," 2012, www.cancer.gov; M. P. Little et al., "Mobile Phone Use and Glioma Risk: Comparison of Epidemiological Study Results with Incidence Trends in the United States," *British Medical Journal* 344 (2012): e1147, doi: 10.1136/bmj.e1147; D. Aydin et al., "Mobile Phone Use and Brain Tumors in Children and Adolescents: A Multicenter Case-Control Study," *Journal of the National Cancer Institute* 103, no. 16 (2011): 1264–1276, doi: 10.1093/jnci/djr244.

molecular structure. Examples of nonionizing radiation are radio waves, TV signals, microwaves, infrared waves, and visible light. Concerns have been raised about the safety of radio-frequency waves generated by cell phones, discussed in the **Tech & Health** box.

Ionizing Radiation

Ionizing radiation is caused by the release of particles and electromagnetic rays from atomic nuclei during the normal process of disintegration. This type of radiation has enough energy to remove electrons from the atoms it passes through. Some naturally occurring elements, such as uranium, emit ionizing radiation. The sun is another source of ionizing radiation, in the form of high-frequency ultraviolet rays.

Radiation exposure is measured in **radiation absorbed doses**, or **rads** (also called *roentgens*). Radiation can cause damage at doses as low as 100 to 200 rads. At this level, signs of radiation sickness include nausea, diarrhea, fatigue, anemia, sore throat, and hair loss. At 350 to 500 rads, these symptoms become more severe, and death may result as production of the white blood cells we need to fight disease is hindered. Doses above 600 to 700 rads are fatal.

Recommended maximum "safe" exposure ranges from 0.05 to 5 rads per year.[52] Approximately 50 percent of the radiation to which we are exposed comes from natural and human-made sources. Natural sources include radon gas in the air and cosmic radiation. Human-made sources include, but are not limited to, manufactured building materials. Another 45 percent comes from medical and dental X-rays. The remaining 5 percent is nonionizing radiation that comes from sources such as computer monitors, microwave ovens, televisions, and radar screens.[53] Most of us are exposed to far less radiation than the safe maximum dosage per year. The effects of long-term exposure to relatively low levels of radiation are unknown. Some scientists believe that such exposure can cause lung cancer, leukemia, skin cancer, bone cancer, and skeletal deformities.

Nuclear Power Plants

Although nuclear power plants account for less than 1 percent of the total radiation to which we are exposed, the number of U.S. plants may increase in the next decade.

ionizing radiation Electromagnetic waves and particles having short wavelengths and energy high enough to ionize atoms.

radiation absorbed dose (rad) Unit of measure of radiation exposure.

Proponents of nuclear energy believe that it is a safe and efficient way to generate electricity. Initial costs of building nuclear power plants are high, but actual power generation is relatively inexpensive. A 1,000-megawatt reactor produces enough energy for 650,000 homes and saves 420 million gallons of fossil fuels each year. In some areas where nuclear power plants were decommissioned, electricity bills tripled when power companies turned to hydroelectric or fossil fuel sources to generate electricity. Nuclear reactors discharge fewer carbon oxides into the air than do fossil fuel–powered generators. Advocates believe that converting to nuclear power could help slow global warming.

The advantages of nuclear energy must be weighed against the disadvantages. Disposal of nuclear waste is extremely problematic. In addition, a reactor core meltdown could pose serious threats to the immediate environment and to the world in general. A **nuclear meltdown** occurs when the temperature in the core of a nuclear reactor increases enough to melt both the nuclear fuel and its containment vessel. Most modern facilities seal the reactors and containment vessels in concrete buildings with pools of cold water on the bottom. If a meltdown occurs, the building and the pool are supposed to prevent radiation from escaping.

One serious nuclear accident in particular contributed to a steep decline in public support for nuclear energy: the 1986 reactor core fire and explosion at the Chernobyl nuclear power plant in Russia, which killed thousands of people and left the area uninhabitable for decades.[54] The damage to the Fukushima Daiichi Nuclear Power Station in northern Japan caused by the March 2011 earthquake and tsunami has newly awakened worldwide fears about nuclear energy. Even so, the use of nuclear power worldwide is expected to double in the next 20 to 25 years.[55]

Noise Pollution

Our bodies have definite physiological responses to noise, and it can become a source of physical and mental distress. Sounds are measured in decibels. A sound with a decibel level of 110 is 10 times louder than one at 100 decibels (dB). A jet takeoff from 200 feet has a noise level of approximately 140 dB, whereas the human voice in normal conversation has a level of about 60 dB (Figure 15.6). Short-term exposure to loud noise reduces concentration and productivity and may affect mental and emotional health. Symptoms of noise-related distress include disturbed sleep patterns, headaches, and tension. Prolonged exposure to loud noise can lead to hearing loss, although risks depend on both the decibel level and the length of exposure.

Despite increasing awareness that noise pollution is more than just a nuisance, noise control programs have received low budgetary priority in the United States. According to the National Institute for Occupational Safety and Health, 30 million Americans are exposed to hazardous noise at work, and 10 million suffer from permanent hearing loss.[56] Here are some steps you can take to protect your hearing:

- Use headphones that go over, rather than inside, your ears, and don't crank up the volume on any sound system.
- Always use ear protection when using power equipment or firearms.
- Close windows to establish a barrier between yourself and outside noise.
- Wear earplugs when attending concerts, athletic events, races, and clubs, and avoid seats near speakers.

nuclear meltdown Accident that results when the temperature in the core of a nuclear reactor increases enough to melt the nuclear fuel and breach the containment vessel.

Threshold of pain

130 — Rock concert, Jet airplane
120 — Jackhammer, Stereo at max
110 — MP3 player at max
100 — Chainsaw
90 — Motorcycle, Snowmobile
80 — Diesel truck
70 — Lawnmower
60
50 — Vacuum cleaner
40
30 — Quiet office
20
10
0 — Rustling leaves, Whisper

Risk of injury and gradual hearing loss at 85 dB and higher

Threshold of hearing

FIGURE 15.6 **Noise Levels of Various Sounds (in Decibels)**
Decibels increase logarithmically, thus each increase of 10 dB represents a tenfold increase in loudness.
Source: Adapted from National Institute on Deafness and Other Communication Disorders, "How Loud Is Too Loud? Bookmark," 2011, www.nidcd.nih.gov

Are You Doing All You Can to Protect the Environment?

Environmental problems often seem too big for the actions of one person to make a difference. Each day, however, there are things you can do. For each statement below, indicate how often you follow the described behavior.

		Always	Usually	Sometimes	Never
1.	Whenever possible, I walk or ride my bicycle rather than drive a car.	1	2	3	4
2.	I carpool to school or work.	1	2	3	4
3.	I follow the manufacturer's recommended maintenance schedule for my car.	1	2	3	4
4.	When the oil in my car is changed, I make sure that used oil is properly recycled, rather than dumped on the ground or into a floor drain.	1	2	3	4
5.	I use air conditioning only as needed on very hot days and open windows for air circulation when possible.	1	2	3	4
6.	I turn off the lights when a room is not being used.	1	2	3	4
7.	I take a shower rather than a bath most of the time.	1	2	3	4
8.	I have water-saving devices installed on my shower, toilet, and sinks.	1	2	3	4
9.	I make sure faucets and toilets do not leak.	1	2	3	4
10.	I use bath towels more than once before putting them in the wash.	1	2	3	4
11.	I wear my clothes more than once between washings, when appropriate.	1	2	3	4
12.	I limit my use of the clothes dryer and line dry my clothes as often as possible.	1	2	3	4
13.	I purchase biodegradable soaps and detergents.	1	2	3	4
14.	I use biodegradable trash bags.	1	2	3	4
15.	At home, I use dishes and utensils rather than Styrofoam or plastic.	1	2	3	4
16.	When I buy prepackaged foods, I choose the ones with the least packaging.	1	2	3	4
17.	I do not subscribe to newspapers and magazines that I can view online.	1	2	3	4
18.	I use an energy-efficient hair dryer.	1	2	3	4
19.	I bring my own reusable bags to the grocery store.	1	2	3	4
20.	I don't run water continuously when washing the dishes, shaving, or brushing my teeth.	1	2	3	4
21.	I use unbleached or recycled paper whenever possible.	1	2	3	4
22.	I use both sides of printer paper and other paper when possible.	1	2	3	4
23.	I donate items I'm no longer using to charity.	1	2	3	4
24.	I use a refillable mug for coffee or tea instead of a new paper cup each time I buy a hot beverage.	1	2	3	4
25.	I use a refillable water bottle instead of buying bottled water.	1	2	3	4
26.	I clean up after myself after picnicking, camping, etc.	1	2	3	4
27.	I volunteer for clean-up days in my community.	1	2	3	4
28.	I consider candidates' positions on environmental issues before casting my vote.	1	2	3	4

For Further Thought

Review your scores. Are your responses mostly 1s and 2s? If not, what actions can you take to become more environmentally responsible? Are there ways to help the environment on this list that you had not thought of before? Are there behaviors not on the list that you are already doing?

YOUR PLAN FOR CHANGE

The **Assess** yourself activity gave you the chance to look at your behavior and consider ways to conserve energy, save water, reduce waste, and otherwise help protect the planet. Now that you have considered these results, you can take steps to become more environmentally responsible.

Today, you can:

◯ Find out how energy savvy you are and how much energy you are using. Visit www.carbonfund.org, www.carbonoffsets.org, or www.greatestplanet.org to find out what your carbon footprint is and to learn about projects you can support to offset your own emissions and energy usage. New carbon offset programs and organizations are popping up all the time, so watch for other opportunities to counter your carbon usage.

◯ Reduce the amount of paper waste in your mailbox. You can stop junk mail, such as credit card offers and unwanted catalogs, by visiting the Direct Marketing Association's Mail Preference Service site at www.dmachoice.org. You can also call 1-888-5 OPT OUT to put an end to unwanted mail, and www.catalogchoice.org lets you decline paper catalogs you no longer want to receive.

O Go paperless whenever possible. Invest in secure, cloud-based storage instead of having hard copies of everything.

Within the next 2 weeks, you can:

◯ Look into joining a local environmental group, attending a campus environmental event, or taking an environmental science course.

◯ Take part in a local clean-up day or recycling drive to meet like-minded people while benefiting the planet.

By the end of the semester, you can:

◯ Come up with a plan for using less and only buying what you really need. Buy groceries with less packaging. Think long shelf life with products, including your clothing.

◯ Interview and talk with your campus's dining hall director about initiating a compost recycling program.

◯ Make a habit of recycling everything you can. Find out what items can be recycled in your neighborhood and designate a box or bin to hold recyclable materials—cans, bottles, plastic, newspapers,

junk mail, and so on—until you can transport them to a curbside bin or drop-off center.

◯ Work to influence the environment on a larger scale. Take part in an environmental activism group on campus or in your community. Listen carefully to what political candidates say about the environment. Let your legislators know how you feel about environmental issues and that you will vote according to their record on the issues.

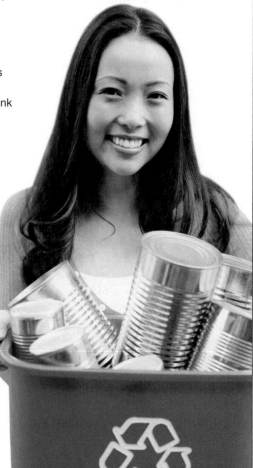

MasteringHealth™

Build your knowledge—and health!—in the Study Area of MasteringHealth with a variety of study tools.

Summary

* Population growth is the single largest factor affecting the environment. Demand for more food, water, and energy—as well as places to dispose of waste—places great strain on Earth's resources.

* Climate change is a major environmental threat and is caused by a wide range of factors. Air, water, and solid waste pollution are key contributors, as is our growing dependence on fossil fuels. Sustainable development should be an international goal.

* The primary constituents of air pollution are sulfur dioxide, particulate matter, carbon monoxide, nitrogen dioxide, ozone, carbon dioxide, and hydrocarbons. Indoor air pollution is caused primarily by tobacco smoke, woodstove smoke, furnace emissions, asbestos, formaldehyde, radon, lead, and mold.

* Air pollution is depleting Earth's protective ozone layer and contributing to global warming by enhancing the greenhouse effect.

* Water pollution can be caused by either point sources (direct entry) or nonpoint sources (runoff or seepage). Major contributors to water pollution include petroleum products, organic solvents, PCBs, dioxins, pesticides, and lead.

* Limited landfill space creates problems in dealing with growing volumes of municipal solid waste. Hazardous waste is toxic; improper disposal creates health hazards.

* Nonionizing radiation comes from electromagnetic fields like those around power lines. Ionizing radiation results from the natural erosion of atomic nuclei. The disposal and storage of radioactive waste

from nuclear power plants pose potential public health problems.

* Noise pollution can affect concentration and productivity and can also lead to hearing loss.

Pop Quiz

1. The United States is responsible for what percentage of total global resource consumption?
   a. 10 percent
   b. 25 percent
   c. 50 percent
   d. 70 percent
2. Human fertility rates go down when
   a. there is poverty and people can't afford to feed their families.
   b. governments subsidize families in the form of tax breaks.
   c. women have more education and power.
   d. environmental threats influence people to have fewer children.
3. The air pollutant that originates primarily from motor vehicle emissions is
   a. particulates.
   b. nitrogen dioxide.
   c. sulfur dioxide.
   d. carbon monoxide.
4. What substance separates into stringy fibers, embeds itself in lungs, and causes mesothelioma?
   a. Asbestos
   b. Particulate matter
   c. Radon
   d. Formaldehyde
5. One source of indoor air pollution is a gas present in some carpets called
   a. lead.
   b. asbestos.
   c. radon.
   d. formaldehyde.

6. Which gas could become cancer causing when it seeps into a home?
   a. Carbon monoxide
   b. Radon
   c. Hydrogen sulfide
   d. Ozone
7. The barrier that protects us from the sun's harmful ultraviolet rays is
   a. photochemical smog.
   b. the ozone layer.
   c. gray air smog.
   d. the greenhouse effect.
8. The terms *point source* and *nonpoint source* are used to describe the two general sources of
   a. water pollution.
   b. air pollution.
   c. noise pollution.
   d. ozone depletion.
9. Some herbicides contain toxic substances called
   a. THMs.
   b. PCPs.
   c. dioxins.
   d. PCBs.
10. Intensity of (exposure to) sound is measured in
    a. foot candles.
    b. noise volume.
    c. hertz.
    d. decibels.

Answers to these questions can be found on page A-1.

Think about It!

1. How are the rapid increases in global population and consumption of resources related? Is population control the best solution? Why or why not?
2. What are the primary sources of air pollution? What can be done to reduce air pollution?
3. What are the causes and consequences of global warming? What can individuals do to reduce the threat of global warming?
4. What are point and nonpoint sources of water pollution? What can be done to reduce or prevent water pollution?

5. How do you think communities and governments could encourage recycling efforts?
6. What are the physiological consequences of noise pollution? How can you lessen your exposure to it?

Accessing Your Health on the Internet

The following websites explore further topics and issues related to personal health. For links to the websites, visit the Study Area in MasteringHealth.

1. *Environmental Literacy Council.* This website is an excellent source of information about environmental issues in general. Topics range from how the ozone layer works to why the rain forests are important ecosystems. www.enviroliteracy.org
2. *Environmental Protection Agency (EPA).* The EPA is the government agency responsible for overseeing environmental regulation and protection issues in the United States. Information on these subjects is available on their website. www.epa.gov

3. *National Center for Environmental Health (NCEH).* This site provides information on a wide variety of environmental health issues, including a series of helpful fact sheets. www.cdc.gov/nceh
4. *National Environmental Health Association (NEHA).* This organization provides educational resources and opportunities for environmental health professionals. www.neha.org

Making Smart Health Care Choices

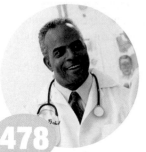

478

What questions should I ask my health care provider?

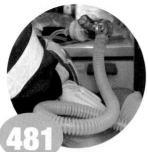

481

What happens if I don't have insurance and I need medical care?

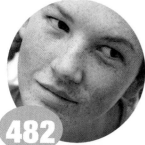

482

Can I count on my school's health care plan to cover my medical needs?

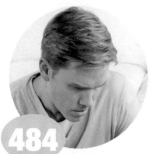

484

What should I consider when choosing health insurance?

LEARNING OUTCOMES

✻ Explain why it is important to be a responsible, knowledgeable, and proactive health care consumer.

✻ Identify important factors to consider when making health care decisions.

✻ Outline the appropriate uses of prescription and over-the-counter drugs.

✻ Describe the U.S. health care system in terms of types and availability of insurance and the changes related to health care reform.

✻ Discuss issues facing our health care system today, including those related to cost, quality, and access to services.

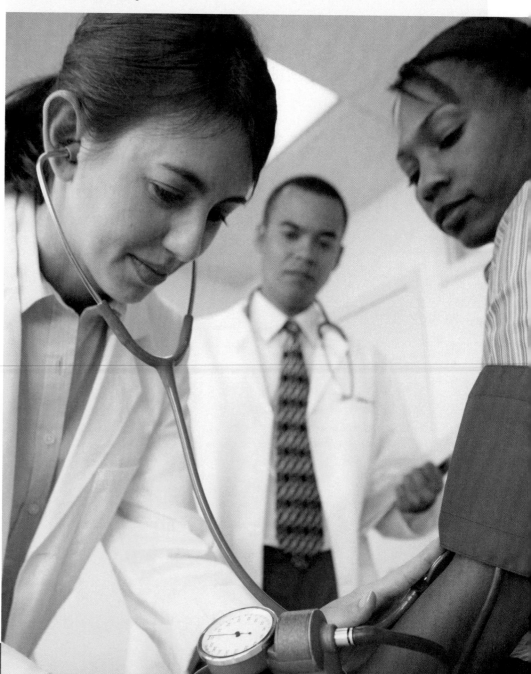

For many, college is the first time they will be responsible for making personal health care decisions. While most students enjoy relatively good health at this stage of life, there are still occurrences such as acquiring a virus or becoming injured that require decisions about whether self-care or medical intervention is most appropriate. About 90 percent of students have some sort of health insurance, but it's important to understand your particular coverage in terms of practitioners and facilities before you make an appointment for medical care. Being a savvy health care consumer can not only get you better care in the long run, but also can help you spend less. Learning how to navigate the health care system is an important part of taking charge of your health.

Taking Responsibility for Your Health Care

Acting responsibly in times of illness can be challenging. If you are not feeling well, you must first decide whether you really need to seek medical advice. For minor ailments such as colds or minor injuries, self-care may be the best course of action. In more serious cases, not seeking treatment, whether because of high costs or limited insurance coverage, or trying to self-medicate when more rigorous methods of treatment are needed, is potentially dangerous. It's important to know the benefits and limits of self-care.

Self-Care

Individuals can practice behaviors that promote health and reduce the risk of disease as well as treat minor afflictions without seeking professional help. Self-care consists of knowing your body, paying attention to its signals, and taking appropriate action to stop the progression of illness or injury. Common forms of self-care include the following:

● Diagnosing symptoms or conditions that occur frequently but may not require physician visits (e.g., the common cold, minor abrasions)
● Using over-the-counter remedies to treat minor pains, scrapes, stomach upsets, or cold or allergy symptoms
● Performing monthly breast or testicular self-examinations
● Learning first aid for common, uncomplicated injuries and conditions

● Checking vital signs: blood pressure, pulse, and temperature
● Using home pregnancy tests and ovulation kits

See It! Videos
How do you avoid misdiagnosed medical advice online? Watch **Misdiagnosis on the Web** in the Study Area of MasteringHealth™

In addition, there are health-related websites, DVDs, and books, as well as home kits that test for HIV, genetic disorders, and other conditions. Caution is in order here: Diagnoses from these sources and kits may not always be accurate, or you may not have the ability to understand the ramifications of what you learn without professional interpretations.

Many people also use self-care treatments inappropriately. Taking someone else's prescription drugs, taking drugs given to you for a previous illness, or using treatments that may not be scientifically proven should all be avoided.

When to Seek Help

Effective self-care also means understanding when to seek medical attention rather than treating a condition yourself. Generally, you should consult a physician if you experience *any* of the following:

● A serious accident or injury
● Sudden or severe chest pains, especially if they cause breathing difficulties
● Trauma to the head or spine accompanied by persistent headache, blurred vision, loss of consciousness, vomiting, convulsions, or paralysis
● Sudden high fever or recurring high temperature (over 102°F for children and 103°F for adults) and/or sweats

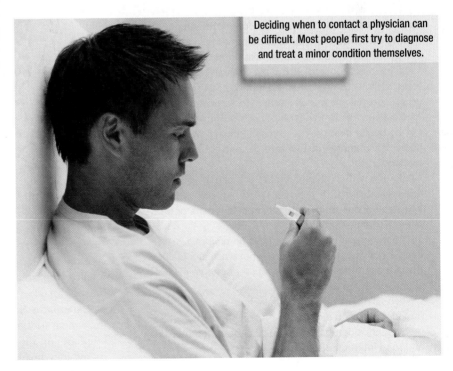

Deciding when to contact a physician can be difficult. Most people first try to diagnose and treat a minor condition themselves.

Hear It! Podcasts
Want a study podcast for this chapter? Download the podcast **Consumerism: Selecting Health Care Products and Services** in the Study Area of MasteringHealth™

- Tingling sensation in the arm accompanied by slurred speech or impaired thought processes
- Adverse reactions to a drug or insect bite (shortness of breath, severe swelling, or dizziness)
- Unexplained bleeding or loss of body fluid from any body opening
- Unexplained sudden weight loss
- Persistent or recurrent diarrhea or vomiting
- Blue-tinted lips, eyelids, or nail beds
- Any lump, swelling, thickness, or sore that does not subside or that grows for over a month
- Any marked change or pain in bowel or bladder habits
- Yellowing of the skin or the whites of the eyes
- Any symptom that is unusual and recurs over time
- Pregnancy

Keep in mind that home health tests are no substitute for regular, complete examinations by a trained practitioner.

See the **Skills for Behavior Change** box for pointers on taking an active role in your own health care.

Choosing a Conventional Health Care Provider

Conventional health care, also known as **allopathic medicine**, is traditional Western medical practice, generally believed to be based on scientifically validated methods. But be aware that not all allopathic treatments have had the benefit of the extensive clinical trials and long-term studies of outcomes that would conclusively prove effectiveness in various populations. Even when studies appear to support the benefits of a particular treatment or product, other studies with equal or better scientific validity often refute earlier claims. Also, recommended treatments may change dramatically as new technologies and medical advances replace older practices. Like other professionals, medical doctors must keep up with new research and changing practices in their field(s) of specialty.

Selecting a **primary care practitioner (PCP)**—a physician you visit for routine ailments, preventive care, general medical advice, and referrals to specialists—is not an easy task. Most people select a family practitioner, internist, or an obstetrician/gynecologist (OB/GYN) as their PCP.

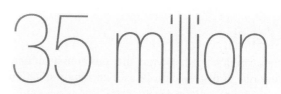

35 million

Americans are admitted to the hospital each year.

Pediatricians serve as PCPs for children and teens. As a college student, you may opt to visit a PCP at your campus health center. The reputation of health care providers on college campuses is excellent. In national surveys, students have indicated that the health center medical staff is their most trusted source of health information.[1]

Doctors undergo rigorous training before they can begin practicing. After 4 years of undergraduate work, students typically spend 4 additional years studying for their doctor of medicine degree (MD). Some students choose a specialty, such as pediatrics, cardiology, oncology, radiology, or surgery, and spend another year in an internship and several years doing a residency. Some specialties also require a fellowship, so additional training after receiving a medical degree can take up to 8 years.

Osteopaths are general practitioners who receive training similar to that of a medical doctor but who place special emphasis on the skeletal and muscular systems. Their treatments may involve manipulation of the muscles and joints. Osteopaths receive the degree of doctor of osteopathy (DO).

Eye care specialists can be either ophthalmologists or optometrists. An **ophthalmologist** holds a medical degree and can perform surgery and prescribe medications. An **optometrist** is trained to evaluate vision problems and prescribe corrective lenses but is not a physician. If you have an eye infection or some other eye condition requiring diagnosis and treatment, you need to see an ophthalmologist.

Dentists diagnose and treat diseases of the teeth, gums, and oral cavity. They attend dental school for 4 years and receive the title of doctor of dental surgery (DDS) or doctor of medical dentistry (DMD). They must also pass both state and national board examinations before receiving their licenses to practice. The field of dentistry includes specialties; for example, *orthodontists* specialize in the alignment of teeth, *periodontists* treat diseases of the gums and other tissues surrounding the teeth, and *oral surgeons* perform surgical procedures to correct problems of the mouth, face, and jaw.

Nurses are highly trained and strictly regulated health professionals who provide a wide range of services for patients and their families, including patient education, counseling, community health and disease prevention information, and administration of medications. Registered nurses (RNs) in the United States complete either a 4-year program leading to a bachelor of science in nursing (BSN) degree or a 2-year associate degree program, and they must also pass a national certification exam.

Lower-level licensed practical or vocational nurses (LPN or LVN) complete a 1- to 2-year training program, which may be based in either a community college or hospital, and take a licensing exam.

Nurse practitioners (NPs) are nurses with advanced training obtained through either a master's degree program or a specialized nurse practitioner program. Nurse practitioners have the training and authority to conduct diagnostic tests and prescribe medications (in some states). They work in a variety of settings, including clinics and student health centers, and can specialize in areas such as pediatrics or acute care. Nurses and nurse practitioners may also earn the clinical doctor of nursing degree (ND), doctor of nursing science (DNS and DNSc degrees), or a research-based PhD in nursing.

Physician assistants (PAs) are licensed to examine and diagnose patients, offer treatment, and write prescriptions under a physician's supervision. An important difference between a PA and an NP is that the PA must practice under a physician's supervision. Like other health care providers, PAs are licensed by state boards of medicine.

ophthalmologist Physician who specializes in the medical and surgical care of the eyes, including prescriptions for lenses.

optometrist Eye specialist whose practice is limited to prescribing and fitting lenses to correct vision problems.

dentist Physician who diagnoses and treats diseases of the teeth, gums, and oral cavity.

nurse Health professional who provides patient care in a variety of settings.

nurse practitioner (NP) Nurse with advanced training obtained through either a master's degree program or a specialized nurse practitioner program.

physician assistant (PA) Health care practitioner trained to handle most routine care under the supervision of a physician.

Assessing Health Professionals

Once you decide that you need medical help, finding a health care provider is the next step. Selecting a professional may seem simple, yet many people have no idea how to evaluate a provider's qualifications. Numerous studies document the importance of good communication skills: The most satisfied patients are those who feel their health care provider explains diagnosis and treatment options thoroughly and involves them in decisions regarding their own care.[2]

When evaluating health care providers, be sure to consider the following questions:

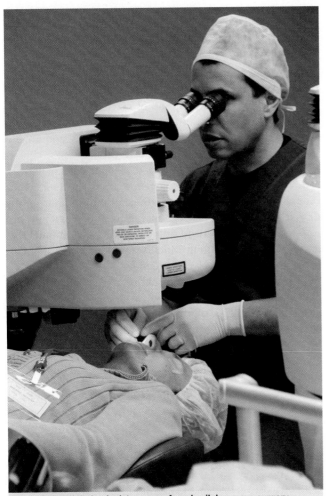

Only ophthalmologists can perform Lasik laser eye surgery.

> **what do you think?**
> Do you believe that patients should have access to information about practitioners' and facilities' malpractice records?
> ● What about information on success and failure rates or outcomes of various procedures?

● What professional education and training have they had? What license or board certification(s) do they hold? Note an important difference: *Board certified* indicates that the physician has passed the national board examination for his or her specialty (e.g., pediatrics) and has been certified as competent in that specialty. In contrast, *board eligible* merely means that the physician is eligible to take the exam, but not that he or she has passed it.

● Are they affiliated with an accredited medical facility or institution? The Joint Commission is an independent nonprofit organization that evaluates and accredits more than

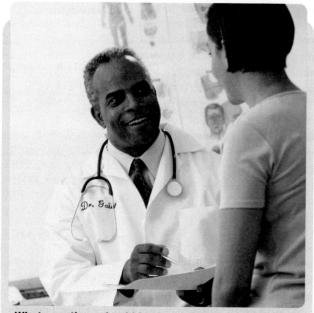

What questions should I ask my health care provider?

It's important to understand recommendations made by your health care provider. Questions to ask include why a test has been ordered, how often the practitioner has performed a procedure, the percentage of successful outcomes for the proposed treatment or procedure, any side effects and whether they can be treated or reduced, and whether a hospital stay will be required.

20,000 health care organizations and programs in the United States. Accreditation requires that these institutions verify all education, licensing, and training claims of their affiliated practitioners.[3]

● Are they open to complementary or alternative strategies? Would they refer you for different treatment modalities if appropriate?

● Do they indicate clearly how long a given treatment may last, what side effects you might expect, and what problems you should watch for?

● Are their diagnoses, treatments, and general statements consistent with established scientific theory and practice?

● Do they make alternate arrangements for your care when on vacation or off call?

● Do they listen, respect you as an individual, and give you time to ask questions? Do they return your calls, and are they available to answer questions?

malpractice Improper or negligent treatment by a health practitioner that results in loss, injury, or harm to the patient.

placebo Inactive substance used as a control in a clinical test to determine the effectiveness of a particular drug; the *placebo effect* occurs when patients given a placebo drug or treatment experience an improved state of health owing to the belief that they are receiving something that will be of benefit.

Being prepared for appointments and asking the right questions at the right time allow you to work in partnership with your health care provider. Many patients find that writing down their questions before an appointment helps in getting the answers they need. You should not accept a defensive or hostile response; if you are not satisfied with how a practitioner

communicates with you, go elsewhere. It is also important that you provide honest answers to his or her questions about your symptoms, condition, lifestyle, and medical history.

Active participation in your treatment is the only sensible course in a health care environment that encourages *defensive medicine*, in which providers take certain actions primarily to avoid a **malpractice** claim. In a recent survey of physicians, 58 percent indicated that they have ordered a test or procedure for primarily defensive medicine reasons.[4] Unnecessary drugs and procedures are not likely to improve health outcomes and, in some cases, may create new health problems.

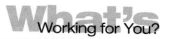
Working for You?

Maybe you already have your health care under control. Below is a list of some things you can do to manage your health care successfully. Which of these are you already incorporating into your life?

☐ I research any condition that I have using periodicals, texts, research articles, and reliable websites.

☐ I have a health care provider with whom I discuss all of my health care decisions.

☐ Before I proceed with any treatment, I try to find out as much as I can about it so I know the risks and benefits.

☐ I have health insurance, and I understand what it covers.

Being a proactive consumer of health care services also means being aware of your rights as a patient:[5]

1. The *right of informed consent* means that before receiving care, you should be fully informed of what is planned; risks and potential benefits; and possible alternative forms of treatment, including the option of no treatment. Your consent must be voluntary and without any form of coercion. It is critical that you read consent forms carefully and amend them as necessary before signing.

2. You are entitled to know whether the treatment you are receiving is *standard* or *experimental*. In experimental conditions, you have the legal and ethical right to know if any drug is being used as part of a research project for a purpose not approved by the Food and Drug Administration (FDA) and if the study is one in which some people receive treatment while others receive a **placebo**.

3. You have the *right to make decisions* regarding the health care that is recommended by the physician.

4. You have the *right to confidentiality*, which includes the source of payment for treatment and care. It also includes protecting your right to make personal decisions concerning all reproductive matters.

5. You have the *right to receive adequate health care*. You also have the legal right to refuse treatment at any time and to cease treatment at any time.

6. You are entitled to have *access to all of your medical records* and to have those records remain confidential.

7. You have the *right to continuity of health care*.

See It! Videos

Knowing your medical history can keep you informed of health risks. Watch **Your Medical History** in the Study Area of MasteringHealth™

8. You have the *right to continuity of health care.*

9. You have the *right to seek the opinions of other health care professionals* regarding your condition.

10. You have the *right to courtesy, respect, dignity, responsiveness, and timely* attention to health needs.

Choosing Health Products

Prescription drugs can be obtained only with a written prescription from a physician, while over-the-counter drugs can be purchased without a prescription (see **Chapter 7**). Just as making wise decisions about providers is an important aspect of responsible health care, so is making wise decisions about medications.

Prescription Drugs

In about two thirds of doctor visits, the physician administers or prescribes at least one medication.[6] In fact, prescription drug use has risen by 25 percent over the past decade.[7] Even though these drugs are administered under medical supervision, the wise consumer still takes precautions. Hazards and complications arising from the use of prescription drugs are common.

Consumers have a variety of resources available to help them determine the risks of various prescription medicines and make educated decisions about whether to take a certain drug. One of the best resources is the U.S. FDA Center for Drug Evaluation and Research website (www.fda.gov/drugs), which provides current information for consumers on risks and benefits of prescription drugs. Being knowledgeable can help ensure your safety. Common types of

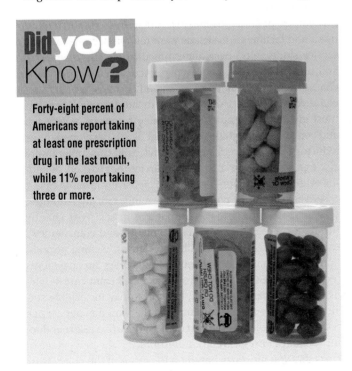

Did you Know?

Forty-eight percent of Americans report taking at least one prescription drug in the last month, while 11% report taking three or more.

prescription drugs discussed in this text include antidepressants and antianxiety drugs, hormonal contraceptives, weight-loss aids, smoking-cessation aids, stimulants and sedatives, statins and other cholesterol-lowering drugs, and antibiotics.

generic drugs Medications marketed by chemical names rather than brand names.

Generic drugs, medications sold under a chemical name rather than a brand name, contain the same active ingredients as brand-name drugs but are usually much less expensive. Not all drugs are available as generics. If your doctor prescribes medication, always ask if a generic equivalent exists and if it would be safe and effective for you to try.

Be aware, though, that there is some controversy about the effectiveness of generic drugs; substitutions sometimes are made in minor ingredients that can affect the way the drug is absorbed, potentially causing discomfort or even allergic reactions in some patients. Always note any reactions you have to medications and tell your doctor about them.

Over-the-Counter Drugs

Over-the-counter (OTC) drugs are nonprescription substances used in the course of self-diagnosis and self-medication. More than one third of the time, people treat their routine health problems with OTC medications. In fact, U.S. consumers spend billions of dollars yearly on OTC preparations for relief of everything from runny noses to ingrown toenails.

The FDA has categorized 26 types of OTC preparations. Those most commonly used are analgesics (pain relievers); medications for cough, cold, and allergy symptoms; stimulants; sleeping aids; weight loss aids; laxatives; and antacids.

Despite a common belief that OTC products are safe and effective, indiscriminate use and abuse can occur with these drugs as with all others. For example, people who frequently use eye drops to "get the red out" or pop antacids after every meal are likely to become dependent. Many people also experience adverse side effects because they ignore warnings on drug interactions and other cautions that are clearly printed on labels. The FDA has developed a standard label that appears on most OTC products (see **Figure 16.1** on the following page). It provides directions for use, warnings, and other important information. Diet supplements, which are regulated as food products, have their own type of label that includes a Supplement Facts panel.

Health Insurance

Whether you're visiting your regular doctor, consulting a specialist, or preparing for a hospital stay, chances are that you'll be using some form of health insurance to pay for your care. Insurance typically allows you, the consumer, to pay into a pool of funds and then bill the insurance carrier for covered charges you incur. The fundamental principle of insurance underwriting is that the cost of health care can be predicted for large populations. This is how health care **premiums** are determined. Policyholders pay premiums into

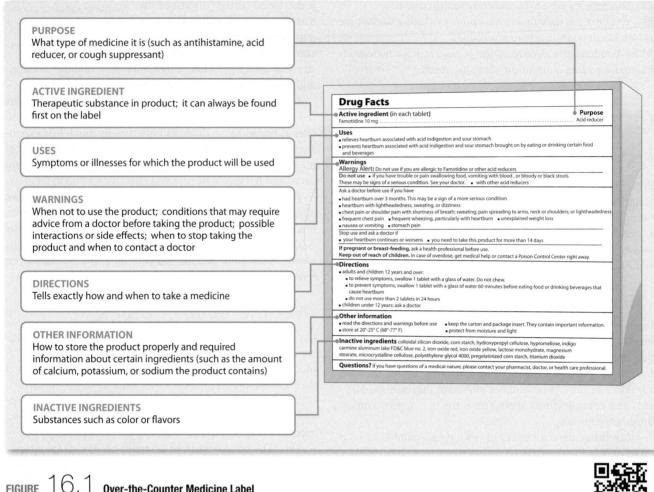

PURPOSE
What type of medicine it is (such as antihistamine, acid reducer, or cough suppressant)

ACTIVE INGREDIENT
Therapeutic substance in product; it can always be found first on the label

USES
Symptoms or illnesses for which the product will be used

WARNINGS
When not to use the product; conditions that may require advice from a doctor before taking the product; possible interactions or side effects; when to stop taking the product and when to contact a doctor

DIRECTIONS
Tells exactly how and when to take a medicine

OTHER INFORMATION
How to store the product properly and required information about certain ingredients (such as the amount of calcium, potassium, or sodium the product contains)

INACTIVE INGREDIENTS
Substances such as color or flavors

Drug Facts

Active ingredient (in each tablet)   **Purpose**
Famotidine 10 mg .... Acid reducer

Uses
- relieves heartburn associated with acid indigestion and sour stomach
- prevents heartburn associated with acid indigestion and sour stomach brought on by eating or drinking certain food and beverages

Warnings
Allergy Alert: Do not use if you are allergic to Famotidine or other acid reducers
Do not use ■ if you have trouble or pain swallowing food, vomiting with blood , or bloody or black stools. These may be signs of a serious condition. See your doctor. ■ with other acid reducers
Ask a doctor before use if you have
- had heartburn over 3 months. This may be a sign of a more serious condition.
- heartburn with lightheadedness, sweating, or dizziness
- chest pain or shoulder pain with shortness of breath; sweating; pain spreading to arms, neck or shoulders; or lightheadedness
- frequent chest pain ■ frequent wheezing, particularly with heartburn ■ unexplained weight loss
- nausea or vomiting ■ stomach pain
Stop use and ask a doctor if
- your heartburn continues or worsens ■ you need to take this product for more than 14 days
If pregnant or breast-feeding, ask a health professional before use.
Keep out of reach of children. In case of overdose, get medical help or contact a Poison Control Center right away.

Directions
- adults and children 12 years and over:
  - to relieve symptoms, swallow 1 tablet with a glass of water. Do not chew.
  - to prevent symptoms, swallow 1 tablet with a glass of water 60 minutes before eating food or drinking beverages that cause heartburn
  - do not use more than 2 tablets in 24 hours
- children under 12 years: ask a doctor

Other information
- read the directions and warnings before use ■ keep the carton and package insert. They contain important information.
- store at 20°-25° C (68°-77° F) ■ protect from moisture and light

Inactive ingredients colloidal silicon dioxide, corn starch, hydroxypropyl cellulose, hypromellose, indigo carmine aluminum lake FD&C blue no. 2, iron oxide red, iron oxide yellow, lactose monohydrate, magnesium stearate, microcrystalline cellulose, polyethylene glycol 4000, pregelatinized corn starch, titanium dioxide

Questions? If you have questions of a medical nature, please contact your pharmacist, doctor, or health care professional.

FIGURE 16.1 Over-the-Counter Medicine Label
Source: Consumer Healthcare Products Association, OTC Label. Courtesy of CHPA Educational Foundation, www.otcsafety.org

Video Tutor: Being a Good Health Care Consumer

---

premium Payment made to an insurance carrier, usually in monthly installments, that covers the cost of an insurance policy.

a pool from which companies pay claims. When you are sick or injured, the insurance company pays out of the pool, regardless of your total contribution. If you require a great deal of medical care, you may never pay anything close to the actual cost of that care. Or, if you are basically healthy, you may pay more in insurance premiums than the total cost of your medical bills. Health insurance is based on the idea that policyholders pay affordable premiums so they never have to face catastrophic bills. In today's profit-oriented system, insurers prefer to cover healthy people who pay more into risk pools than is needed to cover the cost of their health care claims.

Private Health Insurance

Originally, health insurance consisted solely of coverage for hospital costs (it was called *major medical*), but was gradually extended to cover things such as routine physician treatment, dental and vision services, and pharmaceuticals. These payment mechanisms laid the groundwork for today's steadily rising health care costs as hospitals were reimbursed for the costs of providing care plus an amount for profit. This system

provided no incentive to contain costs, limit the number of procedures, or curtail capital investment in redundant equipment and facilities. Physicians were reimbursed on a fee-for-service (indemnity) basis determined by "usual, customary, and reasonable" fees. This system encouraged physicians to charge high fees, raise them often, and perform as many procedures as possible. Until the mid- to late-twentieth century, most insurance did not cover routine or preventive services, and consumers generally waited until illness developed to see a doctor instead of seeking preventive care. Consumers were also free to choose any provider or service they wished, including even inappropriate—and often expensive—levels of care.

Private insurance companies have increasingly employed several mechanisms to limit potential losses: cost sharing (in the form of deductibles, co-payments, and coinsurance), exclusions, "preexisting condition" clauses, waiting periods, and upper limits on payments. *Deductibles* are payments (commonly $250 to $1,000) you make for health care services before insurance coverage kicks in to pay for eligible services. *Co-payments* are set amounts that you pay per service received, regardless of the cost of the service (e.g., $20 per doctor visit or per prescription). *Coinsurance* is the percentage of costs that you must pay based on the terms of the policy (e.g.,

20 percent of the total bill). Because health insurance policies may include a combination of these mechanisms, keeping track of the costs you are responsible for can become difficult.

Some plans specify a *waiting period* such as 6 or 12 months before they will provide coverage for preexisting conditions. All insurers set limits on the types of services they cover (e.g., most exclude cosmetic surgery, private hospital rooms, and experimental procedures).

Managed Care

Managed care describes a health care delivery system consisting of the following:

- A network of physicians, hospitals, and other providers and facilities linked contractually to deliver comprehensive health benefits within a predetermined budget and sharing economic risk for any budget deficit or surplus
- A budget based on an estimate of the annual cost of delivering health care for a given population
- An established set of administrative rules regarding how services are to be obtained from participating health care providers under the terms of the health plan

Types of managed care plans include health maintenance organizations (HMOs), preferred provider organizations (PPOs), and point of service (POS). Approximately 66 million Americans are enrolled in HMOs, the most common type of managed care.[8]

Many managed care plans pay their contracted health care providers through **capitation**, a fixed monthly amount paid for each enrolled patient without regard for the type or number of services provided, and some are still fee-for-service plans. Doctors participating in managed care networks are motivated to keep their patient pool healthy and avoid preventable catastrophic ailments, and they may receive incentives for doing so. Prevention and health education to reduce risk and intervene early to avoid major problems are often capstone components of such plans.

Managed care plans have grown steadily over the past several decades and there has been a proportionate decline of enrollment in traditional indemnity plans. The reason for this shift is that indemnity insurance, which pays providers and hospitals on a fee-for-service basis with no built-in incentives to control costs, has become unaffordable or unavailable for most Americans.

Health Maintenance Organization

Health maintenance organizations (HMOs) provide a wide range of covered health benefits (e.g., physician visits, lab tests, surgery)

for a fixed amount prepaid by the patient, the employer, Medicaid, or Medicare. Usually, HMO premiums are the least expensive form of managed care, but they are also the most restrictive (offering more limited choices of staff and health care facilities). There are low or no deductibles or coinsurance payments, and co-payments are small.

The downside of HMOs is that patients are required to use the plan's doctors and hospitals. Within an HMO, the PCP serves as a *gatekeeper*, coordinating the patient's care and providing referrals to specialists and other services. As more and more people enroll in HMOs, concerns have arisen about care allocation and access to services, profit-motivated medical decision making, and the degree of focus on prevention and intervention.

Preferred Provider Organization
Preferred provider organizations (PPOs) are networks of independent doctors and hospitals that contract to provide care at discounted

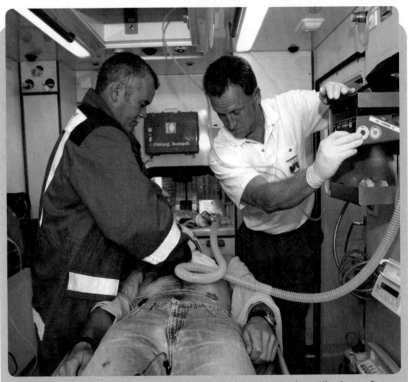

What happens if I don't have insurance and I need medical care?

People without health insurance can only access preventive care if they are willing or able to pay out of pocket. Lower-income individuals who are uninsured tend to seek care only in emergency or crisis situations. Because emergency care is extraordinarily expensive, they often are unable to pay, and the cost is absorbed by those who can pay—the insured or taxpayers. Using the emergency room for anything other than a real crisis contributes to higher health care costs and reduces access to emergency care for those who truly need it. If you need nonemergency health care, there are often community-based resources, such as free or low-cost clinics, that can provide checkups and treatment for common ailments and injuries.

managed care Type of health insurance plan based on coordination of care and cost-reduction strategies; emphasizes health education and preventive care.

capitation Fixed payment made at regular intervals (usually monthly) to a medical provider by a managed care organization for each enrolled patient without regard to the type or number of services provided.

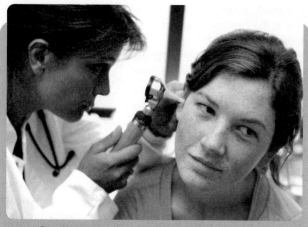

Can I count on my school's health care plan to cover my medical needs?

Most university insurance plans are short term and noncatastrophic and have low upper limits of benefits, all of which are problematic in the event of an emergency illness or accident. If you are covered only under your school's health care plan, you may want to consider also purchasing a high-deductible catastrophic plan or asking your parents if you are eligible to become a dependent on their plan. If you are enrolled in your parents' health insurance plan, under the Affordable Care Act of 2010 you can continue this coverage until age 26 if you are not able to obtain coverage from an employer.

Medicare A federal health insurance program that covers people over the age of 65, permanently disabled people, and people with end-stage kidney failure.

Medicaid A federal–state matching funds program that provides health insurance to low-income people, including pregnant women, the blind, the disabled, the elderly, or needy families.

rates. Although they often offer more choices of providers than do HMOs, they are less likely to coordinate a patient's care. Members may choose to see doctors who are not on the preferred list, and this choice involves having to pay a higher percentage of out-of-pocket costs.

Point of Service Point of service (POS)—a hybrid of HMO and PPO plans—provides a more familiar form of managed care for people used to traditional indemnity insurance, which may explain why it is among the fastest growing of managed care plans. Under POS plans, members select an in-network PCP, but they can go to non-network providers for care without a referral and must pay the extra cost.

No matter what type of plan you have, a special savings account for health-related expenses could save you money. See the **Money & Health** box on the following page for details.

Government-Funded Programs

The federal government, through programs such as Medicare and Medicaid, currently funds 45 percent of total U.S. health spending.[9]

Medicare **Medicare** is a federal insurance program that covers a broad range of services, except long-term care. Medicare covers 99 percent of Americans over age 65, all totally and permanently disabled people (after a waiting period), and all people with end-stage kidney failure. Taken together, these groups comprise over 45 million people, or 1 in 7 Americans.[10] By 2030, it is estimated that 1 in 5—or 77 million—Americans will be insured by Medicare. As the costs of medical care have continued to increase, Medicare has placed limits on the amount of reimbursement to providers. As a result, some providers no longer accept Medicare patients.

To control hospital costs, the federal government set up a prospective payment system based on *diagnosis-related groups (DRGs)* for Medicare. Nearly 500 groupings were created to establish how much a hospital would be reimbursed for caring for a patient diagnosed with a particular condition or combination of conditions. DRGs are based on the assumption that patients with similar health status and conditions will require a similar amount of hospital resources. If the costs of treating a patient are less than the predetermined amount, the hospital can keep the difference. However, if a patient's care costs more than the set amount, the hospital must absorb the difference (with a few exceptions, this must be reviewed by a panel). This system motivates hospitals to discharge patients quickly, to provide more ambulatory care, and to admit patients classified into the most favorable (profitable) DRGs. Many private health insurance companies have also adopted reimbursement rates based on DRGs. In 1998, the federal Health Care Financing Administration (HCFA) expanded the prospective payment system to include payments for outpatient surgery and skilled nursing care.

In its continuing effort to control rising costs, HCFA, now known as the Centers for Medicare and Medicaid Services (CMS), has encouraged the growth of HMO plans for Medicare-eligible persons. Under this system, commercial managed care insurance plans receive a fixed per capita premium from CMS and then offer more preventive services with lower out-of-pocket co-payments. These managed care plans encourage providers and patients to use health care resources under administrative rules similar to commercial HMO plans.

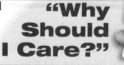

"Why Should I Care?"

The ultimate choice about health care remains with you. In order to make sound decisions about what is best for your health, you need to understand as much as you can about your options.

Medicaid In contrast to Medicare, **Medicaid** is a federal–state matching funds program that provides health insurance for people defined as low income, including many who are pregnant, blind, disabled, elderly, or eligible for Temporary Assistance for Needy Families (TANF).[11] Medicaid relies on funds provided by both federal and state sources, and covers approximately 52 million people.[12] Because each state determines income eligibility, covered services, and payments to providers, there are vast differences in the way Medicaid operates from state to state.

The Children's Health Insurance Program (CHIP) provides health insurance coverage to more than 8 million uninsured

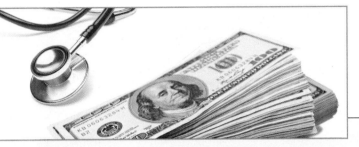

Money&Health

HEALTH CARE SPENDING ACCOUNTS

A Flexible Spending Account (FSA) for health care and a Health Savings Account (HSA) are savings plans that give you the opportunity to save money tax free to be used toward qualified health care expenses. As long as you're not claimed as a dependent on someone else's tax return, you can open either an FSA through your employer or an HSA through your bank.

If you're an employee, upon enrollment you identify the amount you want diverted from your paycheck into your FSA before taxes are withheld. The maximum you can contribute varies with different employers and health plans. One drawback to the FSA is that any funds still in the account at the end of the plan year are forfeited. This is known as the "use it or lose it" rule. Therefore, you need to estimate carefully what your out-of-pocket health expenses will be during the plan year.

With an HSA, there is no time limit on when the funds have to be used. Contributions to the account can be made from your paycheck by your employer as pre-tax deductions, or you can make them yourself, in which case you can claim them as an "above-the-line" deduction (a deduction from your gross income) when you file your tax return.

What expenses can you pay for with the money in your account? Deductibles, co-payments, eyeglasses, contact lenses, and prescription drugs are all allowed. Visits to approved health care providers, including dentists and optometrists, are also payable from your account if you have no health insurance coverage for them. You can even use the funds to pay for OTC drugs such as pain relievers or allergy medications as long as you have a written statement from your care provider that the item is being purchased for a specific medical condition.

Does a health care spending account make sense for you? If you currently pay out of pocket for more than one or two health care visits a year, for a few prescriptions, contact lenses, etc., and the money you use for these expenses comes from taxable income, then a health care savings plan might be worth a closer look. Contact your employee benefits specialist, your tax preparer, or a customer service provider at your bank.

---

children.[13] Like Medicaid, it is jointly funded by federal and state funds and is administered by state governments.

Insurance Coverage by the Numbers

In 2013, the average family's annual health insurance premium was more than $13,000.[14] For workers employed in organizations that offer health care insurance, most of this cost is covered by the employer. A worker typically pays 15 to 25 percent of the full premium, usually as a paycheck deduction. However, people who are self-employed or work in companies that do not provide group health insurance must pay their premiums independently, and millions of employed but uninsured Americans do not find them affordable. In total, over 46 million Americans—15 percent—are completely uninsured; that is, they have no private health insurance and are not eligible for Medicare, Medicaid, or other government health programs.[15] The vast majority of the uninsured work or are dependents of employed people.

Lack of health insurance has been associated with delayed health care and increased mortality. *Underinsurance* (i.e., the inability to pay out-of-pocket expenses despite having insurance) also may result in adverse health consequences. Among young adults ages 18 to 24, 26 percent do not have health insurance coverage.[16] However, for young adults who are college students, the statistics are different. In a 2012 national survey of college students, 7 percent of respondents said they did not have health insurance.[17] People without adequate health care coverage are less likely than other Americans to have their children immunized, seek early prenatal care, obtain annual blood pressure checks and other screenings, and seek attention for symptoms of health problems. Forgoing preventative care because of cost, they tend to rely on emergency care at later stages of illness. Because emergency care is far more expensive than other types of care, uninsured and underinsured patients are often unable to pay, and the cost is absorbed by "the system" in the form of higher hospital costs, insurance premiums, and taxes for all.

Issues Facing Today's Health Care System

In recent decades the number of Americans without health insurance increased dramatically as costs and restrictions on eligibility for coverage rose. In 2010, Congress passed the Patient Protection and Affordable Care Act (ACA), otherwise known as Obamacare, to provide a means for all Americans to obtain affordable heath care. In addition to increasing access to care, the ACA is expected to address the United States' high cost of care and to improve the overall quality of care. Here we examine these three key issues, as well as the potential impact of the ACA.

Access

The most significant factors in determining access to health care are the supply and proximity of providers and facilities and insurance coverage.

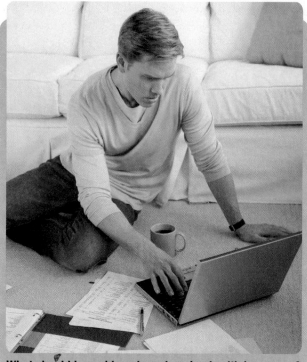

What should I consider when choosing health insurance?

Choosing a health insurance plan can be confusing. Some things to think about include how comprehensive your coverage needs to be; how far are you willing to travel to obtain care; how much can you spend on premiums, deductibles, and co-payments; and will services offered by the plan meet your needs?

Access to Providers, Facilities, and Treatments In 2012, there were almost 700,000 physicians in the United States.[18] However, there is an oversupply of higher-paid specialists and a shortage of lower-paid primary care physicians (family practitioners, internists, pediatricians, etc.). The majority of nongovernment hospitals in the United States are also located in urban areas, leaving many rural communities with a lack of facilities.[19]

Managed care health plans determine access on the basis of participating providers, health plan benefits, and administrative rules, which means that consumers have little say in who treats them or what facility they can use.

Access to Quality Health Insurance Not everyone has the same insurance (or any at all), and unfortunately that means not everyone gets the same level of care. Patients with excellent insurance may be encouraged to undergo expensive tests and treatments (a practice that can lead to useless or even harmful overtreatment), whereas patients with poor insurance may not be informed of the full variety of diagnostic and treatment options.[20]

Key provisions in the ACA aim to increase access to quality health insurance among Americans. These include the following:

● Insurers are now required to cover preventive services, such as screenings for cancer, mammograms and colonoscopies, tests of blood glucose and blood pressure, and counseling on topics such as losing weight, quitting smoking, treating depression, and reducing alcohol use.

● Insurers are required to cover young adults on a parent's plan through age 26.

● Coverage for prescription medications, including psychotropic medications, is required.

● Americans with preexisting conditions cannot be denied coverage.

● No annual and lifetime limits on benefits are allowed.

● Affordable Insurance Exchanges (AIEs) will facilitate consumer shopping and enrollment in plans with the same kinds of choices that members of Congress have.

● Small businesses, which typically paid as much as 18 percent more than large businesses for health insurance coverage for their employees, now qualify for special tax credits to help fund insurance plans.

Even before passage of the ACA, Congress provided assistance with insurance coverage for employees who change jobs. Under the Consolidated Omnibus Budget Reconciliation Act (COBRA), former employees, retirees, spouses, and dependents have the option to continue their insurance for up to 18 months at group rates. People who enroll in COBRA do pay a higher amount than they did when they were employed because they are covering both the personal premium and the amount previously covered by the employer.

Cost

The United States spends more on health care than any other nation. In 2011, our national health expenditures reached $2.7 trillion, over $8,600 for every man, woman, and child—17.9 percent of our gross domestic product (GDP).[21] Health care expenditures are projected to grow by 6.2 percent each year, reaching over $4.7 trillion annually by 2021—nearly 20 percent of our projected GDP (see **Figure 16.2** on the following page).[22]

Why are the United States' health care costs so high? Many factors are involved: duplication of services; an aging population; growing rates of obesity, inactivity, and related health problems; demand for new diagnostic and treatment technologies; an emphasis on crisis-oriented care instead of prevention; physician overtreatment, whether to avoid malpractice suits or to increase income; and inappropriate use of services by consumers, including use of emergency services for routine care, and family demands for futile and expensive procedures for patients who are dying.

Our insurance system is also to blame. Currently, more than 2,000 companies provide health insurance in the United States, each with different coverage structures and administrative

The estimated cost of medical errors each year is

$17.1 billion.

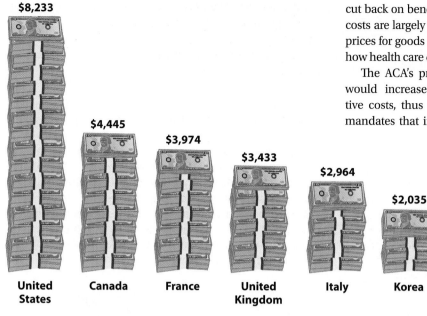

FIGURE 16.2 **Health Care Spending per Person, 2010 (in thousands of U.S. dollars)**

$8,233 — United States
$4,445 — Canada
$3,974 — France
$3,433 — United Kingdom
$2,964 — Italy
$2,035 — Korea

Source: Data from Organization for Economic Co-operation and Development, *OECD Health Data 2012*, 2012, www.oecd.org

cut back on benefits, and drop some benefits altogether. These costs are largely passed on to consumers in the form of higher prices for goods and services. See Figure 16.3 for a breakdown of how health care dollars are spent.

The ACA's provision for Affordable Insurance Exchanges would increase bulk purchasing and reduce administrative costs, thus achieving some savings. Moreover, the ACA mandates that insurance companies that spend less than 80 percent of premium dollars on medical care in a given year now must send enrollees a rebate. All insurance companies now have to publicly justify their actions if they plan to raise rates by 10 percent or more, and tougher screening procedures and penalties are helping to reduce health care fraud, which should also cut down on ballooning costs.

Quality

requirements. This lack of uniformity prevents our system from achieving the *economies of scale* (bulk purchasing at a reduced cost) and administrative efficiency realized in countries in which there is a single-payer delivery system. According to the Health Insurance Association of America, commercial insurance companies commonly experience administrative costs greater than 10 percent of the total health care insurance premium, whereas the administrative cost of the government's Medicare program is less than 4 percent. These administrative expenses contribute to the high cost of health care and force companies to require their employees to share more of the costs,

In the United States, health care providers are assessed according to education, licensure, certification/registration, accreditation, peer review, and the legal system of malpractice litigation. Over-the-counter and prescription medications, as well as medical devices, must be approved by the Food and Drug Administration. Insurance companies and government payers may also require a higher level of quality by linking payment to whether a practitioner is board certified, a facility is accredited, or a treatment is an approved therapy. Although our health care spending far exceeds that of any other nation, we rank far below many other nations in key indicators of quality. For example, in 2011, life expectancy in the United States (78.49 years) was lower than that of 49 other nations of the world.[23]

Additionally, our infant mortality rate—5.98 deaths per every 1,000 live births—is higher than that of 48 other nations.[24] The ACA is intended to improve the quality of health care in the United States by emphasizing preventative and effective care.[25] Despite this, many health experts feel that our system has failed, and an entirely new system must be put in its place. See the Points of View box

Total expenditures = $2.5 trillion

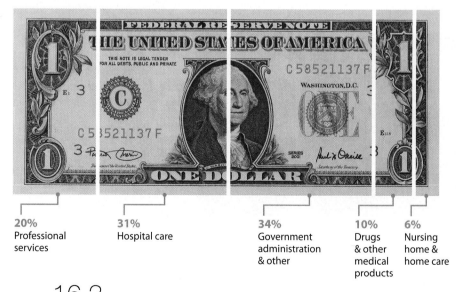

20% Professional services
31% Hospital care
34% Government administration & other
10% Drugs & other medical products
6% Nursing home & home care

FIGURE 16.3 **Where Do We Spend Our Health Care Dollars?**

Source: Data from National Center for Health Statistics, *Health, United States, 2011, with Special Feature on Medical Technology* (Hyattsville, MD: National Center for Health Statistics, 2012.

what do you think?

Why is it important that private insurance cover preventive or lower-level care as well as hospitalization and high-tech interventions?

● What kinds of incentives would cause you to seek care early rather than delay care?

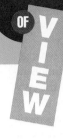
National Health Care:
IS IT A GOVERNMENT RESPONSIBILITY?

Whether universal health care coverage will—or should—be achieved in the United States and through what mechanism remain hotly debated topics. Proponents of reform argue that health care is a basic human right and should be available and affordable for everyone. They point to other Western countries like Canada, the United Kingdom, and France that currently provide health care to all citizens through a national service funded through taxes. Opponents of health care reform feel that health care is not a right, but a commodity. They contend that the high cost of changing the system is more than the United States can afford and that the government should not interfere in what has been largely a free-market industry. In addition, lobbying efforts by the insurance industry, pharmaceutical manufacturers, the medical community, and special interest groups have all played a role in thwarting comprehensive reform.

In 2010, Congress passed the Patient Protection and Affordable Care Act (ACA), known as Obamacare. This act does not provide for a system of national health care but is merely a set of initial steps toward increasing the number of insured Americans. Still, it has been subjected to intense and often rancorous debate. The reforms mandated by the ACA are currently being implemented, and their actual effects are uncertain.

Arguments for National Health Insurance

○ Health care is a human right. The United Nations Universal Declaration of Human Rights states that "everyone has the right to a standard of living adequate for the health and well-being of oneself and one's family, including . . . medical care."

○ Americans would be more likely to engage in preventive health behaviors and clinicians would be encouraged to practice preventive medicine; people without insurance often avoid preventive care checkups and inquiring early about suspected symptoms because of cost concerns.

○ Medical professionals could concentrate on the care of patients rather than on insurance procedures, malpractice liability, and other administrative distractions.

○ Taxes already pay for a substantial amount of our health care expenditures.

○ Providing all citizens the right to health care is good for economic productivity because it allows them to live longer and healthier lives, thus contributing to society for a longer time.

Arguments against National Health Insurance

○ Health care is not a right, because it is not in the Bill of Rights in the U.S. Constitution, which lists rights that the government cannot infringe upon, not services or goods that the government must ensure for the people. Amending the U.S. Constitution to acknowledge a right to health care would be bad for economic productivity.

○ It is the individual's responsibility, not the government's, to ensure personal health. Diseases and health problems can often be prevented by individuals choosing to live healthier lifestyles.

○ Expenses for health care would have to be paid for with higher taxes or spending cuts in other areas, such as defense and education.

○ Profit motives, competition, and individual ingenuity have always led to greater cost control and effectiveness. These concepts should be brought to health care reform.

Where Do You Stand?

○ Do you think that all Americans should have the right to health care?

○ Is health insurance a personal responsibility?

○ Do you currently have health insurance? If you don't, what are the barriers that prevent you from having health insurance?

○ If you do have health insurance, are you currently paying for it? If you are not paying for it, who is?

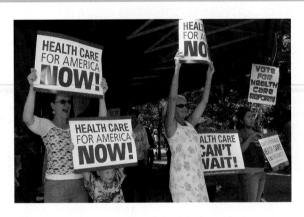

○ Do you have a family member or close friend who lives in a country with a national health care system? If so, does this person support national health care or not, and why?

Sources: "The Universal Declaration of Human Rights" from The United Nations, 1948; Right to Health Care ProCon.org, "Should All Americans Have the Right (Be Entitled) to Health Care?" Updated October 2010, http://healthcare.procon.org; The White House, "Health Care Reform: The Affordable Care Act," 2010, www.whitehouse.gov

for a discussion of the pros and cons of a system of national health insurance that advocates believe would address these key concerns.

On a personal level, perhaps the most important measurement is how you and your loved ones experience the health care provided.

Are You a Smart Health Care Consumer?

Answer the following questions to determine what you might do to become a better health care consumer.

	Yes	No
1. Do you have health insurance, and if so, do you understand the coverage available to you under your plan?	○	○
2. Do you know which health care services are available for free or at a reduced cost at your student health center or local clinic? If so, what are they?	○	○
3. When you receive a prescription, do you ask the doctor or pharmacist if a generic brand could be substituted?	○	○
4. When you receive a prescription, do you ask the doctor or pharmacist about potential side effects, including possible food and drug interactions?	○	○
5. Do you report any unusual drug side effects to your health care provider?	○	○
6. Do you take medication as directed?	○	○

	Yes	No
7. When you receive a diagnosis, do you seek more information about the diagnosis and treatment?	○	○
8. If your health care provider recommends surgery or an invasive type of treatment, do you seek a second opinion?	○	○
9. Do you seek health information only from reliable and credible sources? Can you name three examples of such sources?	○	○
10. Do you read labels carefully before buying over-the-counter (OTC) medications?	○	○
11. Do you have a primary health care provider?	○	○
12. How much of a role do you think advertising plays in your decision to purchase health care products and services?		

None ○   Some ○   A lot ○

YOUR PLAN FOR CHANGE

Once you have considered your responses to the **Assess yourself** questions, you may want to change or improve certain behaviors to get the best treatment from your health care provider and the heath care system.

Today, you can:

○ Research the insurance plan under which you are covered. Find out which health care providers and hospitals you can visit, the amounts of any co-payments and premiums you will be responsible for, and the drug coverage of your plan.

○ Clean out your medicine cabinet. Get rid of any expired prescriptions or OTC medications and take stock of what you have. Keep on hand a supply of basic items, such as pain relievers, antiseptic cream, bandages, cough suppressants, and throat lozenges, and replenish the supply if you are running low.

Within the next 2 weeks, you can:

○ Find a regular health care provider if you do not have one and make an appointment for a general checkup.

○ Think about health conditions that you should know more about—such as those that run in your family or that you've experienced in the past—and do some research on them. Write down any unanswered questions so that you can discuss them with your health care provider.

By the end of the semester, you can:

○ Ask if a generic version is appropriate and available when filling your next prescription.

○ Become informed about health care issues both in your state and the country. Write to your state and congressional legislators to express your opinions about needed reforms.

MasteringHealth™

Build your knowledge—and health!—in the Study Area of MasteringHealth with a variety of study tools.

Summary

* Self-care and individual responsibility are key factors in reducing health care costs and improving health status. Advance planning can help you navigate health care treatment in unfamiliar situations or emergencies. Assess health professionals by considering their qualifications, their record of treating conditions similar to yours, and their willingness to answer questions and respect you as an educated consumer.

* In theory, allopathic (conventional Western) medicine is based on scientifically validated methods and procedures. General physicians, specialists, nurses, and physician assistants are examples of health professionals who practice allopathic medicine.

* Prescription drugs are administered under medical supervision. Generic drugs can often be substituted for more expensive brand-name products. Over-the-counter (OTC) drugs include analgesics (pain relievers); medications for cough, cold, and allergy symptoms; stimulants; sleeping aids; weight loss aids; laxatives; and antacids. Consumers should be aware of the potential side effects and interactions of both prescription and OTC drugs.

* Health insurance is based on the concept of spreading risk. Insurance is provided by private insurance companies and several government-funded programs: Medicare, Medicaid, and CHIP. Managed care plans (in the form of HMOs, PPOs, and POS plans) attempt to control costs by streamlining administrative procedures and stressing preventive care, among other initiatives.

* Issues facing the U.S. health care system today include the increasing cost of care, access to appropriate care, and ensuring the quality of care.

Pop Quiz

1. Which of the following is a condition that does not warrant a visit to a physician?
   a. Recurring high temperature (over 103°F in adults)
   b. Persistent or recurrent diarrhea
   c. The common cold
   d. Yellowing of the skin or the whites of the eyes

2. Which medical practice is based on treating the patient's symptoms using scientifically validated methods?
   a. Allopathic medicine
   b. Nonallopathic medicine
   c. Osteopathic medicine
   d. Chiropractic medicine

3. Jack evaluates visual problems and fits glasses but is not a trained physician. Jack is an
   a. osteopath.
   b. ophthalmologist.
   c. optometrist.
   d. orthopedist.

4. A specialist who diagnoses and treats diseases of the teeth, gums, and oral cavity is a(n)
   a. dentist.
   b. orthodontist.
   c. oral surgeon.
   d. periodontist.

5. Which is a common type of over-the-counter drug?
   a. Antibiotics
   b. Hormonal contraceptives
   c. Antidepressants
   d. Antacids

6. What is the term for an amount paid directly to a provider by a patient before his or her insurance carrier will begin paying for services?
   a. Coinsurance
   b. Cost sharing
   c. Co-payment
   d. Deductible

7. Which of the following is true under the Affordable Care Act (ACA)?
   a. Young adults can remain on their parents' health insurance plan until they're 30.
   b. Insurance providers cannot deny coverage for preexisting health conditions.
   c. Insurance providers can set annual and lifetime spending limits.
   d. Only HMO health plans are available through the Affordable Insurance Exchanges.

8. The most restrictive type of managed care is
   a. fee-for-service.
   b. health maintenance organizations.
   c. point of service.
   d. preferred provider organizations.

9. The federal health insurance program that covers 99 percent of adults over 65 years of age is
   a. Medicare.
   b. Medicaid.
   c. COBRA.
   d. HMO.

10. Deborah, 28, is a low-income single parent who receives Temporary Assistance for Needy Families (TANF). Her health insurance coverage is provided by a federal program known as
    a. CHIP.
    b. Social Security.
    c. Medicaid.
    d. Medicare.

Answers to these questions can be found on page A-1.

Think about It!

1. List several conditions (resulting from illness or accident) for which you wouldn't need to seek medical help. When would you consider each condition to be bad enough to require medical attention? How would you decide where to go for treatment?
2. Describe your rights as a patient. Have you ever received treatment that violated these rights? If so, what action, if any, did you take?
3. What are the inherent benefits and risks of managed care health insurance plans?
4. Explain the differences between traditional indemnity insurance and managed health care. Should insurance companies dictate reimbursement rates for various medical tests and procedures in an attempt to keep prices down? Why or why not?
5. Discuss how pharmaceutical waste has a negative impact on the environment. What are two ways that you personally can reduce such waste?

Accessing Your Health on the Internet

The following websites explore further topics and issues related to personal health. For links to the websites below, visit the Study Area in MasteringHealth.

1. *Agency for Healthcare Research and Quality (AHRQ).* This gateway to consumer health information provides links to sites that can address health care concerns and provide information on what questions to ask, what to look for, and what you should know when making critical decisions about personal care. www.ahrq.gov
2. *Food and Drug Administration (FDA).* This website provides news on the latest government-approved home health tests and other health-related products. www.fda.gov
3. *HealthGrades.* This company provides quality reports on physicians as well as hospitals, nursing homes, and other health care facilities. www.healthgrades.com

4. *The Leapfrog Group.* A nationwide coalition of more than 150 public and private organizations, the Leapfrog Group focuses on identifying problems in the U.S. hospital system that can lead to medical errors and on devising solutions. www.leapfroggroup.org
5. *National Committee for Quality Assurance (NCQA).* The NCQA assesses and reports on the quality of managed care plans, including HMOs. www.ncqa.org
6. *National Library of Medicine.* The library supports Medline/Pubmed information retrieval systems in addition to providing public health information for consumers. www.nlm.nih.gov
7. *Healthcare.gov.* This website provides up-to-date information regarding health care reform in the United States. www.healthcare.gov
8. *Physician Compare.* The Affordable Care Act mandated this website be established to provide basic information on physicians for consumers to use to assist them in finding a doctor. www.medicare.gov/find-a-doctor

Understanding Complementary and Alternative Medicine

LEARNING OUTCOMES

✱ Explain the difference between complementary, alternative, and integrative medicine.

✱ Describe the main alternative medical systems available in the United States.

✱ Identify the key features of chiropractic medicine, massage therapy, and movement therapy.

✱ Compare and contrast acupuncture, acupressure, qigong, Reiki, and therapeutic touch.

✱ Explain how mind-body therapies counteract the negative effects of stress.

✱ Describe functional foods and dietary supplements and explain why caution is important when using these products.

✱ Discuss the future of complementary and alternative medicine.

493
Why are so many people using complementary and alternative medicine?

494
What does chiropractic medicine do?

496
How does acupuncture work?

497
Do herbal remedies have any risks or side effects?

Increasingly popular in self-care and health promotion, **complementary and alternative medicine (CAM)** is a group of diverse medical and health care systems, practices, and products not generally considered part of conventional medicine.[1] CAM offers consumers a broad range of choices and an opportunity for greater control over their health.

complementary and alternative medicine (CAM) Group of diverse medical and health care systems, practices, and products that are not considered part of conventional medicine.

Distinguishing between Complementary and Alternative Medicine

Although the terms are often used interchangeably, there is a distinction between *complementary* and *alternative* *medicine*. **Complementary medicine** is used *along with* conventional medicine, as when a patient combines acupuncture treatments with prescription medication to reduce chronic pain.[2] **Alternative medicine** is used *in place of* conventional medicine. Using an herbal remedy to treat cancer instead of relying on radiation, surgery, or other conventional treatments is an example of alternative medicine. As discussed in the chapter on health care choices, doctors of medicine (MDs), doctors of osteopathy (DOs), nurses, and various allied health professionals practice conventional medicine. However, some conventional practitioners also employ CAM therapies in a practice known as **integrative medicine**.[3]

A survey conducted by the National Center for Complementary and Alternative Medicine (NCCAM) revealed that 38 percent of U.S. adults use some form of CAM.[4] Figure 1 identifies the therapies most commonly used. Why do so many people find CAM appealing? CAM therapies incorporate a **holistic** approach that focuses on treating the mind and the whole body, rather than just an isolated symptom or body part. CAM users are often seeking a less invasive, more natural, gentle approach to healing, one that gives them greater control over their health care. People are most likely to use CAM therapies for back, neck, head, or joint pain. Research suggests that therapies such as acupuncture, spinal manipulation, and massage are indeed beneficial in treating such conditions.[5]

Practitioners of most CAM therapies spend many years in training. Some types of CAM are even being taught in U.S. medical schools. Similar

to conventional medicine, there is no national training or licensure standard, and states differ in their requirements and regulations. Each type of CAM practice has a different set of training standards, guidelines for practice, and licensure procedures.

Before you consider using any form of CAM, visit the website of the National Center for Complementary and Alternative Medicine (NCCAM), which is a division of the National Institutes of Health (NIH). Its mission is to explore CAM practices using rigorous scientific methods and build an evidence base regarding their safety and effectiveness. The organization serves as an information clearinghouse and conducts research, education, and outreach programs.

NCCAM groups the various forms of CAM into five general categories of practice. These are identified in Figure 2 on the following page.

> More and more people are opting for complementary and alternative treatments. What are the potential benefits and risks of these treatments?

complementary medicine Treatment used in conjunction with conventional medicine.

alternative medicine Treatment used in place of conventional medicine.

integrative medicine Medical practice that combines conventional medicine with complementary and alternative therapies.

holistic Relating to or concerned with the whole body and the interactions of systems, rather than treatment of individual parts.

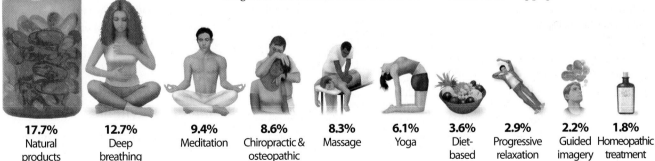

17.7%	12.7%	9.4%	8.6%	8.3%	6.1%	3.6%	2.9%	2.2%	1.8%
Natural products	Deep breathing	Meditation	Chiropractic & osteopathic	Massage	Yoga	Diet-based therapies	Progressive relaxation	Guided imagery	Homeopathic treatment

FIGURE 1 The 10 Most Common CAM Therapies among U.S. Adults

Source: Data from P. M. Barnes, B. Bloom, and R. Nahin, "Complementary and Alternative Medicine Use among Adults and Children: United States, 2007," *CDC National Health Statistics Report,* no. 12 (2008).

alternative (whole) medical systems Specific theories of health, balance, and practice that have developed outside the influence of conventional medicine.

traditional Chinese medicine (TCM) Ancient comprehensive system of healing that uses herbs, acupuncture, massage, and qigong to bring vital energy, qi, into balance and to remove blockages of qi that lead to disease.

Ayurveda A comprehensive system of medicine, originating in ancient India, that places equal emphasis on the body, mind, and spirit and strives to restore the body's innate harmony through diet, exercise, meditation, herbs, massage, sun exposure, and controlled breathing.

Alternative Medical Systems

Alternative (whole) medical systems reflect specific theories of health, balance, and practice that have developed outside the influence of conventional medicine. Many have been practiced by various cultures throughout the world for centuries. For example, Native American, aboriginal, African, Middle Eastern, South American, and Asian cultures have their own unique healing systems. Here, we discuss only a few of the most commonly available options.

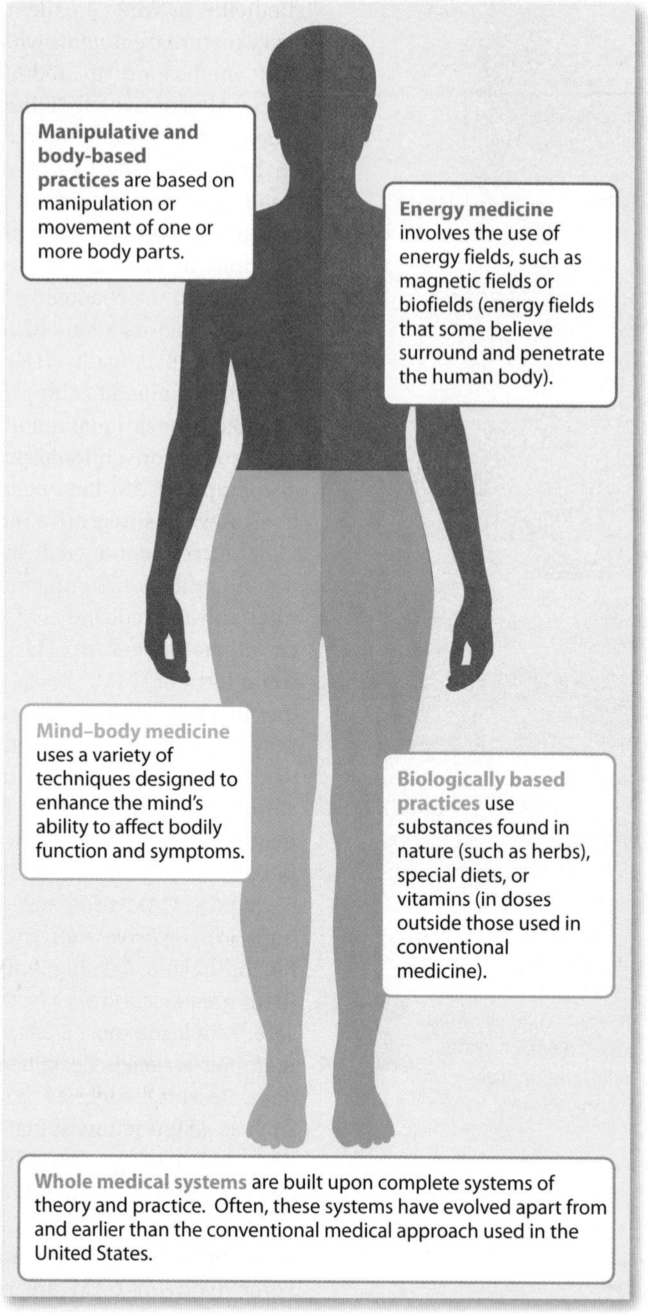

Manipulative and body-based practices are based on manipulation or movement of one or more body parts.
Energy medicine involves the use of energy fields, such as magnetic fields or biofields (energy fields that some believe surround and penetrate the human body).
Mind–body medicine uses a variety of techniques designed to enhance the mind's ability to affect bodily function and symptoms.
Biologically based practices use substances found in nature (such as herbs), special diets, or vitamins (in doses outside those used in conventional medicine).
Whole medical systems are built upon complete systems of theory and practice. Often, these systems have evolved apart from and earlier than the conventional medical approach used in the United States.

FIGURE 2 Types of Complementary and Alternative Medicine
NCCAM groups CAM practices into five major categories, recognizing that there can be some overlap.
Source: National Center for Complementary and Alternative Medicine, "What Is CAM?," NCCAM Publication no. D347, Updated May 2012, http://nccam.nih.gov

Traditional Chinese Medicine

The concept of *qi* (pronounced "chee"), or vital energy, is foundational to **traditional Chinese medicine (TCM)**. When qi is in balance, the person is in a state of health; imbalance of qi results in disease. Diagnosis is based on personal history, observation of the body (especially the tongue), palpation, and pulse diagnosis, a detailed procedure requiring considerable skill. Techniques such as acupuncture, herbal medicine, massage, and qigong (a form of energy therapy) are among the TCM approaches to health and healing.

Traditional Chinese medicine practitioners within the United States must have completed a graduate program at an approved college or university. Graduate programs usually involve an extensive 3- or 4-year clinical internship. In addition, the student must pass a certification and licensing examination. Acupuncture and qigong, two TCM techniques, are discussed later in the chapter.

Ayurveda

The "science of life," **Ayurveda** (or *ayurvedic medicine*) is an alternative medical system that has evolved over thousands of years in India. Ayurveda seeks to integrate and balance the body, mind, and spirit and to restore

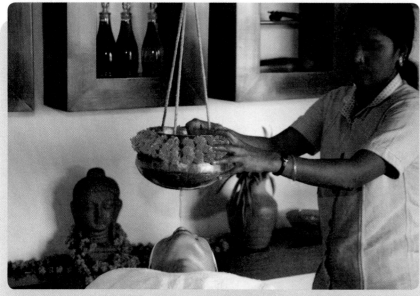

Why are so many people using complementary and alternative medicine?

People use CAM for multiple reasons, and many treatments can relieve a variety of symptoms. For example, *shirodhara*—a traditional ayurvedic treatment in which warm herb-infused oil is poured over the forehead in rhythmic patterns—is said to relieve stress and anxiety, treat insomnia and chronic headaches, and improve memory.

harmony in the individual.[6] Ayurvedic practitioners use various techniques, including questioning, observation, and pulse palpation, to determine which of three vital energies, or *doshas,* is dominant in the patient. They then establish a treatment plan to bring the doshas into balance, thereby reducing the patient's symptoms. Dietary modification and herbal remedies drawn from the botanical wealth of the Indian subcontinent are common. Treatments may also include certain yoga postures, meditation, massage, steam baths, changes in sleep patterns and sun exposure, and controlled breathing.

Training of ayurvedic practitioners varies. There is no national standard for certification, although professional groups are working toward creating licensing guidelines.

36%
of 18- to 29-year-olds report having used some form of CAM.

Homeopathy

Homeopathy is an unconventional Western system of medicine based on the principle that "like cures like." In other words, the same substance that in a large dose produces the symptoms of an illness—and may even be fatal—will in a small dose prompt the body's own defenses to cure the illness. Developed in the late 1700s by Samuel Hahnemann, a German physician, homeopathy follows the "law of minimum dose," which asserts that the lower the dose of a remedy, the greater its effectiveness. Thus, homeopathic remedies, which are derived from a wide range of natural, sometimes toxic, substances such as arsenic and belladonna, may be so diluted that no molecules of the original substance remain.[7] Although homeopathic physicians use certain standard remedies for certain common conditions, they also classify patients by type and work within each patient's type to heal ever-deeper layers of disturbance.

Homeopathic training varies considerably and is offered through diploma programs, certificate programs, short courses, and correspondence courses. Laws that detail requirements to practice vary from state to state.

Naturopathy

Naturopathy is a system of medicine that works with nature to restore people's health.[8] Naturopathic physicians view disease as a manifestation of the body's effort to ward off impurities and harmful substances from the environment. Naturopathic physicians emphasize prevention of disease and restoration of health through methods that encourage the person's inherent self-healing process. They employ an array of healing practices, including diet and clinical nutrition; homeopathy; acupuncture; herbal medicine; spinal and soft-tissue manipulation; physical therapies involving electric currents, ultrasound, water, magnets, and light therapy; therapeutic counseling; and pharmacology.

Several major naturopathic schools in the United States and Canada provide training, conferring the *naturopathic doctor (ND)* degree on students who have completed a 4-year graduate program that emphasizes humanistically oriented family medicine.

Manipulative and Body-Based Practices

The CAM domain of **manipulative and body-based practices** includes methods that are based on manipulation or movement of the body.

Chiropractic Medicine

Chiropractic medicine has been practiced for more than 100 years and focuses on manipulation of the spine and other neuromuscular structures.[9] A century ago, allopathic medicine and chiropractic medicine were in direct competition. Today, many health care organizations work closely with chiropractors, and many insurance companies pay for chiropractic treatment, particularly if it is recommended by a medical doctor.

Chiropractic medicine is based on the idea that a life-giving energy flows through the nervous system, including the spinal cord. If the spine is partly misaligned or dislocated, that force is disrupted. Chiropractors use a variety of techniques to manipulate the spine back into proper alignment so the energy can flow unimpeded. It has been established that their treatment can be effective for back pain, neck pain, and headaches.

The average chiropractic training program includes intensive courses in biochemistry, anatomy, physiology, diagnostics, pathology, nutrition, and related topics, combined with hands-on clinical training. Most state licensing boards require a 4-year course of study after completing at least a 3-year undergraduate program. Although states vary, increasing numbers require a 4-year undergraduate degree prior to entrance into chiropractic colleges. After completion of these requirements, applicants must pass an extensive licensing examination. The practice of chiropractic is licensed and regulated in all 50 states.[10]

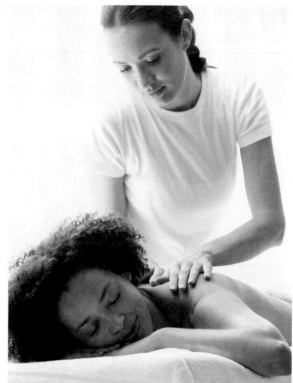

Evidence from over 20 years of research shows that massage therapy reduces anxiety, pain perception, and levels of stress hormones; increases weight gain and growth in preterm infants; enhances immune function; and reduces the frequency of migraine and tension headaches.

Massage Therapy

Massage therapy is soft tissue manipulation by trained therapists for relaxation and healing. References to massage have been found in ancient writings from many cultures, including ancient Greece, ancient Rome, Japan, China, Egypt, and the Indian subcontinent.[11] Today, massage therapy is used to treat painful conditions, relax tired and overworked muscles, reduce stress and anxiety, rehabilitate sports injuries, and promote general health. Therapists manipulate the patient's muscles and connective tissues to loosen the fibers, break up adhesions, and improve circulation. The following are some of the more popular types of massage therapy:

- *Swedish massage* uses long strokes, kneading, and friction on the muscles and moves the joints to aid flexibility.
- *Sports massage* is performed to prevent athletic injury and to help athletes recover from injuries.

- *Trigger point massage* uses a variety of strokes but applies deeper, more focused pressure on "knots" that can form in the muscles.
- *Shiatsu massage,* from Japan, applies firm finger pressure to specified points on the body that are believed to be important for the flow of vital energy.

There are about 1,500 massage therapy schools and training programs in the United States.[12] The course of study typically includes anatomy and physiology; kinesiology; therapeutic evaluation; massage techniques; first aid; business, ethical, and legal issues; and hands-on practice. For licensing, many states require a minimum of 500 hours of training and a passing grade on a national certification exam. Massage therapists work in private studios and health spas and in medical and chiropractic offices, hospitals, nursing homes, and fitness centers.[13]

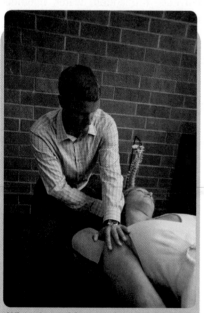

What does chiropractic medicine do?

Chiropractic medicine is often used to treat pain. Chiropractors manipulate the alignment of the spine, allowing energy to flow freely throughout the body.

Movement Therapies

CAM encompasses a broad range of Eastern and Western movement-based approaches used to promote physical, mental, emotional, and spiritual well-being. Examples include movement re-education techniques, exercise modalities, and techniques in which the therapist induces movement of the patient's body. According to the NCCAM, 1.5 percent of adults use movement therapies. Some commonly available approaches include the following:

- The *Alexander technique* is designed to release harmful tension in the body and improve ease of movement, balance, and coordination.
- The *Feldenkrais method* is a system of gentle movements and exercises that enhance awareness and retrain the nervous system to improve movement, flexibility, coordination, and overall functioning.
- *Pilates* is a popular exercise method focused on improving flexibility, strength, and body awareness. It involves a series of controlled movements, some of which are performed using special equipment.

Energy Medicine

Energy medicine therapies focus either on energy fields thought to originate within the body (biofields) or on fields from other sources (electromagnetic fields). The existence of these

Acupuncture practitioners use over

365

points along 14 meridians on the human body to treat a variety of conditions.

fields has not been demonstrated. Most forms of energy therapy manipulate biofields by applying pressure and/or manipulating the body by placing the hands in, or through, these fields.[14] The best-known forms of energy medicine include acupuncture and acupressure, qigong, Reiki, and therapeutic touch.

Acupuncture and Acupressure

Acupuncture, one of the oldest and most popular TCM therapies, is used to relieve a wide variety of health conditions, from musculoskeletal dysfunction to depression. The therapist stimulates various points on the body with a series of precisely placed and extremely fine needles. The stimulation of these acupuncture points is thought to increase the flow of qi through the *meridians,* or energy pathways, in the body (Figure 3).

Most participants in clinical studies report high levels of satisfaction following acupuncture treatment, improved quality of life, improvement in or cure of the condition, and reduced reliance on prescription drugs and surgery. Results have been promising in the treatment of headaches, fibromyalgia, low back pain, and nausea associated with chemotherapy.[15] Although there has been long-standing debate over the effectiveness of acupuncture, newer research provides

energy medicine Therapies using energy fields, such as electromagnetic fields or biofields.

acupuncture Technique of traditional Chinese medicine that involves the placement of fine needles to affect energy (qi) flow along meridians (energy pathways) within the body.

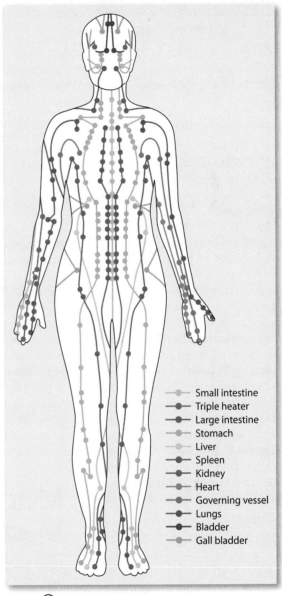

- Small intestine
- Triple heater
- Large intestine
- Stomach
- Liver
- Spleen
- Kidney
- Heart
- Governing vessel
- Lungs
- Bladder
- Gall bladder

FIGURE 3 **The Main Meridians**
Acupuncture and acupressure are two forms of traditional Chinese methods based on the belief that vital energy, qi, flows through meridians (energy pathways) in the body.
Source: Courtesy of the Association for Energy and Meridian Therapies, East Sussex, UK, http://theamt.com

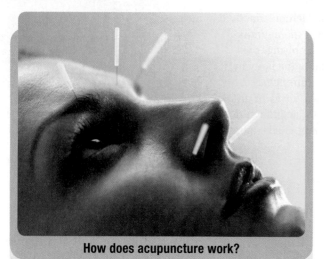

How does acupuncture work?

Fine needles are placed into specific points along meridians (energy pathways) in the body. This is thought to balance and increase the flow of vital energy (*qi*), providing many physical and mental benefits.

strong evidence for using acupuncture in chronic pain reduction, particularly for people who believe it will work and when needles are used in a specific way.[16]

Most U.S. acupuncturists are state licensed; however, the licensing requirements vary by state. Many have completed a 2- to 3-year postgraduate program. In addition, many conventional physicians and dentists practice acupuncture.[17]

Acupressure is based on the same principles of energy flow as acupuncture. Instead of inserting needles, however, the therapist applies pressure to the acupuncture points. The goal of the therapy is for qi to be evenly distributed and flow freely throughout the body. Practitioners typically have the same basic training and understanding of meridians and acupuncture points as do acupuncturists.

acupressure Technique of traditional Chinese medicine that uses application of pressure to selected points along meridians to balance energy.

mind-body medicine Techniques designed to enhance the mind's ability to affect bodily functions and symptoms and promote health.

Other Forms of Energy Therapy

Qigong, a traditional Chinese medicine technique, combines postures—whether stationary or moving—with meditation and focused breathing to regulate the flow of qi. Recent research shows that qigong, and the related practice tai chi, are effective for promoting bone health, cardiopulmonary fitness, and balance.[18]

Reiki is a hands-on energy therapy that originated in Japan. The name is derived from the Japanese words representing "universal" and "vital energy," or *ki*. Reiki is based on the belief that by channeling ki to the patient, the practitioner facilitates healing.

Therapeutic touch and a related therapy called *healing touch* are based on the premise that the therapist has the ability to perceive, through his or her hands held just above the patient's body, imbalances in the patient's energy. The therapist is said to promote healing by manipulating the patient's energy field and bringing it into balance. Research supporting the effectiveness of these therapies is limited.[19]

Mind-Body Medicine

Mind-body medicine employs a variety of techniques to enhance the mind's capacity to affect bodily functions and symptoms and to promote health. At present, mind-body techniques include deep breathing, meditation, yoga, progressive relaxation, and guided imagery—all among the ten most commonly used CAM thera-

pies in the United States. Mind-body medicine also includes certain uses of hypnosis, dance, music and art therapies, and prayer.

Research on *psychoneuroimmunology* (*PNI*) supports the effectiveness of mind-body therapies. *PNI* studies interrelationships among behavioral, neural, endocrine, and immune processes.[20] Many researchers have postulated that excessive stress and maladaptive coping can lead to immune system dysfunction and increase the risk of disease. Scientists are exploring ways in which relaxation, biofeedback, meditation, yoga, tai chi, and other activities that involve either conscious or unconscious mind "quieting" may counteract the negative effects of stressors. For example, a recent review study found that psychological support—including relaxation therapies—can improve wound healing.[21] In other research, inflammatory molecules such as C-reactive protein, a risk factor for heart disease, were found to be reduced in older adults after 16 weeks of tai chi.[22] Studies have also shown promising positive effects of mind-body techniques that encourage relaxation and other stress-reduction strategies for people with cancer.[23]

Dietary Products

Dietary products, including specially formulated foods and dietary supplements, are perhaps the most controversial domain of CAM therapies because of the sheer number of options available and the many claims that are made about their effects. Many of these claims have not been thoroughly investigated, and many of the products are not currently regulated.

Functional Foods

Dietary changes are often part of CAM therapies and commonly involve increased intake of certain *functional foods*—foods said to improve some specific aspect of physical or mental functioning beyond the contribution of their specific nutrients. Both whole foods, such as broccoli and nuts, and modified foods, such as an energy bar said to enhance memory, are classified as functional foods.[24] Food producers sometimes refer to their functional foods as **nutraceuticals** to emphasize their combined nutritional and pharmaceutical benefits. For example, the label on a bar of dark chocolate may state that modest consumption helps to reduce the risk of heart disease. The claim is backed up by research: Plant compounds called flavonoids found in chocolate improve several risk factors for heart disease.[25] The FDA regulates claims made on food labels; however, the FDA does not test functional foods before they come to market and can only remove a product from the market if it is found to be unsafe.

In recent years, functional foods containing *antioxidants* have received the most attention. Antioxidants are chemicals that combat free radicals and oxidative damage in cells. They include vitamins C and E, the mineral selenium, and a variety of phytochemicals, naturally occurring compounds present in many plant foods, from fruits and vegetables to coffee and tea.

Other common functional foods and their purported benefits include the following:

- **Plant stanols/sterols.** Can lower "bad" low-density lipoprotein (LDL) cholesterol.
- **Oat fiber.** Can lower LDL cholesterol; serves as a natural soother of nerves; stabilizes blood sugar levels.
- **Sunflower seeds and oil.** Can lower risk of heart disease; may prevent angina.
- **Soy protein.** May lower heart disease risk by reducing LDL cholesterol and triglycerides.
- **Garlic.** Lowers cholesterol and reduces clotting tendency of blood; lowers blood pressure; may serve as a form of antibiotic.
- **Ginger.** May prevent motion sickness, stomach pain, and stomach upset; discourages blood clots; may relieve rheumatism.

- **Probiotics.** Yogurt and other fermented dairy foods that are labeled "live and active cultures" contain active, friendly bacteria called *probiotics*. Normal residents of the large intestine, probiotics in foods are thought to reduce the risk for certain types of infections, including opportunistic yeast infections and those associated with acute diarrhea. The NIH is currently funding extensive research into the therapeutic effects of probiotics on human health.[26]

Herbal Remedies and Other Dietary Supplements

The Office of Dietary Supplements, part of the NIH, defines a *dietary supplement* as a "product (other than tobacco) that is intended to supplement or add to the diet; contains one or more dietary ingredients (including vitamins, minerals, herbs or other botanicals, amino acids, and other substances) or their constituents; is intended to be taken by mouth as a pill, capsule, tablet, or liquid; and is labeled on the front panel as being a dietary supplement."[27] Typically, people take dietary supplements—often without guidance from any CAM practitioner—to improve health, prevent disease, or enhance mood.

Herbal remedies, often referred to as *botanicals*, are among the most common dietary supplements sold. People have been using herbal remedies for thousands of years. Herbs were the original sources for compounds found in approximately 25 percent of the pharmaceutical drugs we use today, including

aspirin (white willow bark), the heart medication digitalis (foxglove), and the cancer treatment Taxol (Pacific yew tree). In addition, scientists continue to make pharmacological advances by studying the herbal remedies used in cultures throughout the world.

It's tempting to assume herbal remedies are safe because they are natural, but natural does not mean safe. For example, in recent years, the NCCAM has warned that certain herbal products containing kava may be associated with severe liver damage.[28] Even rigorously tested products can be risky. Many plants are poisonous, and some can be toxic if ingested in high doses. Others may be dangerous when combined with prescription or over-the-counter drugs, could disrupt the normal action of the drugs, or could cause unusual side effects.[29]

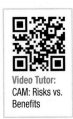

Video Tutor: CAM: Risks vs. Benefits

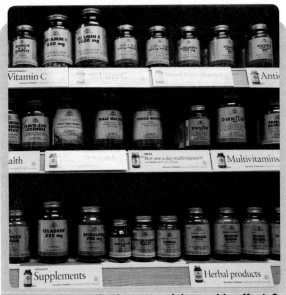

Do herbal remedies have any risks or side effects?

Herbs have the potential to cause negative side effects. St. John's wort, for example, has potentially harmful interactions with several prescription medications, including antidepressants, birth control pills, and heart drugs. Other herbs, such as kava, which can cause liver damage, can have negative effects even when taken alone.

In general, herbal medicines tend to be milder than synthetic medications and produce their effects more slowly. But too much of any herb, particularly from nonstandardized extracts, can cause problems. Table 1 on the following page gives an overview of some of the most common herbal supplements on the market.

Not all the supplements on the market today are directly derived from plant sources. In recent years, there have been increasing media claims about the health benefits of various hormones, enzymes, and other biological and synthetic compounds. Although a few products, such as melatonin (a hormone) or zinc lozenges (a mineral), have been widely studied, there is little quality research to support the claims of many others.

Consumer Protection

The burgeoning popularity of functional foods and dietary supplements concerns many scientists and consumers. Dietary supplements can currently be sold without FDA approval. This raises issues of consumer safety. Even when products are dispensed by CAM practitioners, the situation can be risky. Some homeopaths and herbalists who mix their own tonics may not use standardized measures and may not fully understand the potential interactions of their preparations. Products sold in "health food" stores and over the Internet may have varying levels of the active ingredient or may contain additives to which the consumer may have an adverse reaction.

As a result of such concerns, pressure has mounted to establish an approval process for dietary supplements similar to the process the FDA uses for drugs. In the meantime, if you're considering purchasing a dietary supplement, look for the USP Verified Mark on the label. The USP (United States Pharmacopeial Convention) is a nonprofit, scientific organization. It does not evaluate safety or effectiveness, but dietary supplement products must meet stringent quality and manufacturing criteria to earn the USP Verified Mark.[30] Visit their website at www.usp.org to learn more and see a list of USP verified products.

In addition, it is important to gather whatever information you can on both the safety and efficacy of any CAM treatment you are considering. Start your research with NCCAM (www.nccam.nih.gov) and the Cochrane Collaboration's review on complementary and alternative medicine (www.cochrane.org).

The Future of CAM Therapy

U.S. consumers are choosing CAM therapies in record numbers, and many pay out of pocket for these therapies. However, health insurance providers are increasingly likely to cover at least one form of CAM. Payments for chiropractic, acupuncture, and massage therapy are the most common.

Support from professional organizations, such as the American Medical Association, is also increasing as more medical schools are educating doctors about the pros and cons of CAM and are offering training in integrative practices. As health care providers and consumers learn more, we will be better able to integrate conventional treatments and CAM to improve health and combat disease.

Individuals must take an active role in their health care, which means staying educated. CAM can offer new avenues toward better health, but you must make sure that you are on the right path. See the Skills for Behavior Change box for tips on how to make smart decisions about integrating CAM therapies into your health care.

CAM and Self-Care

To help you make the best decisions about CAM, consider these pointers:

> Do your homework. Look into scientific studies on the safety and effectiveness of the CAM product or treatment you're considering. Consult only reliable sources such as established journals and periodicals and government resources such as the NCCAM, the Cochrane Collaboration, and the FDA.

> Consult your health care provider. If you use any CAM therapy, inform your primary health care provider. It is particularly important to talk with your provider if you are currently taking a prescription drug, have a chronic medical condition, are planning to have surgery, or are pregnant or nursing.

> If you use a CAM therapy such as acupuncture, choose the practitioner with care and make sure he or she has appropriate credentials for the area of specialty. Check with your insurer to see if services will be covered.

> Remember that *natural* and *safe* are not synonymous. Many people have become seriously ill after using "natural" products. Be cautious about combining supplements, just as you should be cautious about combining prescription and/or OTC drugs. Seek help if you notice any unusual side effects.

> Look out for your own health. Regulations regarding the quality and purity of dietary supplements are minimal. Check for the word *standardized* or the USP Verified Mark on supplement products and look for reputable manufacturers.

TABLE

1

Common Supplements: Benefits, Research, and Risks

	Herb	Claims of Benefits	Research Findings	Potential Risks
	Echinacea (purple coneflower, *Echinacea purpurea, E. angustifolia, E. pallida*)	Stimulates the immune system and increases the effectiveness of white blood cells that attack bacteria and viruses. Useful in preventing and treating colds or the flu.	Many studies in Europe have provided preliminary evidence of its effectiveness in preventing or treating a cold, but studies in the United States are mixed as to whether echinacea is more effective than a placebo.	Allergic reactions, including rashes, increased asthma, gastrointestinal problems, and anaphylaxis (a life-threatening allergic reaction). Pregnant women and those with diabetes, autoimmune disorders, or multiple sclerosis should avoid it.
	Flaxseed (*Linum usitatissimum*)	Useful as a laxative and for hot flashes and breast pain; the oil is used for arthritis; both flaxseed and flaxseed oil have been used for cholesterol level reduction and cancer prevention.	May have a laxative effect. Study results are mixed on whether flaxseed decreases hot flashes or lowers cholesterol levels.	Delays absorption of medicines, but otherwise has few side effects. Should be taken with plenty of water. In high amounts, may cause diarrhea.
	Ginkgo (*Ginkgo biloba*)	Useful for depression, impotence, premenstrual syndrome, dementia and Alzheimer's disease, diseases of the eye, and general vascular disease.	An NCCAM-funded study found it ineffective for Alzheimer's disease and dementia. Study results are mixed on its ability to enhance memory and reduce the incidence of cardiovascular disease.	Gastric irritation, headache, nausea, dizziness, and allergic reactions.
	Ginseng (*Panax ginseng*)	Useful for boosting immune system, reducing blood glucose, aiding skin, muscle tone, and sex drive; improving concentration and muscle strength.	Studies are inconclusive. Ginseng may boost immune response and reduce blood glucose, but most trials have been small.	Insomnia, high blood pressure, headaches, and allergic reactions.
	Green tea (*Camellia sinensis*)	Useful for lowering cholesterol and risk of some cancers, protecting the skin from sun damage, bolstering mental alertness, and boosting heart health.	Although some studies have shown possible links between green and white tea consumption and cancer prevention, recent research questions the ability of tea to significantly reduce the risk of any type of cancer in humans.	In high doses, insomnia, liver problems, anxiety, irritability, upset stomach, nausea, diarrhea, or frequent urination.
	Zinc (mineral)	Supports immune system; used to lessen duration and severity of cold symptoms; aids wound healing.	Research results are mixed, but zinc lozenges or syrup may lessen duration and severity of a cold. May also promote wound healing.	Excessive intake associated with nausea, vomiting, diarrhea, reduced immune function, and reduced levels of high-density lipoproteins ("good" cholesterol).

Sources: National Center for Complementary and Alternative Medicine, "Herbs at a Glance," November 2012, http://nccam.nih.gov; Office of Dietary Supplements, National Institutes of Health, "Dietary Supplement Fact Sheets," 2011, http://ods.od.nih.gov; American Cancer Society, "Green Tea," May 2012, www.cancer.org

Are You a Savvy CAM Consumer?

If you are like millions of Americans, you've already tried one or more CAM therapies (including supplements) or may be considering one. Take this quiz to assess your knowledge of complementary and alternative medicine. For each item, indicate whether you believe the statement is true or false.

1. When considering a CAM technique, it is important to do some research and identify scientific findings on the specific CAM therapy. **T F**

2. Researching the credentials of a CAM practitioner is an important step to take before receiving any type of CAM treatment. **T F**

3. CAM therapies can be used with traditional medical treatments. **T F**

4. I should inform new practitioners of all treatments I am currently receiving, including all CAM and traditional therapies. **T F**

5. If my friend or family member didn't have success with a CAM therapy, then it probably won't work for me either. **T F**

6. I should ask if the CAM therapy is covered by insurance before receiving the treatment. **T F**

7. Learning about CAM therapies can be a proactive way to maintain good health. **T F**

8. Taking supplements is a good idea because even if a product isn't helpful, it isn't likely to be harmful. **T F**

9. The word *natural* on a supplement package means that the product is effective and safe. **T F**

10. When buying supplements, I should choose those with the USP (U. S. Pharmacopeia) Verified Mark on their labels. **T F**

11. The FDA routinely analyzes the content of dietary supplements. **T F**

12. A recall of a harmful product guarantees that all such harmful products will be immediately and completely removed from the marketplace. **T F**

13. There is no reason for me to consult a physician before taking a supplement. **T F**

14. Fewer than 10 percent of Americans use dietary supplements. **T F**

Scoring Key

1. *True.* Scientific evidence on a particular CAM therapy can help to verify or disprove its effectiveness.

2. *True.* CAM techniques require rigorous training, and it is important to receive treatment from only those practitioners who have received extensive training and are licensed. Inadequate training can result in injury, transmission of disease, and improper balancing of energy.

3. *True.* CAM techniques can be used with traditional medical treatment and can provide additional benefits as part of a comprehensive treatment plan.

4. *True.* Any new practitioner, whether CAM or traditional, should be aware of all therapies you are receiving to prevent any complications if a new therapy is introduced and to allow providers to communicate with one another to provide the best overall care.

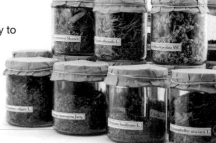

5. *False.* Individuals respond differently to CAM therapies. You should consult your physician when considering CAM therapies.

6. *True.* Many CAM therapies are not covered by insurance. If the procedure is covered, you may still have to pay a percentage of the total amount. It is important to find this out before pursuing the treatment.

7. *True.* A recent study showed that those who inquired about CAM therapies were more health conscious than those who did not.

8. *False.* When consumed in high-enough amounts, for a long-enough time, or in combination with certain other substances, all chemicals can be toxic, including nutrients, plant components, and other biologically active ingredients.

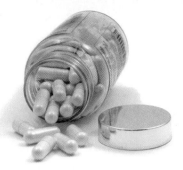

9. *False.* The word *natural* on labels is not well defined and is sometimes used ambiguously to imply unsubstantiated benefits or safety. For example, many weight-loss products claim to be "natural" or "herbal," but this doesn't necessarily make them safe. Their ingredients may interact with drugs or may be dangerous for people with certain medical conditions.

10. *True.* The USP symbol is currently the best way to tell if a supplement has been tested, contains the listed ingredients, and dissolves properly in the body.

11. *False.* The FDA has very limited resources to routinely analyze the contents of all supplements currently on the market.

12. *False.* A product recall of a dietary supplement is voluntary, and although many manufacturers do their best, a recall does not necessarily remove all harmful products from the marketplace.

13. *False.* Supplements can interact with prescription medications, so if you are on any medications, telling your doctor what you intend to take can help him or her check for any potentially harmful interactions.

14. *False.* National surveys indicate that about half of all Americans use dietary supplements. Research shows that people who take supplements tend to have better diets and generally healthier habits than those who don't. They also tend to have higher levels of both education and income.

Interpreting Your Score

Add up the number of items you got right: The higher your score, the better your knowledge of the potential risks and benefits of supplements and CAM techniques. Incorrect responses indicate areas you need to learn more about to be an informed consumer. Ultimately, you are the one responsible for your health and safety, so think about ways to increase your understanding of the CAM methods you use or are considering using.

Sources: Adapted from NCCAM, "Are You Considering Complementary Medicine?" Modified March 2012, http://nccam.nih.gov; NCCAM, "Selecting a CAM Practitioner," Updated January 2012, http://nccam.nih.gov; NCCAM, "CAM Use in America: Up Close," *CAM at the NIH: Focus on Complementary and Alternative Medicine* 15, no. 1 (2008): 8–9, Available at http://nccam.nih.gov

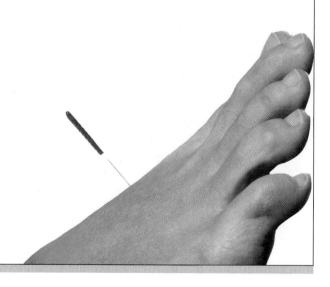

YOUR PLAN FOR CHANGE

The **Assess**Yourself activity gave you the chance to evaluate your understanding of responsible use of CAM treatments. Depending on the results of the assessment, and your own interest in CAM therapies, you may consider investigating CAM further.

Today, you can:

○ Close your eyes and think of a calm place or activity you enjoy for a few minutes. Perhaps you are lying on a beach or are curled up in front of a fireplace. Clear your mind of everything else and use relaxation to improve your health.

○ Go to a credible website and look up information on a CAM therapy. What are the scientific findings? What are the benefits?

Within the next 2 weeks, you can:

○ Review your insurance documents or check with your carrier to see what CAM therapies are covered. Ask which expenses you'll be responsible for, and if you are limited to a certain network of practitioners.

○ Check with your college's health clinic and find out what types of CAM it offers.

By the end of the semester, you can:

○ Schedule an appointment with your health care provider to discuss any CAM therapies you are considering.

○ Make relaxation and mind-body stress-reduction techniques a part of your everyday life. This can mean practicing meditation, deep breathing, or even taking long walks in nature. You don't need to visit a CAM practitioner or follow a specific therapeutic practice to benefit from methods of relaxation, meditation, and spiritual awakening.

References

Chapter 1: Accessing Your Health

1. Centers for Disease Control and Prevention, "Table A," *National Vital Statistics Report* 61, no. 6 (2012), Available at www.cdc.gov

2. Centers for Disease Control and Prevention, "Achievements in Public Health, 1900–1999: Control of Infectious Diseases," *Morbidity and Mortality Weekly Report* 48, no. 29 (1999): 621–629, www.cdc.gov

3. H. L. Walls, K. Backholer, J. Proietto, and J. J. McNeil, "Obesity and Trends in Life Expectancy," *Journal of Obesity*, 2012, doi: 10.1155/2012/107989.

4. G. Danaei et al., "The Promise of Prevention: The Effects of Four Preventable Risk Factors on National Life Expectancy and Life Expectancy Disparities by Race and County in the United States," *PLoS Medicine* 7, no. 3 (2010): e1000248, www.plosmedicine.org

5. U. S. Department of Health and Human Services, *Healthy People 2020*, (Washington, DC: U.S. Government Printing Office, 2011), www.healthypeople.gov

6. R. A. Hammond, "Obesity, Prevention, and Health Care Costs," 2012, Brookings Institution, 2012, www.brookings.edu

7. S. Drenkard, "Overreaching on Obesity: Governments Consider New Taxes on Soda and Candy," *Tax Foundation Special Report* no. 196, October 31, 2011, Available at http://taxfoundation.org

8. World Health Organization (WHO), "Constitution of the World Health Organization," *Chronicles of the World Health Organization* (Geneva: WHO, 1947), www.who.int

9. R. Dubos, *So Human an Animal: How We Are Shaped by Surroundings and Events* (New York: Scribner, 1968), 15. Copyright © 1998 Transaction Publishers.

10. U.S. Department of Health and Human Services, *Healthy People 2020*, U.S. Government Printing Office, Washington, DC: 2011.

11. Centers for Disease Control and Prevention, "Chronic Disease Prevention and Health Promotion," August 2012, www.cdc.gov

12. G. Danaei et al., "The Preventable Causes of Death in the United States: Comparative Risk Assessment of Dietary, Lifestyle, and Metabolic Risk Factors," *PLoS Medicine* 6, no. 4 (2009): e1000058, www.plosmedicine.org; Centers for Disease Control and Prevention, "Chronic Disease"; Centers for Disease Control and Prevention, "Alcohol and Public Health Fact Sheets," October 2012, www.cdc.gov; I-Min Lee et al., "Effect of Physical Inactivity on Major Non-Communicable Diseases Worldwide: An Analysis of Burden of Disease and Life Expectancy," *The Lancet* 380, no. 9838 (2012): 219–229, doi: 10.1016/S0140-6736(12)61031-9; Centers for Disease Control and Prevention, "Smoking and Tobacco Use Fast Facts," December 2012, www.cdc.gov

13. E. Kvaavik et al., "Influence of Individual and Combined Health Behaviors on Total and Cause-Specific Mortality in Men and Women: The United Kingdom Health and Lifestyle Survey," *Archives of Internal Medicine* 170, no. 8 (2010): 711–718.

14. U.S. Department of Health and Human Services, *Healthy People 2020*, 2011.

15. American College Health Association, *American College Health Association-National College Health Assessment II: Reference Group Executive Summary Fall 2012* (Hanover, MD: American College Health Association, 2013), www.acha-ncha.org

16. D. Ding et al., "Neighborhood Environment and Physical Activity among Youth: A Review," *American Journal of Preventive Medicine* 41, no. 4 (2011): 442–455; J. Sallis et al., "Role of Built Environments in Physical Activity, Obesity, and Cardiovascular Disease." *Circulation* 125 (2012): 729–737, Available at www.med.upenn.edu

17. W.C. Willett and A. Underwood, "Crimes of the Heart," *Newsweek*, February 5, 2010, www.newsweek.com

18. R. A. Cohen and M. E. Martinez, National Center for Health Statistics, "Health Insurance Coverage: Early Release of Estimates from the National Health Interview Survey," June 2012, www.cdc.gov

19. U.S. Department of Health and Human Services, *Healthy People 2020*.

20. I. Rosenstock, "Historical Origins of the Health Belief Model," *Health Education Monographs* 2, no. 4 (1974): 328–335.

21. J. O. Prochaska and C. C. DiClemente, "Stages and Processes of Self-Change of Smoking: Toward an Integrative Model of Change," *Journal of Consulting and Clinical Psychology* 51 (1983): 390–395.

22. D. Hammond et al., "The Impact of Cigarette Warning Labels and Smoke-Free Bylaws on Smoking Cessation Evidence from Former Smokers," *Canadian Journal of Public Health* 95, no. 3 (2004): 201–204; L. Winerman, "New Labels, New Attitudes," *Monitor on Psychology* 42, no. 11 (2011): 54, Available at www.apa.org

23. C. Nigg, K. Geller, and R. Moti, "A Research Agenda to Examine the Efficacy and Relevance of the Transtheoretical Model for Physical Activity Behavior," *Psychology of Sport and Exercise* 12, no. 1 (2011): 12; M. Backer, K. Simpson, and B. Lloyd, "Behavioral Strategies in Diabetes Prevention Programs: A Systematic Review of Randomized Controlled Trials," *Diabetes Research in Clinical Practice* 91, no. 1 (2011): 1–12.

24. H. Gagnon et al., "Psychosocial Factors and Beliefs Related to Intentions to Not Binge Drink among Young Adults," *Alcohol and Alcoholism* 47, no. 5 (2012), doi: 10.1093/alcalc/ags049; J. Macy et al., "Applying the Theory of Planned Behavior to Explore the Relation between Smoke-Free Air Laws and Quitting Intention," *Health Education and Behavior* no. 39 (2012): 27–34.

25. K. Simmen-Janevska, V. Brandstatter, and A. Maercker, "The Overlooked Relationship between Motivational Abilities and Posttraumatic Stress: A Review," *European Journal of Psychotraumatology* 10, no. 3 (2012), doi: 10.3402/ejpt.v3i0.18560.

26. A. Ellis and M. Benard, *Clinical Application of Rational Emotive Therapy* (New York: Plenum, 1985).

Pulled statistics:

page 3, Centers for Disease Control and Prevention, "Health Insurance Coverage," August 2012, www.cdc.gov

page 16, M. E. Martinez and R. A. Cohen, "Health Insurance Coverage: Early Release of Estimates from the National Health Interview Survey, January–September 2012," *Division of Health Interview Statistics, National Center for Health Statistics* (June 2013), www.cdc.gov

Focus On: Improving Your Financial Health

1. Centers for Disease Control and Prevention (CDC), "Obesity and Socioeconomic Status in Adults: United States, 2005–2008," NCHS Data Brief, no. 50 (December 2010), www.cdc.gov

2. G. Georgiadis, F.R. Rodriguea, and J. Pineda, "Has the Preston Curve Broken Down?" *United Nations Development Programme Human Development Reports, Research Paper 2010/32* (October 30, 2010), dx.doi.org/10.2139/ssrn.2031504

3. State Higher Education Executive Officers Association, "The Economic Value of Post Secondary Degrees," December 2012, www.sheeo.org

4. National Survey of Student Engagement, *NSSE Annual Results 2012: Promoting Student Learning and Institutional Improvement: Lessons from NSSE at 13* (Bloomington, IN: Indiana University Center for Postsecondary Research, 2012), http://nsse.iub.edu

5. American College Health Association, *American College Health Association-National College Health Assessment II (ACHA-NACHA II): Undergraduate Students, Reference Group Data Report Fall 2012* (Hanover, MD: American College Health Association, 2013), www.acha-ncha.org

6. Sallie Mae and Ipsos, *How America Pays for College 2012: A National Study*, 2012, www1.salliemae.com

7. Ibid.

8. *Bankruptcy Abuse Prevention and Consumer Protection Act of 2005*. Full text available at www.govtrack.us

9. Federal Reserve Bank of New York, Research and Statistics Group, Microeconomic Studies, "Quarterly Report on Household Debt and Credit," November 2012, www.newyorkfed.org

10. Federal Trade Commission, "Equal Credit Opportunity: Understanding Your Rights under the Law," May 2009, www.ftc.gov

11. *Credit Card Accountability Responsibility and Disclosure Act, The CARD Act of 2009*, www.gpo.gov

12. Javelin Strategy & Research, "The 2011 Identity Fraud Report: Social Media and Mobile Forming the New Fraud Frontier," February 2012, www.javelinstrategy.com

13. Ibid.

14. Federal Trade Commission, "Avoiding Identity Theft," January 2013, www.consumer.gov

15. Federal Trade Commission, Consumer Information, "Medical Identity Theft," January 2013, www.consumer.ftc.gov

16. Javelin Strategy & Research, "The 2011 Identity Fraud Report," February 2012.

Pulled statistics:

page 27, Nerd Wallet, "American Household Credit Card Debt Statistics through 2012," www.nerdwallet.com

page 32, Sallie Mae and Ipsos, "How America Pays for College 2012: A National Study," 2012, www1.salliemae.com

page 33, Javelin Strategy & Research, "The 2011 Identity Fraud Report: Social Media and Mobile Forming the New Fraud Frontier," February 2012.

Chapter 2: Promoting and Preserving Your Psychological Health

1. A. H. Maslow, *Motivation and Personality,* 2nd ed. (New York: Harper and Row, 1970).

2. U.S. Department of Health and Human Services, *Mental Health: A Report of the Surgeon General—Executive Summary* (Rockville, MD: U.S. Department of Health and Human Services, Substance Abuse and Mental Health Services Administration, National Institute of Mental Health, 1999), Available at www.surgeongeneral.gov

3. M. A. Brackett, S. E. Rivers, and P. Salovey, "Emotional Intelligence: Implications for Personal, Social, Academic, and Workplace Success," *Social and Personality Psychology Compass* 5, no. 1 (2011): 88–103.

4. Helpguide.org, Improving Emotional Health, Strategies and Tips for Good Mental Health, 2012, http://helpguide.org

5. D. Umberson and J. K. Montez, "Social Relationships and Health: A Flashpoint for Health Policy," *Journal of Health and Social Behavior* 51, no. 1, Supplement (2010): S54–S66; J. Holt-Lunstad, T. B. Smith, and J. B. Layton, "Social Relationships and Mortality Risk: A Meta-Analytic Review," *PLoS Medicine* 7, no. 7 (2010): e1000316.

6. K. Karren et al., *Mind/Body Health,* 4th ed. (San Francisco: Benjamin Cummings, 2010).

7. S. Dowshen, "How Can Spirituality Affect Your Family's Health," 2011, http://kidshealth.org; National Center for Cultural Competence, Georgetown University. "Definitions and Discussion of Spirituality and Religion," 2011, http://nccc.georgetown.edu

8. C. Carter, *Raising Happiness: 10 Simple Steps for More Joyful Kids and Happier Parent*s (New York: Ballantine Publishing, 2010); M. Bundick et al., "Thriving Across the Life Span," in *The Handbook of Life-Span Development,* eds. R. Lerner, M. Lamb, and M. Freund (Hoboken, NJ: John Wiley & Sons, 2010), 882–923.

9. J. Mattanah, J. Ayers, B. Brand, and L. Brooks, "A Social Support Intervention to Ease the College Transition: Exploring Main Effects and Moderators," *Journal of College Student Development* 51, no. 1 (2010): 93–108.

10. M. Seligman, *Helplessness: On Depression, Development, and Death* (New York: W.H. Freeman, 1975).

11. M. Seligman, *Learned Optimism: How to Change Your Mind and Your Life* (New York: Free Press, 1998); M. Seligman, *Flourish* (New York: Free Press, 2011).

12. E. H. Erikson, *Childhood and Society,* (New York: W. W. Norton & Company, 1950).

13. R. Curtis, *"Post-Graduation Advising: Needed More Now Than Ever,"* The Mentor, Penn State's Division of Undergraduate Studies, January 13, 2010, http://dus.psu.edu

14. S. Rimer, Harvard School of Public Health, "The Biology of Emotion—And What It May Teach Us about Helping People to Live Longer," 2011, www.hsph.harvard.edu

15. Ibid; M. Miller and W. F. Fry, "The Effect of Mirthful Laughter on the Human Cardiovascular System," *Medical Hypotheses* 73, no. 5 (2009): 636–639; S. Horowitz, "The Effect of Positive Emotions on Health: Hope and Humor," *Alternative and Complementary Therapies* 15, no. 4 (2009): 196–202.

16. E. Diener, "Subjective Well-Being," in *Social Indicators Research Series* 37 (2009): 11–58.

17. J. De Neve, "Functional Polymorphism (*5-HTTLPR*) in the Serotonin Transporter Gene Is Associated with Subjective Well-Being: Evidence from a U.S. Nationally Representative Sample," *Journal of Human Genetics* 56 (2011): 456–459, doi: 10.1038/jhg.2011.39.

18. C. Carter, "Raising Happiness," 2010; R. I. Dunbar et al., "Social Laughter Is Correlated with an Elevated Pain Threshold," *Proceedings of the Royal Society* 279, no. 1731 (2011): 1161–1167, doi: 10.1098/rspb.2011.1373.

19. Mayo Clinic Staff, MayoClinic.com, "Mental Illness: Causes," 2010, www.mayoclinic.com

20. Ibid.

21. Substance Abuse and Mental Health Services Administration, Results from the 2011 National Survey on Drug Use and Health: Mental Health Findings, NSDUH Series H-45, HHS Publication no. (SMA) 12-4725 (Rockville, MD: Substance Abuse and Mental Health Services Administration, 2012); R. C. Kessler et al., "Twelve-Month and Lifetime Prevalence and Lifetime Morbid Risk of Anxiety and Mood Disorders in the United States," *International Journal of Methods in Psychiatric Research* 21, no. 3 (2012): 169–184, doi: 10.1002/mpr.1359.

22. The World Health Organization (WHO), "Annex Table 3: Burden of Disease in DALYs by Cause, Sex, and Mortality Stratum in WHO regions, Estimates for 2002" *The World Health Report 2004: Changing History* A126–A127 (Geneva: WHO, 2004); T. L. Mark et al., "Changes in U.S. Spending on Mental Health and Substance Abuse Treatment, 1986–2005, and Implications for Policy," *Health Affairs* 30, no. 2 (2011): 284–292, www.healthaffairs.org, doi: 10.1377/hlthaff.2010.0765.

23. J. Hunt and D. Eisenberg, "Mental Health Problems and Help-Seeking Behavior among College Students," *Journal of Adolescent Health* 46, no. 1 (2010): 3–10.

24. American College Health Association, *American College Health Association–National College Health Assessment II (ACHA–NCHA II): Reference Group Data Report Fall 2012* (Hanover, MD: American College Health Association, 2013), www.acha-ncha.org

25. American Psychological Association, "College Students Exhibiting More Severe Mental Illness, Study Finds," *ScienceDaily,* August 12, 2010, www.sciencedaily.com

26. R. C. Kessler et al., "Twelve-Month and Lifetime Prevalence," 2012.

27. Ibid; Substance Abuse and Mental Health Services Administration, "Results from the 2011 National Survey on Drug Use and Health," 2012.

28. National Institute of Mental Health, "Depression," Revised 2011, www.nimh.nih.gov

29. American College Health Association, *American College Health Association–National College Health Assessment II (ACHA–NCHA II): Reference Group Data Report Fall 2012,* 2013.

30. C. Blanco et al., "The Epidemiology of Chronic Major Depressive Disorder and Dysthymic Disorder: Results from the National Epidemiologic Survey on Alcohol and Related Conditions," *Journal of Clinical Psychiatry* 71, no. 12 (2012): 1645–1656, doi: 10.4088/JCP.09m05663gry.

31. R. C. Kessler et al., "Twelve-Month and Lifetime Prevalence," 2012.

32. WebMD, "Seasonal Depression (Seasonal Affective Disorder)", 2012, www.webmd.com

33. Mayo Clinic Staff, MayoClinic.com, "Depression: Causes," 2010, www.mayoclinic.com

34. R. C. Kessler et al., "Twelve-Month and Lifetime Prevalence," 2012.

35. K.R. Merikangas et al., "Lifetime Prevalence of Mental Disorders in U.S. Adolescents: Results from the National Comorbidity Survey Replication—Adolescent Supplement (NCS-A)," *Journal of the American Academy of Child and Adolescent Psychiatry* 49, no. 10, (2010): 980–989, doi: 10.1016/j.jaac.2010.05.017.

36. American College Health Association, *American College Health Association–National College Health Assessment II (ACHA–NCHA II): Reference Group Data Report Fall 2012,* 2013.

37. National Institute of Mental Health, "Generalized Anxiety Disorder, GAD," January 2013, www.nimh.nih.gov

38. R. C. Kessler et al., "Twelve-Month and Lifetime Prevalence," 2012.

39. Mayo Clinic Staff, MayoClinic.com, "Panic Attacks and Panic Disorder: Symptoms," 2012, www.mayoclinic.com

40. R. C. Kessler et al., "Twelve-Month and Lifetime Prevalence," 2012.

41. Ibid.

42. Ibid.

43. R. C. Kessler et al., "Prevalence, Severity, and Comorbidity of Twelve-Month DSM-IV Disorders in the National Comorbidity Survey Replication (NCS-R)," *Archives of General Psychiatry* 62, no. 6 (2005): 617–627.

44. Ibid; R. C. Kessler et al., "Twelve-Month and Lifetime Prevalence," 2012.

45. Congressional Budget Office, "The Veterans Health Administration's Treatment of PTSD and Traumatic Brain Injury among Recent Combat Veterans," Congress of the United States, Pub. No. 4097, (Washington, DC: Governmental Printing Office, 2012); J. Gradus, United States Department of Veterans Affairs, National Center for PTSD, "Epidemiology of PTSD," December 2011, www.ptsd.va.gov

46. National Institute of Mental Health, "Generalized Anxiety Disorder (GAD): When Worry Gets out of Control," 2010, www.nimh.nih.gov

47. American Psychiatric Association, *Diagnostic and Statistical Manual of Mental Disorders, (DSM-5),* 5th ed. (Washington, DC: American Psychiatric Association, 2013).

48. M.F. Lenzenweger, et al., "DSM-IV Personality Disorders in the National Comorbidity Survey Replication," *Biological Psychiatry* 62, no. 6, (2007): 553–564.

49. A.D.A.M. Medical Encyclopedia, "Antisocial Personality Disorder," PubMed Health (Bethesda MD: U.S. National Library of Medicine, 2012).

50. About Recovery, "Personality Disorders," 2012, http://aboutrecovery.com

51. J. Cole, "Facts," BPDWORLD, 2011, www.bpdworld.org

52. D. A. Regier et al., "The De Facto Mental and Addictive Disorders Service System. Epidemiologic Catchment Area Prospective 1-Year Prevalence Rates of Disorders and Services," *Archives of General Psychiatry* 50, no. 2 (1993): 85–94; National Institute of Mental Health, "The Numbers Count," 2013.

53. National Institute of Mental Health, "Schizophrenia," January 2013, www.nimh.nih.gov

54. Ibid.

55. D. L. Hoyert and J. Xu, "Deaths: Preliminary Data for 2011, Table 7," *National Vital Statistics Reports* 61, no. 6 (Hyattsville, MD: National Center for Health Statistics, 2012).

56. J. C. Turner, "Leading Causes of Mortality among American College Students at 4-year Institutions," Poster presented at the American Public Health Association 139th Annual Conference, October 2011, www.apha.org

57. I. H. Rockett et al., "Leading Causes of Unintentional and Intentional Injury Mortality: United States, 2000–2009," *American Journal of Public Health* 102, no. 11 (2012):. e84–e92, doi: 10.2105/AJPH.2012.300960.

58. D.L. Hoyert and J. Xu, "Deaths: Preliminary Data for 2011, 2012.

59. National Institute of Mental Health, "Suicide in the U.S.: Statistics and Prevention," 2010.

60. American Foundation for Suicide Prevention, "Warning Signs of Suicide," About Suicide, 2013, www.afsp.org

61. National Institute of Health, "Suicide in the U.S.," 2010.

62. American Association of Suicidology, "Understanding and Helping the Suicidal Individual," January 2012, www.suicidology.org

63. Substance Abuse and Mental Health Services Administration, "Results from the 2011 National Survey on Drug Use and Health," 2012.

64. Mayo Clinic Staff, "Mental Health: Overcoming the Stigma of Mental Illness," 2011; "Mental Health America, Stigma: Building Awareness and Understanding," 2012, www.nmha.org

65. American Psychological Association, "Psychodynamic Psychotherapy Brings Lasting Benefits through Self-Knowledge," 2010, www.apa.org

66. CRC Health Group, "Interpersonal Therapy What Is It?," 2011, www.crchealth.com

67. Mayo Clinic, "Cognitive Behavioral Therapy," 2010, www.mayoclinic.com

68. U.S. Food and Drug Administration, "Antidepressant Use in Children, Adolescents, and Adults," 2010, www.fda.gov

Pulled statistics:

page 42, Bureau of Labor Statistics, "Economic News Release: Volunteering in the United States, 2011," U.S. Department of Labor, 2012.

page 52, National Institute of Mental Health, Suicide in the U.S.: Statistics and Prevention, U.S. Department of Health and Human Services, 2010, www.nimh.nih.gov

Focus On: Cultivating Your Spiritual Health

1. A. Asten, H. Asten, and J. Lindholm, *Cultivating the Spirit: How College Can Enhance Students' Inner Lives* (San Francisco: Jossey-Bass, 2010).

2. J. H. Pryor, et al., *The American Freshman: National Norms Fall 2011,* (Los Angeles: Higher Education Research Institute, UCLA), Available at http://heri.ucla.edu

3. Ibid.

4. National Cancer Institute, "General Information on Spirituality," June 2012, www.cancer.gov

5. H. G. Koenig, "Religion, Spirituality and Health: The Research and Clinical Implications," *ISRN Psychiatry*, 2012, doi: 10.5402/2012/27830.

6. Ibid.

7. Pew Forum, "Religion Among the Millennials," February 2010, www.pewforum.org

8. Ibid.

9. B. Seaward, *Managing Stress: Principles and Strategies for Health and Well Being,* 7th ed. (Sudbury, MA: Jones and Bartlett, 2012).

10. D. Zohar, "Learn the Qs," 2010, DanahZohar.com

11. National Institutes of Health, National Center for Complementary and Alternative Medicine, "Exploring the Science of Complementary and Alternative Medicine: Third Strategic Plan: 2011–2015," NIH Publication No. 11-7643, D458, February 2011, http://nccam.nih.gov

12. M. Javnbakht, R. Hejazi Kenari, and M. Ghasemi, "Effects of Yoga on Depression and Anxiety of Women," *Complementary Therapies in Clinical Practice* 15, no. 2 (2009); V. Conn, "The Power of Being Present: The Value of Mindfulness Interventions in Improving Health and Well-Being," *Western Journal of Nursing Research* 33 (2011): 993–995; Y. Matchim, J. Armer, and B. Stewart, "Breast Cancer Survivors Benefit from Practicing Mindfulness-Based Stress Reduction," *Western Journal of Nursing Research* 33, no. 8 (2011): 996–1016, first published on October 18, 2010.

13. National Institutes of Health, "Exploring the Science of Complementary and Alternative Medicine," February 2011.

14. B. K. Hölzel et al., "Mindfulness practice leads to increases in regional brain gray matter density," *Psychiatry Research: Neuroimaging,* 191, no. (2011): 36–43, doi: 10.1016/j.pscychresns.2010.08.006.

15. National Cancer Institute (NCI), "Spirituality in Cancer Care," September 2012, www.cancer.gov

16. C. Lysne and A. Wachholtz, "Pain, Spirituality and Meaning Making: What Can We Learn from the Literature?" *Religions,* no. 2 (2011): 1–16, doi:10.3390/rel2010001; H. Koenig and A. Bussing, "Spiritual Needs of Patients with Chronic Diseases," *Religions* 1, no. 1 (2010): 18–27.

17. R. E. Wells et al., "Complementary and Alternative Medicine Use among U. S. Adults with Common Neurological Conditions," *Journal of Neurology* 257, no. 11 (2010): 1822–1831, Available at www.ncbi.nlm.nih.gov

18. G. Lucchetti, A. Lucchetti, and H. Koenig, "Impact of Spirituality/Religiosity on Mortality: Comparison with Other Health Interventions." *EXPLORE: The Journal of Science and Healing* 7, no. 4 (2011): 234–238.

19. National Cancer Institute (NCI), "Spirituality in Cancer Care," September 2012, www.cancer.gov

20. Ibid; National Center for Complementary and Alternative Medicine (NCCAM), "Prayer and Spirituality in Health: Ancient Practices, Modern Science," CAM at the NIH 12, no. 1 (2005): 1–4.

21. G. G. Ano and E. B. Vasconcelles, "Religious Coping and Psychological Adjustment to Stress: A Meta-Analysis," *Journal of Clinical Psychology* 61, no. 4 (2005): 461–480; U. Winter et al., "The Psychological Outcome of Religious Coping with Stressful Life Events in a Swiss Sample of Church Attendees," *Psychotherapy and Psychosomatics* 78, no. 4 (2009): 240–244; G. Lucchetti, Lucchetti, and Koenig, "Impact of Spirituality/Religiosity," 2011; Y. Matchim, Armer, and Stewart, "Breast Cancer Survivors Benefit," 2011.

22. A. Chiesa and A. Serretti, "Mindfulness-Based Stress Reduction for Stress Management in Healthy People: A Review and Meta-Analysis," *Journal of Alternative and Complementary Medicine* 15, no. 5 (2009): 593–600. G. Lucchetti, Lucchetti, and Koenig, "Impact of Spirituality/Religiosity," 2011; Y. Matchim, Armer, and Stewart, "Breast Cancer Survivors Benefit," 2011.

23. R. Jahnke, L. Larkey, C. Rogers, et al., "A Comprehensive Review of Health Benefits of Qigong and Tai Chi," *American Journal of Health Promotion* 24, no. 6 (2010): e1–e25, doi.org/10.4278/ajhp.081013-LIT-248

24. G. Lucchetti, A. Lucchetti, and H. Koenig "Impact of Spirituality/Religiosity," 2011; Y. Matchim, Armer, and Stewart, "Breast Cancer Survivors Benefit," 2011.

25. G. Desbordes et al., "Effects of Mindful-Attention and Compassion Meditation Training on Amygdala Response to Emotional Stimuli in an Ordinary, Non-meditative State," *Frontiers in Human Neuroscience* 6, no. 292(2012). doi: 10.3389/fnhum.2012.00292.

26. National Center for Complementary and Alternative Medicine (NCCAM), "Research Spotlight: Meditation May Increase Empathy," January 2012, http://nccam.nih.gov

27. G. Desbordes et al., "Effects of Mindful-attention and Compassion," 2012.

28. Ibid; B. K. Hölzel, et al., "Mindfulness Practice Leads to Increases," 2011; E. Luders et al., "Enhanced Brain Connectivity in Long-term Meditation Practitioners," *NeuroImage* 57, 2011, doi: 10.1016/j.neuroimage.2011.05.075.

29. National Institutes of Health, National Center for Complementary and Alternative Medicine, "Meditation: An Introduction," 2010, http://nccam.nih.gov

30. C. Carter, *Raising Happiness: 10 Simple Steps for More Joyful Kids and Happier Parents* (New York: Ballantine Publishing, 2010); R. I. Dunbar et al., "Social Laughter Is Correlated with an Elevated Pain Threshold," *Proceedings of the Royal Society* 279, no. 1731 (2011), doi: 10.1098/rspb.2011.1373.

Pulled statistics:

page 61, A. W. Astin et al., Cultivating the Spirit: How College Can Enhance Students' Inner Lives (San Francisco: Jossey-Bass, 2011).

page 69, The Pew Forum on Religion and Public Life, "Religion Among the Millennials," June 2010, www.pewforum.org

Chapter 3: Managing Stress and Coping with Life's Challenges

1. American Psychological Association, "Stress in America: Our Health at Risk," *Monitor on Psychology* 43, no. 3 (2012): 18, www.apa.org

2. S. Cohen and D. Janicki-Deverts, "Who's Stressed? Distributions of Psychological Stress in the United States in Probability Samples from 1983, 2006, and 2009," *Journal of Applied Social Psychology* 42, no. 6 (2012): 1320–1334, doi:10.1111/j.1559-1816.2012.00900.

3. American Psychological Association, "Stress in America," 2012.

4. K. Glanz and M. Schwartz, "Stress, Coping and Health Behavior," in *Health Behavior and Health Education: Theory, Research and Practice*, 4th ed., eds. K. Glanz, B. Rimer, and K. Viswanath (San Francisco: Jossey Bass, 2002), 210–236.

5. American Psychological Association, "Stress: The Different Kinds of Stress," 2012, www.apa.org

6. B. L. Seaward, *Managing Stress: Principles and Strategies for Health and Well-Being*, 7th ed. (Sudbury, MA: Jones and Bartlett, 2012); National Institute of Mental Health (NIMH), "Stress Fact Sheet," December, 2012, www.nimh.nih.gov

7. H. Selye, *Stress without Distress* (New York: Lippincott Williams & Wilkins, 1974), 28–29.

8. W. B. Cannon, *The Wisdom of the Body* (New York: Norton, 1932).

9. B. S. McEwen and P. Tucker, "Critical Biological Pathways for Chronic Psychosocial Stress and Research Opportunities to Advance the Consideration of Stress in Chemical Risk Assessment," *American Journal of Public Health* 101, no. 1, Supplement (2011): S131–S139; S. Cohen, et al., "Chronic Stress, Glucocorticoid Receptor Resistance, Inflammation and Disease Risk," *Proceedings of the National Academy of Sciences of the United States of America* 109, no. 16 (2012): 5995–5999, doi: 10.1073/pnas.1118355109.

10. P. Thoits, "Stress and Health: Major Findings and Policy Implications," *Journal of Health and Social Behavior* 51, no. 1 supplement (2010): 554–555, doi: 10.1177/0022146510383499.

11. E. Backe et al., "The Role of Psychosocial Stress at Work for the Development of Cardiovascular Disease: A Systematic Review," *International Archives of Occupational and Environmental Health* 85, no. 1 (2011): 67–79; A. Steptoe, A. Rosengren, and P. Hjemdahl, "Introduction to Cardiovascular Disease, Stress, and Adaptation" in *Stress and Cardiovascular Disease,* eds. A. Steptoe, A. Rosengren, and P. Hjemdahl (New York: Springer, 2012), 1–14.

12. S. Richardson et al., "Meta-analysis of Perceived Stress and Its Association with Incident Coronary Heart Disease," *American Journal of Cardiology* 110, no. 12 (2012): 1711–1717; G. Marshall, "The Adverse Effects of Psychological Stress on Immunoregulatory Balance: Applications to Human Inflammatory Disease," *Immunology and Allergy Clinics of North America* 31, no. 1 (2011): 133–140; A. Steptoe and M. Kivimaki, "Stress and Cardiovascular Disease." *Nature Reviews Cardiology* 9, no. 6 (2012) 360–370.

13. M. Kivimaki et al., "Job Strain as a Risk Factor for Coronary Heart Disease: A Collaborative Meta-Analysis of Individual Participants," *The Lancet* 380, no. 9852 (2012): 1491–1497; E. Mostofsky et al., "Risk of Acute Myocardial Infarction after the Death of a Significant Person on One's Life. The Determinants of Myocardial Infarction Onset Study," *Circulation* 125, no. 3 (2012): 491–496, doi: 10.1161/CIRCULATIONAHA.111.061770.

14. K. Scott, S. Melhorn, and R. Sakai. "Effects of Chronic Social Stress on Obesity," *Current Obesity Reports Online First* 1, no. 1 (2012): 16–25, doi: 10.1007/s13679-011-0006-3; V. Vicennati et al., "Cortisol, Energy Intake, and Food Frequency in Overweight/Obese Women," *Nutrition* 27, no. 6 (2011): 677–680; S. Pagota et al., "Association of Post-Traumatic Stress Disorder and Obesity in a Nationally Representative Sample," *Obesity* 20, no. 1 (2012): 200–205.

15. N. Ribertim et al., "Corticotropin Releasing Factor-Induced Amygdala Gamma Aminobutyric Acid Release Plays a Key Role in Alcohol Dependence," *Biological Psychiatry* 67, no. 9 (2010): 831–839.

16. D. K. Hall-Flavin, "Stress and Hair Loss: Are They Related?" Mayo Clinic.com, 2012, www.mayoclinic.com

17. American Diabetes Association, "How Stress Affects Diabetes," 2011, www.diabetes.org; A. Pandy et al., "Alternative Therapies Useful in the Management of Diabetes: A Systematic Review," *Journal of Pharmacy & BioAllied Sciences* 3, no. 4 (2011): 504–512.

18. National Digestive Diseases Information Clearinghouse (NDDIC), "What I Need to Know about Irritable Bowel Syndrome," December, 2012, www.digestive.niddk.nih.gov

19. H.F. Herlong, "Digestive Disorders White Paper-2013," *Johns Hopkins Health Alerts*, 20123, www.johnshopkinshealthalerts.com; C. Fang et al., "Enhanced Psychosocial Well-Being Following Participation in a Mindfulness-Based Stress Reduction Program Is Associated with Increased Natural Killer Cell Activity," *Journal of Alternative and Complementary Medicine* 16, no. 5 (2010): 531–536.

20. G. Marshall, ed., "Stress and Immune-Based Diseases," *Immunology and Allergy Clinics of North America* 31, no. 1 (2011): 1–148; L. Christian, "Psychoneuroimmunology in Pregnancy: Immune Pathways Linking Stress with Maternal Health, Adverse Birth Outcomes and Fetal Development," *Neuroscience and Biobehavioral Reviews* 36, no. 1 (2012): 350–361, doi: 10.1016/j.neubiorev.2011.07.005; A. Pedersen et al., "Influence of Psychological Stress on Upper Respiratory Infection: A Meta-Analysis of Prospective Studies," *Psychosomatic Medicine* 72, no. 8 (2010): 823–832.

21. M. Kondo, "Socioeconomic Disparities and Health: Impacts and Pathways," *Journal of Epidemiology* 22, no. 1 (2012): 2–6; T. Theorell, "Evaluating Life Events and Chronic Stressors in Relation to Health: Stressors and Health in Clinical Work," *Advances in Psychosomatic Medicine* 32 (2012): 58–71; J. Gouln and J. Kiecolt-Glaser, "The Impact of Psychological Stress on Wound Healing: Methods and Mechanisms," *Immunology and Allergy Clinics of North America* 31, no. 1 (2011): 81–93.

22. American College Health Association, *American College Health Association-National College Health Assessment II: Reference Group Executive Summary Fall 2012* (Hanover, MD: American College Health Association, 2013), www.acha-ncha.org

23. M. Marin et al., "Chronic Stress, Cognitive Functioning and Mental Health," *Neurobiology of Learning and Memory* 96, no. 4 (2011): 583–595; L. Schwabe, T. Wolf, and M. Oitzi, "Memory Formation under Stress: Quantity and Quality," *Neuroscience and Biobehavioral Reviews* 34, no. 4 (2009): 584–591.

24. E. Dias-Ferreira et al., "Chronic Stress Causes Frontostriatal Reorganization and Affects Decision-Making," *Science* 325, no. 5940 (2009): 621–625; D. de Quervain et al., "Glucocorticoids and the Regulation of Memory in Health and Disease," *Frontiers in Neuroendocrinology* 30, no. 3 (2009): 358–370.

25. J. Fox et al., "Stressful Life Events and the Tripartite Model: Relations to Anxiety and Depression in Adolescent Females," *Journal of Adolescence* 33, no. 1 (2010): 43–54; K. Scott et al., "Association of Childhood Adversities and Early-Onset Mental Disorders with Adult-Onset Chronic Physical Conditions," *Archives of General Psychiatry* 68, no. 8 (2011): 833–844.

26. J. Hunt and D. Eisenbe, "Mental Health Problems and Help Seeking Behaviors among College Students—Review Article," *Journal of Adolescent Health* 46, no. 1 (2010): 3–10; C. Segrin and S. Passalacqua, "Functions of Loneliness, Social Support, Health Behaviors, and Stress in Association with Poor Health," *Health Communication* 25, no. 4 (2010): 312; R. C. Chao, "Managing Perceived Stress Among College Students: The Role of Social Support and Dysfunctional Coping," *Journal of College Counseling* 1, no. 15 (2012): 5–21.

27. American Psychological Association, "Stress in America," 2012.

28. R. Lazarus, "The Trivialization of Distress," in *Preventing Health Risk Behaviors and Promoting Coping with Illness*, eds. J. Rosen and L. Solomon (Hanover, NH: University Press of New England, 1985), 279–298.

29. D. Hellhammer et al., "Measuring Stress," *Encyclopedia of Behavioral Neurosciences* 3, eds. G. Koob, M. Le Moal, R. F. Thompson (San Diego: Elsevier, 2010), 186.

30. A. Nixon et al., "Can Work Make You Sick? A Meta-Analysis of the Relationships between Job Stressors and Physical Symptoms," *Work and Stress* 25, no. 1 (2011): 1–22.

31. S. Schwartz et al., "Acculturation and Well-Being among College Students from Immigrant Families," *Journal of Clinical Psychology* (2012): 1–21, doi: 10.1002/jclp21847; A. Pieterse et al., "An Exploratory Examination of the Associations among Racial and Ethnic Discrimination, Racial Climate, and Trauma-Related Symptoms in a College Student Population," *Journal of Counseling Psychology* 57, no. 3 (2010): 255–263; A. McAleavey, L. Castonguay, and B. Locke, "Sexual Orientation Minorities in College Counseling: Prevalence, Distress, and Symptom Profiles," *Journal of College Counseling* 14, no. 2 (2011): 127–142.

32. D. Iwamoto, L, Kenji, and W. Ming, "The Impact of Racial Identity, Ethnic Identity, Asian Values and Race-Related Stress on Asian Americans and Asian International College Students' Psychological Well-Being," *Journal of Counseling Psychology* 57, no. 1 (2010): 79–91.

33. E. Brondolo et al., "Racism and Hypertension: A Review of the Empirical Evidence and Implications for Clinical Practice," *American Journal of Hypertension* 24, no. 5 (2011): 518–524; F. Fuchs, "Editorial: Why Do Black Americans Have Higher Prevalence of Hypertension?"

Hypertension 57 (2011): 379–380, Available at http://hyper.ahajournals.org

34. K. Karren et al., *Mind/Body Health: The Effect of Attitudes, Emotions, and Relationships*, 4th ed. (San Francisco: Pearson Education, 2010).

35. B.L. Seaward, *Managing Stress*, 2012.

36. K. Brown, *Predictors of Suicide Ideation and the Moderating Effects of Suicide Attitudes*, Master's thesis, University of Ohio, 2011, http://etd.ohiolink.edu; J. Gomez, R. Miranda, and L Polanco, "Acculturative Stress, Perceived Discrimination and Vulnerability to Suicide Attempts among Emerging Adults," *Journal of Youth and Adolescence* 40, no. 11 (2011): 1465–1476.

37. K. Glanz, B. Rimer, and F. Levis, eds., *Health Behavior and Health Education: Theory, Research, and Practice*, 4th ed. (San Francisco: Jossey-Bass, 2008).

38. S. Abraham, "Relationship between Stress and Perceived Self-Efficacy among Nurses in India," International Conference on Technology and Business Management, 2012, www.ictbm.org; Seaward, *Managing Stress*, 2012.

39. I. Bragard et al., "Efficacy of a Communication and Stress Management Training on Medical Resident's Self Efficacy, Stressful Communication and Burnout." *Journal of Health Psychology* 15, no. 7 (2010): 1075–1084.

40. M. Friedman and R. H. Rosenman, *Type A Behavior and Your Heart* (New York: Knopf, 1974).

41. M. Whooley and J. Wong, "Hostility and Cardiovascular Disease," *Journal of the American College of Cardiology* 58, no. 12 (2011): 1228–1230; J. Newman et al., "Observed Hostility and the Risk of Incident Ischemic Heart Disease: A Perspective Population Study from the 1995 Canadian Nova Scotia Health Survey," *Journal of the American College of Cardiology* 58, no. 12 (2011): 1222–1228; T. Smith et al., "Marital Discord and Coronary Artery Disease: A Comparison of Behaviorally Defined Discrete Groups," *Journal of Consulting and Clinical Psychology* 80, no. 1 (2012): 87–92.

42. G. Mate, *"When the Body Says No: Understanding the Stress-Disease Connection"* (Hoboken, NJ: John Wiley and Sons, 2011).

43. H. Versteeg, V. Spek, and S. Pedersen, "Type D Personality and Health Status in Cardiovascular Disease Populations: A Meta-Analysis of Prospective Studies," *European Journal of Cardiovascular Prevention and Rehabilitation* 19, no. 6 (2011): 1373–380, doi: 10.1177/1741826711425338; F. Mols and F. J. Denollet, "Type D Personality in the General Population: A Systematic Review of Health Status, Mechanisms of Disease and Work-Related Problems," *Health and Quality of Life Outcomes* 8, no. 9 (2010): 1–10, Available from www.hqlo.com

44. S. Kobasa, "Stressful Life Events, Personality, and Health: An Inquiry into Hardiness," *Journal of Personality and Social Psychology* 37, no. 1 (1979): 1–11.

45. C. D. Schetter and C. Dolbier, "Resilience in the Context of Chronic Stress and Health in Adults," *Social and Personality Psychology Compass* 5, no. 9 (2011): 634–652, doi: 10.1111/j.1751-9004.2011.00379.x.

46. C. Ryff et al., "Psychological Resilience in Adulthood and Later Life: Implications for Health," *Annual Review of Gerontology and Geriatrics* 32, no. 1 (2012): 73–92.

47. The American Psychological Association Help Center, "What Is Resilience?" *The Road to Resilience* (Washington, DC: American Psychological Association, 2012), 2. Available at www.apa.org

48. E. Chen et al., "Protective Factors for Adults from Low-Childhood Socioeconomic Circumstances: The Benefits of Shift-and-Persist for Allostatic Load," *Psychosomatic Medicine* 74, no. 2 (2012): 178–186, doi:10.1097/PSY. 0B013e31824206fd.

49. J. H. Pryor et al., *The American Freshman: National Norms Fall 2011* (Los Angeles: Higher Education Research Institute, 2012), Available at http://heri.ucla.edu; J. Pryor, "The Changing First-Year Student: Challenges for 2011," Higher Education Research Institute at UCLA, Presented at AAC&U 2011 Annual Meeting (San Francisco, CA).

50. J. Pryor, "The Changing First-Year Student," 2011.

51. A. Hubs, E. Doyle, and R. Bowden, "Relationships among Self-Esteem, Stress and Physical Activity in College Students," *Psychological Reports* 110, no. 2 (2012): 46–74; H. Morrell, L. Cohen, and D. McChargue, "Depression Vulnerability Predicts Cigarette Smoking among College Students: Gender and Negative Reinforcement Expectancies as Contributing Factors," *Addictive Behavior* 35, no. 6 (2010): 607–611; J. Tomaka, S. Morales-Monks, and A. Shamaley, "Stress and Coping Mediate Relationships between Contingent and Global Self-Esteem and Alcohol-Related Problems among College Drinkers," *Stress and Health* (2012), doi:10.1002/smi.2448.

52. J. Boardman and K. Alexander, "Stress Trajectories, Health Behaviors and the Mental Health of Black and White Young Adults," *Social Science and Medicine* 72, no. 10 (2011): 1659–1666; E. Avant, J. Davis, and C. Cranston, "Posttraumatic Stress Symptom Clusters, Trauma History, and Substance Use among College Students," *Journal of Aggression, Maltreatment and Trauma* 20, no. 5 (2011): 539–555.

53. B. L. Seaward, *Managing Stress*, 2012.

54. J. Moskowitz et al., "A Positive Affect Intervention for People Experiencing Health-related Stress: Development and Non-randomized Pilot Test," *Journal of Health Psychology* 17, no. 5 (2012): 676–692, doi: 10.1177/1359105311425275; P. Thoits, "Mechanisms Linking Social Ties and Support to Physical and Mental Health," *Journal of Health and Social Behavior* 52, no. 2 (2011): 145–161; B. Lake and E. Oreheck, "Relational Regulation Theory: A New Approach to Explain the Link between Perceived Social Support and Mental Health," *Psychological Review* 118, no. 3 (2011): 482–495.

55. B. L. Seaward, *Managing Stress*, 2012.

56. G. Colom et al., "Study of the Effect of Positive Humour as a Variable That Reduces Stress. Relationship of Humour with Personality and Performance Variables," *Psychology in Spain* 15, no. 1 (2011): 9–21.

57. L. Poole et al., "Associations of Objectively Measured Physical Activity with Daily Mood Ratings and Psychophysiological Stress Responses in Women," *Psychophysiology* 48, no. 8 (2011): 1165–1172, doi: 10.1111/j.1469-8986.2011.01184.x;

D. A. Girdano, D. E. Dusek, and G. S. Everly, *Controlling Stress and Tension*, 9th ed. (San Francisco: Benjamin Cummings, 2013), 375.

58. A. Dalton and S. Spiller, "Too Much of a Good Thing: The Benefits of Implementation Intentions Depend on the Number of Specific Goals," *Journal of Consumer Research* 39, no. 3 (2012): 600–614; P. Gollwitzer and P. Sheeran, "Implementation Intentions," 2009, National Cancer Institute, http://cancercontrol.cancer.gov

59. H. Benson and M. Klipper, *The Relaxation Response, 25th Anniversary Edition* (New York: Harper Torch, 2000).

60. A. Grant, "Yoga Teaching Increasingly Popular as Second Career," *U.S. News & World Report*, Money, 2012, http://money.usnews.com

61. J. Kiecolt-Glaser et al., "Stress, Inflammation, and Yoga Practice," *Psychosomatic Medicine* 72, no. 2 (2010): 113–121.

62. V. Barnes and D. Orme-Johnson, "Prevention and Treatment of Cardiovascular Disease in Adolescents through the Transcendental Meditation Program," *Current Hypertension Reviews* 8, no. 3 (2012): 1573–1621.

63. M. Rapaport, P. Schettler, and C. Bresee, "A Preliminary Study of the Effects of a Single Session of Swedish Massage on Hypothalamic-Pituitary-Adrenal and Immune Function in Normal Individuals," *The Journal of Alternative and Complementary Medicine* 16, no. 10 (2010): 1–10.

Pulled statistics:

page 72, S. Cohen and D. Janicki-Deverts, "Who's Stressed? Distributions of Psychological Stress in the United States in Probability Samples from 1983, 2006, and 2009," *Journal of Applied Social Psychology* 42, no. 6 (2012): 1320–1334, doi:10.1111/j.1559-1816.2012.00900.

page 75, C. Aldwin et al., "Do Stress Trajectories Predict Mortality in Older Men? Longitudinal Findings from the VA Normative Aging Study," *Journal of Aging Research* (2011): 1–10, doi: 10.4061/2011/896109.

page 88, American College Health Association, *American College Health Association-National College Health Assessment II: Reference Group Executive Summary Fall 2012*, 2013.

Focus On: Improving Your Sleep

1. M. F. Bear, B.W. Connors, and M. A. Paradiso, *Neuroscience*, 3rd ed. (Philadelphia: Lippincott, Williams & Wilkins, 2007), 594.

2. The Philips Center for Health and Well-being, "Philips Index for Health and Well-being: A Global Perspective Report 2010," October 2011, www.philips-thecenter.org

3. American College Health Association, *American College Health Association-National College Health Assessment II: Reference Group Data Report Fall 2012* (Hanover, MD: American College Health Association, 2013), www.acha-ncha.org

4. J. Gaultney, "The Prevalence of Sleep Disorders in College Students: Impact on Academic Performance," *Journal of American College Health* 59, no. 2 (2010): 91–97; H. Lund et al., "Sleep Predictors of Disturbed Sleep in a Large Population of College Students," *Journal of Adolescent Health* 46, no. 2 (2010): 124–132; D. Taylor and A. Bramoweth, "Patterns and Consequences of Inadequate Sleep in College Students:

Substance Abuse and Motor Vehicle Accidents," *Journal of Adolescent Health* 46, no. 6 (2010): 610–612; Central Michigan University, "College Student Sleep Patterns Could Be Detrimental," May 2008, *Science Daily*, www.sciencedaily.com

5. National Sleep Foundation, "Sleep in America Poll: Communications Technology and Sleep," (Washington, DC: The Foundation, 2011), www.sleepfoundation.org

6. J. Gaultney, "The Prevalence of Sleep Disorders in College Students: Impact on Academic Performance," *Journal of American College Health* 59, no. 2 (2010): 91–97; K. Ahrberg, et al., "Interaction between Sleep Quality and Academic Performance," *Journal of Psychiatric Research* 46, no. 12 (2012): 1618–1622.

7. L.R. McKnight-Eily et al., "Unhealthy Sleep-Related Behaviors–2009," *Morbidity and Mortality Weekly Report* 60, no. 8 (2011): 233–238; National Sleep Foundation, Sleep in America Poll, 2011.

8. Ibid.

9. F. Cappuccio et al., "Sleep Duration and All-Cause Mortality: A Systematic Review and Meta-Analysis of Prospective Studies," *Sleep* 33, no. 5 (2010): 585–592.

10. Ibid.

11. J. M. Krueger and J. A. Majde, "Sleep and Host Defense," in *Principles and Practice of Sleep Medicine*, eds. M. H. Kryger, T. Roth, and W. C. Dement (St. Louis, MO: Saunders 2011), 261–290; M. Manzer and M. Hussein, "Sleep-Immune System Interaction: Advantages and Challenges of Human Sleep Loss Model," *Frontiers of Neurology* 3, no. 2 (2012), doi: 10.3389/fneur.2012.00002.

12. T. Bollinger et al., "Sleep, Immunity and Circadian Clocks: A Mechanistic Model," *Gerontology* 56, no. 6 (2010): 574–580, doi: 10.1159/000281827.

13. R. Lanfranchi et al., "Sleep Deprivation Increases Blood Pressure in Healthy Normotensive Elderly and Attenuates the Blood Pressure Response to Orthostatic Challenges," *Sleep* 34, no. 3 (2010): 335–339; F. Cappuccio, D. Cooper, and D. Lanfranco, "Sleep Duration Predicts Cardiovascular Outcomes: A Systematic Review and Meta-analysis of Prospective Studies," *European Heart Journal,* February (2011), doi: 10.1093/eurheart.

14. S. Agarwal, N. Bajaj, and C. Bae, "Association between Sleep Duration and Cardiovascular Disease: Results from the National Health and Nutrition Examination Survey (NHANES 2005–2008), "*Journal of the American College of Cardiology* 59, no. 13 Supplement 1, (2012): E1514; F. Sofi et al., "Insomnia and Risk of Cardiovascular Disease: A Meta-analysis. *European Journal of Preventive Cardiology,* 2047487312460020, (2012), doi: 10.1177/2047487312460020.

15. M. P. St-Onge et al., "Short Sleep Duration, Glucose Dysregulation and Hormonal Regulation of Appetite in Men and Women," *Sleep* 35, no. 11 (2012): 1503–1510, doi: 10.5665/sleep.2198; American Academy of Sleep Medicine, "Sleep Duration Affects Hunger Differently in Men and Women," October 2012, www.aasmnet.org; J. Broussard et al., "Impaired Insulin Signaling in Human Adipocytes After Experimental Sleep Restriction: A Randomized, Crossover

Study," *Annals of Internal Medicine* 157, no. 8 (2012): 549–557, doi: 10.7326/0003-4819-157-8-201210160-00005; K. Hairston et al., "Sleep Duration and Five-Year Fat Accumulation in a Minority Cohort: The IRAS Family Study," *Sleep* 33, no. 3 (2010): 289–295; L. Nielson, T. Danielson, and A. Serensen, "Short Sleep Duration as a Possible Cause of Obesity: Critical Analysis of the Epidemiological Evidence," *Obesity Reviews* 12, no. 2 (2011): 78–92.

16. National Sleep Foundation, "Sleep Apnea and Diabetes, 2010, www.sleepfoundation.org

17. National Institutes of Health (NIH), "Information about Sleep," 2011, http://science.education.nih.gov; C. Peri and M. Smith, "What Lack of Sleep Does to Your Mind," WebMD, January 2013, www.webmd.com

18. E. Fortier-Brochu et al., "Insomnia and Daytime Cognitive Performance: A Meta-Analysis," *Sleep Medicine Reviews* 16, no. 1, (2011): 83–94, doi: 10-1016/j.smrv.2011.03.008

19. A. Gomes, J. Tavares, and M. Azevedo. "Sleep and Academic Performance in Undergraduates: A Multi-Measure, Multi-Predictor Approach." *Chronobiology* 28, no. 9 (2011): 786–801, doi: 10.3109/07420528.2011.606518; P. V. Thatcher, "University Students and the 'All-Nighter': Correlates and Patterns of Students' Engagement in a Single Night of Total Sleep Deprivation," *Behavioral Sleep Medicine* 6, no. 1 (2008): 16–31.

20. M. Tucker, S. McKinley, and R. Stickgold, "Sleep Optimizes Motor Skill in Older Adults," *Journal of the American Geriatrics Society* 59, no. 4 (2011): 603–609, doi: 10.1111/j.1532-5415.2011.03324.x; L. Genzel et al., "Complex Motor Sequence Skills Profit from Sleep," *Neuropsychobiology* 66, no. 4 (2012): 237–243, doi: 10.1159/000341878.

21. Centers for Disease Control and Prevention (CDC), "Drowsy Driving: Asleep at the Wheel," CDC Features (blog), 2013, www.cdc.gov

22. AAA Foundation for Traffic Safety, "Asleep at the Wheel: The Prevalence and Impact of Drowsy Driving," (Washington, DC: AAA, 2010), Available at www.aaafoundation.org; Centers for Disease Control and Prevention, "Drowsy Driving-19 States and the District of Columbia. 2009-2010," *Morbidity and Mortality Weekly Report* 61, no. 51 (2013): 1033–1037, Available at www.cdc.gov

23. National Institutes of Health (NIH), "Teacher's Guide-Information about Sleep," January 2012, http://science.education.nih.gov

24. H. Oster, "Does Late Sleep Promote Depression?" *Expert Reviews of Endocrinology and Metabolism* 7, no. 1, (2012): 27–29, Available at www.expert-reviews.com; C. Baglioni et al., "Insomnia as a Predictor of depression: A Meta-Analytic Evaluation of Longitudinal Epidemiological Studies," *Journal of Affective Disorders* 135, no. 1 (2011): 10–19, doi: 10.1016/j.jad.2011.01.011.

25. "Circadian Rhythms Fact Sheet," National Institute of General Medical Sciences, Science Education (blog), 2012, www.nigms.nih.gov

26. E. Carlson et al., "Tick Tock: New Clues About Biological Clocks and Health." Inside Life Science (blog), National Institute of General Medical Science, November 2012, http://publications.nigms.nih.gov; M. Vitaterna,

J. Takahashi, and F. Turek, "Overview of Circadian Rhythms," National Institute on Alcohol Abuse and Alcoholism, 2012, http://pubs.niaaa.nih.gov

27. NIH, "Teacher's Guide: Information about Sleep," 2012.

28. M. Kopasz et al., "Sleep and Memory in Healthy children and Adolescents–A Critical Review," *Sleep Medicine Reviews* 14, no. 3 (2010): 167–177, doi: 10.1016/j.smrv.2009.10.006; M. Fantini et al., "Longitudinal Study of Cognitive Function in Idiopathic REM Sleep Behavior Disorder," *Sleep* 34, no. 5 (2011): 619–625, www.ncbi.nlm.nih.gov

29. F. Cappuccio et al., "Sleep Duration and All-Cause Mortality" 2010; F. Cappuccio, L. D'Elia, P. Strazzullo, and M. Miller, "Quantity and Quality of Sleep and Incidence of Type 2 Diabetes: A Systematic Review and Meta-Analysis," *Diabetes Care* 33, no. 2 (2009): 414–420.

30. NIH, "Teacher's Guide: Information about Sleep," 2012.

31. E. Carlson et al., "Tick Tock: New Clues about Biological Clocks and Health," 2012.

32. N. Marshall et al., "Sleep Apnea as an Independent Risk Factor for All-Cause Mortality: The Busselton Health Study," *Sleep* 31, no. 6 (2008): 1079–1085; F. Cappuccio et al., "Sleep Duration Predicts Cardiovascular Outcomes: A Systematic Review and Meta-Analysis of Prospective Studies," *European Heart Journal* 32, no. 12 (2011): 1484–1492; E. Kronhom et al., "Self-Reported Sleep Duration, All-Cause Mortality, Cardiovascular Mortality and Morbidity in Finland," *Sleep Medicine* 12, no. 3 (2011): 215–221; F. Cappuccio et al., "Sleep Duration and All-Cause Mortality," 2010.

33. National Sleep Foundation, "How Much Sleep Do We Really Need?," 2011.

34. National Sleep Foundation, "Napping," (2011), www.sleepfoundation.org; B. Faraut et al., "Benefits of Napping and an Extended Duration of Recovery Sleep on Alertness and Immune Cells After Acute Sleep Restriction," *Brain, Behavior, and Immunity* 25, no. 1 (2011): 18–24, doi: 10.1016/j.bbi.2010.08.001.

35. National Sleep Foundation, "Caffeine and Sleep," 2011, www.sleepfoundation.org

36. E. Carlson et al., "Tick Tock" 2012.

37. American College Health Association, *National College Health Assessment II: Undergraduate Students Reference Group Data Report Fall 2012*, 2013.

38. National Sleep Foundation, "Can't Sleep? What to Know About Insomnia," 2011, www.sleepfoundation.org

39. American College Health Association, *National College Health Assessment II: Undergraduate Students Reference Group Data Report Fall 2012*, 2013.

40. National Sleep Foundation, "Obstructive Sleep Apnea and Sleep," 2011, www.sleepfoundation.org

41. Sleep Disorders Guide, "Sleep Apnea Statistics," January 2012, www.sleepdisordersguide.com

42. National Sleep Foundation, "Sleep Apnea and Sleep," 2011, www.sleepfoundation.org

43. Ibid.

44. National Institute of Neurological Disorders and Stroke, "Restless Legs Syndrome Fact Sheet," November 2011, www.ninds.nih.gov

45. Ibid.
46. Narcolepsy Patient Information Fact Sheet, January, 2012. www.empr.com

Pulled statistics:

page 100, American College Health Association, *American College Health Association-National College Health Assessment II: Reference Group Executive Summary Fall 2012* (Hanover, MD: American College Health Association, 2013), www.acha-ncha.org

Chapter 4: Preventing Violence and Injury

1. Voltaire, *Semiramis, V. 1,* trans. by J. K. Hoyt from *The Cyclopaedia of Practical Quotations,* 1896.
2. World Health Organization, "Violence: A Public Health Priority," *WHO Global Consultation on Violence and Health,* 1996.
3. Centers for Disease Control and Prevention, Injury Prevention and Control, "Ten Leading Causes of Injury and Deaths—2010" and "10 Leading Causes of Injury Deaths by Age Highlighting Violence-Related Injury Deaths, United States—2010," October 2012, www.cdc.gov
4. U.S. Department of Justice, Federal Bureau of Investigation, "Crime in the United States, Preliminary Semiannual Uniform Crime Report for 2011," July 2012, www.fbi.gov
5. Terry Frieden, "U.S. Violent Crime Down for Fifth Straight Year," *CNN,* October 29, 2012, www.cnn.com
6. J. Rudolph, "Violent Crime Up in the U.S. for the First Time in Nearly 2 Decades, Despite FBI Claims," *Huffington Post,* October 17, 2012, www.huffingtonpost.com
7. Bureau of Justice Statistics, "The Nation's Two Crime Measures," March 13, 2013, http://bjs.ojp.usdoj.gov
8. Bureau of Justice Statistics, "Criminal Victimization, 2011," October 2012, http://bjs.ojp.usdoj.gov
9. American College Health Association, *American College Health Association—National College Health Assessment II: Reference Group Data Report Fall 2012* (Hanover, MD: American College Health Association, 2013), www.acha-ncha.org
10. National Criminal Justice Reference Service, "Section 6: Statistical Overviews," *NCVRW Resource Guide,* 2012, http://bjs.ojp.usdoj.gov
11. Center for Public Integrity, "Sexual Assault on Campus: A Frustrating Search for Justice," Updated February 2013, www.publicintegrity.org
12. K. Jones, "Barriers Curb Reporting on Campus Sexual Assault," Center for Public Integrity, June 2012, www.publicintegrity.org
13. World Health Organization Violence Prevention Alliance, "The Ecological Framework," 2010, www.who.int; Centers for Disease Control and Prevention, National Center for Injury Prevention and Control, "Understanding Youth Violence: Fact Sheet," 2012, www.cdc.gov
14. Substance Abuse and Mental Health Services Administration, "The NSDUH Report: Violent Behaviors and Family Income among Adolescents," August 19, 2010, Newsletter, www.oas.samhsa.gov
15. D. M. Capaldi et al., "A Systematic Review of Risk Factors for Intimate Partner Violence," *Partner Abuse* 2, no. 2 (2012) 231–280, www.ncbi.nlm.nih.gov
16. J. H. Derzon, "The Correspondence of Family Features with Problem, Aggressive, Criminal and Violent Behaviors: A Meta-Analysis," *Journal of Experimental Criminology* 6, no. 3 (2010): 263–292, doi: 10.1007/s11292-010-9098-0; D. Bernat et al., "Risk and Direct Protective Factors for Youth Violence: Results from the National Longitudinal Study of Adolescent Health," *American Journal of Preventive Medicine* 1, no. 43 (2012): 557–566.
17. J. W. White, M. P. Kossand, and A. E. Kazdin, eds., *Violence Against Women and Children: Mapping the Terrain,* (Vols. 1 and 2) (Washington, D. C.: American Psychological Association, 2011); L. Kiss et al., "Gender-based Violence and Socioeconomic Inequalities: Does Living in More Deprived Neighborhoods Increase Women's risk of Intimate Partner Violence?" *Social Science and Medicine* 8, no. 74 (2012): 1172–1179.
18. M. L. Hunt, A. W. Hughey, and M. G. Burke, "Stress and Violence in the Workplace and on Campus: A Growing Problem for Business, Industry and Academia," *Industry and Higher Education* 1, no. 26 (2012): 43–51; Centers for Disease Control and Prevention, "Understanding Intimate Partner Violence Fact Sheet, 2012," www.cdc.gov
19. T. Frisell et al., "Violent Crime Runs in Families: A Total Population Study of 12.5 Million Individuals," *Psychological Medicine* 41, no. 1 (2010): 97–105, doi:10.1017S0023329170000462.
20. K. Makin-Byrd and K. L. Bierman, "Individual and Family Predictors of the Perpetration of Dating Violence and Victimization in Late Adolescence," *Journal of Youth Adolescence* 4, no. 42 (2013): 536–550, doi: 10.1007/s10964-012-9810-7; J. H. Derzon, "The Correspondence of Family Features," 2010; C. Cook et al., "Predictors of Bullying and Victimization in Childhood and Adolescence: A Meta-Analytic Investigation," *School Psychology Quarterly* 25, no. 2 (2010): 65–83.
21. R. Kendra, K. Bell, and J. Guimond, "The Impact of Child Abuse History, PTSD and Anger Arousal on Dating Violence Perpetrators Among College Women," *Journal of Family Violence* 27, no. 3 (2012): 165–175.
22. D. Matsumoto, S. Yoo, and J. Chung, "The Expression of Anger across Culture," in *International Handbook of Anger,* eds. M. Potegal, et al. (New York: Springer, 2010).
23. M. M. Ttofi, D. Farrington, and F. Losel, "School Bullying as a Predictor of Violence," 2012.
24. A. Abbey, "Alcohol's Role in Sexual Violence Perpetration: Theoretical Explanations, Existing Evidence and Future Directions," *Drugs and Alcohol Review* 30, no. 5 (2012): 481–485; J. M. Boden, D. M. Fergusen, and L. J. Horwood, "Alcohol Misuse and Violent Behavior: Findings from a 30-Year Longitudinal Study," *Drugs and Alcohol Dependence* 122, (2012): 135–141; United Nations Office on Drugs and Crime, "World Drug Report," 2012, www.unodc.org
25. P. H. Smith et al., "Intimate Partner Violence and Specific Substance Use Disorders: Findings from the National Epidemiological Survey on Alcohol and Related Conditions," *Psychology of Addictive Behaviors* 26, no. 2 (2012): 236–245.
26. A. Abbey, "Alcohol's Role in Sexual Violence Perpetration" 2012.
27. M. McMurran ed., *Alcohol-Related Violence Prevention and Treatment* (West Sussex, U.K: John Wiley and Sons, 2013); K. Graham et al., "Alcohol-Related Negative Consequences among Drinkers Around the World," *Addiction* 106, (2011): 1391–1405; A. Abbey, "Alcohol's Role in Sexual Violence Perpetration," 2012; J. M. Boden, D. M. Fergusen, and L. J. Horwood, "Alcohol Misuse and Violent Behavior," 2012.
28. W. Gunter and K. Daley, "Causal or Spurious? Using Propensity Score Matching to Detangle the Relationship between Violent Video Games and Violent Behavior," *Computers in Human Behavior* 4, no. 28 (2012): 1348–1355.
29. T. Niederkrotenthaler et al., "Changes in Suicide Rates Following Media Reports of Celebrity Suicide: A Meta-Analysis," *Journal of Epidemiology and Community Health* (2012), doi: 10.1136/jech-2011-200707.
30. R. A. Ramos et al., "Comfortably Numb or Just Yet Another Movie? Media Violence Exposure Does NOT Reduce Viewer Empathy for Victims of Real Violence Among Primarily Hispanic Viewers," *Psychology of Popular Media Culture* 1, no. 2 (2013): 210, Available at www.tamiu.edu
31. ChildStats.Gov, "America's Children in Brief: Key National Indicators of Well-Being, 2012," http://childstats.gov
32. World Health Organization, *World Report on Violence and Health,* 2002.
33. World Health Organization, "Definition and Typology of Violence," March 2013, www.who.int
34. Centers for Disease Control and Prevention, National Center for Injury Prevention and Control, Division of Violence Prevention, "Youth Violence: Definitions," 2011; L. L. Dahlberg and E. G. Krug, "Violence: A Global Public Health Problem," in *World Report on Violence and Health,* eds. E. G. Krug et al. (Geneva: World Health Organization, 2002), 1–21.
35. Centers for Disease Control and Prevention, Injury Prevention and Control, "Ten Leading Causes of Injury and Death," October 2012, www.cdc.gov
36. D. Hoyert and J. Xu, Centers for Disease Control and Prevention, "Deaths: Preliminary Data for 2011," *National Vital Statistics Reports* 61, no. 6 (2012), www.cdc.gov
37. Centers for Disease Control and Prevention, National Center for Injury Prevention and Control, Web-Based Injury Statistics Query and Reporting System (WISQARS), 2011, www.cdc.gov; U. S. Department of Justice, Federal Bureau of Investigation, *Crime in the United States 2011,* 2012, www.fbi.gov
38. Ibid.
39. Federal Bureau of Investigation, "Hate Crime Statistics, 2011," February 2013, www.fbi.gov
40. Ibid.
41. Ibid.
42. Ibid.
43. The Federal Bureau of Investigation, "2011 National Gang Threat Assessment Issued," October 2011, www.fbi.gov
44. U.S. Department of Justice, National Drug Intelligence Center, *National Gang Threat Assessment 2011* (Washington, DC: National Drug Intelligence Center, 2013), www.fbi.gov

45. National Youth Violence Prevention Resource Center, "Straight Talk about Gangs: Facts for Educators," February 6, 2013, www.ncpc.org

46. U.S. Code of Federal Regulations, Title 28CFRO.85.

47. P. Lin and J. Gill, "Homicides of Pregnant Women," *Journal of Forensic Medicine and Pathology*, (2010), doi: 10-1097/PAF. obo13e3181d3dc3b.

48. Violence Policy Center, *American Roulette: Murder-Suicide in the United States*, 4th ed. (Washington, DC: Violence Policy Center, 2012), Available at www.vpc.org

49. M. C. Black et al., "The National Intimate Partner and Sexual Violence Survey (NISVS): 2010 Summary Report," (Atlanta, GA: National Center for Injury Prevention and Control, Centers for Disease Control and Prevention, 2011), Available at www.cdc.gov

50. L. Walker, *The Battered Woman* (New York: Harper and Row, 1979).

51. L. Walker, *The Battered Woman Syndrome*, 3rd ed. (New York: Springer, 2009).

52. L. Rosen and J. Fontaine, *Compendium of Research on Violence against Women, 1993–Present* (Washington, DC: National Institute of Justice, 2009), DOJ (US) NCJ223572, www.ojp.usdoj.gov

53. U. S. Department of Health and Human Services, Administration for Children and Families, "*Definitions of Child Abuse and Neglect*," February 2011, www.childwelfare.gov

54. Childhelp, National Child Abuse Statistics, "Child Abuse in America," 2012, www.acf.hhs.gov

55. National Center for Injury Prevention and Control, Division of Violence Prevention, "Elder Maltreatment Prevention," June 11, 2012; U.S. Department of Health and Human Services, National Institute on Aging, "Elder Abuse," 2012, www.nia.nih.gov

56. Bureau of Justice Statistics, "Criminal Victimization, 2008," September 2, 2009, http://bjs.ojp.usdoj.gov

57. Ibid; M. C. Black et al., "The National Intimate Partner and Sexual Violence Survey," 2011.

58. D. G. Kilpatrick et al., "Drug-Facilitated, Incapacitated, and Forcible Rape: A National Study," 2007, Available at www.ncjrs.gov

59. J. Carr, *American College Health Association Campus Violence White Paper* (Baltimore: American College Health Association, 2005), Available at www.acha.org

60. National Criminal Justice Reference Service, "School and Campus Crime," *Resource Guide*, 2013, http://ovc.ncjrs.gov

61. Centers for Disease Control and Prevention, National Center for Injury Prevention and Control, "Understanding Sexual Violence Fact Sheet," 2012, www.cdc.gov

62. R. Bergen and E. Barnhill, National Online Resource Center on Violence against Women, "Marital Rape: New Research and Directions," February 2006, www.vawnet.org

63. L. P. Chen et al., "Sexual Abuse and Lifetime Diagnosis of Psychiatric Disorders: Systematic Review and Meta-Analysis," *Mayo Clinic Proceedings* 85, no. 7 (2010): 618–629; Childhelp, National Child Abuse Statistics, 2012; U.S. Department of Health and Human Services, Children's Bureau, "Child Maltreatment," February 2013, www.acf.hhs.gov

64. Ibid; Childhelp, National Child Abuse Statistics, 2012.

65. L. P. Chen et al., "Sexual Abuse and Lifetime Diagnosis of Psychiatric Disorders" 2010; T. Hilberg, C. Hamilton-Giachrtsis, and L. Dixon, "Review of Meta-Analyses on the Association between Child Sexual Abuse and Adult Mental Health Difficulties: A Systematic Approach," *Trauma, Violence, Abuse* 12, no. 1 (2011): 38–49.

66. Childhelp, National Child Abuse Statistics, 2013.

67. Oregon State University, Sexual Harassment Policy, February 2013. http://oregonstate.edu

68. Centers for Disease Control and Prevention, "Sexual Violence, Stalking, and Intimate Partner Violence Widespread in the US," NISVS 2010 Summary Report, Press Release, December 2011.

69. Ibid; NCVRW Resource Guide-2012, "Crime Victimization in the United States: Statistical Overviews," 2012, http://ovc.ncjrs.gov

70. Ibid.

71. J. Carr, *American College Health Association Campus Violence White Paper*, 2005.

72. S. L. Murphy, J. Q. Xu, and K. D. Kochanek, "Deaths: Preliminary Data for 2010," *National Vital Statistics Reports* 60, no. 4 (2012), www.cdc.gov

73. Ibid.

74. Ibid.

75. National Highway Traffic Safety Administration, *Traffic Safety Facts 2010 Motor Vehicle Crashes: Overview* (Washington, DC: NHTSA's National Center for Statistics and Analysis, February, 2012), DOT HS 811 552, www.nhtsa.gov

76. National Highway Traffic Safety Administration, "Traffic Safety Facts 2010: Bicyclists and Other Cyclists," June 2012, www.nhtsa.gov

77. Ibid.

78. Insurance Institute for Highway Safety, *Fatality Facts: Bicycles 2010*, 2010, www.iihs.org

Pulled statistics:

page 112, D. Drysdale, W. Modzeleski, and A. Simons, Campus Attacks: Targeted Violence Affecting Institutions of Higher Education (Washington, DC: U.S. Secret Service, U.S. Department of Homeland Security, Office of Safe and Drug-Free Schools, U.S. Department of Education, and Federal Bureau of Investigation, U.S. Department of Justice, 2010), www.fbi.gov

page 117, M. C. Black et al., "The National Intimate Partner and Sexual Violence Survey (NISVS): 2010 Summary Report" (Atlanta, GA: National Center for Injury Prevention and Control, Centers for Disease Control and Prevention, 2011), Available at www.cdc.gov

page 120, Ibid.

Chapter 5: Building Healthy Relationships and Understanding Sexuality

1. J. Holt-Lunstad, T. Smith, and J. Layton, "Social Relationships and Mortality Risk: A Meta-Analytic Review," *PLoS Medicine* 7, no. 7 (2010); Y. Luo, L. Hawkley, L. Waite, and J. Cacioppo, "Loneliness, Health, and Mortality in Old Age: A National Longitudinal Study," *Social Science and Medicine* 74, no. 6 (2012): 907–914.

2. Ibid.

3. Ibid.

4. S. R. Braithwaite, R. Delevi, and F. D. Fincham, "Romantic Relationships and the Physical and Mental Health of College Students," *Personal Relationships* 17, no. 1 (2010): 1–12.

5. D. Akst, "America: Land of Loners?" *The Wilson Quarterly*, Summer 2010, www.wilsonquarterly.com

6. N. Christakis and J. Fowler, *Connected: The Surprising Power of Our Social Networks and How They Shape Our Lives* (New York: Little, Brown and Company, 2009).

7. R. Sternberg, "Construct Validation of a Triangular Love Scale," *European Journal of Social Psychology* 27, no. 3 (1997): 313–335, doi: 10.1002/(SICI)1099-0992(199705)27:3<313: AID-EJSP824>3.0.CO;2-4.

8. H. Fisher, *Why We Love* (New York: Henry Holt, 2004); H. Fisher et al., "Defining the Brain System of Lust, Romantic Attraction, and Attachment," *Archives of Sexual Behavior* 31, no. 5 (2002): 413–419.

9. Ibid.

10. S. A. Rathus, J. Nevid, and L. Fichner-Rathus, *Human Sexuality in a World of Diversity*, 8th ed. (Boston: Allyn & Bacon, 2010).

11. C. R. Rogers, "Interpersonal Relationship: The Core of Guidance" in *Person to Person: The Problem of Being Human*, eds. C. R. Rogers and B. Stevens (Lafayette, CA: Real People Press, 1967).

12. J. Wood, *Interpersonal Communication: Everyday Encounters*, 7th ed. (Belmont, CA: Cengage, 2012).

13. Ibid.

14. D. Cohn et al., "Barely Half of U.S. Adults Are Married," Pew Research Center, Social and Demographic Trends, December 14, 2011, www.pewsocialtrends.org

15. E. Marquardt et al., "The President's Marriage Agenda for the Forgotten Sixty Percent," *The State of Our Unions: Marriage in America, 2012* (Charlottesville, VA: National Marriage Project and the Institute for American Values, 2012).

16. U.S. Census Bureau, "Table MS-2, Estimated Median Age at First Marriage, by Sex: 1890 to the Present," Families and Living Arrangements: 2012, www.census.gov

17. K. McCoy, "Can Marriage Help You Live Longer?" HealthLibrary, EBSCO Publishing, April 2010, http://healthlibrary.epnet.com; I. Siegler, B. Brummett, P. Martin, and M. Helms, "Consistency and Timing of Marital Transitions and Survival During Midlife: The Role of Personality and Health Risk Behaviors," *Annals of Behavioral Medicine* (2013), doi: 10.1007/s12160-012-9457-3. (Epub ahead of print).

18. U.S. Department of Health and Human Services, Vital and Health Statistics, *Health Behaviors of Adults: United States, 2005-2007*, DHHS Pub No. (DHS) 2010-1573. Washington, D.C.: U.S. Government Printing Office.

19. National Center for Health Statistics, Division of Vital Statistics, "First Marriages in the United States: Data from the 2006–2010 National Survey of Family Growth," 2012, www.cdc.gov

20. P. Y. Goodwin, W. D. Mosher, and A. Chandra, "Marriage and Cohabitation in the United States: A Statistical Portrait Based on Cycle 6 (2002) of the National Survey of Family Growth, National Center for Health Statistics," *Vital Health Statistics* 23, no. 28 (2010), Available at www.cdc.gov

21. U.S. Census Bureau, "Census Bureau Releases Estimates of Same-Sex Married Couples," September 27, 2011, www.census.gov

22. National Gay and Lesbian Task Force, "Relationship Recognition Map for Same-Sex Couples in the U.S.," January 2013, www.thetaskforce.org

23. D. Masci et al., "Gay Marriage Around the World," The Pew Forum on Religion & Public Life, Blog, Pew Research Center, February 8, 2013, www.pewforum.org

24. U.S. Census Bureau, "2011 American Community Survey, Marital Status," Table S1201, 2012, www.census.gov

25. U.S. Census Bureau, "Table C2. Household Relationship And Living Arrangements Of Children Under 18 Years, By Age And Sex: 2012," America's Families and Living Arrangements: 2012, www.census.gov

26. M. Lino, *Expenditures on Children by Families, 2011* (Alexandria, VA: U.S. Department of Agriculture, Center for Nutrition Policy and Promotion, 2012), www.cnpp.usda.gov

27. U.S. Bureau of Labor Statistics, "Women in the Labor Force: A Databook 2011 Edition," 2012, http://data.bls.gov

28. National Association of Child Care Resource and Referral Agencies, "Parents and the High Cost of Child Care, 2012 Report," 2012, www.naccrra.org

29. Guttmacher Institute, "Facts on Unintended Pregnancy in the United States," January 2012, www.guttmacher.org

30. M. Gatzeva and A. Paik, "Emotional and Physical Satisfaction in Noncohabiting, Cohabiting, and Marital Relationships: The Importance of Jealous Conflict," *Journal of Sex Research* 48, no. 1 (2010): 29–42, doi: 10.1080/00224490903370602; B. Sagarin et al., "Sex Differences in Jealousy: A Meta-Analytic Examination," *Evolution & Human Behavior* 33, no. 6 (2012): 595–614.

31. United States Department of Labor, Bureau of Labor Statistics, "American Time Use Survey Summary—2011 Results," June 2012, www.bls.gov

32. United States Department of Labor, Bureau of Labor Statistics, "Labor Force Statistics from the Current Population Survey—Wives Who Earn More than Their Husbands, 1987–2011," November 20, 2012, www.bls.gov; R. Fry and D. Cohn, "New Economics of Marriage: The Rise of Wives," Pew Research Center, January 19, 2010, http://pewresearch.org

33. K. Heller, "The Myth of the High Rate of Divorce," Family & Parenting, Blog, Psych Central, 2012, http://psychcentral.com

34. G. F. Kelly, *Sexuality Today,* 10th ed. (New York: McGraw-Hill, 2010).

35. Intersex Society of North America, "How Common Is Intersex?," 2008, www.isna.org

36. W. J. Jenkins, "Can Anyone Tell Me Why I'm Gay? What Research Suggests Regarding the Origins of Sexual Orientation," *North American Journal of Psychology* 12, no. 2 (2010): 279–296.

37. G. M. Herek, "Sexual Stigma and Sexual Prejudice in the United States: A Conceptual Framework," in *Contemporary Perspectives on Lesbian, Gay, and Bisexual Identities, Nebraska Symposium on Motivation,* ed. D.A. Hope (New York City: Springer, 2009), 65–111.

38. Federal Bureau of Investigation, "Hate Crime Statistics, 2011," December 10, 2012, www.fbi.gov

39. C. Currie et al., "Is Obesity at Individual and National Level Associated with Lower Age at Menarche? Evidence from 34 Countries in the Health Behaviour in School-Aged Children Study," *Journal of Adolescent Health* 50, no. 6 (2012): 621–626, doi: 10.1016/j.jadohealth.2011.10.254.

40. Mayo Clinic Staff, "Premenstrual Syndrome (PMS)," 2012, www.mayoclinic.com

41. Mayo Clinic Staff, "Premenstrual Dysphoric Disorder (PMDD): Different from PMS," 2012, www.mayoclinic.com

42. Mayo Clinic Staff, "Menstrual Cramps," 2011, www.mayoclinic.com/Health/Menstrual-Cramps/Ds00506

43. WebMD, "Women's Health Initiative (WHI): Risks and Benefits of Hormone Replacement Therapy (HRT) and Estrogen Replacement Therapy (ERT)," 2011, http://women.webmd.com

44. M. Beck, "Benefits of Hormone-Replacement Therapy Outweigh Risks, Reviews of Studies Show," Health Blog, Blog, *The Wall Street Journal,* May 22, 2012, http://blogs.wsj.com

45. Mayo Clinic Staff, "Circumcision (Male): Why It's Done," September 2012, www.mayoclinic.com; American Academy of Pediatrics, "2012 Technical Report, Male Circumcision," *Pediatrics* 130, no. 3 (2012) e756–e785, doi: 10.1542/peds.2012-1990.

46. G. F. Kelly, *Sexuality Today,* 10th ed. (New York: McGraw-Hill, 2010).

47. Ibid.

48. J. A. Higgins, J. Trussell, N. B. Moore, and J. K. Davidson, "Young Adult Sexual Health: Current and Prior Sexual Behaviours among Non-Hispanic White U.S. College Students," *Sexual Health* 7, no. 1 (2010): 35–43, doi: 10.1071/SH09028.

49. American College Health Association, *American College Health Association–National College Health Assessment II:) Reference Group Data Report Fall 2012* (Hanover, MD: American College Health Association, 2013), www.acha-ncha.org

50. Ibid.

51. Ibid.

52. G. F. Kelly, *Sexuality Today,* 2010.

53. Cleveland Clinic, "An Overview of Sexual Dysfunction," Updated October 2012.

54. A. Mullens et al., "The Amyl Nitrite Expectancy Questionnaire for Men Who Have Sex with Men (AEQ-MSM): A Measure of Substance-Related Beliefs," *Substance Use & Misuse* 46, no. 13 (2011): 1642–1650.

Pulled statistics:

page 144, K. Hymowitz et al., "Other Consequences of Delayed Marriage," *The Knot Yet Report: The Benefits and Costs of Delayed Marriage in America,* The National Marriage Project at the University of Virginia, The National Campaign to Prevent Teen and Unplanned Pregnancy, and The Relate Institute, 2013, http://twentysomethingmarriage.org

page 158, American College Health Association, *National College Health Assessment II: Undergraduate Reference Group Executive Summary Fall 2012,* 2013.

Chapter 6: Considering Your Reproductive Choices

1. American College Health Association, *American College Health Association-National College Health Assessment II: Undergraduate Students Reference Group Data Fall 2012* (Hanover, MD: American College Health Association, 2013), www.acha-ncha.org

2. Centers for Disease Control and Prevention, "Incidence, Prevalence and Cost of Sexually Transmitted Infections in the United States," 2013, www.cdc.gov

3. The National Campaign to Prevent Teen and Unplanned Pregnancy, "Unplanned Pregnancy among Unmarried Young Women," 2012, www.thenationalcampaign.org

4. J. Trussell, "Contraceptive Efficacy," in *Contraceptive Technology,* 20th rev. ed., eds. R. A. Hatcher et al. (New York: Ardent Media, 2011).

5. Ibid.

6. Ibid.

7. Ibid.

8. Ibid.

9. Ibid.

10. Ibid.

11. J. Trussell, "Contraceptive Efficacy," in *Contraceptive Technology,* 2011.

12. Ibid.

13. Ibid.

14. Ibid.

15. American College Health Association, *National College Health Assessment II: Undergraduate Students Reference Group Data Fall 2012,* 2013.

16. Drug Information Online Drugs.com, "Seasonale," April 2012, www.drugs.com; Drug Information Online Drugs.com, "Seasonique," March 2013, www.drugs.com

17. J. Trussell, "Contraceptive Efficacy," in *Contraceptive Technology,* 2011.

18. R. A. Hatcher et al., *Contraceptive Technology,* 20th rev. ed. (New York: Ardent Media, 2011).

19. O. Lidegaard et al., "Thrombotic Stroke and Myocardial Infarction with Hormonal Contraception," *New England Journal of Medicine* 366 (2012): 2257–2266, doi: 10.1056/NEJMoa1111840

20. Associated Press, "Free Birth Control: Insurance Now Covers It with No Copay," *The Times-Picayune,* August 1, 2011, www.nola.com; Planned Parenthood, "Key Facts on Birth Control Coverage," 2012, www.plannedparenthood.org

21. J. Trussell, "Contraceptive Efficacy," in *Contraceptive Technology,* 2011.

22. E. G. Raymond, "Progestin-Only Pills," in R. A. Hatcher et al., *Contraceptive Technology,* 20th rev. ed. (New York: Ardent Media, 2011).

23. Janssen Pharmaceuticals, "Ortho Evra," www.orthoevra.com, last modified October 17, 2012.

24. J. Trussell, "Contraceptive Efficacy," in *Contraceptive Technology,* 2011.

25. Janssen Pharmaceuticals, "Important Safety Update for U.S. Health Care Professionals ORTHO EVRA," March 2011, www.orthoevra.com

26. J. Trussell, "Contraceptive Efficacy," in *Contraceptive Technology,* 2011.

27. Ibid.

28. Pfizer, "Depo-subQ Provera," 2011, www.depo-subqprovera104.com

29. J. Trussell, "Contraceptive Efficacy," in *Contraceptive Technology,* 2011.

30. N. V. Organon-Merck & Co., Inc., "Implanon," 2012, www.implanon-usa.com

31. J. Jones, W. Mosher, and K. Daniels, "Current Contraceptive Use in the United States,

2006–2010, and Changes in Pattern of Use Since 1995," *National Health Statistics Reports*, No. 60 November 2012.

32. The American Congress of Obstetricians and Gynecologists, "ACOG Committee Opinion-Adolescents and Long-Acting Reversible Contraception: Implants and Intrauterine Devices," No. 539, October 2012, www.acog.org

33. J. Trussell, "Contraceptive Efficacy," in *Contraceptive Technology*, 2011.

34. Office of Population Research & Association of Reproductive Health Professionals, "Answers to Frequently Asked Questions about Effectiveness," The Emergency Contraception Website, updated November 2012, http://ec.princeton.edu

35. Ibid.

36. American College Health Association, *National College Health Assessment II: Undergraduate Students Reference Group Data Fall 2012*, 2013.

37. Ibid.

38. J. Trussell, "Contraceptive Efficacy," in *Contraceptive Technology*, 2011.

39. Ibid.

40. Guttmacher Institute, *Facts on Contraceptive Use in the United States*, June 2010, www.guttmacher.org; J. Jones, W. Mosher, and K. Daniels, "Current Contraceptive Use in the United States, 2006–2010, and Changes in Patterns of Use Since 1995," *National Health Statistics Reports*, no. 60 (Hyattsville, MD: National Center for Health Statistics, 2012).

41. J. Trussell, "Contraceptive Efficacy," in *Contraceptive Technology*, 2011.

42. R. A. Hatcher et al., *Contraceptive Technology*, 2011.

43. Guttmacher Institute, Facts on Induced Abortion in the United States, January 2011, www.guttmacher.org

44. American Psychological Association, Task Force on Mental Health and Abortion, *Report of the Task Force on Mental Health and Abortion* (Washington, DC: American Psychological Association, 2008), Available at www.apa.org

45. *Roe v. Wade*, 410 U.S. 113 (1973).

46. L.B. Finer and M. R. Zolna, "Unintended Pregnancy in the United States: Incidence and Disparities, 2006," *Contraception* 84, no. 5 (2011): 475–485, doi: 10.1016/j.contraception.2011.07.013.

47. L. Saad, "Abortion," Gallup Politics, blog, March, 2013, www.gallup.com

48. American Psychological Association, Task Force on Mental Health and Abortion, *Report of the Task Force on Mental Health and Abortion*, 2008.

49. Ibid.

50. Ibid.

51. Guttmacher Institute, Facts on Induced Abortions in the United States, August 2011.

52. Ibid.

53. Ibid.

54. Planned Parenthood, "The Abortion Pill (Medication Abortion)," Health Info & Services, March 2013, www.plannedparenthood.org

55. Ibid.

56. American College of Obstetricians and Gynecologists (ACOG), "Medical Management of Abortion, ACOG Practice Bulletin No. 67," *Obstetrics and Gynecology* 106, no. 4 (2005): 871–882.

57. M. Lino, *Expenditures on Children by Families, 2011* (Alexandria, VA: U.S. Department of Agriculture, Center for Nutrition Policy and Promotion, 2012), Available at www.cnpp.usda.gov

58. National Association of Child Care Resource and Referral Agencies, *Parents and the High Cost of Child Care, 2012 Report*, (2012), www.naccrra.org

59. Truven Health Analytics, "The Cost of Having a Baby in the United States," January 2013, http://transform.childbirthconnection.org

60. D. Wigle et al., "Epidemiologic Evidence of Relationships between Reproductive and Child Health Outcomes and Environmental Chemical Contaminants," *Journal of Toxicology and Environmental Health, Part B, Critical Reviews* 11, no. 5–6 (2008): 373–517, doi: 10.1080/10937400801921320.

61. Centers for Disease Control and Prevention, "Preconception Care and Health Care: Women," May 2012, www.cdc.gov

62. Ibid.

63. Planned Parenthood, "Pregnancy Tests," 2013, www.plannedparenthood.org

64. Committee on Obstetric Practice, "Weight Gain During Pregnancy," Committee Opinion no. 548, American Congress of Obstetricians and Gynecologists, *Obstetrics and Gynecology* 121, no. 1 (2013): 210–212, doi: 10.1097/01.AOG.0000425668.87506.4c.

65. The American Congress of Obstetricians and Gynecologists, "Alcohol and Women," FAQ068, American College of Obstetricians and Gynecologists, August 2011, www.acog.org

66. National Center for Chronic Disease Prevention and Health Promotion, "Tobacco Use and Pregnancy," Reproductive Health, updated April 2013, www.cdc.gov; U.S. Department of Health and Human Services, *How Tobacco Smoke Causes Disease: The Biology and Behavioral Basis for Smoking-Attributable Disease: A Report of the Surgeon General* (Atlanta: Centers for Disease Control and Prevention, National Center for Chronic Disease Prevention and Health Promotion, Office on Smoking and Health, 2010), Available at www.surgeongeneral.gov

67. U.S. Department of Health and Human Services, Health Resources and Services Administration, Maternal and Child Health Bureau, *Child Health USA 2010* (Rockville, MD: U.S. Department of Health and Human Services, 2010), Available at http://mchb.hrsa.gov

68. American Pregnancy Association, "Miscarriage," Pregnancy Complications, blog, updated November 2011, http://americanpregnancy.org

69. March of Dimes, "In Depth: Down Syndrome," Birth Defects, blog, 2009, www.marchofdimes.com

70. Medline Plus, "Quadruple Screen Test," updated February 2012, www.nlm.nih.gov

71. Centers for Disease Control and Prevention, "Percent of Births by Cesarean Delivery, by State 2011," National Vital Statistics System, www.cdc.gov

72. E. Puscheck, "Early Pregnancy Loss," *Medscape Reference: Drugs, Diseases & Procedures*, updated April 2013, http://reference.medscape.com

73. K. W. Hoover, G. Tao, and C. K. Kent, "Trends in the Diagnosis and Treatment of Ectopic Pregnancy in the United States," *Obstetrics and Gynecology* 115, no. 3 (2010): 495–502; V. P. Sepilian et al., "Ectopic Pregnancy," *Medscape Reference: Drugs, Diseases & Procedures*, updated August 2012, http://emedicine.medscape.com

74. March of Dimes, "Stillbirth Fact Sheet," Baby: Loss and Grief, 2010, www.marchofdimes.com

75. K. L. Wisner et al., "Onset Timing, Thoughts of Self-Harm, and Diagnoses in Postpartum Women with Screen-Positive Depression Findings," *JAMA Psychiatry* (2013): 1–9, doi:10.1001/jamapsychiatry.2013.87

76. American Academy of Pediatrics, "Benefits of Breastfeeding for Mom," Ages & Stages, updated June 2012, www.healthychildren.org

77. Centers for Disease Control and Prevention, "Sudden Unexpected Infant Death and Sudden Infant Death Syndrome," March 2013, www.cdc.gov

78. Ibid.

79. Centers for Disease Control and Prevention, "Infertility FAQs," Reproductive Health, updated February 2013, www.cdc.gov

80. Mayo Clinic Staff, MayoClinic.com, "Infertility: Causes," September 2011, www.mayoclinic.com

81. U.S. Department of Health and Human Services, "Polycystic Ovary Syndrome (PCOS) Fact Sheet," July 2012, www.womenshealth.gov

82. B. Kumbak, E. Oral, and O. Bukulmez, "Female Obesity and Assisted Reproductive Technologies," *Seminars in Reproductive Medicine* 30, no. 6 (2012), 507–516, doi: 10.1055/s-0032-1328879.

83. Centers for Disease Control and Prevention, "Pelvic Inflammatory Disease CDC Fact Sheet," Sexually Transmitted Diseases, updated September 2011, www.cdc.gov

84. Centers for Disease Control and Prevention, "Infertility FAQ's," *Reproductive Health*, updated February 2013, www.cdc.gov

85. S. S. Du Plessis et al., "The Effect of Obesity on Sperm Disorders and Male Infertility," *Nature Reviews Urology* 7, no. 3 (2010): 153–161, doi:10.1038/nrurol.2010.6.

86. Centers for Disease Control and Prevention, "Infertility: FAQs," 2013.

87. Ibid.

88. WebMD Medical Reference, "Fertility Drugs," reviewed July 2012, www.webmd.com

89. American Society for Reproductive Medicine, "Fertility Drugs and the Risk for Multiple Births," ReproductiveFacts.org, 2012, www.asrm.org

90. M. Gugucheva, "Surrogacy in America," Council for Responsible Genetics, 2010 www.councilforresponsiblegenetics.org

91. J. Jones, "Who Adopts? Characteristics of Women and Men Who Have Adopted Children," *NCHS Data Brief*, no. 12 (Hyattsville, MD: National Center for Health Statistics, 2009): DHHS Publication No. (PHS) 2009-1209, Available at www.cdc.gov

92. Intercountry Adoption, U.S. Department of State, "Statistics: Adoptions by Year," February 2012, http://adoption.state.gov

93. Ibid.

Pulled statistics:

page 167, W. D. Mosher and J. Jones, "Use of Contraception in the United States: 1982–2008," *Vital and Health Statistics* 23, no. 29 (Hyattsville, MD: National Center for Health Statistics, 2010), www.cdc.gov

page 175, American College Health Association, *American College Health Association-National College Health Assessment II: Undergraduate Students Reference Group Data Report Fall 2012* (Hanover, MD: American College Health Association, 2013), www.acha-ncha.org

page 183, Guttmacher Institute, "Facts on Unintended Pregnancy in the United States," *In Brief: Fact Sheet*, 2012, www.guttmacher.org

Chapter 7: Recognizing and Avoiding Addiction and Drug Abuse

1. J. Grant et al., "Introduction to Behavioral Addictions," *American Journal of Behavioral Addictions* 36, no. 5 (2010): 233–241; National Institute on Drug Abuse, National Institutes of Health, U.S. Department of Health and Human Services, *Drugs, Brains, and Behavior: The Science of Addiction*, NIH Publication no. 07-5605 (Bethesda, MD: National Institute on Drug Abuse, Revised 2010), Available at www.drugabuse.gov

2. Ibid.

3. National Council on Problem Gambling, "FAQs—Problem Gamblers," September 28, 2011, www.ncpgambling.org

4. C. Holden, "Behavioral Addictions Debut in Proposed DSM-5," *Science* 347, no. 5968 (2010): 935.

5. College Gambling.org, "Fact Sheet: Gambling on College Campuses," National Center for Responsible Gaming, 2012, www.collegegambling.org

6. Ibid.

7. M. Lejoyeux and A. Weinstein, "Compulsive Buying," *The American Journal of Drug and Alcohol Issues* 36, no.5 (2010): 248–253.

8. B. Cook and H. A. Hausenblas, "The Role of Exercise Dependence for the Relationship between Exercise Behavior and Eating Pathology: Mediator or Moderator?" *Journal of Health Psychology* 13, no. 4 (2008): 495–502.

9. The Center for Internet Addiction, "The Growing Epidemic," 2010, www.netaddiction.com

10. American College Health Association, *American College Health Association—National College Health Assessment: Executive Summary Fall 2012* (Hanover, MD: American College Health Association, 2013), www.acha-ncha.org

11. Substance Abuse and Mental Health Services Administration, *Results from the 2011 National Survey on Drug Use and Health: Summary of National Findings*, NSDUH Series H-44, HHS Publication No. (SMA) 12-4713 (Rockville, MD: Substance Abuse and Mental Health Services Administration, 2012).

12. J. Swendsen et al., "Use and Abuse of Alcohol and Illicit Drugs in the US Adolescents: Results of the National Comorbidity Survey-Adolescent Supplement," *Archives of General Psychiatry* 69, no. 4 (2012): 390–398.

13. L. D. Johnston et al., *Monitoring the Future National Results on Drug Use: 2012 Overview, Key Findings on Adolescent Drug Use* (Ann Arbor: Institute for Social Research, The University of Michigan, 2013).

14. National Institute of Drug Abuse, Drug Abuse at Highest Level in Nearly a Decade. *NIDA Notes* 23, no. 3 (2010), Available at www.nida.nih.gov

15. National Drug Intelligence Center, "National Drug Threat Assessment 2011," 2011, Available at www.justice.gov

16. Centers for Disease Control and Prevention, National Center for Health Statistics, Office of Analysis and Epidemiology, "Table 99: Prescription Drug Use in the Past 30 Days, by Sex, Age, Race and Hispanic Origin: United States Selected Years 1988–1994 through 2007–2010," Health, United States, 2011, www.cdc.gov

17. Consumer Health Care Products Association, "The Value of OTC Medicine to the United States," January 2012, www.yourhealthathand.org

18. Ibid.

19. L. D. Johnston et al., *Monitoring the Future National Results on Adolescent Drug Use*, 2011.

20. Erowid, The DXM Vault, 2011, www.erowid.org

21. Substance Abuse and Mental Health Services Administration, *Results from the 2011 National Survey*, 2012.

22. Ibid.

23. Ibid.

24. Ibid.

25. American College Health Association, *American College Health Association–National College Health Assessment Fall 2012*, 2013.

26. A. Garnier-Dykstra et al., "Nonmedical Use of Prescription Stimulants During College: Four-Year Trends in Exposure Opportunity, Use, Motives, and Sources," *Journal of American College Health* 30, no. 3 (2012): 226–234.

27. Substance Abuse and Mental Health Services Administration, *Results from the 2011 National Survey on Drug Use and Health*, 2012.

28. L. D. Johnston et al., *Monitoring the Future National Results on Adolescent Drug Use*, 2011.

29. A. Arria, et al., "Drug Use Patterns and Continuous Enrollment in College: Results from a Longitudinal Study," *Journal of Studies on Alcohol and Drugs* 74, (2013): 71–83.

30. A. Arria et al., "Drug Use Patterns in Young Adulthood and Post-College Employment," *Drug and Alcohol Dependence* 127, no. 1–3, (2013): 23–30.

31. National Center on Addiction and Substance Abuse at Columbia University, "Wasting the Best and the Brightest: Substance Abuse at America's Colleges and Universities" (New York: National Center on Addiction and Substance Abuse at Columbia University, 2007), Available at www.casacolumbia.org

32. L. D. Johnston et al., *Monitoring The Future National Results on Adolescent Drug Use*, 2011.

33. Substance Abuse and Mental Health Services Administration, *Results from the 2011 National Survey on Drug Use and Health*, 2012.

34. CPDD Community Website, "Methamphetamine Abuse and Parkinson's Disease," July 31, 2011, www.cpddblog.com

35. Harvard Health Letter, "What Is It about Coffee," January 2012, www.health.harvard.edu

36. Substance Abuse and Mental Health Services Administration, Results from the 2011 National Survey on Drug Use and Health: Detailed Tables, NSDUH Series H-44, HHS Publication no. (SMA) 12-4713 (Rockville, MD: Substance Abuse and Mental Health Services Administration, 2012).

37. Ibid.

38. U.S. Department of Health and Human Services, "Marijuana: Facts for Teens," 2010, http://teens.drugabuse.gov

39. M. Asbridge et al., "Acute Cannabis Consumption and Motor Vehicle Collision Risk: Systematic Review of Observational Studies and Meta-analysis," *British Medical Journal* 344 (2012): 1–9, doi:10.1136/bmj.e536.

40. National Institute on Drug Abuse, "NIDA InfoFacts: Marijuana," Revised July 2012, http://drugabuse.gov

41. Ibid.

42. Alcohol and Drug Abuse Institute, "Marijuana: Science-Based Information for the Public," University of Washington, December 2012, http://adai.washington.edu

43. National Institute on Drug Abuse, Marijuana: Facts for Teens," updated March 2011, www.drugabuse.gov; Science Daily, "Marijuana Use Prior to Pregnancy Doubles Risk of Premature Birth," July 17, 2012, www.sciencedaily.com

44. Substance Abuse and Mental Health Services Administration, *Results from the 2011 National Survey on Drug Use and Health,* 2012.

45. The Partnership at Drugfree.org, "GHB" 2012, www.drugfree.org

46. Substance Abuse and Mental Health Services Administration, *Results from the 2011 National Survey on Drug Use and Health,* 2012.

47. L. D. Johnston et al., *Monitoring the Future National Results on Adolescent Drug Use,* 2012.

48. National Institute on Drug Abuse, "NIDA InfoFacts: MDMA (Ecstasy)," Revised March 2010, www.drugabuse.gov

49. The National Collegiate Athletic Association, "Substance Use: National Study of Substance Use Trends among NCAA College Student-Athletes," 2012, www.ncaapublications.com; American College Health Association, *American College Health Association–National College Health Assessment Fall 2012*, 2013.

50. National Institute on Drug Abuse, NIDA for Teens, "Anabolic Steroids," 2010, http://teens.drugabuse.gov

51. Substance Abuse and Mental Health Services Administration, *Results from the 2011 National Survey on Drug Use and Health,* 2012.

Pulled statistics:

page 207, American College Health Association. *American College Health Association—National College Health Assessment II: Undergraduate Reference Group Executive Summary, Fall 2012,* 2013.

page 213, Substance Abuse and Mental Health Services Administration, *Results from the 2011 National Survey on Drug Use and Health: Summary of National Findings,* NSDUH Series H-44, HHS Publication No. (SMA) 12-4713 (Rockville, MD: Substance Abuse and Mental Health Services Administration, 2012), 27.

Chapter 8: Drinking Alcohol Responsibly and Ending Tobacco Use

1. Centers for Disease Control and Prevention, "Alcohol-Related Disease Impact (ARDI)," 2008, http://apps.nccd.cdc.gov

2. Centers for Disease Control and Prevention, "Current Cigarette Smoking Among Adults—United States, 2011," *Morbidity and Mortality Weekly Report* 61, no. 44 (2012): 88994.

3. J. Marrone et al., "Moderate Alcohol Intake Lowers Biochemical Markers of Bone Turnover in Postmenopausal Women," *Journal of the North American Menopause Society* 19, no. 9 (2012): 974–979; C. Stockley, "Is It Merely a Myth That Alcoholic Beverages Such as Red Wine Can Be Cardioprotective?" *Society of Chemical Industry* 92 (2012): 1815–1821, doi: 10.1002/jsfa.5696; A. Klatsky, "Alcohol and Cardiovascular Health," *Physiology and Behavior* 100, no. 1 (2010): 76–81, doi: 10.1016/j.physbeh.2009.

4. National Center for Health Statistics, "Summary Health Statistics for U.S. Adults: National

Health Interview Survey, 2010," *Vital and Health Statistics* 10, no. 252 (2012): 94, Available at www.cdc.gov

5. Ibid.

6. American College Health Association, *American College Health Association—National College Health Assessment II: Reference Group Executive Summary Fall 2012* (Hanover, MD: American College Health Association, 2013), www.acha-ncha.org

7. Substance Abuse and Mental Health Services Administration, "Results from the 2011 National Survey on Drug Use and Health: Summary of National Findings 2012," September 2012, www.samhsa.gov

8. National Institute on Alcohol Abuse and Alcoholism, "Moderate and Binge Drinking," 2012, www.niaaa.nih.gov

9. C. Neighbors et al., "Event Specific Drinking among College Students," *Psychology of Addictive Behaviors* 25, no. 4 (2011): 702–707, doi: 10.1037/a0024051.

10. M. A. Lewis et al., "Use of Protective Behavioral Strategies and Their Association to 21st Birthday Alcohol Consumption and Related Negative Consequences:A Between and Within Person Evaluation," *Psychology of Addictive Behaviors* 26, no. 2 (2012), 179–186, doi: 10.1037/a0023797.

11. National Institute on Alcohol Abuse and Alcoholism, "Fall Semester: A Time for Parents to Revisit Discussions about College Drinking," June 2012, www.collegedrinkingprevention.gov

12. American College Health Association, *National College Health Assessment II: Reference Group Executive Summary Fall 2012*, 2013.

13. S. Omyper et al., "Class Start Times, Sleep and Academic Performance in College: A Path Analysis," *Chronobiology* 29, no. 3 (2012): 318–335, doi: 10.3109/07420528.2012.655868; S. Kenney et al., "Global Sleep Quality as a Moderator of Alcohol Consumption and Consequences in College Students," *Addictive Behaviors* 37 (2012): 507–512, doi: 10.1016/j.addbeh.2012.01.006.

14. R. Hingson et al., "Magnitude of Alcohol-Related Mortality and Morbidity among U.S. College Students Ages 18–24: Changes from 1998 to 2005," *Journal of Studies on Alcohol and Drugs* (2009): 12–20.

15. Ibid.

16. S. Wells, K. Graham, and J. Purcell, "Policy Implications of the Widespread Practice of 'Pre-drinking' or 'Pre-gaming' before Going to Public Drinking Establishments—Are Current Prevention Strategies Backfiring?" *Addiction* 104, no 1 (2008): 4–9, doi: 10.1111/j.1360-0443.2008.02393.x; L.D. Johnston et al., "Monitoring the Future national Survey Results on Drug Use, 1975–2011: Volume II, College Students and Adults Ages 19–50," 2012, www.monitoringthefuture.org

17. N. R. Ahern et al., "Youth in Mind: Drinking Games and College Students," *Journal of Psychosocial Nursing and Mental Health Services* 48, no. 2 (2010): 17–20, doi: 10.3928/02793695-20100108-03.

18. J. M. Cameron et al., "Drinking Game Participation among Undergraduate Students Attending National Alcohol Screening Day," *Journal of American College Health* 58, no. 5 (2010): 499–506, doi: 10.1080/07448481003599096.

19. R. Hingson et al., "Magnitude of Alcohol-Related Mortality and Morbidity among U.S. College Students Ages 18–24: Changes from 1998 to 2005," 2009.

20. A. Barry et al., "Drunkorexia: Understanding the Co-occurrence of Alcohol Consumption and Eating/Exercise Weight Management Behaviors," *Journal of American College Health Association* 60, no. 3 (2012): 236–243, doi: 10.1080/07448481.2011.587487.

21. S. Burke et al., "Drunkorexia: Calorie Restriction Prior to Alcohol Consumption among College Freshmen," *Journal of Alcohol Drug Education* 54 (2010): 17–34.

22. S. Giles et al., "Calorie Restriction on Drinking Days: An Examination of Drinking Consequences among College Students," *Journal of American College Health* 57, no. 6 (2009): 603–610, doi: 10.3200/JACH.57.6.603-610.

23. G. DiFulvio et al., "Effectiveness of the Brief Alcohol and Screening Intervention for College Students (BASICS) Program for Mandated Students," *Journal of American College Health* 60, no. 4 (2012): 269–280, doi: 10.1080/07448481.2011.599352.

24. D.J. Rohsenow et al., "Hangover Sensitivity after Controlled Alcohol Administration as Predictor of Post-College Drinking," *Journal of Abnormal Psychology* 121, no. 1 (2012): 270–275, doi: 10.1037/a0024706.

25. K. Jackson et al., "Role of Tobacco Smoking in Hangover Symptoms among University Students," *Journal of Studies on Alcohol and Drugs* 74 (2013): 41–49.

26. M. A. White et al., "Hospitalizations for Alcohol and Drug Overdoses in Young Adults Ages 18–24 in the United States, 1999–2008: Results from the Nationwide Inpatient Sample," *Journal of Studies on Alcohol and Drugs* 72, no. 5 (2011): 774–876.

27. National Institute on Alcohol Abuse and Alcoholism, "Drinking Can Put a Chill on Your Summer Fun," 2012, http://pubs.niaaa.nih.gov; Centers for Disease Control and Prevention, "Unintentional Drowning: Get the Facts," November 2012, www.cdc.gov

28. Centers for Disease Control and Prevention, "Injury Prevention and Control: Home and Recreational Safety: Fire Deaths and Injuries: Fact Sheet," October 2011, www.cdc.gov

29. U.S. Department of Health and Human Services (HHS) Office of the Surgeon General and National Action Alliance for Suicide Prevention, "2012 National Strategy for Suicide Prevention: Goals and Objectives for Action," September 2012, http://www.surgeongeneral.gov

30. K. Davis, "College Women's Sexual Decision Making: Cognitive Mediation of Alcohol Expectancy Results," *American Journal of College Health* 58, no. 5 (2010): 481–490, doi: 10.1080/07448481003599112.

31. S. Lawyer et al., "Forcible, Drug-Facilitated, and Incapacitate Rape and Sexual Assault among Undergraduate Women," *Journal of American College Health* 58, no. 5 (2010): 453–460, doi: 10.1080/07448480903540515.

32. C. Stappenbeck, "A Longitudinal Investigation of Heavy Drinking and Physical Dating Violence in Men and Women," *Addictive Behaviors* 35, no. 5 (2010): 479–485, doi: 10.1016/j.addbeh.2009.12.027.

33. S. J. Nielsen et al., "Calories Consumed from Alcoholic Beverages by U.S. Adults, 2007–2010," *NCHS Data Brief*, no. 110 (2012), Available at www.cdc.gov

34. M. Silveri, "Adolescent Brain Development and Underage Drinking in the United States: Identifying Risks of Alcohol Use in College Populations," *Harvard Review of Psychiatry* 20, no. 4 (2012): 189–200, doi: 10.3109/10673229.2012.714642.

35. Ibid.

36. L. Arriola et al., "Alcohol Intake and the Risk of Coronary Heart Disease in Spanish EPIC Cohort Study," *Heart* 96, no. 10 (2010): 124–130, doi:10.1136/hrt.2009.173419; T. Wilson et al., "Should Moderate Alcohol Consumption Be Promoted?" *Nutrition and Health: Nutrition Guide for Physicians* (2010): 107–114, doi: 10.1007/978-1-60327-431-9_9; The American Heart Association, "Alcohol and Cardiovascular Disease," 2011, www.heart.org

37. Ibid.

38. The American Heart Association, "Alcohol and Cardiovascular Disease," 2011, www.heart.org

39. H. K. Seitz and P. Becker, "Alcohol Metabolism and Cancer Risk," *NIAAA Publications* 30, no. 1 (2007): 38–47, Available at http://pubs.niaaa.nih.gov

40. W. Y. Chen et al., "Moderate Alcohol Consumption during Adult Life, Drinking Patterns, and Breast Cancer Risk," *Journal of the American Medical Association* 306, no. 17 (2011): 1884–1890, doi:10.1001/jama.2011.1590.

41. C. S. Berkey et al., "Prospective Study of Adolescent Alcohol Consumption and Risk of Benign Breast Disease in Young Women," *Pediatrics* 125, no. 5 (2010): e1081–1087, doi: 10.1542/peds.2009-2347.

42. Centers for Disease Control and Prevention, "Alcohol Use and Binge Drinking Among Women of Childbearing Age-United States, 2006–2010," *Morbidity and Mortality Weekly* 61, no. 28 (2012): 534–538.

43. S. Lewis et al. "Fetal Alcohol Exposure and IQ at Age 8: Evidence from a Population-Based Birth-Cohort Study," *PLOS One* 7, no. 11 (2012): e49407, Available at www.plosone.org

44. Centers for Disease Control and Prevention, "Fetal Alcohol Spectrum Disorders (FASDs) Data and Statistics," May 2010, www.cdc.gov

45. Fetal Alcohol Spectrum Disorders (FASD) Center for Excellence, "What Is FASD?" March 2013, www.fasdcenter.samhsa.gov

46. Centers for Disease Control and Prevention, "Ten Leading Causes of Death by Age Group," October 2012, www.cdc.gov

47. National Highway Traffic Safety Administration, "2010 Motor Vehicle Crashes: Overview," February 2012, www.nhtsa.gov

48. American College Health Association, *National College Health Assessment II: Reference Group Executive Summary Fall 2012*, 2013.

49. National Highway Traffic Safety Administration, "Traffic Safety Facts: 2010 Data Alcohol-Impaired Driving," April 2012, at www.nhtsa.gov

50. Ibid.

51. Insurance Institute for Highway Safety, "Fatality Facts 2010: Alcohol," 2012, www.iihs.org

52. Ibid.

53. Ibid.

54. Medline Plus, "Alcoholism and Alcohol Abuse," March 2011, www.nlm.nih.gov

55. Center of Behavioral Health Statistics and Quality, "Nearly Half of College Student Treatment Admissions Were for Primary Alcohol Abuse," *Data Spotlight* (2012), www.samhsa.gov

56. A. Arria, "College Student Success: The Impact of Health Concerns and Substance Abuse," Lecture presented at NASPA Alcohol and Mental Health Conference (Fort Worth, TX: January 19, 2013).

57. National Institute on Alcohol Abuse and Alcoholism, "A Family History of Alcoholism: Are You at Risk?," 2007, http://pubs.niaaa.nih.gov

58. A. Levin, "Determining Alcoholism Proves Complicated Endeavor," *Psychiatric News* 47, no. 24 (2012): 20, doi: 10.1176/appi.pn.2012.12b13.

59. D. Stacey, "RASGRF2 Regulates Alcohol-Induced Reinforcement by Influencing Mesolimbic Dopamine Neuron Activity and Dopamine Release," *Proceedings of the National Academy of Sciences* 109, no. 51 (2012): 21128–21133, doi: 10.1073/pnas.1211844110.

60. J. Niels Rosenquist et al., "The Spread of Alcohol Consumption Behavior in a Large Social Network," *Annals of Internal Medicine* 152, no. 7 (2010): 426–433, doi: 10.7326/0003-4819-152-7-201004060-00007.

61. Centers for Disease Control and Prevention, "Fact Sheet: Excessive Alcohol Use and Risks to Women's Health: 2010," October 2012, www.cdc.gov

62. Centers for Disease Control and Prevention, "Excessive Drinking Costs U.S. $233.5 Billion," October 2011, www.cdc.gov

63. Ibid.

64. T. R. Miller et al., "Societal Costs of Underage Drinking," *Journal of Studies on Alcohol* 67, no. 4 (2006): 519–528.

65. Underage Drinking Enforcement Training Center, "Underage Drinking Costs," September 2011, www.udetc.org

66. Substance Abuse and Mental Health Services Administration, "The NSDUH Report—Alcohol Treatment: Need, Utilization, and Barriers," April 2009, www.samhsa.gov

67. Center of Behavioral Health Statistics and Quality, "Nearly Half of College Student Treatment Admissions Were for Primary Alcohol Abuse," 2012.

68. Centers for Disease Control and Prevention, "Adult Cigarette Smoking in the United States: Current Estimate," December 2012, www.cdc.gov

69. Centers for Disease Control and Prevention, "Morbidity and Mortality Weekly Report: Current Cigarette Smoking Among Adults – United States, 2011," November 2012, http://www.cdc.gov

70. Ibid.

71. Campaign for Tobacco-Free Kids, "Tobacco Company Marketing to Kids," March 2012, Available at www.tobaccofreekids.org

72. American Lung Association, "General Smoking Facts," June 2011, www.lung.org

73. Tobacco Free Providence, "Sweet Deceit Survey Results," January 2012, www.tobaccofreeprovidence.org

74. American Cancer Society, "Cancer Facts & Figures 2013," 2013, Available at www.cancer.org

75. American Lung Association, "General Smoking Facts," 2011.

76. Centers for Disease Control and Prevention, "Tobacco Control State Highlights 2010," 2010, Available at www.cdc.gov; Centers for Disease Control and Prevention, "Smoking-Attributable Mortality, Years of Potential Life Lost, and Productivity Losses, 2000–2004," *Morbidity and Mortality Weekly Report* 57, no. 45 (2008): 1226–1228.

77. Campaign for Tobacco-Free Kids, "State Cigarette Excise Tax Rates & Rankings," December 2012, www.tobaccofreekids.org

78. L. D. Johnston et al., "Monitoring the Future National Survey Results on Drug Use, 1975–2011: Volume II, College Students and Adults Ages 19–50," 2012, Available at www.monitoringthefuture.org

79. Ibid.

80. E. Sutfin et al., "Tobacco Use by College Students: A Comparison of Daily and Nondaily Smokers," *American Journal of Health Behavior* 36, no. 2 (2012): 218–229, doi: 10.5993/AJHB.36.2.7.

81. U.S. Department of Health and Human Services, "How Tobacco Smoke Causes Disease: The Biology and Behavioral Basis for Smoking Attributable Disease: A Report of the Surgeon General," 2010, Available at www.ncbi.nlm.nih.gov

82. C. Quintero-Lopez et al., "Probability and Predictors of Transition from First Use to Dependence on Nicotine, Alcohol, Cannabis, and Cocaine: Results of the National Epidemiologic Survey on Alcohol and Related Conditions (NESARC)," *Drug and Alcohol Dependence* 115, no. 1–2, (2011): 120–130, doi: 10.1016/j.drugalcdep.2010.11.004.

83. National Institute on Drug Abuse Research Report Series, "Tobacco Addiction," *NIH Publication no. 12-4342*, 2012, Available at www.drugabuse.gov

84. American Cancer Society, "Cancer Facts & Figures 2013," 2013.

85. K. Sterling et al., "Factors Associated with Small Cigar Use Among College Students," *American Journal of Health Behavior* 37, no. 3 (2013): 325–333.

86. Centers for Disease Control and Prevention, "Smoking and Tobacco Use: Bidis and Kreteks," June 2011, www.cdc.gov

87. Ibid.

88. American Cancer Society, "Questions about Smoking, Tobacco, and Health: What about More Exotic Forms of Smoking Tobacco, Such as Clove Cigarettes, Bidis, and Hookahs?" January 2013, www.cancer.org

89. Centers for Disease Control and Prevention, "Youth and Tobacco Use," Smoking and Tobacco, November 2012, www.cdc.gov

90. Campaign for Tobacco Free Kids, "The Toll of Tobacco Use in the USA," February 2013, Available at www.tobaccofreekids.org

91. American Cancer Society, "Cancer Facts & Figures 2013," 2013.

92. Ibid.

93. Ibid.

94. International Agency for Research on Cancer. "Smokeless tobacco and some tobacco specific n-nitrosamines," *IARC Monographs on the Evaluation of Carcinogenic Risks to Humans* 89, 2007, Available at http://monographs.iarc.fr

95. J. Zhao et al., "Tobacco Smoking and Colorectal Cancer: A Population-Based Case-Control Study in Newfoundland and Labrador," *Canadian Journal of Public Health* 101, no. 4 (2010): 281–289.

96. American Heart Association, "AHA Statistical Update: Heart Disease and Stroke Statistics —2013 Update," *Circulation* 127, (2013): e6-e245, Available at http://circ.ahajournals.org

97. Ibid.

98. Ibid.

99. American Heart Association, "Stroke Risk Factors," October 2012, www.strokeassociation.org; Centers for Disease Control and Prevention, "Health Effects of Cigarette Smoking," January 2012, www.cdc.gov

100. American Cancer Society, "Cancer Facts & Figures, 2013," 2013

101. Johns Hopkins Health Alerts, "Emphysema: Symptoms and Remedies," March 2012, www.johnshopkinshealthalerts.com

102. C. B. Harte et al., "Association between Cigarette Smoking and Erectile Tumescence: The Mediating Role of Heart Rate Variability," *International Journal of Impotence Research* (2013): doi: 10.1038/ijir.2012.43.

103. Centers for Disease Control and Prevention, "Pregnant? Don't Smoke! Learn How and Why to Quit for Good," November 2012, www.cdc.gov

104. Centers for Disease Control and Prevention, "Tobacco Use and Pregnancy," January 2013, www.cdc.gov

105. M. Thun et al., "50-Year Trends in Smoking-Related Mortality in the United States," *The New England Journal of Medicine* 368 (2013): 351–364, doi: 10.1056/NEJMsa1211127.

106. Ibid.

107. American Academy of Periodontology, "Gum Disease Risk Factors," 2013, www.perio.org

108. J. Cataldo et al., "Cigarette Smoking Is a Risk Factor of Alzheimer's Disease: An Analysis Controlling for Tobacco Industry Affiliation," *Journal of Alzheimer's Disease* 19, no. 2 (2010): 465–480, doi: 10.3233/JAD-2010-1240.

109. Centers for Disease Control and Prevention, "Smoking and Tobacco Use Facts: Secondhand Smoke (SHS) Facts," March 2012, www.cdc.gov

110. Ibid.

111. Ibid.

112. Ibid.

113. Ibid.

114. Centers for Disease Control and Prevention, "2006 Surgeon General's Report—The Health Consequences of Involuntary Exposure to Tobacco Smoke," April 2012, Available at www.cdc.gov

115. Centers for Disease Control and Prevention, "CDC Health Disparities and Inequalities Report–United States, 2011, Supplement: Cigarette Smoking—United States, 1965–2008," *Morbidity and Mortality Weekly Report* 60, Supplement (2011): 109–113.

116. Tobacco-Free Kids, "1998 Tobacco Settlement: Decade of Broken Promises," 2011, www.tobaccofreekids.org

117. 111th Congress of the United States of America, *Family Smoking Prevention and Tobacco Control Act of 2009*, HR 1256, www.govtrack.us

118. Centers for Disease Control and Prevention, "Tobacco Use: Smoking Cessation," November 2011, www.cdc.gov

119. P. Jha et al., "21st Century Hazards of Smoking and Benefits of Cessation in the United States," *The New England Journal of Medicine* 368 (2013): 341–350, doi: 10.1056/NEJMsa1211128.

120. American Cancer Society, "Guide to Quitting Smoking," July 2010, Available at www.cancer.org

121. Everyday Health, "A Guide to Using the Nicotine Patch," May 2011, www.everydayhealth.com

122. U.S. Food and Drug Administration, "Public Health Advisory: FDA Requires New Boxed Warnings for the Smoking Cessation Drugs Chantix and Zyban," July 2009, http://www.fda.gov

123. American Lung Association, "Benefits of Quitting," March 2012, www.lungusa.org

124. K. Pirie et al., "The 21st Century Hazards of Smoking and Benefits of Stopping: A Prospective Study of One Million Women in the UK," *The Lancet* 81, no. 9861 (2013): 133–141, doi: 10.1016/S0140-6736(12)61720-6.

125. Campaign for Tobacco-Free Kids, "State Cigarette Excise Tax Rates & Rankings," December 2012, www.tobaccofreekids.org

Pulled statistics:

page 228, National Institute on Alcohol Abuse and Alcoholism, "Drinking Statistics," 2012, www.niaaa.nih.gov

page 238, California Department of Alcohol and Drug Programs, "Frequently Asked Questions: General," 2012, www.adp.ca.gov

Chapter 9: Eating for a Healthier You

1. L. L. Wilkinson et al., "Attachment Anxiety, Disinhibited Eating and Body Mass Index in Adulthood," *Appetite* 57, no. 2 (2011): 543.

2. U. S. Department of Agriculture, "Part D: Section 6: Sodium, Potassium, and Water," *Report of the Dietary Guidelines Advisory Committee on the Dietary Guidelines for Americans, 2010* (Washington, DC: U.S. Department of Agriculture, Agricultural Research Service, 2010), Available at www.cnpp.usda.gov; E. Jéquier and F. Constant, "Water as an Essential Nutrient: The Physiological Basis of Hydration," *European Journal of Clinical Nutrition* 64, no. 2 (2010): 115–123.

3. U. S. Department of Agriculture, "Part D: Section 6: Sodium, Potassium, and Water," 2010.

4. Institute of Medicine of the National Academies, Food and Nutrition Board, *Dietary References for Water, Potassium, Sodium, Chloride, and Sulfate* (Washington, DC: The National Academies Press, 2005), Available at www.nal.usda.gov

5. American College of Sports Medicine, "American College of Sports Medicine Position Stand: Exercise and Fluid Replacement," *Medicine and Science in Sports and Exercise* 39, no. 2 (2007): 377–390, doi: 10.1249/mss.0b013e31802ca597.

6. U. S. Department of Agriculture, Agricultural Research Service, Beltsville Human Nutrition Research Center, Food Surveys Research Group and Centers for Disease Control and Prevention, National Center for Health Statistics, *What We Eat in America, NHANES 2009–2010,* Data: Table 1. "Nutrient Intakes from Food: Mean Amounts Consumed per Individual by Gender and Age, in the United States, 2009–2010," www.ars.usda.gov

7. Institute of Medicine of the National Academies, "Dietary, Functional, and Total Fiber," in *Dietary Reference Intakes for Energy, Carbohydrate, Fiber, Fat, Fatty Acids, Cholesterol, Protein, and Amino Acids* (Washington, DC: The National Academies Press, 2005), 339–421. Available at www.nap.edu

8. Ibid.

9. L. Gillingham, S. Harris-Janz, and P. Jones, "Dietary Monounsaturated Fatty Acids Are Protective against Metabolic Syndrome and Cardiovascular Disease Risk Factors," *Lipids* 46, no. 3 (2011): 209–228, doi: 10.1007/s11745-010-3524-y; N. D. Riediger et al., "A Systemic Review of the Roles of n-3 Fatty Acids in Health and Disease," *Journal of the American Dietetic Association* 109, no. 4 (2009): 668–679, doi: 10.1016/j.jada.2008.12.022; B. McKevith, "Review: Nutritional Aspects of Oilseeds," *Nutrition Bulletin* 30, no. 1 (2005): 13–26, doi: 10.1111/j.1467-3010.2005.00472.x.

10. A. H. Stark, M. A. Crawford, and R. Reifen, "Update on Alpha-Linolenic Acid," *Nutrition Reviews* 66, no. 6 (2008): 326–332, doi: 10.1111/j.1753-4887.2008.00040.x; C. E. Ramsden et al., "Use of Dietary Linoleic Acid for Secondary Prevention of Coronary Heart Disease and Death: Evaluation of Recovered Data from the Sydney Diet Heart Study and Updated Meta-Analysis," *British Medical Journal* 346 (2013): e8707, doi: http://dx.doi.org/10.1136/bmj.e8707.

11. W. Stonehouse et al., "Consumption of Salmon v. Salmon Oil Capsules: Effects on n-3 PUFA and Selenium Status," *British Journal of Nutrition* 106, no. 8 (2011): 1231–1239, doi: http://dx.doi.org/10.1017/S000711451100153X.

12. W. Willet, "Dietary Fats and Coronary Heart Disease," *Journal of Internal Medicine* 272, no. 1 (2012): 13–24, doi: 10.1111/j.1365-2796.2012.02553.x; N. Bendson et al., "Consumption of Industrial and Ruminant Trans Fatty Acids and Risk of CHD: A Systemic Review and Meta-Analysis of Cohort Studies," *European Journal of Clinical Nutrition* 65, no. 7 (2011): 773–783, doi: 10.1038/ejcn.2011.34.

13. F. Sacks et al., "Comparison of Weight-Loss Diets with Different Compositions of Fat, Protein, and Carbohydrates," *New England Journal of Medicine* 360, no. 9 (2009): 859–873, doi: 10.1056/NEJMoa0804748; M. Hession et al., "Systematic Review of Randomized Controlled Trials of Low-carbohydrate vs. Low-fat/Low-calorie Diets in the Management of Obesity and Its Comorbidities," *Obesity Reviews* 10, no. 1 (2008): 36–50, doi: 10.1111/j.1467-789X.2008.00518.x.

14. H. D. Sesso et al., "Multivitamins in the Prevention of Cardiovascular Disease in Men: The Physicians' Health Study II Randomized Controlled Trial," *Journal of the American Medical Association* 308, no 17 (2012): 1751–1760, doi: 10.1001/jama.2012.14805.

15. H. J. Fulan et al., "Retinol, Vitamins A, C, and E and Breast Cancer Risk: A Meta-Analysis and Meta-Regression," *Cancer Causes & Control* 22, no. 10 (2011): 1382–1396, doi: 10.1007/s10552-011-9811-y.

16. N. Mikirova et al., "Effect of High-Dose Intravenous Vitamin C on Inflammation in Cancer Patients," *Journal of Translational Medicine* 10, no. 1 (2011): 189, doi: 10.1186/1479-5876-10-189.

17. E. A. Klein et al., "Vitamin E and the Risk of Prostate Cancer: The Selenium and Vitamin E Cancer Prevention Trial (SELECT)," *Journal of the American Medical Association* 306, no. 14 (2011): 1549–1556, doi: 10.1001/jama.2011.1437.

18. J. Chan and E. Giovannucci, "Vegetables, Fruits, Associated Micronutrients and Risk of Prostate Cancer," *Epidemiology Review* 23, no. 1 (2001): 82–86.

19. H. D. Sesso et al., "Tomato-Based Foods Products Are Related to Clinically Modest Improvements in Selected Coronary Biomarkers in Women," *Journal of Nutrition* 142, no. 2 (2012): 326–333, doi: 10.3945/jn.111.150631.

20. National Institutes of Health, Office of Dietary Supplements, "Dietary Supplement Fact Sheet: Vitamin D," Updated June 2011, http://ods.od.nih.gov

21. C. L. Wagner and F. R. Greer, American Academy of Pediatrics Section on Breastfeeding, American Academy of Pediatrics Committee on Nutrition, "Prevention of Rickets and Vitamin D Deficiency in Infants, Children, and Adolescents," *Pediatrics* 122, no. 5 (2008): 1142–1152, doi: 10.1542/peds.2008-1862.

22. A. Ross et al., eds., Institute of Medicine Committee to Review Dietary Reference Intakes for Vitamin D and Calcium, *Dietary Reference Intakes for Calcium and Vitamin D* (Washington DC: National Academies Press US, 2011), Available at www.iom.edu

23. L. J. Appel and C. A. Anderson, "Compelling Evidence for Public Health Action to Reduce Salt Intake," *New England Journal of Medicine* 362, no. 7 (2010): 650–652, doi: 10.1056/NEJMe0910352.

24. U. S. Department of Agriculture, "What We Eat in America, NHANES 2009–2010 Data: Table 1," 2010, www.ars.usda.gov; C. Ayala et al., "Application of Lower Sodium Intake Recommendations to Adults—United States, 1999–2006," *Morbidity and Mortality Weekly* 58, no. 11 (2009): 281–283.

25. Q. Yang et al., "Sodium and Potassium Intake and Mortality among US Adults: Prospective Data from the Third National Health and Nutrition Examination Survey," *Archives of Internal Medicine* 171, no. 13 (2011): 1183–1191, doi: 10.1001/archinternmed.2011.257.

26. R. L. Bailey et al., "Estimation of Total Usual Calcium and Vitamin D Intakes in the United States," *Journal of Nutrition* 140, no. 4 (2010): 817–822, doi: 10.3945/jn.109.118539.

27. S. A. McNaughton et al., "An Energy-Dense, Nutrient-Poor Dietary Pattern Is Inversely Associated with Bone Health in Women," *Journal of Nutrition* 141, no. 8 (2011): 1516–1523, doi: 10.3945/jn.111.138271.

28. World Health Organization, "Micronutrient Deficiencies: Iron Deficiency Anemia," 2013, www.who.int

29. Centers for Disease Control and Prevention, "Iron and Iron Deficiency," Nutrition for Everyone, Updated February 23, 2011, www.cdc.gov

30. C. Geissler and M. Singh. "Iron, Meat, and Health," *Nutrients* 3, no. 3 (2011): 283–316, doi: 10.3390/nu3030283.

31. U. S. Department of Agriculture, Economic Research Service, "Loss-Adjusted Food

Availability Documentation: Overview: Calories," November 2, 2012, www.ers.usda.gov

32. D. Grotto and E. Zied, "The Standard American Diet and Its Relationship to the Health Status of Americans," *Nutrition in Clinical Practice* 25, no. 6 (2010): 603–612, doi: 10.1177/0884533610386234.

33. U. S. Department of Agriculture and U. S. Department of Health and Human Services, *Dietary Guidelines for Americans, 2010,* 7th ed. (Washington, DC: U.S. Government Printing Office, December, 2010), Available at www.cnpp.usda.gov

34. U. S. Department of Agriculture, "Empty Calories: How Do I Count the Empty Calories I Eat?" Updated June 4, 2011, www.choosemyplate.gov

35. U. S. Food and Drug Administration, "Labeling & Nutrition Food Labeling and Nutrition Overview," Updated November 2012, www.fda.gov

36. The Vegetarian Resource Group, "How Often Do Americans Eat Vegetarian Meals? And How Many Adults in the U.S. Are Vegetarian?" Vegetarian Resource Group Blog, May 18, 2012, www.vrg.org

37. Vegetarian Times, "Vegetarian Times Study Shows 7.3 Million Americans Are Vegetarians," Press Release, April 15, 2008, www.vegetariantimes.com

38. American Dietetic Association, "Position of the American Dietetic Association: Vegetarian Diets," *Journal of the American Dietetic Association* 109, no. 7 (2009): 1266–1282, www.eatright.org

39. National Institutes of Health Office of Dietary Supplements, "Frequently Asked Questions," Reviewed June 6, 2011, http://ods.od.nih.gov

40. A. L. Rogovik, S. Vohra, and R. D. Goldman, "Safety Considerations and Potential Interactions of Vitamins: Should Vitamins Be Considered Drugs?" *Annals of Pharmacotherapy* 44, no. 2 (2010): 311–324, doi: 10.1345/aph.1M238.

41. Academy of Nutrition and Dietetics, "Dietary Supplements," It's About Eating Right, Last reviewed January 2013, www.eatright.org

42. The Organic Trade Organization, "Consumer-Driven U.S. Organic Market Surpasses $31 Billion in 2011," 2012, www.organicnewsroom.com

43. A. D. Dangour et al., "Nutrition-Related Health Effects of Organic Foods: A Systematic Review," *American Journal of Clinical Nutrition* 92, no.1 (2010): 203–210, doi: 10.3945/ajcn.2010.29269.

44. U.S. Department of Agriculture, *Pesticide Data Program: Annual Summary, Calendar Year 2011,* (Washington, DC: Agricultural Marketing Service, February 2013), Available at www.ams.usda.gov

45. U.S. Department of Health and Human Services, "Food Safety Modernization Act (FSMA)," 2011, www.fda.gov

46. Centers for Disease Control and Prevention, "Estimates of Food-Borne Illnesses in the United States," Updated February 6, 2013, www.cdc.gov

47. Centers for Disease Control and Prevention, "Improvements in 2011 Estimates," Updated April 21, 2011, www.cdc.gov

48. R. Johnson, "The U.S. Trade Situation for Fruit and Vegetable Products," Congressional Research Service, January 2012, www.crs.gov

49. S. Clark et al., "Frequency of US Emergency Department Visits for Food-Related Acute Allergic Reactions," *Journal of Allergy Clinical Immunology* 127, no. 3 (2011): 682–683, doi: 10.1016/j.jaci.2010.10.040.

50. R. S. Gupta et al., "The Prevalence, Severity, and Distribution of Childhood Food Allergy in the United States," *Journal of Pediatrics* 128, no. 1 (2011): e9–e17, doi: 10.1542/peds.2011-0204.

51. U. S. Food and Drug Administration, "Food Allergies: What You Need to Know," Updated April 2013, www.fda.gov

52. M. Hahn and M. McKnight, "Answers to Frequently Asked Questions about FALCPA," Food Allergy Research and Education, 2010, www.foodallergy.org

53. University of Chicago Celiac Disease Center, "Celiac Disease Facts and Figures," 2010, www.cureceliacdisease.org

54. A. Ranciaro and S. A. Tishkoff, "Population Genetics: Evolutionary History of Lactose Intolerance in Africa," NIH Consensus Development Conference: Lactose Intolerance and Health, February 2010, http://consensus.nih.gov

55. U. S. Department of Agriculture, Economic Research Service, "Adoption of Genetically Engineered Crops in the U.S.," Updated July 2012, www.ers.usda.gov

56. Center for Food Safety, "Food Safety Fact Sheet," April 2013, www.centerforfoodsafety.org

57. A. Coghlan, "Engineered Maize Toxicity Claims Roundly Rebuffed," *New Scientist* 2744, January 22, 2010.

58. R. E. Goodman et al., "Allergenicity Assessment of Genetically Modified Crops—What Makes Sense?," *Nature Biotechnology* 26, no. 1 (2008): 73–81, doi: 10.1038/nbt1343.

59. World Health Organization, "20 Questions on Genetically Modified Foods," www.who.int

Pulled statistics:

page 264, C. Ogden et al., "Consumption of Sugar Drinks in the United States, 2005–2008," NCHS data brief, no. 71 (Hyattsville, MD: National Center for Health Statistics, 2011), Available at www.cdc.gov

page 281, K. Heidal et al., "Cost and Calorie Analysis of Fast Food Consumption in College Students," *Food and Nutrition Sciences* 3, no. 7 (2012): 942–946. doi:10.4236/fns.2012.37124.

Chapter 10: Reaching and Maintaining a Healthy Weight

1. C. L. Ogden et al., "Prevalence of Obesity in the United States, 2009-2010," *NCHS Data Brief*, no. 82 (2012): 1–7.

2. U.S. Department of Health and Human Services, "The Surgeon General's Vision for a Healthy and Fit Nation," January 2010, www.surgeongeneral.gov

3. K. M. Flegal et al., "Prevalence of Obesity and Trends in the Distribution of Body Mass Index among U.S. Adults, 1999–2010," *Journal of the American Medical Association* 307, no. 5 (2012), doi: 10.1001/jama.2012.39.

4. Ibid.

5. Ibid.

6. A. Go et al., "Heart Disease and Stroke Statistics, 2013. Update—A Report from the American Heart Association," *Circulation* (2013): doi: 10.1161/CIR.0b013e31828124ad. (Epub ahead of print.)

7. Ibid.

8. American Diabetes Association, "Diabetes Statistics," January 2011, www.diabetes.org

9. American Diabetes Association, "Diabetes Statistics: Cost of Diabetes," March 6, 2013, www.diabetes.org

10. Ibid.

11. C. L. Himes and S. L. Reynolds, "Effect of Obesity on Falls, Injury, and Disability" *Journal of the American Geriatrics Society* 60, no. 1 (2012): 124–129; K. Froehlich-Grobe and D. Lollar, "Obesity and Disability: Time to Act," *American Journal of Preventive Medicine* 41, no. 5 (2011): 541–545; L. A. Schaap, A. Koster, and M. Visser, "Adiposity, Muscle Mass, and Muscle Strength in Relation to Functional Decline in Older Persons," *Epidemiologic Reviews* 35, no. 1 (2013): 51–65, doi:10.1093/epirev/mxs006.

12. World Health Organization, "Obesity and Overweight Fact Sheet," 2011, www.who.int; International Obesity Taskforce, "Obesity—The Global Epidemic," 2011, www.iaso.org

13. D. Spruijt-Metz, "Etiology, Treatment, and Prevention of Obesity in Childhood and Adolescence: A Decade in Review," *Journal of Research on Adolescence* 21 (2011): 129–152, doi: 10.1111/j.1532–7795.2010.00719.x; S.A. Affenito et al., "Behavioral Determinants of Obesity: Research Findings and Policy Implications," *Journal of Obesity* 2012 (2012), Available at www.hindawi.com

14. Ibid.

15. D. Cummings and M. Schwartz, "Genetics and Pathophysiology of Human Obesity," *Annual Review of Medicine* 54 (2003): 453–471.

16. K. Silventoinen et al., "The Genetic and Environmental Influences on Childhood Obesity: A Systematic Review of Twin and Adoption Studies," *International Journal of Obesity* 34, no. 1 (2010): 29–40.

17. S. Li et al., "Cumulative and Predictive Value of Common Obesity—Susceptibility Variants Identified by Genome-wide Association Studies," *American Journal of Clinical Nutrition* 91, no. 1 (2010): 184–190; J. M. McCaffery et al., "Obesity Susceptibility Loci and Dietary Intake in the Look AHEAD Trial," *American Journal of Clinical Nutrition* 95, no. 6 (2012):1477, doi: 10.3945/ajcn. 111.026955.

18. J. M. McCaffery et al., "Obesity Susceptibility Loci and Dietary Intake," 2012.

19. C. Bouchard, "Defining the Genetic Architecture of the Predisposition to Obesity: A Challenging but Not Insurmountable Task," *American Journal of Clinical Nutrition* 91, no. 1 (2010): 5–6; T. O. Kilpelainen et al., "Physical Activity Attenuates the Influence of FTO Variants on Obesity Risk: A Meta-Analysis of 218,166 Adults and 19,268 Children," *PLoS Medicine* 8, no.11 (2012): e1001116, doi:10.1371/journal.pmed.1001116; S. Li et al., "Cumulative Effects and Predictive Value of Common Obesity-Susceptibility Variants," 2010; B. Herera and C. Lindgren, "The Genetics of Obesity," *Current Diabetes Report* 10, no. 6 (2010): 498–505.

20. J. C. Wells. "The Evolution of Human Adiposity and Obesity: Where did it All Go Wrong?" *Disease Models and Mechanisms* 5, no. 5 (2012): 595–607, doi:10-1242/dmm.009613; J. R. Speakman et al., "Set Points, Settling Points and Some Alternative Models: Theoretical Options to Understand How Genes and Environments Combine to Regulate Body Adiposity," *Disease*

Models and Mechanisms 4, no. 6 (2011): 733–745, Available at http://intl-dmm.biologists.org

21. U. Baig et al., "Can Thrifty Gene(s) or Predictive Fetal Programming for Thriftiness Lead to Obesity?" *Journal of Obesity* 2011 (2011), doi: 10.1155/2011/861049; J. Wells, "The Thrifty Phenotype: An Adaptation in Growth or Metabolism?" *American Journal of Human Biology* 23, no. 1 (2011): 65–75.

22. B. Biondi, "Thyroid and Obesity: An Intriguing Relationship," *Journal of Clinical Endocrinology and Metabolism* 95, no. 8 (2010): 3614–3617; T. Reinehr, "Obesity and Thyroid Function," *Molecular and Cellular Endocrinology* 316, no. 2 (2010): 165–171.

23. M. Rotondi, F. Magri, and L. Chiovato, "Thyroid and Obesity: Not a One Way Interaction," *The Journal of Clinical Endocrinology and Metabolism* 96, no. 2 (2011): 344–356.

24. D. E. Cummings et al., "Plasma Ghrelin Levels after Diet-Induced Weight Loss or Gastric Bypass Surgery," *New England Journal of Medicine* 346, no. 21 (2002): 1623–1630.

25. C. DeVriese et al., "Focus on the Short- and Long-Term Effects of Ghrelin on Energy Homeostasis," *Nutrition* 26, no. 6 (2010): 579–584; T. Castaneda et al., "Ghrelin in the Regulation of Body Weight and Metabolism," *Frontiers in Neuroendocrinology* 31, no. 1 (2010): 44–60.

26. P. Marzullo et al., "Investigations of Thyroid Hormones and Antibodies in Obesity: Leptin Levels Are Associated with Thyroid Autoimmunity Independent of Bioanthropometric, Hormonal and Weight-Related Determinants," *The Journal of Clinical Endocrinology and Metabolism* 95, no. 8 (2010): 3965–3972; Y. Friedlander et al., "Leptin, Insulin, and Obesity-Related Phenotypes: Genetic Influences on Levels and Longitudinal Changes," *Obesity* 17, no. 7 (2009): 1458–1460.

27. L. K. Mahan and S. Escott-Stump, *Krause's Food, Nutrition, and Diet Therapy*, 13th ed. (New York: W. B. Saunders, 2012).

28. W. Dietz et al., "Despite Obesity Rise, U.S. Calories Trending Downward," *American Journal of Clinical Nutrition*, March 6, 2013, Available at www.nlm.nih.gov

29. Centers for Disease Control and Prevention, "Overweight and Obesity—A Growing Problem," April 2012, www.cdc.gov; Centers for Disease Control and Prevention, "Overweight and Obesity: Facts about Physical Activity," January 2013, www.cdc.gov

30. L. Poston, L. F. Harthoorn, and E. M. Van Der Beek, "Obesity in Pregnancy: Implications for the Mother and Lifelong Health of the Child—A Consensus Statement," *Pediatric Research* 69, no. 2 (2011): 175–180; K. L. Connor et al., "Nature, Nurture or Nutrition? Impact of Maternal Nutrition on Maternal Care, Offspring Development and Reproductive Function," *Journal of Physiology* 590, no. 9 (2012): 2167–2180.

31. M. A. Schuster et al., "Racial and Ethnic Health Disparities among Fifth-Graders in Three Cities," *The New England Journal of Medicine* 367, no. 8 (2012): 735–745; C. L. Odgen et al., "Prevalence of Obesity and Trends in Body Mass Index among U.S. Children and Adolescents. 1999–2010." *Journal of the American Medical Association* 307 (2012): 483–490.

32. R. M. Puhl and K. M. King, "Weight Discrimination and Bullying: A Review," *Best Practices and Research Clinical Endocrinology and Metabolism,* January 2013, http://dx.doi.org/10.1016/j.beem.2012.12.002 (Epub ahead of print.); M. H. Schafer and K. F. Ferraro, "The Stigma of Obesity: Does Perceived Weight Discrimination Affect Identity and Physical Health?" *Social Psychology Quarterly* 74 (2011): 76–97, doi: 10.1177/0190272511398197.

33. C. Gillespie et al., "The Growing Concern of Poverty in the United States: An Exploration of Food Prices and Poverty on Obesity Rates for Low-income Citizens," *Undergraduate Economic Review* 8, no. 1 (2012): 1–38.

34. J. F. Sallis et al., "Role of Built Environments in Physical Activity, Obesity and Cardiovascular Disease," *Circulation* 125, no. 5 (2012): 729–737.

35. A. Go et al., "Heart Disease and Stroke Statistics, 2013 Update," 2013.

36. Centers for Disease Control and Prevention, "Prevalence of Underweight among Adults Aged 20 and Over: United States, 1960–1962 through 2007–2010," September 2012, www.cdc.gov; Centers for Disease Control and Prevention, "Prevalence of Underweight among Children and Adolescents Aged 2–19 Years: United States, 1963–1965 through 2007–2012," September 2012, www.cdc.gov

37. Centers for Disease Control and Prevention, "About BMI for Adults," March 2013, www.cdc.gov

38. Centers for Disease Control and Prevention, "Defining Overweight and Obesity," April 2012, www.cdc.gov

39. K. M. Flegal et al., "Prevalence and Trends in Obesity among U.S. Adults, 1999–2010," *Journal of the American Medical Association* 307, no. 5 (2012): 491–497.

40. Centers for Disease Control and Prevention, "Defining Overweight and Obesity," 2012.

41. American Heart Association, "Body Composition Tests," May 2010, www.heart.org; S. J. Mooney, A. Baecker, and A. G. Rundel, "Comparison of Anthropometric and Body Composition Measures as Predictors of Components of the Metabolic Syndrome in the Clinical Setting," *Obesity Research and Clinical Practice* 7, no. 1 (2013): e55–e66.

42. Centers for Disease Control and Prevention, "Data and Statistics," 2012, www.cdc.gov

43. R. Puhl, "Weight Stigmatization toward Youth: A Significant Problem in Need of Societal Solutions," *Childhood Obesity* 7, no. 5 (2011): 359–363; R. Puhl and C. Heuer, "Obesity Stigma: Important Considerations for Public Health," *American Journal of Public Health* 100, no. 6 (2010): 1019–1028.

44. J. Kizer et al., "Measures of Adiposity and Future Risk of Ischemic Stroke and Coronary Heart Disease in Older Men and Women," *American Journal of Epidemiology* 173, no. 1 (2010): 10–25; A. Taylor, S. Ebrahim, and Y. Ben-Shlomo, "Comparison of the Associations of Body Mass Index and Measures of Central Adiposity and Fat Mass with Coronary Heart Disease, Diabetes, and All-Cause Mortality: A Study Using Data from 4 UK Cohorts," *American Journal of Clinical Nutrition* 91, no. 3 (2010): 547–556, doi: 10.3945/ajcn.2009.28757.

45. National Heart, Lung, and Blood Institute, "Classification of Overweight and Obesity by BMI, Waist Circumference and Associated Disease Risks," 2012, www.nhlbi.nih.gov

46. University of Maryland Medical Center, "Waist to Hip Ratio Calculator," www.healthcalculators.org

47. L. Gray et al., "A Systematic Review and Mixed Treatment Comparison of Pharmacological Interventions for the Treatment of Obesity," *Obesity Reviews* 13, no. 6 (2012): 483–498.

48. U.S. Food and Drug Administration, "Fen-Phen Safety Update Information," July 2012, www.fda.gov

49. Mayo Clinic, "Gastric Bypass Surgery," October 2011, www.mayoclinic.com

50. F. Rubino et al., "Metabolic Surgery to Treat Type 2 Diabetes: Clinical Outcomes and Mechanisms of Action," *Annual Review of Medicine* 61 (2010): 393–411; E. Karra et al., "Mechanisms Facilitating Weight Loss and Resolution of Type 2 Diabetes Following Bariatric Surgery," *Trends in Endocrinology and Metabolism* 21, no. 6 (2010): 227–344; C. Mottin et al., "Behavior of Type 2 Diabetes Mellitus in Morbid Obese Patients Submitted to Gastric Bypass," *Obesity Surgery* 18, no. 2 (2008): 179–182.

Pulled statistics:

page 295, C. D. Fryar and R. B. Ervin, "Caloric Intake From Fast Food Among Adults: United States, 2007–2010," *NCHS Data Brief* no. 114 (2013), www.cdc.gov

page 304, ABC News, "100 Million Dieters, $20 Billion: The Weight Loss Industry By the Numbers," May 2012, http://abcnews.go.com

Focus On: Enhancing Your Body Image

1. University of the West of England, "30% of Women Would Trade at Least One Year of Their Life to Achieve Their Ideal Body Weight and Shape," Press Release, March 31, 2011, info.uwe.ac.uk

2. M. Bucchianeri et al., "Body Dissatisfaction from Adolescence to Young Adulthood: Findings from a 10-year Longitudinal Study," *Body Image* 10, no. 1 (2013): 1–7.

3. National Institute of Diabetes and Digestive and Kidney Diseases, Weight Control Information Network, "Overweight and Obesity Statistics," 2012, win.niddk.nih.gov

4. V. Swami et al., "The Attractive Female Body Weight and Female Body Dissatisfaction in 26 Countries across 10 World Regions: Results of the International Body Project I," *Personality and Social Psychology Bulletin* 36, no. 3 (2010): 309–325.

5. Ibid.

6. Mayo Clinic Staff, "Body Dysmorphic Disorder," November 2010, www.mayoclinic.com

7. J. D. Feusner et al., "Abnormalities of Object Visual Processing in Body Dysmorphic Disorder," *Psychological Medicine* 41, no. 11 (2011): 2385–2397, doi: 10.1017/S0033291711000572.

8. K. Kater, *Healthy Bodies: Teaching Kids What They Need to Know* (St. Paul, MN: BodyImageHealth, 2012), Available at http://bodyimagehealth.org

9. I. Ahmed, L. Genen, and T. Cook, "Psychiatric Manifestations of Body Dysmorphic Disorder," *Medscape*, February 11, 2011, http://emedicine.medscape.com

10. Mayo Clinic Staff, "Body Dysmorphic Disorder," 2010, www.mayoclinic.com; "Body Dysmorphic Disorder," October 2010, http://kidshealth.org

11. I. Ahmed, L. Genen, and T. Cook, "Psychiatric Manifestations of Body Dysmorphic Disorder," 2011.

12. O. Mülazimoğlu-Balli, C. Koka, and F. H. Asci, "An Examination of Social Physique Anxiety with Regard to Sex and Level of Sport Involvement," *Journal of Human Kinetics* 26, (2010): 115–122; S. R. Bratrud et al., "Social Physique Anxiety, Physical Self-Perceptions and Eating Disorder Risk: A Two-Sample Study," *Pamukkale Journal of Sport Sciences* 1, no. 3 (2010): 1–10.

13. F. Smink, D. van Hoeken, and H. Hoek, "Epidemiology of Eating Disorders: Incidence, Prevalence and Mortality Rates," *Current Psychiatry Reports* 14, no. 4 (2012): 406–414, doi: 10.1007/s11920-012-0282-y, Available at www.ncbi.nlm.nih.gov

14. Danielle A. Gagne et al., "Eating Disorder Symptoms and Weight and Shape Concerns in a Large Web-based Convenience Sample of Women Ages 50 and Above: Results of the Gender and Body Image (GABI) Study," *International Journal of Eating Disorders* 45, no. 7 (2012): 832–844, doi: 10.1002/eat.22030.

15. American College Health Association, *American College Health Association-National College Health Assessment II: Reference Group Executive Summary Fall 2012* (Hanover, MD: American College Health Association, 2013), www.acha-ncha.org

16. L. M. Gottschlich, "Female Athlete Triad," *Medscape Reference, Drugs, Diseases & Procedures,* January 25, 2012, http://emedicine.medscape.com

17. The Alliance for Eating Disorders Awareness, "What Are Eating Disorders?" 2013, www.allianceforeatingdisorders.com

18. T. Wade and M. Tiggemann, "The Role of Perfectionism in Body Dissatisfaction," *Journal of Eating Disorders* 1, no. 2 (2013): e1–e6, doi: 10.1186/2050-2974-1-2.

19. S. A. Swanson, S. J. Crow, D. Le Grange et al., "Prevalence and Correlates of Eating Disorders in Adolescents: Results from the National Comorbidity Survey Replication Adolescent Supplement," *Archives of General Psychiatry,* March 7, 2011, doi: 10.1001/archgenpsychiatry. 2011.22.

20. American Psychiatric Association, *Diagnostic and Statistical Manual of Mental Disorders,* 5th Edition (Washington, DC: 2013).

21. National Eating Disorders Association, "Anorexia Nervosa," www.nationaleatingdisorders.org

22. A.D.A.M. Medical Encyclopedia, U.S. National Library of Medicine, "Anorexia Nervosa," February 13, 2012, www.ncbi.nlm.nih.gov; B. Suchan et al., "Reduced Connectivity Between the Left Fusiform Body Area and the Extrastriate Body Area in Anorexia Nervosa Is Associated with Body Image Distortion," *Behavioural Brain Research* 241 (2013): 80–85, doi: 10.1016/j.bbr.2012.12.002; G. Frank et al., "Anorexia Nervosa and Obesity Are Associated with Opposite Brain Reward Response," *Neuropsychopharmacology* 37, no. 9 (2012): 2031–2046, doi: 10.1038/npp.2012.51.

23. R. Kessler et al., "The Prevalence and Correlates of Binge Eating Disorder in the World Health Organization World Mental Health Surveys," *Biological Psychiatry* (2013), doi: 10.1016/j.biopsych.2012.11.020 (Epub ahead of print.).

24. American Psychiatric Association, *Diagnostic and Statistical Manual of Mental Disorders,* 5th Edition (Washington, DC: 2013).

25. National Institute of Mental Health, "Eating Disorders," January 3, 2013, www.ncbi.nlm.nih.gov

26. Mayo Clinic, Mayo Foundation for Medical Education and Research, "Binge-Eating Disorder," (2012), www.mayoclinic.com

27. R. Kessler et al., "The Prevalence and Correlates of Binge Eating Disorder," 2013.

28. Castlewood Treatment Center for Eating Disorders, "Binge Eating Disorder DSM-V," Blog, January 2012, www.castlewoodtc.com

29. K. N. Franco, Cleveland Clinic Center for Continuing Education, "Eating Disorders," 2011; Mirasol Eating Disorder Recovery Centers, "Eating Disorder Questions and Answers," 2012, www.mirasol.net

30. M. Smith, L. Robinson, and J. Segal, "Helping Someone with an Eating Disorder," Helpguide.org, November 2012, www.helpguide.org; C. Biggs, "On the Outside: Helping a Friend through an Eating Disorder," Act: Every Action Counts, Blog, February 28, 2013, http://act.mtv.com

31. H. Goodwin, E. Haycraft, and C. Meyer, "The Relationship between Compulsive Exercise and Emotion Regulation in Adolescents," *British Journal of Health Psychology* 17, no. 4, (2012): 699–710.

32. J. J. Waldron, "When Building Muscle Turns into Muscle Dysmorphia," Association for Applied Sport Psychology, 2012, http://appliedsportpsych.org

33. M. Silverman, "What Is Muscle Dysmorphia?" Massachusetts General Hospital, February 18, 2011, http://mghocd.org; J. J. Waldron, "When Building Muscle Turns into Muscle Dysmorphia," 2012.

34. L. M. Gottschlich, "Female Athlete Triad," *Medscape Reference,* 2012, http://emedicine.medscape.com

Pulled statistics:
page 319, C. Ross, "Why Do Women Hate Their Bodies?" World of Psychology (blog), *Psych Central,* June 2, 2012, http://psychcentral.com

Chapter 11: Improving Your Personal Fitness

1. Centers for Disease Control and Prevention, " Behavioral Risk Factor Surveillance System Prevalence and Trends Data," Updated January 2013, www.cdc.gov

2. C. E. Garber et al., "American College of Sports Medicine Position Stand: Quantity and Quality of Exercise for Developing and Maintaining Cardiorespiratory, Musculoskeletal and Neuromotor Fitness in Apparently Healthy Adults: Guidance for Prescribing Exercise," *Medicine and Science in Sports and Exercise* 33, no. 7 (2011): 1334–1359, doi: 10.1249/MSS.0b013e318213fefb.

3. American College Health Association, *American College Health Association-National College Health Assessment II: Reference Group Executive Summary Fall 2012* (Hanover, MD: American College Health Association, 2013), www.acha-ncha.org

4. P. Kokkinos, H. Sheriff, and R. Kheirbek, "Physical Inactivity and Mortality Risk," *Cardiology Research and Practice,* (2011), doi: 10.4061/2011/924945.

5. D. E. Warburton et al., "Evidence-Informed Physical Activity Guidelines for Canadian Adults," *Canadian Journal of Public Health* 98, Supplement 2 (2007): S16–S68.

6. S. Plowman and D. Smith, *Exercise Physiology for Health, Fitness, and Performance,* 3rd ed. (Philadelphia: Lippincott Williams & Wilkins, 2011).

7. S. Grover et al., "Estimating the Benefits of Patient and Physician Adherence to Cardiovascular Prevention Guidelines: The MyHealthCheckup Survey," *Canadian Journal of Cardiology* 27, no. 2 (2011): 159–166, doi: 10.1016/j.cjca.2011.01.007.

8. American Heart Association, "About Cholesterol," Updated May 1, 2013, www.heart.org

9. A. Mehta, "Management of Cardiovascular Risk Associated with Insulin Resistance, Diabetes, and the Metabolic Syndrome," *Postgraduate Medicine* 122, no. 3 (2010): 61–70, doi: 10.3810/pgm.2010.05.2143.

10. Ibid.

11. D. C. Lee et al., "Changes in Fitness and Fatness on the Development of Cardiovascular Disease Risk Factors Hypertension, Metabolic Syndrome, and Hypercholesterolemia," *Journal of the American College of Cardiology* 59, no. 7 (2012): 665–672, doi: 10.1016/j.jacc.2011.11.013.

12. M. Uusitupa, J. Tuomilehto, and P. Puska, "Are We Really Active in the Prevention of Obesity and Type 2 Diabetes at the Community Level?," *Nutrition and Metabolism in Cardiovascular Diseases* 21, no. 5 (2011): 380–389, doi: 10.1016/j.numecd.2010.12.007.

13. National Diabetes Information Clearinghouse, U.S. Department of Health and Human Services, *Diabetes Prevention Program (DPP),* NIH Publication no. 09–5099 (Bethesda, MD: National Diabetes Information Clearinghouse, 2008), Available at http://diabetes.niddk.nih.gov

14. N. Magné et al., "Recommendations for a Lifestyle Which Could Prevent Breast Cancer and Its Relapse: Physical Activity and Dietetic Aspects," *Critical Review of Oncology and Hematology* 80, no. 3 (2011): 450–459, doi: 10.1016/j.critrevonc.2011.01.013.

15. World Cancer Research Fund/American Institute for Cancer Research, *Policy and Action for Cancer Prevention. Food, Nutrition, and Physical Activity: A Global Perspective* (Washington, DC: American Institute for Cancer Research, 2009), Available at www.dietandcancerreport.org

16. World Cancer Research Fund/American Institute for Cancer Research, *Policy and Action for Cancer Prevention,* 2009 (Washington, DC: American Institute for Cancer Research, 2009); A. Shibata, K. Ishii, and K. Oka, "Psychological, Social, and Environmental Factors of Meeting Recommended Physical Activity Levels for Colon Cancer Prevention among Japanese Adults," *Journal of Science and Medicine in Sport* 12, no. 2 (2010): e155–e156, doi: 10.1016/j.jsams.2009.10.324; K. Y. Wolin et al., "Physical Activity and Colon Cancer Prevention: A Meta-Analysis," *British Journal of Cancer* 100, no. 4 (2009): 611–616, doi: 10.1038/sj.bjc.6604917.

17. C. M. Friedenreich and A. E. Cust, "Physical Activity and Breast Cancer Risk: Impact of Timing, Type, and Dose of Activity and Population Subgroup Effects," *British Journal of Sports Medicine* 42, no. 8 (2008): 636–647, doi: 10.1136/bjsm.2006.029132.

18. M. Nilsson et al., "Increased Physical Activity Is Associated with Enhanced Development of Peak Bone Mass in Men: A Five Year Longitudinal Study," *Journal of Bone and Mineral Research* 27, no. 5 (2012): 1206–1214, doi: 10.1002/jbmr.1549; M. Callréus et al., "Self-Reported Recreational Exercise Combining Regularity and Impact Is Necessary to Maximize Bone Mineral Density in Young Adult Women: A Population-Based Study of 1,061 Women 25 Years of Age," *Osteoporosis International* 23, no. 10 (2012): 2517–2526, doi: 10.1007/s00198-011-1886-5.

19. T. Post et al., "Bone Physiology, Disease and Treatment: Towards Disease System Analysis in Osteoporosis," *Clinical Pharmacokinetics* 49, no. 2 (2010): 89–118, doi: 10.2165/11318150-000000000-00000.

20. V. A. Catenacci et al., "Physical Activity Patterns Using Accelerometry in the National Weight Control Registry," *Obesity* 19, no. 6 (2011): 1163–1170, doi: 10.1038/oby.2010.264.

21. A. Koch, "Immune Response to Resistance Exercise," *American Journal of Lifestyle Medicine* 4, no. 3 (2010): 244–252, doi: 10.1177/1559827609360190.

22. MedLine Plus, National Institutes of Health, "Exercise and Immunity," Updated May 15, 2012, www.nlm.nih.gov

23. N. P. Walsh et al., "Position Statement. Part Two: Maintaining Immune Health," *Exercise and Immunology Review* 17 (2011): 64–103.

24. M. W. Kakanis et al., "The Open Window of Susceptibility to Infection after Acute Exercise in Healthy Young Male Elite Athletes," *Exercise Immunology Review* 16 (2010): 119–137.

25. T. Esch and G. B. Stefano, "Endogenous Reward Mechanisms and Their Importance in Stress Reduction, Exercise and the Brain," *Archives of Medical Science* 6, no. 3 (2010): 447–455, doi: 10.5114/aoms.2010.14269.

26. J. Berry et al., "Lifetime Risks for Cardiovascular Disease Mortality by Cardiorespiratory Fitness Levels Measured at Ages 45, 55, and 65 Years in Men: The Cooper Center Longitudinal Study," *Journal of the American College of Cardiology* 57, no. 15 (2011): 1604–1610, doi: 10.1016/j.jacc.2010.10.056; J. Woodcock, O. Franco, N. Orsini, and I. Roberts, "Non-Vigorous Physical Activity and All-Cause Mortality: Systematic Review and Meta-Analysis of Cohort Studies," *International Journal of Epidemiology* 40, no. 1 (2011): 121–138.

27. American College of Sports Medicine, *ACSM's Guidelines for Exercise Testing and Prescription,* 9th ed. (Baltimore, MD: Lippincott Williams & Wilkins, 2014).

28. C. E. Garber et al., "American College of Sports Medicine Position Stand," 2011.

29. Ibid.

30. W. Micheo, L. Baerga, and G. Miranda, "Basic Principles Regarding Strength, Flexibility, and Stability Exercises," *Physical Medicine & Rehabilitation* 4, no. 11 (2012): 805–811, doi: 10.1016/j.pmrj.2012.09.583; C. E. Garber et al.,

"American College of Sports Medicine Position Stand," 2011.

31. Ibid.

32. D. G. Behm and A. Chaouachi, "A Review of the Acute Effects of Static and Dynamic Stretching on Performance," *European Journal of Applied Physiology* 111, no. 11 (2011): 2633–2651, doi: 10.1007/s00421-011-1879-2.

33. K. Small, L. McNaughton, and M. Matthews, "A Systematic Review into the Efficacy of Static Stretching as Part of a Warm-Up for the Prevention of Exercise-Related Injury," *Research in Sports Medicine* 16, no. 3 (2008): 213–231, doi: 10.1080/15438620802310784.

34. C. E. Garber et al., "American College of Sports Medicine Position Stand," 2011.

35. Ibid.

36. J. R. Fowles, "What I Always Wanted to Know about Instability Training," *Applied Physiology, Nutrition, and Metabolism* 35, no. 1 (2010): 89–90, doi: 10.1139/H09-134; D. G. Behm et al., "The Use of Instability to Train the Core Musculature," *Applied Physiology, Nutrition, and Metabolism* 35, no. 1 (2010): 91–108, doi: 10.1139/H09-127.

37. D. G. Behm et al., "Canadian Society for Exercise Physiology Position Stand: The Use of Instability to Train the Core in Athletic and Nonathletic Conditioning," *Applied Physiology, Nutrition, and Metabolism* 35, no. 1 (2010): 109–112, doi: 10.1139/H09-128.

38. K. B. Fields et al., "Prevention of Running Injuries," *Current Sports Medicine Reports* 9, no. 3 (2010): 176–182, doi: 10.1249/JSR.0b013e3181de7ec5.

39. American Academy of Ophthalmology, "Protective Eyewear," Updated February 2009, www.geteyesmart.org

40. American College Health Association, *American College Health Association-National College Health Assessment II Undergraduate Students Reference Group Executive Summary Fall 2012,* 2013.

41. Insurance Institute for Highway Safety, Highway Loss Data Institute, "Sharing the Road: Communities Try New Ways to Improve Bicycle Safety," *Status Report,* 48, no. 1 (2013), Available at www.iihs.org

42. N. G. Nelson et al., "Exertional Heat-Related Injuries Treated in Emergency Departments in the U.S., 1997–2006," *American Journal of Preventive Medicine* 40, no. 1 (2011): 54–60, doi: 10.1016/j.amepre.2010.09.031.

43. E. E. Turk, "Hypothermia," Forensic Science Medical Pathology 6, no. 2 (2010): 106–115, doi: 10.1007/s12024-010-9142-4.

44. Ibid.

45. American Council on Exercise, "Exercising in the Cold," Fit Facts, Blog, 2010, www.acefitness.org

Pulled statistics:
page 334, Centers for Disease Control and Prevention, "How Much Physical Activity Do Adults Need?" *Physical Activity for Everyone,* Updated December 1, 2011, www.cdc.gov; Office of Disease Prevention and Health Promotion, "Making America Healthier 10 Minutes at a Time," Be Active Your Way, Blog, May 9, 2013, www.health.gov
page 336, U.S. Department of Health and Human Services, "Physical Activity," *HealthyPeople. Gov: 2020 Topics & Objectives,* Updated April 10, 2013, www.healthypeople.gov

page 345, The Physical Activity Council, 2013 Participation Report: *The Physical Activity Council's Annual Study Tracking Sports, Fitness, and Recreation Participation in the USA,* 2013, www.physicalactivitycouncil.com

Chapter 12: Reducing Your Risk of Cardiovascular Disease and Cancer

1. World Health Organization, "Global Atlas on Cardiovascular Disease Prevention and Control," 2011, www.who.int

2. International Agency for Research on Cancer, "World Cancer Fact Sheet," August 2012, http://publications.cancerresearchuk.org

3. A. S. Go et al., "Heart Disease and Stroke Statistics–2013 Update: A Report from the American Heart Association," *Circulation* 127 (2013): e6–e245, doi:10.1161/CIR.0b013e31828124ad

4. Ibid.

5. Ibid.

6. Ibid.

7. D. M. Lloyd-Jones et al., "Defining and Setting National Goals for Cardiovascular Health Promotion and Disease Reduction: The AHA's Strategic Impact Goal through 2020 and Beyond," *Circulation* 121 (2010): e14–e31.

8. Ibid.

9. A. S. Go et al., "Heart Disease and Stroke Statistics–2013," 2013.

10. A. Folsom et al., "Community Prevalence of Ideal Cardiovascular Health, by the American Heart Association Definition, and Relationship with Cardiovascular Disease Incidence," *Journal of the American College of Cardiology* 57, no. 16 (2011): 1690–1696.

11. American Heart Association, "Why Blood Pressure Matters," August 2012, www.heart.org

12. Centers for Disease Control and Prevention, Media Relations, "MMWR-Morbidity and Mortality Weekly Report–News Synopsis for April 4, 2013," April 2013, www.cdc.gov

13. A. S. Go et al., "Heart Disease and Stroke Statistics–2013," 2013.

14. Centers for Disease Control and Prevention, "High Blood Pressure Facts," March 2013, www.cdc.gov

15. A. S. Go et al., "Heart Disease and Stroke Statistics–2013," 2013.

16. Ibid; Centers for Disease Control and Prevention, "High Blood Pressure Facts," March 2013, www.cdc.gov

17. A. S. Go et al., "Heart Disease and Stroke Statistics–2013," 2013.

18. American Heart Association, "Peripheral Artery Disease: Undertreated and Understudied in Women," 2012, http://newsroom.heart.org

19. Ibid.

20. A. S. Go et al., "Heart Disease and Stroke Statistics–2013," 2013.

21. National Heart, Blood, and Lung Institute, "Angina: What Is Angina?" June 2011, www.nhlbi.nih.gov

22. A. S. Go et al., "Heart Disease and Stroke Statistics–2013," 2013.

23. Ibid.

24. B. M. Kissel et al., "Age at Stroke: Temporal Trends in Stroke Incidence in a Large, Biracial Population," *Neurology* 79 (2012): 1781–1787.

25. Ibid.

26. Ibid.

27. A. S. Go et al., "Heart Disease and Stroke Statistics–2013," 2013; S. Saydal, "Early Mortality among Young Adults Linked to Cardiometabolic Risk Factors," *Pediatrics* 131 (2013): e679–e686; L. A. Leiter et al., "Position Statement: Cardiometabolic Risk in Canada–A Detailed Analysis and Position Paper by the Cardiometabolic Risk Working Group," *Canadian Journal of Cardiology* 27 (2011): e1–e33, www.cfpc.ca

28. S. Sharp et al., "Hypertension Is a Potential Risk Factor for Vascular Dementia: Systematic Review," *International Journal of Geriatric Psychiatry* 26, no. 7 (2011): 661–669; F. Testai and P. Gorelick, "Vascular Cognitive Impairment and Alzheimer's Disease: Are These Disorders Linked to Hypertension and Other Cardiovascular Risk Factors?" *Clinical Hypertension and Vascular Diseases* (2011): 195–210.

29. S. Grundy, "Pre-Diabetes, Metabolic Syndrome, and Cardiovascular Risk," *Journal of the American College of Cardiology* 59, no. 7 (2012): 635–643; D. Lee et al., "Changes in Fitness and Fatness on the Development of Cardiovascular Risk Factors Hypertension, Metabolic Syndrome, and Hypercholesterolemia," *Journal of the American College of Cardiology* 59, no. 7 (2012): 665–672; T. Horwich and G. Fonarow, "Glucose, Obesity, Metabolic Syndrome, and Diabetes Relevance to Incidence of Heart Failure," *Journal of the American College of Cardiology* 55, no. 4 (2010): 283–293.

30. A. S. Go et al., "Heart Disease and Stroke Statistics–2013," 2013.

31. S. Grundy et al., "Definition of Metabolic Syndrome. Report of the National Heart, Lung, and Blood Institute/American Heart Association Conference on Scientific Issues Related to Definition," *Circulation* 109, no. 2 (2011): 433–438.

32. A. S. Go et al., "Heart Disease and Stroke Statistics–2013," 2013.

33. Ibid.

34. National Cancer Institute, "Fact Sheet: Harms of Smoking and Benefits of Quitting," January 2011, www.cancer.gov

35. A. Parsons et al., "Influence of Smoking Cessation after Diagnosis of Early Stage Lung Cancer on Prognosis: Systematic Review of Observational Studies with Meta-Analysis," *British Medical Journal* (2010): 340, doi: http://dx.doi.org/10.1136/bmj.b5569

36. Ibid; A. K. Ferketich et al., "Smoking Status and Survival in the National Comprehensive Cancer Network Non–Small Cell Lung Cancer Cohort," *Cancer* 119, no. 4 (2013): 847–853, doi: 10.1002/cncr.27824

37. G. Schwarts et al., "Effects of Dalcetrapib in Patients with a Recent Acute Coronary Syndrome," *New England Journal of Medicine* 367 (2012): 2089–2099; C. Zheng and M. Aikawa, "High Density Lipoproteins: From Function to Therapy," *American College of Cardiology* 60, no. 23 (2012): 2380–2383.

38. A. S. Go et al., "Heart Disease and Stroke Statistics–2013," 2013.

39. National Center For Health Statistics, "Health, United States, 2011: With Special Features on Socioeconomic Status and Health," 2012, www.cdc.gov

40. A. S. Go et al., "Heart Disease and Stroke Statistics–2013," 2013.

41. Ibid.

42. Ibid; Y. Chida and A. Steptoe, "Greater Cardiovascular Responses to Laboratory Mental Stress Are Associated with Poor Subsequent Cardiovascular Risk Status: A Meta-Analysis of Prospective Evidence," *Hypertension* 55 (2010): 1026–1032.

43. T. Kotchen, A. Cowley and E. Frohlich, "Salt in Health and Disease–A Delicate Balance," *New England Journal of Medicine* 368 (2013): 1229–1237.

44. A. Steptoe and M. Kivimaki, "Stress and Cardiovascular Disease: An Update on Current Knowledge," *Annual Review of Public Health* 34 (2013): 337–354, doi: 10.1146/annurev-publhealth-031912-114452; C. Vlachopoulous, P. Xaplanteris, and C. Stefanadis, "Mental Stress, Arterial Stiffness, Central Pressures and Cardiovascular Risk," *Hypertension* 56, no. 3 (2010): e28–e30.

45. Y. Chida and A. Steptoe, "Response to Mental Stress, Arterial Stiffness, Central Pressures, and Cardiovascular Disease," *Hypertension* 56, no. 3 (2010): e29–e34; G. Lambert et al., "Stress Reactivity and Its Association with Increased Cardiovascular Risk: A Role for the Sympathetic Nervous System," *Hypertension* 55 (2010): e20–e23.

46. A. S. Go et al., "Heart Disease and Stroke Statistics–2013," 2013.

47. American Heart Association, "Understand Your Risk of Heart Attack," 2012, www.heart.org

48. T. Ong and L. Perusse, "Impact of Nutritional Epigenomics on Disease Risk and Prevention: Introduction," *Journal of Nutrigenetics and Nutrigenomics* 4, no. 5 (2011): 245–247; A. Angelakopoulou et al., "Comparative Analysis of Genome-Wide Association Studies Signals for Lipids, Diabetes, and Coronary Heart Disease: Cardiovascular Biomarker Genetics Collaboration," *European Heart Journal* 33, no. 3 (2012): 393–407; G. Thanassoulis et al., "A Genetic Risk Score Is Associated with Incident Cardiovascular Disease and Coronary Artery Calcium," *Circulation: Cardiovascular Genetics*, no. 5 (2012): 11321; C. Chow et al., "Parental History and Myocardial Infarction Risk Across the World: The Interheart Study," *Journal of the American College of Cardiology* 57 (2011): 619–627.

49. American Heart Association, "Understand Your Risk of Heart Attack," 2012, www.heart.org

50. Ibid.

51. The Emerging Risk Factors Collaboration, "C-Reactive Protein, Fibrinogen and CVD Prediction," *New England Journal of Medicine* 367 (2012): 1310–1320.

52. The ORIGIN Trial Investigators, "n–3 Fatty Acids and Cardiovascular Outcomes in Patients with Dysglycemia," *New England Journal of Medicine* 367 (2012): 309–318, doi: 10.1056/NEJMoa1203859

53. B. Keavney, "C-reactive Protein and the Risk for Cardiovascular Disease," *British Medical Journal* 342 (2011): d144; The Emerging Risk Factors Collaboration, "C-reactive Protein Concentration and Risk of Coronary Heart Disease, Stroke, and Mortality: An Individual Participant Meta-analysis," *The Lancet* 375, no. 9709 (2010): 132–140.

54. D. Wald, J. Morris, and N. Wald, "Reconciling the Evidence on Serum Homocysteine and Ischemic Heart Disease: A Meta-Analysis," *PLoS ONE* 6(2): e16473; J. Abraham and L. Cho, "The Homocysteine Hypothesis: Still Relevant to the Prevention and Treatment of Cardiovascular Disease?" *Cleveland Clinic Journal of Medicine* 77, no. 12 (2010): 911–918.

55. S. E. Vollset et al., "Effects of Folic Acid Supplementation on Overall and Site-Specific Cancer Incidence During the Randomised Trials: Meta-Analysis of Data on 50,000 Individuals," *The Lancet* 381, no. 9871 (2013): 1029–1036.

56. American Heart Association, "Homocysteine, Folic Acid, and Cardiovascular Disease," January 2012, www.heart.org

57. C. M. Rembold, "ACP Journal Club Review: Aspirin Does Not Reduce CHD or Cancer Mortality But Increases Bleeding," *Annals of Internal Medicine* 156, no. 12 (2012): JC6-3; C. Ling et al., "Aspirin to Prevent Incident Cardiovascular Disease: Is It Causing More Damage Than It Prevents?" *Clinical Practice* 9, no. 3 (2012): 223–225.

58. American Heart Association, "Prevention and Treatment of Heart Attack," January 2013, www.heart.org

59. A. S. Go et al., "Heart Disease and Stroke Statistics–2013," 2013.

60. American Cancer Society, "Cancer Facts and Figures 2013," 2013, www.cancer.org

61. Ibid.

62. Ibid.

63. American Cancer Society, "Staging," June 2012, www.cancer.org

64. American Cancer Society, "Cancer Facts and Figures 2013," 2013

65. Ibid.

66. Ibid.

67. American Cancer Society, "Cancer Facts and Figures 2013," 2013; Centers for Disease Control and Prevention, "Tobacco Use: Targeting the Nation's Leading Killer-At-a-Glance 2011," November 2012, www.cdc.gov

68. Centers for Disease Control, "The Health Consequences of Smoking: A Report of the Surgeon General," May 2004, www.cdc.gov

69. American Cancer Society, "Cancer Facts and Figures 2013," 2013.

70. C. Eheman et al., "Annual Report to the Nation on the Status of Cancer, 1975–2008, Featuring Cancers Associated with Excess Weight and Lack of Sufficient Physical Activity," *Cancer* 118, no. 9 (2012): 2338–2366, doi: 10.1002/cncr.27514/full; American Cancer Society, "Cancer Facts and Figures," 2013.

71. H. R. Harris et al., "Body Fat Distribution and Risk of Premenopausal Breast Cancer in the Nurses' Health Study II," *Journal of the National Cancer Institute* 103, no. 3 (2011): 373–378.

72. C. Eheman et al., "Annual Report to the Nation on the Status of Cancer, 1975–2008," 2012.

73. K. Keikkila et al., "Work Stress and Risk of Cancer: Meta-Analysis of 5700 Incident Cancer Events in 116,000 European Men and Women," *British Medical Journal* 346, (2013): 1165, doi: 10.1136/bmj.1165

74. American Cancer Society, "Cancer Facts and Figures," 2013.

75. American Cancer Society, "Breast Cancer Overview: What Causes Breast Cancer?" February 2013, www.cancer.org

76. L. Hines et al., "Comparative Analysis of Breast Cancer Risk Factors among Hispanic and

Non-Hispanic White Women," *Cancer* 116, no. 13 (2010): 3215–3223.

77. R. Chebowski et al., "Lung Cancer among Postmenopausal Women Treated with Estrogen Alone in the Women's Health Initiative Randomized Trial," *Journal of the National Cancer Institute* 102, no. 18 (2010): 1413–1421; C. Greiser, E. Greiser, and M. Doren, "Menopausal Hormone Therapy and Risk of Lung Cancer–Systematic Review and Meta-Analysis," *Maturitis: The European Menopause Journal* 65, no. 3 (2010): 198–204.

78. W. Chen et al., "Moderate Alcohol Consumption during the Adult Life, Drinking Patterns and Breast Cancer Risk," *Journal of the American Medical Association* 306, no. 17 (2011): 1884–1890; J. Jin et al., "Alcohol Drinking and All-Cause Mortality: A Meta-Analysis," *Annals of Oncology* 24, no. 3 (2013): 807–816; I. Tramacere et al., "A Meta-Analysis on Alcohol Drinking and Gastric Cancer Risk," *Annals of Oncology* 23, no. 1(2011): 28–36.

79. S. Grivennikov, F. Gretan, and M. Karin, "Immunity, Inflammation, and Cancer" *Cell* 140, no. 6 (2010): 883–99, doi: 10.1016/j.cell.2010.01.025; Y. Guo et al., "Association between C-reactive Protein and Risk of Cancer: A Meta-Analysis of Prospective Cohort Studies," *Asian Pacific Journal of Cancer Prevention* 14 (2013) doi: http://dx.doi.org/10.7314/APJCP.2013.14.1.243

80. S. Grivennikov, F. Gretan, and M. Karin, "Immunity, Inflammation, and Cancer" *Cell* 140, no. 6 (2010): 883–899, doi: 10.1016/j.cell.2010.01.025

81. B. Aggarwal et al., "Targeting Inflammatory Pathways for Prevention and Therapy for Cancer: Short Term Friend, Long Term Foe," *Clinical Cancer Research* 15 (2009): 425–430.

82. National Cancer Institute, "Cell Phones and Cancer Risk," March 2013, www.cancer.gov; S. Joachim et al., "Cellular Telephone Use and Cancer Risk: Update of a Nationwide Danish Cohort," *Journal of the National Cancer Institute* 98, no. 23 (2006): 1707–1713.

83. American Cancer Society, "Infectious Agents and Cancer," March 2013, www.cancer.org

84. National Institute of Allergy and Infectious Diseases, "Viral Infections: Treating Cancer as an Infectious Disease," March 2009, www.niaid.nih; American Cancer Society, "Cancer Facts and Figures 2013," 2013.

85. Ibid.; National Cancer Institute, "Cervical Cancer," February 2013, www.cancer.gov

86. American Cancer Society, "Cancer Facts and Figures 2013," 2013.

87. American Cancer Society, "Lung Cancer Also Affects Nonsmokers," November 2011, www.cancer.org

88. J. Samet et al., "Lung Cancer in Never Smokers: Clinical Epidemiology and Environmental Risk Factors," *Clinical Cancer Research* 15, no. 18 (2011): 5626–5645.

89. American Cancer Society, "Cancer Facts and Figures 2013," 2013.

90. American Lung Association, "Benefits of Quitting," 2012, www.lung.org

91. American Cancer Society, "Cancer Facts and Figures 2013," 2013.

92. Ibid.

93. Ibid.
94. Ibid.
95. Ibid.
96. Ibid.
97. Susan G. Komen for the Cure, "Table 11: BRCA1 and BRCA2 Gene Mutations and Cancer Risk," August 2012, www.komen.org
98. R. Patterson, L. Cadmus, and T. Emond, "Physical Activity, Diet, Adiposity and Female Breast Cancer Prognosis: A Review of Epidemiological Literature," *Maturitas* 66 (2010): 5–15.
99. J. Dong et al., "Dietary Fiber Intake and Risk of Breast Cancer: A Meta-Analysis of Prospective Cohort Studies," *American Journal of Clinical Nutrition* 94, no. 3 (2011): 900–905; D. Aune et al., "Dietary Fiber and Breast Cancer Risks: A Systematic Review and Meta Analysis of Prospective Studies," *Annals of Oncology* (2012), doi: 10.1093/annuls/mdr589
100. American Cancer Society, "Cancer Facts and Figures 2013," 2013.
101. Ibid.
102. Ibid.
103. Ibid.
104. Ibid.
105. Ibid.
106. Ibid.
107. Ibid
108. Ibid.
109. Ibid.
110. Ibid.
111. American Cancer Society, "Prostate Cancer," January 2013, www.cancer.org
112. American Cancer Society, "Cancer Facts and Figures 2013," 2013.
113. Ibid.
114. Ibid.
115. Ibid.
116. National Cancer Institute, "Testicular Cancer," 2013, www.cancer.gov

Pulled statistics:

page 356, World Health Organization, "Cardiovascular Diseases," March 2013, www.who.int

page 358, American Heart Association, "Statistical Fact Sheet: 2013 Update," 2013.

page 374, Centers for Disease Control and Prevention, "Lung Cancer Risk Factors," February 2013, www.cdc.gov

Focus On: Minimizing Your Risk for Diabetes

1. Centers for Disease Control and Prevention, *National Diabetes Fact Sheet: 2011*, January 2012, www.cdc.gov
2. Ibid.
3. Ibid.
4. Ibid; American Diabetes Association, "Diabetes Statistics," March 2013, www.diabetes.org
5. American Diabetes Association, "Diabetes Basics: Type 1," 2013, www.diabetes.org
6. The National Diabetes Information Clearinghouse (NDIC), "National Diabetes Statistics: 2011," December 2011, http://diabetes.niddk.nih.gov
7. Centers for Disease Control and Prevention, "National Diabetes Fact Sheet: 2011," 2012.
8. D. Dabelea et al., "Is Prevalence of Type 2 Diabetes Increasing in Youth? The SEARCH for Diabetes in Youth Study," American Diabetes Association 72nd Scientific Sessions. (Philadelphia: June 8–12, 2012).
9. American Heart Association, "Statistical Fact Sheet, 2013 Update: Diabetes," 2013, www.heart.org
10. R. Mihaescu et al., "Genetic Risk Profiling for Prediction of Type 2 Diabetes," *PLoS Currents* 3 (2011), doi: 10.1371/currents.RRN1208; E. Ntzani, K. Evangelia, and F. Kavvoura, "Genetic Risk Factors for Type 2 Diabetes: Insights from the Emerging Genomic Evidence," *Current Vascular Pharmacology* 10, no. 2 (2012): 147–155.
11. J. Logue et al., "Association between BMI Measured within a Year After Diagnosis of Type 2 Diabetes and Mortality," *Diabetes Care* 36, no. 4 (2013): 887–893; M. Ashwell, P. Gunn, and S. Gibson, "Waist-to-Height Ratio is a Better Screening Tool than Waist Circumference and BMI for Adult Cardiometabolic Risk Factors: Systematic Review and Meta-analysis," *Obesity Reviews* 13, no. 3 (2012): 275–286.
12. L. Bromley et al., "*Sleep* Restriction Decreases the Physical Activity of Adults at Risk for Type 2 Diabetes," *Sleep* 35, no. 7 (2012): 977–984, doi:10.5665/sleep.1964.
13. R. Hancox and C. Landlus, "Association between Sleep Duration and Haemoglobin A1C in Young Adults," *Journal of Epidemiology and Community Health* 66, no. 10 (2011): 957–961; H. C. Hung et al., "The Association between Self-Reported Sleep Quality and Metabolic Syndrome," *PLoS One* 8, no. 1: e54304 (2013), doi:10.1371/journal.pone.0054304; T. Ohkuma et al., "Impact of Sleep Duration on Obesity and the Glycemic Level in Patients with Type 2 Diabetes," *Diabetes Care* 36, no. 3 (2013): 611–617.
14. P. Puustinen et al., "Psychological Distress Predicts the Development of Metabolic Syndrome: A Prospective Population-Based Study," *Psychosomatic Medicine* 73, no. 2 (2011): 158–165.
15. Centers for Disease Control and Prevention, "National Diabetes Fact Sheet: 2011," 2012.
16. J. M. Schilter and L. C. Dalleck, "Fitness and Fatness: Indicators of Metabolic Syndrome and Cardiovascular Disease Risk Factors in College Students?" *Journal of Exercise Physiology Online* 13, no. 4 (2010): 29–39.
17. American Heart Association, "Metabolic Syndrome," 2013, www.americanheart.org
18. Ibid; National Heart, Lung, and Blood Institute, "Who Is At Risk for Metabolic Syndrome?" November 2011, www.nhlbi.nih.gov; National Heart, Lung, and Blood Institute, "What Is Metabolic Syndrome?" November 2011, www.nhlbi.nih.gov
19. Ibid.
20. Ibid.
21. Centers for Disease Control, "Awareness of Prediabetes—United States, 2005–2010," March 2013, www.cdc.gov
22. L. S. Geiss et al., "Diabetes Risk Reduction Behaviors among U.S. Adults with Prediabetes," *Journal of Preventive Medicine* 38, no. 4 (2010):403–409; Centers for Disease Control, "National Diabetes Prevention Program: About the Program," October 2012, www.cdc.gov
23. American Diabetes Association, "Diabetes Basics: What Is Gestational Diabetes?", 2013, www.diabetes.org
24. Ibid; C. Kim et al., "Gestational Diabetes and the Incidence of Type 2 Diabetes: A Systematic Review," *Diabetes Care* 25, no.

10 (2002):1862–1868; G. Rice, S. Illanes, and M. Michel, "Gestational Diabetes Mellitus: A Positive Predictor of Type 2 Diabetes?" *International Journal of Endocrinology* (2012), doi:10.1155/2012/721653; C. S. Göbl et al., "Early Possible Risk Factors for Overt Diabetes after Gestational Diabetes Mellitus," *Obstetrics and Gynecology* 118, no. 1 (2011): 71–78.

25. American Diabetes Association, "Living with Diabetes: Complications," 2013, www.diabetes .org; K. Weinspach et al., "Level of Information about the Relationship Between Diabetes Mellitus and Periodontitis—Results from a Nationwide Diabetes Information Program," *European Journal of Medical Research* 18, no. 1 (2013): 6, doi: 10.1186/2047-783X-18-6.

26. K. Behan, "New ADA Guidelines for Diagnosis, Screening of Diabetes," *Advance Laboratory* 20, no. 1 (2011): 22, Available at http:// laboratory-manager.advanceweb.com

27. American Diabetes Association, "Diabetes Basics: Pre-Diabetes FAQs," 2013, www.diabetes.org

28. American Diabetes Association, "Healthy Weight Loss," (2013), www.diabetes.org; W. Knowles et al., "10 Year Follow-Up of Diabetes Incidence and Weight Loss in the DPP Outcomes Study," *The Lancet* 374, no. 9702 (2009): 1677–1686; Diabetes Prevention Program Research Group, "Reduction in the Incidence of Type 2 Diabetes with Lifestyle Intervention or Metformin," *New England Journal of Medicine* 345 (2002): 393–403.

29. Linus Pauling Institute, "Glycemic Index and Glycemic Load," April 2010, http://lpi.oregonstate. edu

30. S. Jonnalagadda et al., "Putting the Whole Grain Puzzle Together: Health Benefits Associated with Whole Grains—Summary of American Society for Nutrition 2010 Satellite Symposium," *Journal of Nutrition* 41, no. 5 (2011): 10115–10125.

31. R. Post et al., "Dietary Fiber for the Treatment of Type 2 Diabetes Mellitus: A Meta Analysis," *Journal of the American Board of Family Medicine* 25, no. 1 (2012): 16–23; J. Tuomilehto, P. Schwarz, and J. Lindstrom, "Long-Term Benefits from Lifestyle Intervention for Type 2 Diabetes Prevention," *Diabetes Care* 34, (2011): 5210S–14S.

32. A. Wallin et al., "Fish Consumption, Dietary Long-Chain N-3 Fatty Acids, and the Risk of Type 2 Diabetes: Systematic Review and Meta Analysis of Prospective Studies," *Diabetes Care* 35, no. 4 (2012): 918–929; L. Djousse et al., "Dietary Omega-3 Fatty Acids and Fish Consumption and Risk of Type 2 Diabetes," *American Journal of Clinical Nutrition* 93, no. 1 (2011): 113–150.

33. C. Jeppesen, K. Schiller, and M. Schultze, "Omega-3 and Omega-6 Fatty Acids and Type 2 Diabetes," *Current Diabetes Reports* 13, no. 2 (2013): 279–288.

34. American Diabetes Association, "Healthy Weight Loss," 2013, www.diabetes.org; National Diabetes Information Clearing House, "Diabetes Prevention Program," November 2012, http://diabetes.niddk.nih.gov

35. P. Poirier et al., "Bariatric Surgery and Cardiovascular Risk Factors: A Scientific Statement from the American Heart Association," *Circulation*, March 2011, doi: 10.1161/ CIR.0b013e3182149099.

Pulled statistics:

page 393, Diabetes Prevention Program Research Group, "Reduction in the Incidence of Type 2 Diabetes with Lifestyle Intervention or Metformin," *New England Journal of Medicine* 345 (2002): 393–403.

Chapter 13: Protecting against Infectious Diseases and Sexually Transmitted Infections

1. F. Dawood et al., "Estimated Global Mortality Associated with the First Months of 2009 Pandemic Influenza *A H1N1* Virus Circulation: A Modelling Study," *The Lancet Infectious Diseases* 12, no. 9 (2012): 687–695, doi:10-1016/ S1473-3099(12)70121-4.

2. J. Remais et al., "Convergence of Non-Communicable and Infectious Diseases in Low- and Middle-Income Countries," *International Journal of Epidemiology* 42, no. 1 (2013): 221–227, doi:10.1093/ije/dys135; Environmental Protection Agency, "Climate Impacts on Human Health," April 2013, www.epa.gov; E. Shuman, "Global Climate Change and Infectious Diseases," *New England Journal of Medicine* 362 (2010): 1061–1063.

3. B. Feingold et al., "A Niche for Infectious Disease in Environmental Health: Rethinking the Toxicological Paradigm," *Environmental Health Perspectives* 118, no. 8 (2010): 1165–1172; L. Martin et al., "The Effects of Anthropogenic Global Changes on Immune Functions and Disease Resistance," *Annals of the New York Academy of Sciences* 1195, no. 1 (2010): 129–148.

4. Association for Professionals in Infection Control and Epidemiology, "CRE: The 'Nightmare Bacteria,'" 2013, http://apic.org; Association for Professionals in Infection Control and Epidemiology, "Infection Prevention and You," 2013, http://apic.org

5. Centers for Disease Control and Prevention, "Birth-18 years and 'Catch-Up' Immunization Schedules," 2013.

6. Centers for Disease Control and Prevention, "Antibiotics: Will They Work When You Really Need Them?" March 2012, www.cdc.gov

7. S. Stefani et al., "Methicillin-Resistant *Staphylococcus Aureus* (MRSA): Global Epidemiology and Harmonization of Typing Methods," *International Journal of Antimicrobial Agents* 39, no. 4 (2012): 273–282, doi: 10.1016/j.ijantimicag.2011.09.030; Centers for Disease Control and Prevention, "MRSA Fact Sheet," April 2013, Available at www. cdc.gov; Centers for Disease Control and Prevention, "MRSA Statistics," 2011, www.cdc.gov

8. W. Jarvis, "Prevention and Control of Methicillin-Resistant *Staphylococcus Aureus:* Dealing with Reality, Resistance, and Resistance to Reality," *Clinical Infectious Diseases* 50, no. 2 (2010): 218–220.

9. Centers for Disease Control and Prevention, "MRSA Statistics," 2011.

10. Centers for Disease Control and Prevention, "Group A Streptococcal (GAS) Disease," March 2012, www.cdc.gov

11. Ibid.

12. Centers for Disease Control and Prevention, "Fast Facts: Group B Strep (GBS)," 2011, www .cdc.gov

13. Centers for Disease Control and Prevention, "Meningitis," 2013, www.cdc.gov; Centers for Disease Control and Prevention, "Factsheet: Meningococcal Disease and Meningococcal Vaccine," April 2013, www.cdc.gov

14. World Health Organization, "Tuberculosis Fact Sheet," February 2013, www.who.int

15. Centers for Disease Control and Prevention, "Tuberculosis (TB): Data and Statistics," September 2012, www.cdc.gov

16. Ibid.

17. Centers for Disease Control and Prevention, "Tuberculosis," April 2013, www.cdc.gov

18. Centers for Disease Control and Prevention, "Tuberculosis (TB): Treatment," August 2012, www.cdc.gov

19. Ibid.

20. National Institute of Allergy and Infectious Diseases, "Common Cold," May 2011, www .niaid.nih.gov

21. Centers for Disease Control and Prevention, "Seasonal Influenza: Key Facts about Influenza (Flu) and Flu Vaccine," February 2013, www .cdc.gov

22. Centers for Disease Control and Prevention, "Selecting the Viruses in the Seasonal Influenza (Flu) Vaccine," March 2011, www.cdc.gov

23. Centers for Disease Control and Prevention, "Viral Hepatitis Surveillance—United States, 2010," June 2012, www.cdc.gov

24. Ibid.

25. Centers for Disease Control and Prevention, "CDC Features: World Hepatitis Day," July 2011, www.cdc.gov

26. Ibid.

27. Centers for Disease Control and Prevention, "Hepatitis C FAQs for Health Professionals," June 2010, www.cdc.gov

28. S. Rajaguru and M. Nettleman, "Hepatitis C," MedicineNet.com, 2010, www.medicinenet.com

29. Centers for Disease Control and Prevention, "vCJD (Variant Creutzfeldt-Jakob Disease)," 2010, www.cdc.gov

30. Centers for Disease Control and Prevention, "Get Smart: Know When Antibiotics Work: Fast Facts," May 2012, www.cdc.gov

31. A. E. Barskey et al., "Mumps Resurgences in the United States: A Historical Perspective on Unexpected Elements," *Vaccine* 27, no. 44 (2009): 6186–6195.

32. Centers for Disease Control and Prevention, "West Nile Virus (WNV) Activity Reported to ArboNET, by State, United States, 2011," April 2012, www.cdc.gov

33. World Health Organization, "Cumulative Number of Confirmed Human Cases of Avian Influenza A (H5N1) Reported to WHO," 2013, www.who.int

34. Ibid.

35. Centers for Disease Control and Prevention, "Avian Influenza A (H7N9) Virus," April 2013, www.cdc.gov; Centers for Disease Control and Prevention, "Avian Influenza in Birds," June 2012, www.cdc.gov; Centers for Disease Control and Prevention, "Avian Influenza A Virus Infections in Humans," June 2012, www.cdc. gov; U.S. Department of Health and Human Services, "H3N2v," 2013, www.flu.gov

36. Centers for Disease Control and Prevention, "Sexually Transmitted Disease Surveillance, 2011," March 2013, www.cdc.gov

37. Ibid.

38. Centers for Disease Control and Prevention, "Chlamydia—CDC Fact Sheet," February 2013, www.cdc.gov

40. Centers for Disease Control and Prevention, "Conjunctivitis (Pink Eye) in Newborns," October 2012, www.cdc.gov

41. Centers for Disease Control and Prevention, "Gonorrhea—CDC Fact Sheet," February 2013, www.cdc.gov

42. Ibid.

43. National Institute of Allergy and Infectious Diseases, "Gonorrhea: Treatment," January 2011, www.niaid.nih.gov

44. Centers for Disease Control and Prevention, "Syphilis—CDC Fact Sheet," February 2013, www.cdc.gov

45. Ibid.

46. Centers for Disease Control and Prevention, "Genital Herpes—CDC Fact Sheet," Modified February 2013, www.cdc.gov

47. American Sexual Health Association, "Learn about Herpes: Fast Facts," 2013, www.ashastd.org

48. Ibid.

49. Centers for Disease Control and Prevention, "Genital HPV Infection—Fact Sheet," March 2013, www.cdc.gov; American Sexual Health Association, "Overview and Fast Stats," 2013, www.ashastd.org

50. National Institute of Cancer, "HPV and Cancer," March 2012, www.cancer.gov

51. National Women's Law Center, "Pap Smears," 2010, http://hrc.nwlc.org; Centers for Disease Control and Prevention, "Cervical Cancer," March 2013, www.cdc.gov

52. Centers for Disease Control and Prevention, "Genital/Vulvovaginal Candidiasis," March 2013, www.cdc.gov

53. Centers for Disease Control and Prevention, "Trichomoniasis: CDC Fact Sheet," August 2012, www.cdc.gov

54. Ibid.

55. UNAIDS, "UNAIDS World AIDS Day Report 2012," 2012, Available at www.unaids.org

56. Centers for Disease Control and Prevention, "HIV in the United States: At a Glance," April 2013, www.cdc.gov

57. Ibid; UNAIDS, "UNAIDS World AIDS Day Report 2012," 2012.

58. AVERT, "Can You Get HIV From …?", July 2010, www.avert.org

59. Ibid.

60. Centers for Disease Control and Prevention, "HIV among Women," April 2013, www.cdc.gov

61. AVERT, "Preventing Mother-to-Child Transmission of HIV (PMTCT)," 2012, www.avert.org

62. AVERT, "HIV Testing," 2012, www.avert.org

Pulled statistics:

page 411, Centers for Disease Control and Prevention, "Incidence, Prevalence and Cost of Sexually Transmitted Infections in the United States," 2013, www.cdc.gov

page 418, UNAIDS, "UNAIDS World AIDS Day Report 2012," 2012.

Focus On: Reducing Risks and Coping with Chronic Diseases and Conditions

1. A. Miniño, "Death in the United States, 2011," Center for Disease Control NCHS Data Brief, no. 115 (2013), Available at www.cdc.gov

2. American Lung Association, "Chronic Obstructive Pulmonary Disease (COPD) Fact Sheet," February 2011, www.lung.org

3. American Lung Association, "Trends in COPD (Chronic Bronchitis and Emphysema): Morbidity and Mortality," March 2013, www.lung.org

4. Ibid.; Centers for Disease Control and Prevention, "Chronic Obstructive Pulmonary Disease Among Adults—United States, 2011," November 2012, www.cdc.gov

5. American Lung Association, "Trends in COPD," 2013.

6. Ibid.

7. Ibid.

8. American Lung Association, "Reduce Asthma Triggers," 2013, www.lung.org

9. Ibid; U. Gohil, A. Modan, and P. Gohil, "Aspirin-Induced Asthma–A Review," Global Journal of Pharmacology 4, no. 1 (2010): 19–30.

10. Centers for Disease Control and Prevention, "FastStats: Asthma," April, 2013, www.cdc.gov

11. Ibid; American Lung Association, "Asthma," 2013, www.lung.org

12. Centers for Disease Control and Prevention, "FastStats: Asthma," 2013.

13. Centers for Disease Control and Prevention, "National Surveillance of Asthma: United States, 2001–2010," Vital and Health Statistics 3, no. 35 (2012), Available at www.cdc.gov

14. Centers for Disease Control and Prevention, "FastStats–Allergies and Hay Fever," January 2013, www.cdc.gov

15. National Institute of Allergy and Infectious diseases, "Pollen Allergy," June 2012, www.niaid.nih.gov

16. J. Lucado, K. Paez, and A. Elixhauser, "Headaches in U.S. Hospitals and Emergency Departments, 2008," HCUP Statistical Brief, no. 111 (2011), Available at www.hcup-us.ahrq.gov

17. National Headache Foundation, "Press Kits: Categories of Headache," 2013, www.headaches.org

18. WebMD, "Migraines and Headache Health Center: Tension Headaches," 2013, www.webmd.com

19. National Headache Foundation, "The Complete Guide to Headache: Migraine," April 2012, www.headaches.org

20. Ibid.

21. Ibid.

22. Ibid.

23. National Headache Foundation, "Cluster Headaches," 2013, www.headaches.org

24. H. F. Herlong, "Digestive Disorders," The Johns Hopkins White Papers (Baltimore, MD: Johns Hopkins Medicine, 2013).

25. National Digestive Diseases Information Clearinghouse, "Irritable Bowel Syndrome," July 2012, http://digestive.niddk.nih.gov

26. H. F. Herlong, "Digestive Disorders," 2013.

27. Ibid.; Centers for Disease Control and Prevention, "Inflammatory Bowel Disease," May 2012, www.cdc.gov

28. E. Quigley and C. Bernstein, "Editorial: 'Irritable Bowel Symptoms' in Inflammatory Bowel Disease: Diagnostic Uncertainty Meets Pathological Reality," The American Journal of Gastroenterology 107 (2012): 1483–1485, doi: 10.1038/ajg.2012.263.

29. Centers for Disease Control and Prevention, "Inflammatory Bowel Disease," May 2012, www.cdc.gov

30. Ibid.

31. H. F. Herlong, "Digestive Disorders," 2013.

32. Ibid.

33. F. Balague et al., "Non-Specific Low Back Pain," The Lancet 379, no. 9814 (2012): 482–491, doi: 10.1016/S0140-6736(11)60610-7.

34. Centers for Disease Control and Prevention, National Institute of Neurological Disorders and Stroke, "Low Back Pain Fact Sheet," Updated January 2010, www.ninds.nih; Centers for Disease Control and Prevention, "47.5 Million U.S. Adults Report a Disability; Arthritis Remains Most Common Cause," June 2011, www.cdc.gov

35. National Institute of Neurological Disorders, "NINDS Repetitive Motion Disorders Information Page," October 2011, www.ninds.nih.gov

Pulled statistics:

page 425, American Lung Association, "Chronic Obstructive Pulmonary Disease (COPD) Fact Sheet," February 2011, www.lung.org

page 430, Anxiety and Depression Association of America, "Irritable Bowel Syndrome (IBS)," 2012, www.adaa.org

Chapter 14: Preparing for Aging, Death, and Dying

1. Central Intelligence Agency, "The World Factbook. Country Comparisons: Life Expectancy at Birth," 2012, www.cia.gov

2. Administration on Aging, "A Profile of Older Americans: 2012," 2013, www.aoa.gov

3. Federal Interagency Forum on Aging-Related Statistics, "Older Americans 2012: Key Indicators of Well-Being," June 2012, www.agingstats.gov

4. Administration on Aging, "A Profile of Older Americans: 2012," 2013.

5. Administration on Aging, "A Profile of Older Americans: 2012, Health and Health Care," 2013, www.aoa.gov

6. Ibid.

7. Ibid.

8. Genworth, "Arizona State-Specific Data from the Genworth 2013, Cost of Care Survey," March 2013, www.genworth.com

9. Administration on Aging, "A Profile of Older Americans: 2012, Health and Health Care," 2013, www.aoa.gov

10. NIH Osteoporosis and Related Bone Diseases National Resource Center, "What Is Osteoporosis?," January 2011, www.niams.nih.gov; NIH Osteoporosis and Related Bone Diseases National Resource Center, "Osteoporosis," May 2009, www.niams.nih.gov; National Osteoporosis Foundation, "Learn About Osteoporosis," 2011, www.nof.org

11. National Association for Continence, "Statistics," 2013, www.nafc.org

12. Ibid.

13. T. E. Howe et al., "Exercise for Improving Balance in Older People," Cochrane Database of Systematic Reviews (2011), at www.summaries.cochrane.org

14. Medline Plus, "Aging Changes in the Senses," March 2013, www.nlm.nih.gov

15. B. J. Cowart, "Smell and Taste in Aging," Perfumer and Flavorist 36, no. 1 (2011): 34–36.

16. L. Fisher, "Sex, Romance, and Relationships: AARP Survey of Midlife and Older Adults," May 2010, http://assets.aarp.org; V. Schick et al., "Sexual Behaviors, Condom Use, and Sexual Health of Americans over 50: Implications for Sexual Health Promotion for Older Adults," The Journal of Sexual Medicine 7 (2010): 315–329, doi: 10.1111/j.1743-6109.2010.02013.x; Center for Sexual Health Promotion, "National Survey of Sexual Health and Behavior," 2010.

17. Alzheimer's Association, "2012 Alzheimer's Disease Facts and Figures," 2012, www.alz.org

18. Ibid.

19. L. Hebert et al., "Alzheimer Disease in the United States (2010–2050) Estimated Using the 2010 Census," *Neurology* 80, no. 19 (2013): doi: 10.1212/WNL.0b013e31828726f5.

20. Ibid.

21. Ibid.

22. Alzheimer's Association, "What Is Alzheimer's?" 2011, www.alz.org

23. National Center for Health Statistics, "Lifetime Alcohol Drinking Status among Adults," Health, United States (2011), www.cdc.gov; National Institute on Aging, "AgePage: Alcohol Use in Older People," April 2012, www.nia.nih.gov

24. Centers for Disease Control and Prevention, "Prescription Drug Use Continues to Increase," *NCHS Data Brief* 42 (2010), www.cdc.gov

25. Centers for Disease Control and Prevention, "Making Physical Activity a Part of an Older Adult's Life," November 2011, www.cdc.gov

26. Ibid.

27. By permission. From Merriam-Webster's Collegiate® Dictionary, 11th Edition © 2013 by Merriam-Webster, Inc., www.Merriam-Webster.com

28. President's Commission on the Uniform Determination of Death, *Defining Death: Medical, Ethical and Legal Issues in the Determination of Death* (Washington, DC: U.S. Government Printing Office, 1981).

29. Ad Hoc Committee of the Harvard Medical School to Examine the Definition of Brain Death, "A Definition of Irreversible Coma," *Journal of the American Medical Association* 205 (1968): 377.

30. Elisabeth Kübler-Ross and David Kessler, "The Five Stages of Grief," 2013, http://grief.com

31. Victorian Government Health Information, "Death and Dying," May 2011, www.health.vic.gov

32. Behavioural Neuropathy Clinic, "Grief and the Grieving Process," Worden's Tasks of Grief, 2012, www.adhd.com

33. American Bar Association Commission on Law and Aging, *Consumer's Tool Kit for Health Care Advance Planning*, 2d ed., (2012), Available at www.abanet.org

34. Aging with Dignity, "Five Wishes," 2013, www.agingwithdignity.org

35. Public Agenda, "Right to Die," 2011, www.publicagendaarchives.org

36. National Hospice and Palliative Care Organization, "NHPCO Facts and Figures: Hospice Care in America, 2012 Edition," 2012, www.nhpco.org

37. MedlinePlus, "Organ Donation," 2012, www.nlm.nih.gov

Pulled statistics:

page 435, U.S. Bureau of Labor Statistics, "The 2012 Statistical Abstract," January 2013, www.census.gov

page 441, U.S. Census Bureau, "2010 Census Shows 65 and Older Population Growing Faster than Total U.S. Population," November 2011, www.census.gov

Chapter 15: Promoting Environmental Health

1. United Nations, "World Population to Reach 10 Billion by 2100 if Fertility in All Countries Converges to Replacement Level," 2011, http://esa.un.org

2. United Nations, "Global Environment Outlook: Environment for Development (GEO-5): Summary for Policy Makers," 2012, www.uncsd2012.org; United Nations, "UNEP Yearbook: Emerging Issues in our Global Environment, 2013," 2013, Available at www.unep.org/yearbook/2013/

3. World Wildlife Report, *Living Planet Report 2012*, 2012, wwf.panda.org; United Nations, "Global Environmental Outlook," 2012, www.unep.org

4. United Nations, "Emerging Issues in our Global Environment, 2013," 2013.

5. Ibid.

6. United Nations, "Global Environmental Outlook," 2012.

7. United Nations Environmental Program, "Towards a Green Economy: Pathways to Sustainable Development and Poverty Eradication," 2011, www.unep.org

8. United Nations, "Emerging Issues in our Global Environment, 2013," 2013.

9. Ibid.

10. U.S. Energy Information Administration, "Independent Statistics and Analysis," 2013, www.eia.gov

11. Central Intelligence Agency, The World Factbook "Country Comparison: Total Fertility Rate," 2013, www.cia.gov

12. U.S. Census Bureau, Population Division, "International Data Base Country Rankings," 2010, http://sasweb.ssd.census.gov

13. U.S. Census Bureau, "Annual Population Estimates," 2013, www.census.gov

14. U.S. Census Bureau, U.S. and World Population Clocks, "U.S. POPClock Projection," 2013, www.census.gov

15. U.S. Environmental Protection Agency, "Air Enforcement," 2013, www.epa.gov

16. U.S. Environmental Protection Agency, "Overview of Greenhouse Gases: Carbon Dioxide Emissions," 2013, www.epa.gov

17. A. Soos, "Acid Rain Change," Environmental News Network, 2013, www.enn.com

18. Ibid; American Lung Association, "Health Effects of Ozone and Particle Pollution," 2013, www.stateoftheair.org

19. U.S. Environmental Protection Agency, "Reducing Acid Rain," 2012, www.epa.gov

20. U.S. Environmental Protection Agency, "Acid Rain: Effects of Acid Rain—Surface Waters and Aquatic Animals," 2012, www.epa.gov

21. Ibid; A. Soos, "Acid Rain Change," 2013.

22. U.S. Environmental Protection Agency, "Acid Rain: Effects of Acid Rain—Human Health," www.epa.gov

23. U.S. Energy Information Administration, "Independent Statistics and Analysis," 2012.

24. U.S. Environmental Protection Agency, "An Introduction to Indoor Air Quality," 2012, www.epa.gov

25. U.S. Environmental Protection Agency, "Health Effects of Exposure to Secondhand Smoke," 2011, www.epa.gov

26. American Nonsmoker's Rights Foundation, "States, Commonwealths and Municipalities with 100 percent Smokefree Laws in Workplaces, Restaurants and Bars," 2013, www.no-smoke.org

27. U.S. Environmental Protection Agency, "Indoor Air Quality: Radon: Health Risks," Updated March 2013, www.epa.gov

28. U.S. Environmental Protection Agency, "U.S. Homes above EPA's Radon Action Level," Updated June 2010, http://cfpub.epa.gov

29. Centers for Disease Control and Prevention, "Lead," 2013, www.cdc.gov; Centers for Disease Control and Prevention, "Blood Lead Levels in Children Aged 1–5 Years—United States, 1999–2010," *Morbidity and Mortality Weekly Report* 62, no. 13 (2013): 245–248, Available at www.cdc.gov

30. U.S. Department of Housing and Urban Development, "Making Homes Healthier for Families," 2013, http://portal.hud.gov

31. National Center for Environmental Health, "Mold: Basic Facts," 2012, www.cdc.gov

32. U.S. Environmental Protection Agency, "Ozone Layer Depletion: Ozone Science: Brief Questions and Answers on Ozone Depletion," Updated February 2010, www.epa.gov; Environment, Health and Safety Online, " Ozone Depletion and UV Radiation," 2013, www.ehso.com; National Aeronautics and Space Administration, "Ozone Hole Watch," 2013, http://ozonewatch.gsfc.nasa.gov

33. Environmental Protection Agency, "Climate Change: Basic Information," 2013, http://epa.gov

34. Environmental Protection Agency, "Climate Change Facts: Answers to Common Questions," 2013, http://epa.gov

35. Ibid.

36. National Aeronautics and Space Administration (NASA), "Global Climate Change: Vital Signs of the Planet," http://climate.nasa.gov

37. U.S. General Accounting Office, "The Quality, Comparability, and Review of Emissions Inventories Vary Between Developed and Developing Nations," 2010, www.gao.gov

38. World Commission on Environment and Development, *Our Common Future* (Oxford: Oxford University Press, 1987): 27.

39. U.S. Geological Survey, "Water Science for Schools: Where Is Earth's Water Located?" 2010, http://ga.water.usgs.gov

40. Department of National Intelligence, "Global Water Security," 2012, www.dni.gov

41. Ibid.

42. A. Hoekstra and M. Mekonnen, "The Water Footprint of Humanity," *Proceedings of the National Academy of Sciences* 109, no. 9 (2012): 3232–3237.

43. U.S. Geological Survey, "Emerging Contaminants in the Environment," 2011, http://toxics.usgs.gov; U.S. Environmental Protection Agency, "Pharmaceuticals and Personal Care Products (PPCPs)," 2010, www.epa.gov

44. J. Donn et al., "AP Probe Finds Drugs in Drinking Water," *Associated Press*, March 10, 2008.

45. Agency for Toxic Substances and Disease Registry (ATSDR), "Polychlorinated Biphenyls (PCBs)," 2011, www.atsdr.cdc.gov

46. U.S. Environmental Protection Agency, "The EPA and Food Security," 2013, www.epa.gov

47. U.S. Environmental Protection Agency, "Municipal Solid Waste Generation, Recycling, and Disposal in the United States: Facts and Figures for 2011," 2013, www.epa.gov

48. United States Environmental Protection Agency Office of Solid Waste, "Municipal Solid Waste in the United States, 2011 Facts and Figures," 2013, www.epa.gov

49. Ibid.

50. U.S. Environmental Protection Agency, "Superfund National Accomplishments Summary Fiscal Year 2012," 2013, www.epa.gov

51. U.S. Environmental Protection Agency, "Frequent Questions," 2013, Available at www.epa.gov

52. U.S. Nuclear Regulatory Commission, "Radiation Basics," 2011, http://nrc.gov

53. National Council on Radiation Protection and Measurements, NCRP Report no. 160, "Section 1 Pie Chart," www.ncrponline.org

54. Reuters, "Factbox: Key Facts on Chernobyl Nuclear Accident," March, 2011, www.reuters.com
55. U.S. Energy Information Administration, "Independent Statistics and Analysis," 2012, www.eia.gov
56. National Institute for Occupational Safety and Health, "Workplace Safety and Health Topics: Noise and Hearing Loss Prevention," 2011, www.cdc.gov

Pulled statistics:
page 454, Population Reference Bureau, "2009 World Population Data Sheet," 2009, www.prb.org
page 464, Safe Bottles, "Plastics and the Environment," 2010, www.safebottles.co.nz

Chapter 16: Making Smart Health Care Choices

1. American College Health Association, *American College Health Association-National College Health Assessment: Reference Group Data Report Fall 2012* (Hanover, MD: American College Health Association, 2013), www.acha-ncha.org
2. V. C. Oliveria et al., "Communication that Values Patient Autonomy Is Associated with Satisfaction with Care," *Journal of Physiotherapy* 58, no. 4 (2012): 215–229, doi: 10.1016/S1836-9553(12)70123-6.
3. The Joint Commission, "About The Joint Commission," 2013, www.jointcommission.org
4. J. Commins, "Defensive Medicine," Health Leaders Media, April 13, 2012, www.healthleadersmedia.com
5. Consumer Health, "Patient Rights: Informed Consent," 2013, www.emedicinehealth.com
6. Centers for Disease Control and Prevention, "Therapeutic Drug Use," 2009, www.cdc.gov
7. Centers for Disease Control and Prevention, "NCHS Data Brief Number 42," September 2010, www.cdc.gov
8. Kaiser Family Foundation, "Total HMO Enrollment, July 2010," 2011, http://kff.org
9. Centers for Medicare & Medicaid Services, "National Health Expenditure Projections 2010–2020," 2012, www.cms.gov
10. Centers for Medicare & Medicaid Services, "Medicare Enrollment: National Trends 1966–2008," 2009, www.cms.hhs.gov
11. Centers for Medicare & Medicaid Services, "Medicaid Information by Topic," http://medicaid.gov
12. Ibid; Centers for Medicare & Medicaid Services, "Medicaid Data Sources," 2008, www.cms.hhs.gov
13. Ibid.
14. National Conference of State Legislators, "Health Insurance: Premiums and Increases," January 2013, www.ncsl.org
15. Centers for Disease Control and Prevention, "Health Insurance Coverage Status, Type, Selected Characteristics, and Age, January–June 2012," 2013, www.cdc.gov
16. Centers for Disease Control and Prevention/National Center for Health Statistics, Early Release of Selected Estimates Based on Data From the 2011 National Health Interview Survey," June 2012, www.cdc.gov
17. American College Health Association, *American College Health Association-National College Health Assessment II: Reference Group Executive Summary Fall 2012*, 2013.
18. Bureau of Labor Statistics, U.S. Department of Labor, "Occupational Outlook Handbook: Physicians and Surgeons," March 2012, www.bls.gov

19. American Hospital Association, "Fast Facts on U.S. Hospitals," 2013, www.aha.org
20. O. W. Brawley, *How We Do Harm: A Doctor Breaks Ranks about Being Sick in America* (New York: St. Martin's Press, 2011).
21. Centers for Medicare & Medicaid Services, "National Health Expenditure Projections 2011–2021," 2012, www.cms.gov
22. Ibid.
23. Central Intelligence Agency, "CIA World Factbook: Country Comparison: Life Expectancy at Birth," 2012, www.cia.gov
24. Central Intelligence Agency, "CIA World Factbook: Country Comparison: Infant Mortality Rate," 2012, www.cia.gov
25. Department of Health and Human Services, "Report to Congress: National Strategy for Quality Improvement in Health Care," 2011, www.healthcare.gov

Pulled statistics:
page 476, Centers for Disease Control and Prevention, "Hospital Utilization," 2013, www.cdc.gov
page 484, J. Van Den Bos, et al., "The $17.1 Billion Problem: The Annual Cost of Measurable Medical Errors," *Health Affairs* 30, no. 4 (2011): 596-603, doi: 10.1377/hlthaff.2011.0084.

Focus On: Understanding Complementary and Alternative Medicine

1. National Center for Complementary and Alternative Medicine, "What Is CAM?," NCCAM Publication no. D347, Updated May 2012, http://nccam.nih.gov
2. Ibid.
3. Ibid.
4. National Center for Complementary and Alternative Medicine, "The Use of Complementary and Alternative Medicine in the United States," 2008, http://nccam.nih.gov
5. National Center for Complementary and Alternative Medicine, "Chronic Pain and CAM: At a Glance," NCCAM Publication no. D456, Updated September 2011, http://nccam.nih.gov
6. National Center for Complementary and Alternative Medicine, "Ayurvedic Medicine: An Introduction," NCCAM Publication no. D287, Modified January 2012, http://nccam.nih.gov
7. National Center for Complementary and Alternative Medicine, "Homeopathy: An Introduction," NCCAM Publication no. D439, updated July 2012, http://nccam.nih.gov
8. American Association of Naturopathic Physicians, "Definition of Naturopathic Medicine," House of Delegates Position paper, Amended 2011, www.naturopathic.org
9. National Center for Complementary and Alternative Medicine, "Chiropractic: An Introduction," NCCAM Publication no. D403, updated June 2012, http://nccam.nih.gov
10. Bureau of Labor Statistics, U.S. Department of Labor, "Chiropractors," in *Occupational Outlook Handbook, 2012–2013 Edition,* March 29, 2012, www.bls.gov
11. National Center for Complementary and Alternative Medicine, "Massage Therapy: An Introduction," NCCAM Publication no. D327, updated January 2012, http://nccam.nih.gov
12. Ibid.
13. Bureau of Labor Statistics, U.S. Department of Labor, "Massage Therapists," in *Occupational Outlook Handbook, 2012–2013 Edition,* April 5, 2012, www.bls.gov
14. Ibid.

15. Agency for Healthcare Research and Quality, U.S. Department of Health and Human Services, "Complementary and Alternative Therapies for Back Pain II," Evidence Report/Technology Assessment no. 194 (October 2010), AHRQ Publication no. 10(11): E007, www.ahrq.gov
16. A. J. Vickers et al., "Acupuncture for Chronic Pain: Individual Patient Data Meta-Analysis," *Archives of Internal Medicine* 172, no. 19 (2012): 1444–1453, Available at http://nccam.nih.gov
17. National Center for Complementary and Alternative Medicine, "Acupuncture: An Introduction," NCCAM Publication no. D404, Modified September 2012, http://nccam.nih.gov
18. R. Jahnke et al., "A Comprehensive Review of Health Benefits of Qigong and Tai Chi," *American Journal of Health Promotion* 24, no. 6 (2010): e1–e25.
19. D. L. Fazzino et al., "Energy Healing and Pain: A Review of the Literature," *Holistic Nursing Practice* 24, no. 2 (2010): 79–88.
20. Psychoneuroimmunology Research Society, "Mission Statement," November 17, 2010, www.pnirs.org
21. E. Broadbent and H. E. Koschwanez, "The Psychology of Wound Healing," *Current Opinions in Psychiatry* 25, no. 2 (2012): 135–140.
22. M. R. Irwin and R. Olmstead, "Mitigating Cellular Inflammation in Older Adults: A Randomized Controlled Trial of Tai Chi Chih," *American Journal of Geriatric Psychiatry* 20, no. 9 (2012): 764–772.
23. J. J. Mao et al., "Complementary and Alternative Medicine Use among Cancer Survivors: A Population-Based Study," *Journal of Cancer Survivorship: Research and Practice* 5, no. 1 (2011): 8–17.
24. Academy of Nutrition and Dietetics, "Functional Foods," *Journal of the American Dietetic Association* 109, no. 4 (2009): 735–746.
25. M. G. Shrime et al., "Flavonoid-Rich Cocoa Consumption Affects Multiple Cardiovascular Risk Factors in a Meta-Analysis of Short-Term Studies," *Journal of Nutrition* 141, no. 11 (2011): 1982–1988.
26. National Center for Complementary and Alternative Medicine, "Oral Probiotics: An Introduction," NCCAM Publication no. D345, Updated January 2013, http://nccam.nih.gov
27. Office of Dietary Supplements, National Institutes of Health, "Dietary Supplements: Background Information," updated June 2011, http://ods.od.nih.gov
28. National Center for Complementary and Alternative Medicine, "Kava," modified November 2012, http://nccam.nih.gov
29. Mayo Clinic Staff, "Herbal Supplements: What to Know before You Buy," updated November 17, 2011, www.mayoclinic.com
30. U.S. Pharmacopeial Convention, "USP & Patients/Consumers," 2012, www.usp.org

Pulled statistics:
page 493, P. M. Barnes, B. Bloom, and R. L. Nahin, "Complementary and Alternative Medicine Use among Adults and Children: United States, 2007," *National Health Statistics Reports*, no. 12 (Hyattsville, MD: National Center for Health Statistics, 2008), Available at www.cdc.gov
page 495, H. Beinfield and E. Korngold, *Between Heaven and Earth* (New York: Ballantine Books, 1991).

Answers to Chapter Review Questions

Chapter 1

1. b; 2. d; 3. b; 4. a; 5. d; 6. a; 7. a; 8. c; 9. a; 10. a

Chapter 2

1. b; 2. c; 3. a; 4. b; 5. a; 6. c; 7. c; 8. b; 9. b; 10. b

Chapter 3

1. c; 2. c; 3. b; 4. c; 5. d; 6. c; 7. d; 8. c; 9. c; 10. d

Chapter 4

1. b; 2. c; 3. d; 4. d; 5. c; 6. a; 7. c; 8. b; 9. c; 10. c

Chapter 5

1. c; 2. b; 3. c; 4. c; 5. c; 6. a; 7. d; 8. c; 9. b; 10. c

Chapter 6

1. b; 2. b; 3. a; 4. c; 5. b; 6. a; 7. c; 8. d; 9. c; 10. a

Chapter 7

1. b; 2. a; 3. b; 4. d; 5. a; 6. c; 7. c; 8. a; 9. d; 10. b

Chapter 8

1. b; 2. d; 3. d; 4. c; 5. c; 6. d; 7. d; 8. c; 9. c; 10. a

Chapter 9

1. a; 2. b; 3. b; 4. a; 5. d; 6. c; 7. b; 8. b; 9. a; 10. b

Chapter 10

1. a; 2. c; 3. b; 4. b; 5. c; 6. c; 7. b; 8. a; 9. d; 10. a

Chapter 11

1. d; 2. c; 3. b; 4. d; 5. c; 6. b; 7. a; 8. c; 9. a; 10. a

Chapter 12

1. d; 2. b; 3. a; 4. c; 5. b; 6. d; 7. b; 8. c; 9. d; 10. c

Chapter 13

1. c; 2. a; 3. d; 4. a; 5. c; 6. b; 7. c; 8. d; 9. a; 10. c

Chapter 14

1. b; 2. b; 3. c; 4. a; 5. d; 6. a; 7. c; 8. d; 9. a; 10. c

Chapter 15

1. b; 2. c; 3. d; 4. a; 5. d; 6. b; 7. b; 8. a; 9. c; 10. d

Chapter 16

1. c; 2. a; 3. c; 4. a; 5. d; 6. d; 7. b; 8. b; 9. a; 10. c

Photo Credits

Fotostock; p. 261 webphotographeer/iStockphoto; p. 263 Pearson Learning Photo Studio/Pearson Education; p. 264 Chris Rout/Alamy; p. 266 Viorel Sima/Shutterstock; p. 267 David R. Frazier Photolibrary, Inc./Alamy; p. 269 top to bottom: Brand X Pictures/AGE Fotostock; Brand X Pictures/AGE Fotostock; Barry Gregg/Spirit/Corbis; C Squared Studios/Getty Images; Barry Gregg/Corbis; Barry Gregg/Corbis; p. 270 top to bottom: Brand X Pictures/AGE Fotostock; Barry Gregg/Keepsake/Corbis; Barry Gregg/Spirit/Corbis; Brand X Pictures/AGE Fotostock; p. 271 top: Fresh Food Images/PhotoLibrary; bottom: matka_Wariatka/iStockphoto; p. 272 Suzannah Skelton/E+/Getty Images; p. 273 top to bottom: Brand X Pictures/AGE Fotostock; Brand X Pictures/AGE Fotostock; Barry Gregg/Corbis; AGE Fotostock America, Inc; Barry Gregg/Spirit/Corbis; p. 274 top to bottom: Barry Gregg/Keepsake/Corbis; Barry Gregg/Spirit/Corbis; Barry Gregg/Corbis; C Squared Studios/Photodisc/Getty Images; p. 275 Image Source/Getty Images; p. 276 top to bottom: Flashon Studio/iStockphoto; Chris Bence/Shutterstock; Westmacott Photograph/Shutterstock; JR Trice/Shutterstock; Stargazer/Shutterstock; JR Trice, Shutterstock; Hurst Photo/Shutterstock; p. 279 Brian Hagiwara/FoodPix/Getty Images; p. 280 Barbara Ayrapetyan/Shutterstock; p. 281 Rolf Bruderer/Blend Images/Photolibrary, Inc.; p. 282 rtyree1/iStockphoto; p. 285 MorePixels/iStockphoto; p. 287 dkapp12/iStockphoto; p. 288 top: alxpin/E+/Getty Images; bottom: PhotoEuphoria/iStockphoto

Chapter 10 Opener: Flashon Studio/Shutterstock; p. 291 top to bottom: bikeriderlondon/Shutterstock; UPI/Brian Kersey/Newscom; Jim Esposito Photography L.L.C/Photodisc/Getty Images; UpperCut Images/Alamy; p. 293 Big Cheese Photo LLC/Alamy; p. 295 bikeriderlondon/Shutterstock; p. 296 UPI/Brian Kersey/Newscom; p. 297 all: Brand X Pictures/Getty Images; p. 298 Stuart Monk/Shutterstock; p. 299 Janine Wiedel Photolibrary/Alamy; p. 300 Jim Esposito Photography L.L.C/Photodisc/Getty Images; p. 303 top to bottom: David Madison/Getty Images; Julie Brown/Custom Medical Stock Photo; May/Science Source; Phanie/Science Source; David Cooper/Toronto Star/Getty Images; p. 304 Edyta Pawlowska/Shutterstock; p. 305 top: Image Source/Getty Images; bottom: EPF/Alamy; p. 308 top: UpperCut Images/Alamy; bottom: Aleksei Potov/Shutterstock; p. 310 Byron Purvis/AdMedia/Newscom; p. 311 Dennis MacDonald/PhotoEdit; p. 313 LeventeGyori/Shutterstock; p. 314 WavebreakmediaMicro/Fotolia; p. 315 Micha Klootwijk/Shutterstock

Focus On: Enhancing Your Body Image Opener: lunamarina/Fotolia; p. 319 left: Pictorial Press Ltd/Alamy; right: Trinity Mirror/Mirrorpix/Alamy; p. 320 left: Custom Medical Stock Photo/Alamy; right: Sakala/Shutterstock; p. 321 Brand X Pictures/Jupiter Images; p. 322 LatitudeStock/Alamy; p. 323 left: Brand X Pictures/Jupiter Images; right: Li Kim Goh/E+/Getty Images; p. 324 Christopher LaMarca/Redux Pictures; p. 325 left: itanistock/Alamy; right: moodboard/Corbis; p. 326 Pascal Broze/ONOKY/Getty Images; p. 327 top: Elena Elisseeva/Shutterstock; bottom: Photodisc/Thinkstock; p. 328 gosphotodesign/Shutterstock

Chapter 11 Opener: Salvatore Siggia/Getty Images; p. 329 top to bottom: Exactostock/SuperStock; Rolf Adlercreutz/Alamy; Ingram Publishing/PhotoLibrary; Dennis Welsh/AGE Fotostock; p. 330 Corbis/PhotoLibrary; p. 332 Miroslav Georgijevic/Vetta/Getty Images; p. 333 George Doyle/Stockbyte/Getty Images; p. 334 Exactostock/SuperStock; p. 335 left to right: Teo Lannie/PhotoAlto Agency/Getty Images; Elena Dorfman/Pearson Education; Photodisc/Getty Images; Exactostock/SuperStock; toxawww/iStockphoto; p. 336 top: John Fryer/Alamy; bottom: Rolf Adlercreutz/Alamy; p. 338 Wave Royalty Free, Inc./Alamy; p. 339 left: Dan Dalton/Digital Vision/Getty Images; center: MIXA/Getty Images; right: daniel grill/Alamy; p. 340 left: Creative Digital Visions/Pearson Education; right: Karl Weatherly/Photodisc/Getty Images; p. 341 top: moodboard/Corbis; bottom left to right: Radu Razvan/Shutterstock; Pearson Education; Pearson Education; Wisky/Fotolia; p. 342 AP Images/Kathy Willens; p. 344 top all: Pearson Education; p. 344 bottom: Masterfile; p. 345 Index Stock Imagery/PhotoLibrary; p. 346 Ingram Publishing/PhotoLibrary; p. 347 morganl/iStockphoto; p. 348 windu/Shutterstock; p. 349 Dennis Welsh/AGE Fotostock; p. 350 top: AleksandrL/iStockphoto; center: Elena Dorfman/Pearson Education; bottom: Elena Dorfman/Pearson Education

Chapter 12 Opener: Vincent Besnault/Getty Images; p. 354 top to bottom: moodboard/Alamy; Thinkstock/Jupiter Images; Philippe Psaila/Science Source; Digital Vision/Thinkstock; p. 356 moodboard/Alamy; p. 361 HA Photos/Alamy; p. 363 Lenets Tan/Fotolia; p. 365 ariusz/iStockphoto; p. 366 top: Thinkstock/Jupiter Images; bottom: stefanphoto/iStockphoto; p. 368 Philippe Psaila/Science Source; p. 371 miws16/iStockphoto; p. 372 Gordo25/iStockphoto; p. 374 Garo/Science Source; p. 376 Digital Vision/Thinkstock; p. 377 left: James Stevenson/

SPL/Science Source; center: Dr. P. Marazzi/SPL/Science Source; right: Dr. P. Marazzi/SPL/Science Source; p. 381: Max Delson Martins Santos/E+/Getty Images; p. 382 Wuka/iStockphoto; p. 383 Denise Bush/iStockphoto

Focus On: Minimizing Your Risk for Diabetes Opener: Chris Fertnig/Getty Images; p. 387 iStockphoto/Bochkarev Photography/evgenyb; p. 388 Kamdyn R Switzer/Cal Sport Media/Newscom; p. 390 John Giustina/Digital Vision/Getty Images; p. 391 ElinaManninen/iStockphoto; p. 392 top: Terry Vine/Blend Images/Corbis; bottom left: VCM/Alamy; bottom right: Paul Parker/Science Source; p. 394 top: Robyn Mackenzie/iStock/Getty Images; bottom: moodboard/SuperStock; p. 395 Andrew Gentry/Shutterstock

Chapter 13 Opener: Andrea Bricco/Stockbyte/Getty Images; p. 396 top to bottom: PhotoAlto/SuperStock; Peter Llewellyn/Alamy; Peter Bernik/Shutterstock; Shashank Bengali/MCT/Newscom; p. 399 Ocean/Corbis; p. 400 nycshooter/iStockphoto; p. 401 Elena Elisseeva/Shutterstock; p. 402 PhotoAlto/SuperStock; p. 404 left to right: Dr. Gary Gaugler/Science Source; Dr. Linda M. Stannard/Science Source; Steve Gschmeissner/Science Source; Eye of Science/Science Source; Medical-on-Line/Alamy; p. 405 Science Photo Library/Photolibrary, Inc.; p. 406 top: Eric Raptosh/Blend Images/Getty Images; bottom: Lezh/E+/Getty Images; 407 Yuli Seperi/ZUMA Press/Newscom; p. 409 Peter Llewellyn/Alamy; p. 410 Peter Bernik/Shutterstock; p. 411 Yuri Arcurs/Age Fotostock; p. 412 Golden Pixels LLC/Alamy; p. 413 top left: Centers for Disease Control and Prevention; top right: SPL/Science Source; center: Martin M. Rotker/Science Source; bottom: Science Source; p. 414 left: NMSB/Custom Medical Stock Photo; right: Centers for Disease Control and Prevention; p. 415 left: Dr. P. Marazzi/Science Source; right: Centers for Disease Control and Prevention; p. 416 left: Eye of Science/Science Source; right: Shashank Bengali/MCT/Newscom; p. 417 Pixtal/Glow Images; p. 419 Kevin Foy/Alamy; p. 420 top: piai/Fotolia; bottom: arturbo/E+/Getty Images; p. 421 top: Vally/Fotolia; bottom: BrandonTBrown/iStockphoto

Focus On: Reducing Risks and Coping with Chronic Diseases and Conditions Opener: Yuri Arcurs/Alamy; p. 426 Ingemar Edfalk/Robert Matton AB/Alamy; p. 427 left: Eric Audras/PhotoAlto sas/Alamy; right: Custom Medical Stock Photo/Alamy; p. 428 IAN HOOTON/SPL/Science Photo Library/Alamy; p. 429 Gladskikh Tatiana/Shutterstock; p. 431 CHASSENET/BSIP SA/Alamy; p. 432 Potapov Alexander/Shutterstock

Chapter 14 Opener: Ariel Skelley/Getty Images; p. 433 top to bottom: Lia Toby/WENN.com/Newscom; Monkey Business Images/Shutterstock; DreamPictures/Blend Images/Corbis; Bodenham, LTH NHS Trust/Science Source; p. 434 Ronnie Kaufman/Blend Images/Getty Images; p. 435 MARKOS DOLOPIKOS/Alamy; p. 437 moodboard/Corbis; p. 438 Jupiterimages/Comstock Images/Getty Images; p. 439 Lia Toby/WENN.com/Newscom; p. 440 Hybrid Images/Getty Images; p. 441 Monkey Business Images/Shutterstock; p. 442 IS770/image Source Plus/Alamy; p. 445 DreamPictures/Blend Images/Corbis; p. 448 Pascal Broze/Science Source; p. 449 Bodenham, LTH NHS Trust/Science Source; p. 450 DanCardiff/iStockphoto

Chapter 15 Opener: Fancy Collection/SuperStock; p. 453 top to bottom: Brianindia/Alamy; Masterfile; Real World People/Alamy; Dorling Kindersley, Inc.; p. 455 Brianindia/Alamy; p. 458 Masterfile; p. 459 Real World People/Alamy; p. 461 Dorling Kindersley, Inc.; p. 466 Image Source/Corbis; p. 467 TonyB/Shutterstock; p. 468 Lawrence Lawry/Photodisc/Getty Images; p. 471 top: Stiv Kahlina/iStockphoto; bottom left: Ju-Lee/iStockphoto; bottom right: Jupiter Images

Chapter 16 Opener: Blend Images/SuperStock; p. 474 top to bottom: Jiang Jin/SuperStock; Jochen Tack/Alamy; Burger/Phanie/Science Source; Tetra Images/Alamy; p. 475 Tom Merton/OJO Images Ltd/Alamy; p. 477 Ilene MacDonald/Alamy; p. 478 Jiang Jin/SuperStock; p. 479 Steve Snowden/Shutterstock; p. 481 Jochen Tack/Alamy; p. 482 Burger/Phanie/Science Source; p. 484 Tetra Images/Alamy; p. 486 Modesto Bee/ZUMAPRESS/Newscom; p. 487 DNY59/E+/Getty Images

Focus On: Understanding Complementary and Alternative Medicine Opener: Phanie/Science Source; p. 493 Thomas Boehm/Alamy; p. 494 top: Monkey Business Images/Shutterstock; bottom: fred goldstein/Shutterstock; p. 496 Rayman/Getty Images; p. 497 Jeffrey Blackler/Alamy; p. 499 top to bottom: Elena Elisseeva/Shutterstock; Shapiso/Shutterstock; joannawnuk/Shutterstock; WEKWEK/iStockphoto; eAlisa/Shutterstock; Astrid & Hanns-Frieder Michler/Science Source; p. 500 left: Paul Merrett/iStockphoto; right: Ivan Ivanov/iStockphoto; p. 501 top: jo unruh/lostinbids/iStockphoto; bottom: Mark Fairey/iStockphoto

Index